Syllabus of Complete Dentures

Syllabus

OF

Complete Dentures

Charles M. Heartwell, Jr., D.D.S., F.A.C.D.
Professor of Denture Prosthodontics, Virginia Commonwealth University, School of Dentistry, Richmond, Virginia

Arthur O. Rahn, D.D.S.
Professor and Chairman, Department of Prosthodontics, Medical College of Georgia, School of Dentistry, Augusta, Georgia

THIRD EDITION

LEA & FEBIGER · 1980 · PHILADELPHIA

Library of Congress Cataloging in Publication Data

Heartwell, Charles M   1901-
  Syllabus of complete dentures.

  Bibliography.
  Includes index.
  1. Complete dentures. I. Rahn, Arthur O.,
1934–   joint author. II. Title.   [DNLM:
RK656.H42   1980   617.6'92   80-10476
ISBN 0-8121-0711-X

First Edition, 1968
  Reprinted, 1972
Second Edition, 1974
  Reprinted, 1975, 1978

Published in Great Britain by Henry Kimpton Publishers, London
PRINTED IN THE UNITED STATES OF AMERICA

Print no. 5 4 3 2 1

Preface to Second Edition

Prior to the publication of the first edition, the *Syllabus of Complete Dentures* was used in mimeographed form for five years in the prosthodontic curriculum at the Virginia Commonwealth University School of Dentistry. During that period the teaching staff and dental students were encouraged to make comments regarding organization and clarity as it applied to clinical procedures. Many of their suggestions and criticisms were incorporated in the text before publication of the first illustrated edition.

In the preface to the first edition the term *complete denture* was defined as a dental prosthesis to replace the lost natural dentition and associated structures of the maxillae and mandible. The hope expressed was that the subject matter and illustrations would aid the general practitioner in dealing with problems encountered in complete denture service, that it would be concise and systematic enough to permit its use in the curriculum of dental students, and that it would have sufficient depth to furnish useful information to the specialist in complete denture prosthodontics.

After publication, a continuous effort to evaluate the fulfillment of the three goals was instituted. First, the publisher presented the book to more than one hundred prosthodontists in the United States, Canada, and Great Britain for critical appraisal and requested suggestions for improvement, especially in factual content and organization. A special effort was made to encourage the members of the prosthodontic staffs of dental schools to comment on the book's value for dental students in the didactic and clinical areas.

The staff and students at the Virginia Commonwealth University School of Dentistry were encouraged to continue their criticisms and to make suggestions. They were asked to make a comparison between the mimeographed form and the illustrated book.

As a result of the appraisals, the acceptance as a teaching text, and the fact that it is being published not only in the United States, but also in Great Britain and Italy, two decisions were made. The first was to find a co-author knowledgeable about the dental profession and dedicated to it, recognized and respected by his peers in the specialty of prosthodontics, and associated with a dental school in a capacity that allows him to get feedback from students and staff as they use textbooks. The second was to collaborate with him in additional study of the contents of each chapter of the *Syllabus,* to review the most recent research projects and publications related to complete denture prosthodontics, and to attend as many courses, seminars, and lectures as possible in preparation for this edition.

The first aim was achieved when Arthur Rahn, D.D.S., Professor and Chairman, Department of Prosthodontics, Medical College of Georgia, School of Dentistry, accepted the challenge.

As a result of the second, the text has been revised. Some of the illustrations have been changed; others have been added. The figures and legends have been designed to reinforce the factual information presented in the text; therefore, it is remembered.

In the first chapter, "Anatomy and Physiology," the section on the neurologic system was rewritten in greater detail to describe the relation of the somatic nervous system and saliva to complete dentures. It is regrettable that much more scientific research is still needed regarding the reaction of the bony support to dentures before the section on the physiology of the bone can be expanded.

In a recent survey conducted by Douglas B. Nuckles, B.S., D.D.S., Associate Professor, Medical University of South Carolina College of Dentistry, it was revealed that of 46 dental schools in the United States approximately one third use Hanau articulators, one third the Whip-Mix articulators, and one third the Denar instruments. As a result of this survey, the chapter on articulators has been revised to include a more in-depth discussion in the use of the Denar articulators.

Of the over thirty million edentulous people in the United States, the majority are in the postmaturational age group.

The chapter "Diagnosis" now includes a section on treating the twenty million people who are 65 years of age or over, the geriatric patients. Dentists must learn proper procedures to be competent in the treatment of these patients.

A new chapter that considers a new philosophy in complete denture prosthodontics has been added. In this chapter the philosophy and procedures involved in the tooth-supported complete denture are presented. Also, there is a new chapter on the single complete denture.

The dental literature has been reviewed, and the reference lists for many chapters have been expanded. As in the first edition the references were chosen for their coverage of the specific subject, their bibliographies, their ready availability, and their up-to-dateness. Although most of the references are in publications in the United States, many have appeared in publications in other countries.

This book relates the sciences of anatomy, physiology, pathology, and psychology with the art and mechanics involved in complete denture service. Both dentists and patients need to realize that when complete denture procedures are carried out by one who has a full knowledge of these sciences and applies this knowledge in each procedure, complete dentures can prevent disease. When dental procedures prevent disease, they may be scientifically classified as a form of preventive dentistry. With the increase in life expectancy the number of edentulous persons in the United States may be expected to increase until procedures to prevent the loss of natural teeth are more widely adopted.

Some of the steps in the procedures for complete dentures, immediate complete dentures, single complete dentures, and tooth-supported complete dentures are similar. Review of procedures is desirable, but often the continuity of thought is disrupted while the reader refers to another chapter in the book. Cross references to earlier discussions of a topic are provided, but usually the procedures are repeated as a convenience to the reader.

The definitions of terminology used in this syllabus come from *The Glossary of Prosthodontic Terms*. Coined terms have been avoided as much as possible. When using terminology not found in the *Glossary*, we have focused attention on the difference and, if possible, have related the term to a corresponding one in the *Glossary*.

The aim of every dentist engaged in complete denture prosthodontics is to preserve, within the limits of normal physiologic processes, the supporting structures. There is no one concept or discipline, no one technique, no one material that will assure this in all situations. For this reason these factors are presented in a manner suitable to change and alterations, provided the dentist knows why.

Richmond, Virginia

Augusta, Georgia

CHARLES M. HEARTWELL, JR.

ARTHUR O. RAHN

Preface

In the preparation of this third edition, we fully realize that there have always been some persons within the dental profession who have attempted to promote the application of the *Why* and *What* in dentistry. The efforts of these people should never be forgotten nor minimized. Members of our profession, particularly those who are active prosthodontists, would have much less problems with the threat from auxiliary persons, i.e., the "taking over" of removable prosthodontics, if the art of *How* had been placed in its proper perspective in both the teaching and practice of prosthodontics. We can become so involved in technique that dentistry as a health science becomes secondary, whereas it should always be primary. Dentists do not construct dentures for patients, but rather they *treat* patients with complete dentures. For this reason much effort and time has been spent consulting with and reviewing the works of oral physiologists, many of whom have a D.D.S. or D.M.D. degree along with a Ph.D. in oral physiology. As a result the section on physiology in the chapter Anatomy and Physiology is revised.

The use of drugs in prosthodontics is presented in the chapter on Diagnosis.

The chapter on the tooth-supported complete denture is revised. This revision is considered necessary, particularly for those who have had limited experience in its use or for those who do not have an efficient recall system. The retention of the vital roots of teeth is briefly discussed. This procedure is in the research stage and is not being advocated in this text as a tried and tested procedure. However, dentists should be aware of the potential of such a treatment.

In this revision many of the requests from practitioners, dental educators, and students, for greater emphasis on certain topics, has been accomplished by expanding the text and adding illustrations as well as redoing some of the old. Even though it has gotten thicker, we have attempted to maintain its simplicity in order that it will continue to aid the general practitioner in his treatment of patients with complete dentures, as well as being useful in the dental school curriculum.

Special thanks are extended to Dr. Marvin Reynolds, Dr. Vincent Urbanek, Dr. James Kaegle, Dr. Al Ciarlone, Dr. Steve Kolas, Dr. P. B. Peters, Dr. Norman Thomas, Dr. Ross Hill,

Dr. Guy Fiebiger, Dr. Barry Goldman, and Dr. Greg Parr, who edited and added their knowledge and writing expertise to various sections of this revision. Their help was immeasurable.

Thanks also should go to Rita Cook who persevered and typed the many re-visions, along with Mr. Lewis Hinely who drew all of the new illustrations.

We express our sincere appreciation to all our esteemed colleagues who assisted in a less direct, but equally valuable way.

Richmond, Virginia

Augusta, Georgia

CHARLES M. HEARTWELL, JR.

ARTHUR O. RAHN

Contents

1. **Anatomy and Physiology**   1
   Anatomy   1
      Osteology   1
      Myology   6
      Oral Mucous Membrane   15
      Temporomandibular
      Articulation   18
   Physiology   26
      Physiology of Bone   26
      Physiology of Muscle   30
      Somatic Nervous System   36
      Salivary Glands and
      Saliva   40
   Summary   43

2. **Articulators**   51
   Uses   51
   Limitations   52
   Precision, Accuracy, and
      Sensitivity   52
   Classification   53
      Articulators of Historic
      Interest   54
      Current Popular
      Articulators   60
   Evaluation   82
      Condyle Path   84
      Lateral Maxillomandibular
      Relations   85

      Mandibular and Articulator
      Movements   86
   Selection   87

3. **Educating The Patient**   91
   Understanding the Patient   92
   Instructing the Patient   92
      Why Replace Teeth   93
      What to Expect from
      Dentures   93
      How to Use Dentures   96
      How to Care for Dentures   97
      Immediate Dentures   98

4. **Diagnosis**   101
   Mental Attitude   101
      Philosophic Patient   102
      Exacting Patient   102
      Indifferent Patient   102
      Hysterical Patient   102
   Systemic Status   102
      Dehabilitating Diseases   103
      Diseases of the Joint   103
      Cardiovascular Diseases   104
      Diseases of the Skin   104
      Neurologic Disorders   104
      Oral Malignancies   104

Climacteric 105
Local Factors 105
The Geriatric Patient 110
  Physiologic Changes 114
  Nutrition and Diet 117
  Psychologic Changes 118
  Pathologic Changes 120
  Intraoral Changes 124
Diagnostic Procedures 125
  Medication 125
  First Appointment 127
  Second Appointment 127

5. Surgical Preparation for Complete Dentures 137
Preoperative Examination 137
Retained Dentition 139
  Clinically Evident Teeth 139
  Root Tips 139
  Unerupted Teeth 140
Nonpathologic Bony Conditions 141
  Alveolectomy 141
  Tori 144
  Generalized Exostosis 145
Soft Tissue 145
  Alveolar Tubercle Area 145
  Frenums 146
  Lingual Frenum 147
Benign Pathologic Soft Tissue 147
  Lips 147
  Hyperplasia of Oral Mucosa 148
  Hyperkeratosis without Dyskeratosis 149
  Lichen Planus 150
  Mucoceles and Retention Cysts 150
  Dermoid Cyst 151
  Papillomas and Fibromas 151
Bony Pathology (Nonmalignant) 152
  Bony Cyst 152
  Cysts of Odontogenic Origin 152
  Cysts of Nonodontogenic Origin 153

Miscellaneous Lesions 153
  Nonodontogenic Benign Lesions 153
  Odontogenic Tumors of the Jaws 153
Other Osteolytic Lesions 154
  Gaucher's Disease; Niemann-Pick Disease 154
  Paget's Disease (Osteitis Deformans) 154
  Hyperparathyroidism 155
  Hyperthyroidism 155
  Fibrous Dysplasia 155
  Other Diseases 155
Procedures for Specialists 155
  Residual Alveolar Ridge 155
  Mandibular Arch 157
  Maxillary Arch 163
Malrelated Jaws 167
Congenital Deformities 167
Postoperative Procedures 167
Prosthodontic Treatment 168

6. Complete Denture Impressions 173
Muscles of Facial Expression 173
Anatomic Landmarks 175
  The Maxillary Arch 175
  The Mandibular Arch 176
  Interpreting Landmarks 177
Impression Objectives 179
  Preservation 179
  Support 179
  Stability 179
  Esthetics 179
  Retention 179
Impression Materials 180
  Gypsum Products 181
  Zinc Oxide-Eugenol Paste 181
  Reversible Hydrocolloid 182
  Irreversible Hydrocolloids 182
  Rubber Impression Materials 183
  Modeling Compound 183
  Impression Waxes 184
Impression Techniques 184

Preliminary Impressions   185
  Equipment   185
  Seating the Patient   185
  Impressions for the
    Mandibular Arch   186
  Impression for the
    Maxillary Arch   186
  Casts for Acrylic Resin
    Impression Trays   188
  Casts and Impression
    Trays of Activated Acrylic
    Resin   189
  Checking Impression Trays   190
Final Impressions   190
  Functional Position   191
  Rest Position   191
  Impression Compound
    Tray and Zinc Oxide-
    Eugenol Paste   192
  Equipment   194
  Refining   194

7. Mandibular Movements, Maxillomandibular Relations, and Concepts of Occlusion

7. Mandibular Movements,
   Maxillomandibular
   Relations, and
   Concepts of Occlusion   203
   Mandibular Movements   204
     Border Positions   205
     Condyle Path   206
   Maxillomandibular Relations   209
     Centric Relation   209
     Eccentric Relation   211
     Physiologic Rest Position   212
     Vertical Dimension   212
     Occlusion   215
   Concepts of Occlusion   216
     Balanced Occlusion   217
     Nonbalanced Occlusion   219

8. Gnathology

8. Gnathology   229

9. Record Bases and Occlusion Rims

9. Record Bases and
   Occlusion Rims   237
   Record Bases   237
     Materials and Methods   237

Occlusion Rims   240
  Maxillary Occlusion Rim   241
  Mandibular Occlusion Rim   243
  Useful Guide Lines   243

10. Hinge Axis and Face-bow

10. Hinge Axis and Face-bow   247
    Hinge Axis   247
      Review of the Literature   247
      Hinge Axis Location
        Technique   249
      Terminal Hinge Axis   250
      Arbitrary Hinge Axis   250
    Face-bow   251
      Review of Face-bows   251
      Discussion of Face-bow
        Use   252
      Face-bow Transfer
        Procedure   255

11. Recording Maxillomandibular Relations

11. Recording Maxillomandibular
    Relations   261
    Vertical Relations   261
      Rest Position   261
      Recording Rest Position   262
      Occlusion Position   264
      Recording Occlusion   264
      Preparing for Evaluation   273
      Evaluating Vertical
        Dimension   273
    Centric Relation Record   273
      Functional ("Chew-in")   274
      Graphic Methods   276
      Tactile or Interocclusal
        Check Record Method   279
    Eccentric Relation Records   285
    Lateral Relation Records   289

12. Tooth Selection

12. Tooth Selection   293
    Anterior Teeth   297
      Size of Anterior Teeth   297
      Form of Anterior Teeth   300
      Color or Shade of Anterior
        Teeth   303
      Composition of Material
        for Anterior Teeth   306

Posterior Teeth 306
   Shade of Posterior Teeth ... 306
   Size and Number of
     Posterior Teeth 306
   Form of Posterior Teeth 307
   Material Composition of
     Posterior Teeth 308

13. Tooth Arrangement 311
Factors Governing the
   Positions of Teeth 311
   Horizontal Positions 312
   Vertical Positions 321

**14. The Arrangement of Teeth
for Esthetics** 327
Age 328
Sex 330
Personality 332
Cosmetic Factor 334
Artistic Reflection 334

**15. Arranging the Artificial
Teeth for the Trial
Denture** 339

**16. Relating Inclinations of
Teeth to Concepts of
Occlusion** 347
Neutrocentric Concept 349
Balanced Occlusion 350

17. Laboratory Procedures 359
Wax Contouring 359
   Requirements 359
   Procedure 359
Flasking of Dentures 361
   Procedure 361
Preparation of Mold 363

Wax Elimination 363
Application of Tinfoil
  Substitute 363
Preparing and Packing
   Acrylic Resin 365
   Mixing the Acrylic Resin 365
   Packing the Acrylic Resin ... 365
Processing of Dentures 366
   Slow Processing 366
Deflasking of Dentures 366
   Removing the Mold 366
   Removing the Denture and
    Cast 366
Laboratory Remount
   Procedure 367
Recovering the Complete
   Denture from the Cast 368
Finishing the Complete
   Denture 369
Polishing the Complete
   Denture 369
Plaster Cast for Denture
   Remount Procedures 370
   Preparation of Remount
    Cast 370

18. Denture Insertion 375
The Insertion Procedures 375
   Reviewing Instructions 375
   Evaluating Tissue Side 375
   Evaluating Borders 377
   Correcting Occlusion 378
Clinical Errors 378
   Errors in Registering Jaw
    Relations 378
   Errors in Mounting Casts ... 379
Correcting Occlusal
   Disharmony 379
   Articulating Paper 379
   Central-bearing Devices 379
   Occlusal Wax 381
   Abrasive Paste 381
   Patient Remount and
    Selective Grinding 381
Selective Grinding
   Procedures 385

19. Treating Problems Associated with Denture Use   391

Review of Denture
    Requirements   391
Incompatibility   391
Problems with Mastication   392
Disharmony   392
Dissatisfaction with Esthetics 392
Deterioration of Supporting
    Tissues   392
Soft Tissue Considerations   393
    Stress-bearing Mucosa   394
    Basal Seat Mucosa   396
    Transitional Submucosa   398
    Lining Mucosa   398
    Specialized Mucosa   398
Problems Involving Bone   399
Treatment Procedures   400
    Problems with Maxillary
        Denture   401
    Problems with Mandibular
        Denture   401
Clicking   402
Commissural Cheilitis   402
Gagging and Vomiting   402
Burning Tongue and Palate   403

20. Treating Abused Tissues   407

Tissue Recovery Routines   408
Tissue Conditioners   409
Rebase and Reline
    Procedures   412
Chairside Procedures for
    Reline or Rebase Impression 414

21. Immediate Complete Dentures   425

Definition   425
Requirements   425
Advantages   426
Disadvantages   429
Diagnosis and Treatment
    Planning   432
    Diagnostic Procedures   432

Systemic Status   436
Past Dental History   438
Surgical Preparation   438

22. Immediate Complete Denture Construction Procedures   441

Preparatory Treatment   441
Treatment   442
    Preliminary Impressions   443
    Final Impression   444
    Record Base   452
    Maxillomandibular
        Relation Records   453
    Selecting and Arranging
        Anterior Teeth   461
    Correcting for Processing
        Error   463
    Plaster Remount Index   464
    Preparation for the
        Insertion Appointment   464
    Surgical Procedures and
        Insertion   464
Postinsertion Treatment   466

23. The Single Complete Denture   471

Mandibular Denture to
    Oppose Natural Maxillary
    Teeth   472
    Preservation of Residual
        Alveolar Ridge   472
    Necessity for Retaining
        Maxillary Teeth   473
    Mental Trauma   473
Single Complete Maxillary
    Denture to Oppose Natural
    Mandibular Teeth   474
Complete Maxillary Denture
    to Oppose a Partially
    Edentulous Mandibular
    Arch with Fixed
    Prosthesis   477
Complete Maxillary Denture
    to Oppose a Partially

Edentulous Mandibular
Arch and a Removable
Partial Denture   478
Single Complete Denture to
Oppose an Existing
Complete Denture   479

**24. Tooth-Supported Complete
Denture**   483
Definitions   483
Classification   484
  Noncoping Abutments   484
  Abutments with Copings   484
  *Abutments with
    Attachments*   485
  Submerged Vital Roots   488
Advantages   488

Indications   490
Contraindications   490
Treatment Planning   491
Preparatory Treatment   491
Preparation of the Retained
  Teeth   492
  *Tooth Preparation for
    Minimal Retention*   492
  *Tooth Preparation to
    Provide Retention*   498

Bibliography   503

Glossary   507

Index   547

Anatomy and Physiology

1

In order to construct a prosthesis a dentist requires an understanding of the foundation: its components, its properties, and its qualities must be analyzed to assure support for the proposed prosthesis. Influences from within and those from without must be evaluated to assure successful results.

Unless the dentist has a thorough knowledge of the anatomy and physiology of the supporting structures, complete dentures become the product of a craftsman who employs only the knowledge of physics and mechanics. A practitioner of a health service, to be classified as such, must know and apply the basic sciences—anatomy, physiology, and psychology—as well as physics and mechanics.

Anatomy

OSTEOLOGY

The osseous structures not only support the dentures, but have a direct bearing on the impression-making procedures, the position of the teeth, and the contours of the finished denture bases.

The maxillary denture is supported by two pairs of bones, the *maxillae* and the *palatine bones*, whereas the mandibular denture is supported by one bone, the *mandible*.

MAXILLA. There are two maxillae, each consisting of a central body and four processes. Areas of the body and two of the processes are involved in the support of the maxillary denture (Fig. 1-1).

The *anterolateral surface* of the body of the maxilla forms the skeleton of the anterior part of the cheek and is termed the malar surface.

The *zygomatico-alveolar crest* starts at the tip of the zygomatic process and continues in an arc inferiorly and laterally in the direction of the first molar, to disappear at the base of the alveolar process. This crest has been likened to the buccal shelf in the mandible as a stress bearing area. The mucosal covering is usually very thin, and even though the bone is in a good position for stress bearing, the mucosa is not considered desirable for this purpose. In some instances the crest is so prominent and the mucosa so thin that the denture base must be relieved, as it is in other hard bony areas. Failure to provide adequate relief in these instances results in poor retention of the denture.

The *posterior convexity* of the maxillary body is termed the maxillary tuberosity or tuber. In the edentulous mouth the alveolar tubercle is frequently referred to erroneously as the maxillary tuberosity. The alveolar tubercle supports the denture, but it is questionable whether the denture would ever extend

1

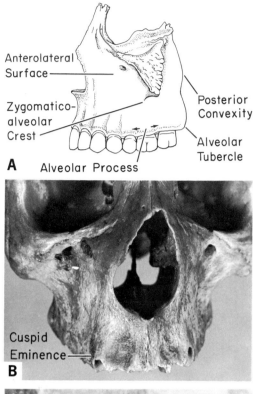

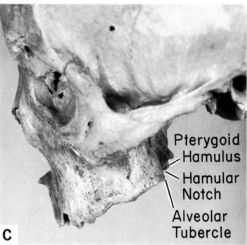

FIG. 1-1. **A.** *The lateral surface of the body of the maxilla. The maxillary tuberosity or tuber is the posterior convexity of the maxillary body; the rough prominence behind the position of the last tooth is the alveolar tubercle.* **B.** *The cortical plate over the cuspid. The cuspid eminence is usually thin.* **C.** *The hamular notch is the space between the pterygoid hamulus and the alveolar tubercle.*

to the height of the maxillary tuberosity.

It is important to preserve the integrity of the tubercles, for they provide resistance against the horizontal movements of the maxillary denture. The medial and lateral walls resist the horizontal and torquing forces which would move the denture base in a lateral or palatal direction. The posterior wall will resist movement in an anterior direction. To take advantage of this resistance to movement, the maxillary denture base should cover the tubercles and fill the hamular notches.

A square arch provides the best form for denture stability. The alveolar tubercles form the posterior corners of the square in the maxillary arch.

The *alveolar process* arises from the lower surface of the maxilla. It consists of two parallel plates of cortical bone, buccolingual or labiolingual, which unite behind the last molar tooth to form the *alveolar tubercle*. When teeth are present, the cortical plates are connected by interalveolar or interdental septa. The bony wall of the tooth socket is the alveolar bone proper (lamina dura), and around the alveolar bone proper is the spongy bone. The labial and buccal cortical plate is relatively thin, especially over the cuspids and central incisors. The alveolar bone proper is often fused with the cortical plate over the cuspids. When teeth are present, the alveolar process could be considered peculiar because then compact bone is found within the plates of compact bone. The alveolar bone proper (lamina dura) is compact bone formed in response to the tensile forces transmitted by the periodontal fibers.

The *palatine processes* (Fig. 1-2) of the maxillary bones arise as horizontal plates from the body of the maxilla. The two horizontal plates unite in the midline forming a suture, the *midpalatal suture*. Quite often a hyperplastic overgrowth of bone, called the *palatal torus,* is seen in this area. This overgrowth usually occurs in the surface of the bone *exostosis*. At times a palatal torus becomes quite large and irregular, presenting unfavorable undercuts. Relief in the denture base is indicated for the less extensive tori, and surgical removal is indicated for the more extensive. If the resiliency of the mucosal covering of the crest of the ridges and the rugae area is the same as that over the torus, very little if any relief is necessary. If the resiliency is more, the relief should be provided at a depth to compensate for the difference. If the torus has undercuts, or is of a magnitude great enough to impede the normal movements of the tongue or to act as a fulcrum area, it should be removed surgically.

The horizontal palatine processes of the maxillary bones appear to resist resorption over a long period. As the bone of the alveolar residual ridges resorb, the pressure of vertical forces is increased over the bone of the palate. When this bone becomes prominent in the mid-palatal suture area, it becomes the fulcrum point around which the maxillary denture will rotate. This in turn results in discomfort to the patient and damage to the soft tissue covering.

The *nasopalatine* or *incisal foramen* is located in the midline of the palate, posterior to the maxillary central incisors or, in the edentulous mouth, slightly to the palatal side of the anterior palatal alveolar plate. The nasopalatine nerve and blood vessels make their exit to the palate at right angles to margins of the bony foramen. It is for this reason, even though the foramen is covered with a protecting pad of fibrous connective tissue, that the denture base should be relieved over the area. Failure to relieve the denture base could result in pressure to the nerve and blood vessels with resultant decrease in blood supply to

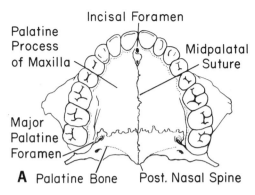

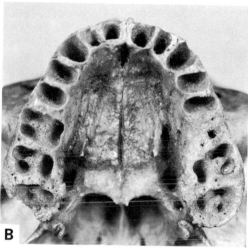

FIG. 1-2. A. *The palatine process. The palatine bone supplements the maxilla. The horizontal plates of the maxilla and the palatine bones form the hard palate. The incisal foramen is an important landmark in denture procedures. The shape of the posterior nasal spine alters the contour of the posterior surface of the palatine bones.* **B.** *The contour of the hard palate is favorable for denture stability. The transverse palatine suture is not visible.*

the anterior part of the palate and nerve irritation with accompanying burning symptoms.

PALATINE BONES (Fig. 1-2). The horizontal plates of the palatine bones articulate with the posterior rough border of the horizontal palatal processes of the maxillae. The posterior border of the horizontal plates of the palatine bones unite at the midline to form a sharp spine, the *posterior nasal spine*. The posterior margins of the hard palate serve as the anterior attachment for the aponeurosis of the soft palate.

The *posterior palatal seal* should follow the contour of the posterior border of the hard palate; this would extend from hamular notch to hamular notch but not in a straight line. The posterior palatal seal is placed in the mucosa of the soft palate, which is movable in speech, respiration, and deglutition. A straight line from hamular notch to hamular notch passes over bone in the area of the posterior nasal spine. The mucosa in this area does not move in speech, respiration, or deglutition. A border seal in this area will result in resorption of the bone and the seal will be lost.

The *major or anterior palatine foramen* is located medial to the third molar at the junction of the maxilla and the horizontal plate of the palatine bone. The bone is notched and from this notch the palatine groove extends anteriorly and houses the anterior palatine nerve and blood vessels. Since the nerve and blood vessels are housed in a groove, rarely would a relief be required in the denture base over the area.

In some instances bony spines are located near the anterior palatine foramen. If these bony projections present problems, the denture base should be relieved over these areas, or the spines should be surgically removed.

The difference between a *low* and *high* palate is expressed not only in quantitative measurements, but also in the changed configuration of the palate. In a flat or low palate the amount of spongy bone is greater than in a high palate. The inner plate of the alveolar process ascends at a moderate angle if the palate is low and then curves without a break into the horizontal roof of the oral cavity. In the high palate the inner plate, particularly in the anterior region, is steep; and there is a fairly sharp angle between the alveolar process and the roof of the mouth. The high palate, because of its configuration, is not conducive to the stability of a denture.

PTERYGOID HAMULUS (Fig. 1-1). Although the pterygoid hamulus does not support a maxillary denture, its position is in the osseous limit of the maxillary denture base posterior to the alveolar tubercle. The pterygoid hamulus is a thin, curved process at the terminal end of the medial plate of the sphenoid bone. Between the pterygoid hamulus and the alveolar tubercles is a notch—the hamular notch.

MANDIBLE (Fig. 1-3). The mandible is the movable member of the stomatognathic system.

The *body of the mandible* is horseshoe-shaped and carries the alveolar process. The distal portion of each side continues upward and backward into the mandibular ramus. The ramus divides superiorly into two processes, *posteriorly* the *condyloid* and *anteriorly* the *coronoid*.

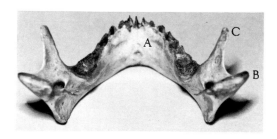

FIG. 1-3. *The mandible—genial tubercles (A); condyle, the head of the mandible (B); coronoid process (C). Note the horseshoe shape and the two vertical ramae.*

The *condyle* (Fig. 1-3B) or capitulum is the articular surface of the condyloid process, the *head* of the *mandible*. The connection of the condyle with the ramus is the slightly constricted mandibular neck. Superior to the neck the condyle is bent anteriorly so that the articulating surface faces upward and forward. It is important to know that the condyles are irregular in size and shape. Variations occur in the same individual between the right and left.

The *coronoid process* (Fig. 1-3C) is a triangular bony plate ending in a sharp corner; the convex anterior border continues into the anterior border of the ramus. When the mandible is protruded, the anterior border of the ramus extends toward the alveolar tuberosity, which is medial to the ramus. If the distobuccal flange of the maxillary denture overfills the vestibule, it will cause discomfort when the mandible is protruded, and if the mandible while in protrusion is moved into left or right lateral, the denture could be dislodged.

The *external oblique line* (Fig. 1-4) is a ridge of dense bone extending from just above the mental foramen superiorly and distally, becoming continuous with the anterior border of the ramus. In most individuals the external oblique line is the anatomic guide for the lateral termination of the buccal flange of the mandibular denture.

The *buccal shelf area* (Fig. 1-4) is bounded externally by the external oblique line and internally by the slope of the residual ridge. The bone is very dense, as the resultant forces of the elevator muscles are directed to this area and the trabeculation is arranged to best resist these forces. The artificial teeth can be arranged so that the long axis can coincide with the direction of the resultant forces. The buccal shelf is designated as the primary stress-bearing area in the mandibular arch, since its density, its

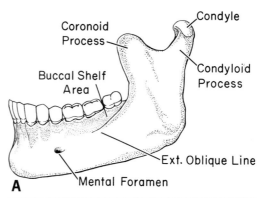

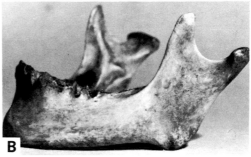

FIG. 1-4. **A.** *Diagram and* **B.** *photograph of the mandible, lateral view. The condyloid and coronoid processes are the upper ends of the ramus. Note that the external oblique line is strong and prominent in its upper part, gradually flattens, and disappears near the lower border below the first molar.*

mucosal covering, and its relation to the vertical closure of the jaws are favorable to best resist the forces generated.

The *mental foramen* (Fig. 1-4) is located on the lateral surface of the mandible, between the first and second bicuspids, halfway between the lower border and the alveolar crest. If the loss of the residual ridge is extensive, the foramen occupies a more superior position and the denture base must be relieved over the foramen, since the force of the denture base could partially occlude the blood vessels and also irritate the mental nerve.

The *mylohyoid line* (Fig. 1-5) is an

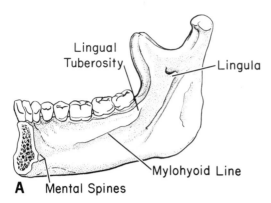

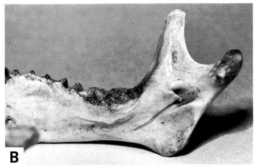

FIG. 1-5. **A.** *Diagram and* **B.** *photograph of section of the mandible showing the mylohyoid line, the lingual tuberosity, and the lingual spines. The mylohyoid muscle takes its origin from the mylohyoid line.*

irregular rough, bony crest extending from the third molar region to the lower border of the mandible in the region of the chin. This rough crest is usually most prominent from the third molar to the area of the second bicuspid. The irregularity of this crest often presents a problem to denture patients. The lingual flange of the mandibular denture should extend inferior but not lateral to the mylohyoid line. If the bony crest is so prominent and sharp that it becomes a stress-bearing surface or fulcrum point, surgical intervention is indicated.

The *lingual tuberosity* is an irregular area of bony prominence at the distal termination of the mylohyoid line. When this area is excessively prominent or rough, it may present an undesirable undercut area. It can be surgically removed or rounded.

The *genial tubercles* or *mental spines* (Fig. 1-5) are situated on the lingual aspect of the mandibular body in the midline slightly above the border. This bony area is often divided into a superior and an inferior section and sometimes into a right and a left prominence. When loss of residual ridge is extensive, these spines are sometimes more superior in position than the crest of the existing ridge. In these cases, surgical procedures are indicated.

MYOLOGY

MUSCLES OF EXPRESSION. The *zygomaticus, quadratus labii superioris, levator anguli oris, mentalis, quadratus labii inferioris, depressor anguli oris, risorius, platysma, upper incisal, lower incisal, orbicularis oris,* and the *buccinator* are responsible for the various expressions seen in the lower half of the face. The action of these muscles is responsible for the facial postures associated with smiling, laughing, frowning, or scowling. When these muscles are relaxed, the face lacks expression. The actions of these muscles often reflect the mental state, the personality, and the well-being of an individual.

The muscles of facial expression do not insert into bone and need support from the teeth for proper function. If the muscles of facial expression are not properly supported, either by the natural teeth or by the artificial substitutes, none of the facial expressions appears normal. The nasolabial sulcus, the philtrum, the commissure of the lips, and the mentolabial sulcus will not have their normal contour (Fig. 1-6A). Incorrectly positioned teeth or an incorrectly contoured denture base will destroy the normal tonicity of the muscles and affect the expression adversely. Lack of support allows sagging; stretching retards the normal contracture of the muscles and results in loss of tonus.

The insertion of the group of muscles about the oral cavity, both superficial and deep, is important. The bundles of muscles insert partly into the skin, partly into the mucous membrane of the lips and the immediate vicinity. In an area situated laterally and slightly above the corner of the mouth is a concentration of the many fibers of this muscle group.

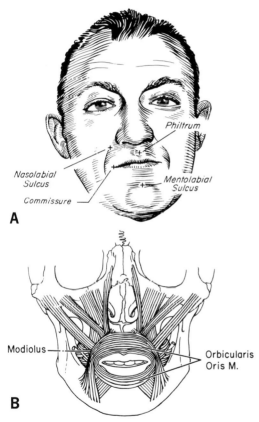

FIG. 1-6. **A.** *The philtrum, nasolabial sulcus, the commissure of the lips, and the mentolabial sulcus, which change in contour when the facial muscles are under- or over-supported by teeth or dentures.* **B.** *Muscles about the oral cavity. The concentration of muscles at the modiolus must be considered when the denture flanges are contoured; the orbicularis must be considered when impressions are made.*

This concentration is known as the muscular node or modiolus (Fig. 1-6B) and continues downward as a tendinous strip of varying lengths. Any muscle that inserts into the mucous membrane of the lips is influenced by the position of the teeth and the contouring of the denture bases. This is particularly true of the maxillary denture. Except in instances of excessive loss of residual ridge, the origins of *most* of this group are removed from the denture-bearing area to the extent that their influence on the denture, except at the modiolus, is negligible. The labial flanges of the maxillary denture frequently need to be reduced lateromedially in the area of the modiolus. When the bundle of muscles is stretched during mouth opening, the vestibular space between the bundle in the cheek and the slopes of the residual alveolar ridges are restricted. To reduce the bulk of the flange to accommodate this muscle action helps to prevent dislodgment of the denture when the mouth is opened. At times, if the tendinous strips extend downward extensively, the mandibular denture base should be reduced lateromedially.

The origins (Fig. 1-7) of several of the muscles of facial expression are near enough to the denture-bearing areas that their actions must be considered as definitely influencing the denture borders; their influence is in proportion to the contour and quantity of residual ridge present in a vertical direction. The higher the residual ridge the less influence will be exerted.

The *mentalis* muscle elevates the skin of the chin and turns the lower lip outward. Since its origin extends to a level higher than that of the fornix of the vestibule, the mentalis muscle, in contracting, renders the lower vestibule shallow. The contraction of this muscle is capable of dislodging a mandibular denture, particularly when the residual

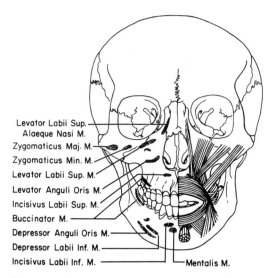

Levator Labii Sup.
Alaeque Nasi M.
Zygomaticus Maj. M.
Zygomaticus Min. M.
Levator Labii Sup. M.
Levator Anguli Oris M.
Incisivus Labii Sup. M.
Buccinator M.
Depressor Anguli Oris M.
Depressor Labii Inf. M.
Incisivus Labii Inf. M.
Mentalis M.

FIG. 1-7. *The origins of the muscles of facial expression. With a few exceptions, they are not in contact with the denture borders when the residual ridges are prominent.*

ridge in its anterior region is nonexistent. One must exercise care in the contouring and extension of the labial flange of the mandibular denture. Surgical repositioning of the mentalis muscle is often advisable.

The *upper incisal* and *lower incisal* muscles arise from the alveolar process. Their action is not well circumscribed; they press upon the vestibular fornix in a manner like that in the mentalis. They are weak muscles and it is doubtful whether their action alone would dislodge a denture. Their presence, in some instances, might present problems associated with flange extension and denture retention.

The *buccinator muscle* (Fig. 1-8) forms the mobile and adaptive substance of the cheeks. It is a wide, rather thin muscle plate which arises from a horseshoe-shaped line, from the outer surface of the maxilla and the mandible opposite the sockets of the first molar teeth. In addition to, and in between these bony attachments, it originates from the ptery-

gomandibular raphe or ligament. The ligament serves as a bond of union between the buccinator and the superior constrictor of the pharynx.

The muscle bundles arising from the *lower jaw* follow the external line to the mesial aspect of the first molar and then ascend slightly toward the corner of the mouth. Most of the fibers insert into the mucous membrane of the cheek in and around the tendinous node and tendinous line. The other fibers terminate in the skin of the upper and lower lips near the commissure.

It is in the lower jaw that the muscle becomes a part of the denture-bearing area. Not only does it become part of the denture-bearing area but where extreme or total loss of residual ridge exists, the buccinator and the mylohyoid have been demonstrated to cover the bony support from the first molar area to the retromolar pad. Fortunately, the action of the fibers of the buccinator does not dislodge the denture. The action is

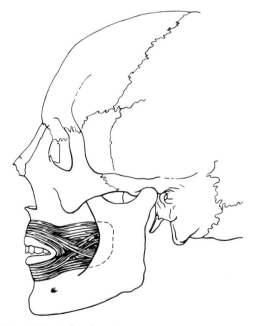

FIG. 1-8. *The buccinator muscle supports the cheek.*

parallel to the plane of occlusion. The fibers parallel to the occlusal plane are at right angles to the fibers of the masseter muscle. When the masseter is activated, it pushes the buccinator medially against the denture border in the area of the retromolar pad. This is a dislodging force and the denture base should be contoured to accommodate this action; this contour in the denture base is termed the *masseter groove*.

The bundle of muscle fibers of the *upper jaw* falls along the base of the residual ridge from the level of the first molar distally to the suture between the maxilla and palatine bone. The position of origin in the upper jaw determines the vertical height of the distobuccal flange of the maxillary denture. The fibers appear to be attached to a thin periosteum and possibly into the bone proper. The action of the buccinator muscles pulls the corners of the mouth laterally and posteriorly. Its main function is to keep the cheeks taut. If this were not so, when the jaws close, the cheeks would collapse and be caught between the teeth. This problem is present in the senile individual where the muscle tonus is diminished or in the individual with facial paralysis.

Another very important function of this muscle is its part in the kinetic chain of swallowing.

The *orbicularis oris muscle* (Fig. 1-6B) is the sphincter muscle of the mouth. It has no skeletal attachment. It is a composite muscle, composed not only of its own fibers but of fibers of all the muscles that converge on the mouth. Owing to the complex arrangement of all different fibers of different origins, the movements of the lips are varied. The upper lip is supported by the six maxillary anterior teeth, not the denture border. When the teeth are in occlusion the superior border of the lower lip is supported by the incisal third of the maxil-

lary anterior teeth; if this were not so, the lower lip would be caught between the anterior teeth during occlusal contacting. When the muscles of the lips are relaxed, the lips become flaccid. This can happen with the jaws open; therefore, it is important to the operator when making impressions for dentures. The angles of the mouth are easily irritated if the lips are stretched taut when an impression tray is inserted.

SUPRAHYOID MUSCLES (Fig. 1-9). The function of this group of muscles is either to elevate the hyoid bone and the larynx or to depress the mandible.

The *digastric, stylohyoid, mylohyoid,* and *geniohyoid* comprise this group of muscles. The *mylohyoid* and the *geniohyoid* influence the borders of the mandibular denture.

The *mylohyoid muscle* is a thin sheet that arises from the whole length of the mylohyoid line. The fibers are directed downward, medially, and forward. The posterior fibers are inserted into the body of the hyoid bone. Most of the

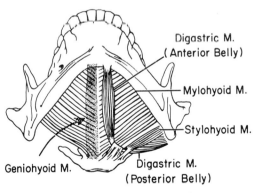

FIG. 1-9. *The suprahyoid muscles—the mylohyoid that forms the muscle floor of the oral cavity; the digastric consisting of two parts; the stylohyoid that aids in elevating and retracting the hyoid bone; and the geniohyoid that pulls the hyoid bone upward and forward or the mandible downward and backward.*

fibers are inserted into a median fibrous raphe extending from the symphysis of the mandible to the hyoid bone. The mylohyoid muscles constitute the muscle floor for the anterior part of the mouth. Its action elevates the hyoid bone, the tongue, and the mucous membrane floor of the mouth during swallowing. If the denture flange is extended below and under the mylohyoid line, it will impinge upon the mylohyoid muscle and will affect its action adversely, or the action of the muscle will unseat the denture. Because the fibers are directed downward, the denture flange can extend below the mylohyoid line but not under. This places the inferior border of the denture in a compatible position with the tongue. In instances of extensive bone loss the mylohyoid can be surgically detached from the periosteal attachment and re-attached more inferiorly on the body of the mandible without apparent impairment of function.

The *geniohyoid muscle* arises above the anterior end of the mylohyoid line from the genial tubercle at or near the midline on the lower surface of the mandible.

This muscle presents no problem in complete denture construction until there is extensive loss of the residual ridge. Like the mylohyoid it can be surgically detached from the periosteum and reattached more inferiorly on the mandible without apparent impairment of function.

INFRAHYOID MUSCLES. The origin and insertion of this group of muscles, which consists of the sternohyoid, omohyoid, sternothyroid, and thyrohyoid, have no particular significance in complete denture prosthodontics insofar as having any influence on the denture borders.

The action of these muscles is important to the prosthodontist, for they are a part of the kinetic chain of the mandibular movement. Their action is to fix the hyoid bone, as it were, to the trunk. It is from this fixed position that the suprahyoid muscles can act upon the mandible.

MUSCLES OF MASTICATION (Fig. 1-10). The muscles that have been designated as the muscles of mastication—the masseter, the temporalis, the internal pterygoid, and the external pterygoid—have their origins from the bones of the skull and are attached to the mandible. These muscles are involved not only in the masticatory movements of the mandible, but also in the nonmasticatory. In complete denture prosthodontics the nonmasticatory movements and the contacting of teeth during these movements are probably of more concern than the masticatory movements.

As a group, the muscles of mastication are very powerful. Only one of these directly influences the contour of the denture base. The contracture of the

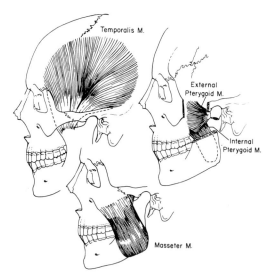

FIG. 1-10. *Muscles of mastication—the temporalis, the external pterygoid, the masseter, and the internal pterygoid.*

masseter forces the buccinator muscle in a medial direction in the area of the retromolar pad. This action can be recorded in the impression, and the denture border can be contoured to accommodate the action. If this is not done, the action will displace the mandibular denture and force it in an anterior direction.

The *masseter muscle* originates from the zygomatic arch and *inserts* to the outer surface of the mandible. The action of this powerful muscle is to elevate the mandible. The magnitude of its force is exerted in the molar region.

The *temporal muscle* is fan-shaped and has its *origin* from the whole of the temporal fossa on the lateral aspect of the skull. The fibers are divided into three groups—the anterior fibers, which form the bulk of the muscle, are vertical; the middle fibers are increasingly oblique; and the posterior fibers run almost horizontally.

The *insertion* occupies the coronoid process and reaches down to the ramus of the mandible. The temporal muscle is built for movement rather than power; the anterior fibers are elevators; and the middle and posterior fibers elevate and play a part in retracting the mandible. The action retracts and elevates the mandible.

The *internal pterygoid* originates from the pterygoid fossa, chiefly from the medial surface of the lateral pterygoid plate; a superficial head springs chiefly from the maxillary tuberosity. The *insertion* is on the medial surface of the angle of the mandible. The internal pterygoid is the synergist of the masseter and its action elevates the mandible.

The *external pterygoid* arises with two heads. The superior and inferior heads are separated by space and are enclosed by separate fascial envelopes, except at their origin. The superior head arises from the infratemporal pterygoid crest and from the adjoining surface of the greater wing of the sphenoid bone. The inferior head arises from the lateral aspect of the lateral plate of the pterygoid bone, the pyramidal portion of the palatal bone, and the maxillary tuberosity. The superior head is the smaller and inserts into the anterior surface of the articular disk with part of its fibers joining the inferior to insert on the anterior surface of the neck of the condyloid process.

The action is to pull the articular disk and the head of the mandible forward, downward, and inward along the posterior slope of the articular eminence.

When one analyzes the action of the muscles that move the mandible, one notes that the depressors are, relatively speaking, weak as compared to the elevators. The muscles which protrude and move the mandible from side to side are much stronger than the retractors. Bruxism (the grinding of teeth) and clenching (the elevating and closing of teeth firmly) are acts that are caused by very powerful muscles, and the results of these actions are damaging to the denture-supporting structures.

In recording the jaw relations, one records centric relation with the aid of the weak posterior fibers of the temporalis. The antagonist to this action is the powerful external pterygoid.

The group of four muscles designated as the muscles of mastication are not the only muscles involved in the masticatory processes; neither is mastication their only function. Mandibular movement or the kinetics of the muscles employed in mandibular movements are quite involved and deserve special study. An example is the kinetics involved in deglutition, the act of swallowing.

By means of Kodachrome motion pictures, Syrop studied the functioning of the intraoral organs involved in mastication and swallowing and reported:

When the tongue determines the proper degree of particle dispersion, the bolus is pushed backward and upward by the tongue against the hard palate. This process is the initial phase of deglutition. The lips close, the mandible elevates, the teeth are clenched and the tip of the tongue is raised and placed against the anterior portion of the palate with a simultaneous contraction of the anterior pillar of the fauces.

At the same time, the nasal cavity is sealed off from the pharynx by the contraction of the posterior pillars of the fauces and the upward and backward elevation of the soft palate and uvula against the upper pharyngeal wall. . . . Breathing is interrupted briefly. [The opening into the trachea is closed off by the action of the epiglottis.] As the bolus is swept backward by the tongue in a sweeping and undulating motion, the hyoid bone is raised upward to provide additional rigidity to the floor of the mouth. . . . The sealing off of the respiratory opening, the nasal cavity and the anterior portions of the mouth allows the bolus no other course save that of going backward and downward along an oblique plane [into the piriform sinus and thus to the esophagus].[45]

When the kinetics of the mandibular muscles and those associated with the oral cavity are understood, the borders of the dentures including the posterior palatal seal, the contour of the polished surfaces, and the positions of the teeth become a part of the individual, not just mechanical artificial substitutes.

TONGUE (Fig. 1-11). The *tongue* is a muscular organ, attached with its base and the central part of its body to the floor of the mouth. The function of the tongue in coordination with the muscles of the lips, cheeks, throat, and palate is associated with mastication, deglutition, and speech. In addition to this muscular function of the tongue, the sensory nerve supply permits taste. The sensory nerve endings permit the tongue to detect not only particle size of food

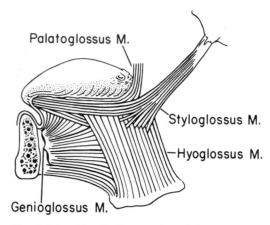

FIG. 1-11. *Extrinsic muscles of the tongue— the palatoglossus, styloglossus, hyoglossus, and genioglossus. The tongue is a protective organ of the body.*

but also defects on teeth or denture base. This sensory acuteness is a protective mechanism, seeking and detecting material that might enter and damage the alimentary tract.

Since the tongue is located in the floor of the mouth, it is intimately in contact with the lingual flanges of the mandibular denture. The denture flanges must be contoured to allow the tongue its normal range of functional movement. The tip of the tongue is used to moisten the lips many times a day; during mastication, the tongue takes the food from the floor of the mouth and the labial and buccal vestibule spaces and places it on the occlusal surfaces of the teeth. The tongue directs the flow of food and liquids to the throat in swallowing.

The muscular activity of the tongue is controlled by two groups of muscles, the intrinsic and extrinsic. The intrinsic muscles, being wholly inside the tongue, can only produce changes of shape in the tongue. The extrinsic group take origin from parts outside the tongue and can move the tongue as well as alter its shape.

The *genioglossus* arises from the genial tubercles on the inner surface of the mandible at its lower border in the midline. The anterior fibers insert into the tip of the tongue, whereas most of the posterior fibers reach the base of the tongue. It acts mainly as a protractor and a depressor of the tongue.

The *styloglossus* muscle arises from the anterior surface of the styloid process and enters the tongue near the base; the fibers continue to the tip of the tongue. Its action is to pull the tongue backward and upward.

The *hyoglossus* muscle arises from the hyoid bone. The muscle forms a thin plate and inserts into the side of the tongue. Its action is to depress the tongue.

The *palatoglossus* draws the tongue and soft palate together. It is described with the palatine musculature.

Investigation shows that 35 per cent of tongues are abnormal in either size, position, or function. The normal tongues are usually quite adaptable to complete dentures, provided the flanges are properly contoured and the teeth placed in a position compatible with the cheek and tongue. The abnormal tongues present problems, do not always readily adapt and must be dealt with individually. It is fortunate that muscle responds to normal function by maintenance or alterations in bulk. This information is valuable in discussions of the use and care of dentures with patients.

MUSCLES OF THE SOFT PALATE (Fig. 1-12). The tensor palati, levator palati, azygos uvulae, palatoglossus, and palatopharyngeus are the muscles of the soft palate, which is a movable curtain extending downward and backward into the pharynx. During deglutition it is raised and helps to shut off the nasal part of the pharynx from the portion below.

The posterior extension of the maxillary denture base rests in the soft palate. This area is the palatine aponeurosis. This tendinous sheet lies in the anterior two-

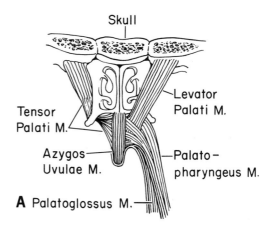

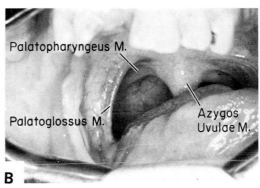

FIG. 1-12. *Muscles of the soft palate.* **A.** *The horizontal part of the tendon of the tensor palati muscle spreads like a fan and is known as the palatine aponeurosis. In the palate the levator palati muscle is situated above and slightly behind the palatine aponeurosis. The azygos uvulae muscle is unpaired and has weak fibers. The palatoglossus muscle arises from the anterior surface of the palatine aponeurosis and descends to the lateral surface of the tongue. The fibers interlace with the transverse fibers of the tongue.* **B.** *When the tongue is moved toward the cheek, the reflection of mucous membrane that overlies the palatoglossus muscle is made taut. The contour of the posterior lingual flange of the mandibular denture must accommodate for this action.*

thirds of the soft palate and is attached to the crest on the lower surface of the bony palate near its posterior end. Near the bony palate the muscle fibers are very scanty, and the aponeurosis is thick and strong at the junction; the anterior part of the soft palate is therefore more horizontal and less movable than the posterior part. The character of the aponeurosis and the overlying mucosa, the activity of the palatine muscles, and the contour of the soft palate determine the extent and the contour of the posterior palatal seal. The seal should be in the soft palate and not over the palatine bone. The placing of the posterior palatal seal is the responsibility of the dentist. The extent, depth, and slope of the extension into the soft palate is determined by visual examination and by palpation (Fig. 1-13). As a general rule, the more acute the angle of attachment between the aponeurosis and the bone, the more active the reflection. The more active the reflection, the less the denture base can extend into the soft palate distally, and the more it must extend vertically. The ac-

tivity is determined by visually watching the attachment action of the aponeurosis when the patient says "Ah." The junction of the soft and hard palate can best be determined by closing both the patient's nostrils and having him blow gently. The air will force the soft palate to flex inferiorly at the junction. The contours of the hamular notch and the palatine bones can best be outlined by palpating with a ball burnisher. The posterior palatal seal, if used, should *follow the contour of the palatine bones* and extend from hamular notch to hamular notch. The pterygomandibular raphe is a strong, narrow ligamentous band which extends from the pterygoid hamulus to the posterior part of the mylohyoid line. When the jaws are separated, this ligamentous band becomes taut, and the placement of a posterior palatal seal in the hamular notch could cause the mucous membrane to be cut or the ligament to dislodge the denture, usually the former (Fig. 1-14B).

Frequently formed at the junction of the aponeurosis and the posterior nasal spine is a narrow bundle similar to a ligament (Fig. 1-14A). The posterior palatal seal is not placed over this narrow area.

The *tensor palati* is a thin, flat triangular muscle that ends inferiorly in a slender tendon that turns around the root of the pterygoid hamulus to enter the palate. This slender tendon, when taut, could influence the denture contour in the hamular notch area.

The *levator palati* is a thick, rounded muscle which arises from the petrous portion of the temporal bone. It has a downward and medial course which flattens as it approaches the midline of the soft palate to interlace with its counterpart from the opposite side. The sling that is formed by the joining of these two muscles causes the soft palate to be elevated during contraction. This action of

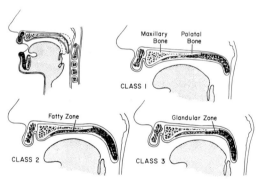

FIG. 1-13. *Schematic illustrations of the three basic slopes of soft palates. Class 1 is considered the most favorable palate for placing an adequate posterior palatal seal. This soft palate would not have to rise far to meet the walls of the throat to obturate the opening to the nasopharynx. Class 2 palate would require more muscle activity than Class 1. Class 3 palate requires considerable muscle activity for closure of the nasopharynx, and this action makes placing a posterior palatal seal difficult. (Suggested by the illustrations in Nagle and Sears: Denture Prosthetics. 2nd ed. St. Louis, The C. V. Mosby Company, 1962.)*

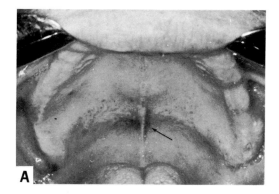

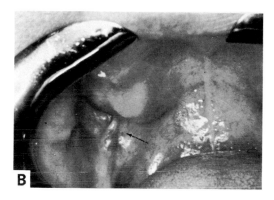

FIG. 1-14. *The soft palate.* **A.** *The arrow points to the band of palatine aponeurosis that is frequently found at the posterior nasal spine.* **B.** *The arrow designates the tight band of tissue that is elevated by the pterygomandibular raphe.*

PHARYNGEAL MUSCLES (Fig. 1-15). The *superior constrictor* is the pharyngeal muscle of most interest in complete denture construction. The superior constrictor has four sites of origin: the pterygoid hamulus, the pterygomandibular raphe, the posterior end of the mylohyoid line, and the mucous membrane of the mouth and side of the tongue. The action of this muscular band exerts pressure against the distal extremity of the mandibular denture. Overextension in this area is very painful to the patient, as the denture will perforate the tissue and cause a sore throat.

ORAL MUCOUS MEMBRANE

The features of the mucous membrane that either supports the complete denture or comes in contact with it must be analyzed, for they determine how this support can best be used.

the muscle is significant in closing off the oral cavity from the nasopharynx during swallowing as well as in the determination of the vibrating line.

The *palatoglossus* muscle forms a thin sheet in the lower part of the soft palate. The fibers converge to form a slender slip that descends in the palatoglossal arch, thence to the side of the tongue, and a small bundle inserts into the capsule of the tonsil. When the two palatoglossi contract, they draw the tongue and soft palate together. This assists in closing the isthmus of the fauces. This action brings lateral pressure to the lingual extension of the mandibular denture (Fig. 1-12B).

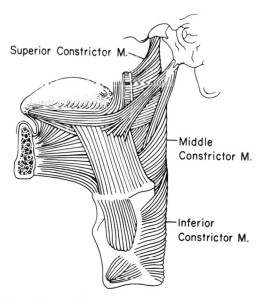

FIG. 1-15. *Pharyngeal muscles. The action of the constrictor muscles is the narrowing of the pharyngeal space. The action of the superior muscle must be evaluated, and the contour of the posterior lingual flange of the mandibular denture must be made to accommodate.*

MAXILLARY ARCH.   The mucosal coverings of the gingiva and the hard palate have in common an epithelium that is thick and hornified; the thickness, firmness, and density of an inelastic lamina propria; and an immovable attachment to the deep structures (Fig. 1-16). These two areas differ in their submucosa. There is no well-differentiated submucous layer in the gingiva; the inelastic connective tissue of the lamina propria fuses with the periosteum of the alveolar process. There is a distinct submucous

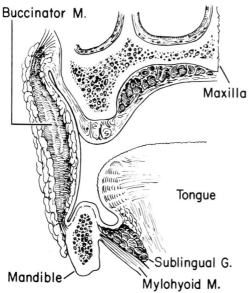

Buccinator M.

Maxilla

Tongue

Sublingual G.

Mandible

Mylohyoid M.

FIG. 1-16.   *Schematic illustration of a frontal section of the maxillary and mandibular arches. The maxilla and mandible provide the bone support for dentures. The positions of the teeth and the contour of the denture flanges should support the buccinator muscle. The mucous membrane floor of the mouth is displaceable. The lingual flange of the mandibular denture is not extended in an inferior direction to trap the sublingual gland between the denture flange and the mylohyoid muscle. The vertical and horizontal positions of the teeth are placed in harmony with the actions of the buccinator muscle and the tongue. (From Nagle and Sears: Denture Prosthetics. 2nd ed. St. Louis, The C. V. Mosby Company, 1962.)*

layer in the covering of the palate, except at its periphery, and a narrow area extending from in front of the incisal papilla over the midpalatal suture. Even though there is a distinct submucosa, the mucous membrane is tightly attached by dense bands and trabeculae of connective tissue to the periosteum of the maxillary and palatine bones.

The submucosa is divided into spaces; the spaces in the middle third of the hard palate are filled with adipose tissue, whereas the spaces in the posterior third contain glands (Fig. 1-17). The presence of fatty or glandular tissue provides a cushioned type of support. The cushioned submucosa in the palate can be compared with the subcutaneous tissue of the palms of the hands and the soles of the feet. Therefore, it appears that the hard palate should be considered the primary stress-bearing area for the maxillary denture. However, the teeth cannot be placed to direct the forces of occlusion to the hard palate. The residual alveolar ridge is, under normal conditions, covered by a tissue which in its structure is identical with normal attached gingiva. It is a firm, thick layer of inelastic, dense connective tissue, immovably attached to the periosteum. Rather recent study by Atwood reveals "no periosteal bone over the crest of the edentulous residual ridges of the mandibles studied."[1] Further study may lead to a better understanding of these tissues as support for a denture.

The mucous membrane that comes in contact with the denture borders has relatively thin, nonhornified epithelium and thin lamina propria. The submucosal structure may be either tightly or loosely attached. On the lips, cheeks, and underside of the tongue the lining mucosa is fixed to the epimysium or the fascia of the muscle. It is highly elastic in character. In the fornix vestibule and in the sublingual sulcus the mucous membrane is loosely and movably attached

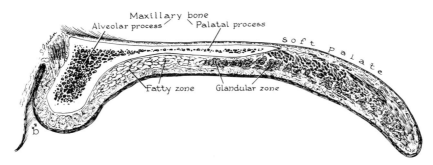

FIG. 1-17. *Schematic illustration of a lower power magnification of a sagittal section through the hard and soft palate (through the lateral incisor region). In an anterior-posterior direction note the (1) loosely attached submucosa in the labial vestibule, (2) tightly attached submucosa on the slopes and crest of the residual ridge, (3) differentiated submucosa in the palate distal to the rugae area. (From Nagle and Sears: Denture Prosthetics. 2nd ed. St. Louis, The C. V. Mosby Company, 1962.)*

to the deep structures. These areas are easily displaced and act as excellent areas to create a seal for the denture borders. The ease of displaceability also accounts for frequent overextension of the denture borders.

SOFT PALATE. The *mucosa of the soft palate* is a transition between the fixed and loosely attached types. For this reason some soft palates afford desirable posterior palatal seal areas and others less desirable.

A *cushion type* of tissue can readily be displaced; however, when displacing forces are relaxed or withdrawn, the tissues will attempt to return to their normal positions. This phenomenon is an important consideration when impressions are being made.

MANDIBULAR ARCH. In the *mandibular arch* the distal end of the gingival area is well marked. After the loss of the last molar, the *retromolar papilla*, a "pear-shaped area" of gingival tissue, remains fused to the scar. This area is firm and pale and easily distinguished from the *retromolar pad*, which is soft, dark red, and usually readily displaceable (Fig. 1-18).

In analyzing the oral mucosa it is readily seen that the soft tissues supporting dentures do not have the same resiliency even when considered normal. This uneven displaceability of the soft tissues is of considerable interest in the

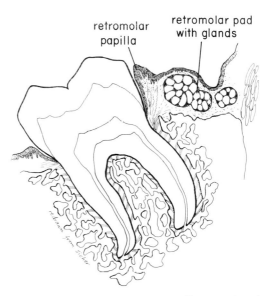

FIG. 1-18. *The retromolar papillae consist of typical gingival tissue. The retromolar pad has a loosely attached submucosa containing glands. (Redrawn after Sicher and Du-Brul: Oral Anatomy. 6th ed. St. Louis, The C. V. Mosby Company, 1975.)*

construction procedures involved in complete dentures. The making of impressions, the recording and verifying of jaw relations, and the harmonizing of the occlusion of the teeth to coincide with jaw movements are greatly influenced by the quantity and quality of soft tissues. Hanau has described this as "realeff," the resiliency and like effects. Much of Hanau's philosophy is based on the resiliency of the supporting soft tissues.

It has been demonstrated that the mucosa supporting the denture bases is not only displaceable, but also compressible, and rather significant findings are applicable to complete denture prosthodontics. Some of the findings are:

1. The tissues in the elderly take many hours to recover from the effect of moderate mechanical force, whereas twenty-five-year-olds need only a short time for complete recovery.

2. The thicker the tissue the more the deformity.

3. The sex of the individual does not appear to affect the results.

4. Small forces can produce distinct compression of the tissues.

5. Light loads over long duration of time deform tissue more than heavy loads for short duration.

When this knowledge is applied in complete denture prosthodontics, several factors appear pertinent:

1. Dentures, particularly for patients over twenty-five years of age, should be removed when making impressions for new dentures: for sufficient time for tissue recovery. This may be twenty-four hours for young persons and several days for the geriatric patient.

2. A low viscosity impression material which will flow freely after the impression material is *seated* should be used. Rubber base and silicone impression materials are not low viscosity materials. Pressure is released after seating.

3. Impression materials should not be confined when making the refined impression. Escape holes should be provided, especially in the maxillary arch.

4. An impression should not be removed and inserted any more repeatedly than necessary. It is advisable to border refine one arch and proceed with border refining the other arch before the refined impression or to border refine at one appointment and make the refined impression the next day.

5. Parafunctional habits produce light loads for long durations, whereas physiological practices occur as heavy loads for short durations. An individual who grinds, doodles, or clinches is a problem patient, regardless of the dentition, natural or artificial. It is the responsibility of the dentist to recognize the problem and institute procedures to correct the source. This may require multidiscipline efforts, for it is recognized that individuals in stress, a state of anxiety, or hypertension develop abnormal muscle habits.

6. Excessively thick mucosa should be evaluated for possible surgical reduction.

TEMPOROMANDIBULAR
ARTICULATION (Fig. 1-19)

Definition: Temporomandibular articulation is the articulation of the condyloid process of the mandible and the interarticular disk with the mandibular fossa of the temporal bone.

The temporomandibular joint, because of its complexity, has received more attention and study than any other joint in the body. Much of the early study was devoted to trying to reproduce the movements in the joint because the development of an instrument was necessary to relate the teeth to these movements. In more recent years, the pathology of the joint, primarily functional disorders, has led to the focusing of attention on the

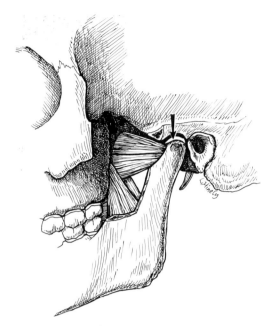

FIG. 1-19. *Schematic illustration of the temporomandibular joint. The arrow points to the articular disk that divides the articular space into two compartments. The component parts are no more complex than other living tissue. (Redrawn after Freese and Scheman: Management of Temporomandibular Joint Problems. St. Louis, The C. V. Mosby Company, 1962.)*

extrinsic influences that are involved in these movements.

To know the anatomy of the joint is to know why the movements are complex. Only by knowing the anatomy is it possible to determine what movements can be duplicated, what movements can be simulated, and what values can be placed on the different entities involved.

OSSEOUS COMPONENTS (Fig. 1-20). The mandibular or glenoid fossae are located anteriorly and inferiorly to the auditory meatus. They are bordered in front by the articular tubercles, and behind they are separated from the external acoustic meatus by the tympanic part of the bone.

The fossae are divided into two parts by a narrow slit, the petrotympanic fissure. The anterior part of the fossae and the articular tubercles are parts of the squamous portion of the temporal bones. The posterior parts, tympanic and petrous, are related structures but do not enter into mandibular articulation.

The articular tubercles or eminences lie at the inferior base of the zygomatic process. The eminence is strongly convex in an anteroposterior direction but somewhat concave in a transverse direction. The anteroposterior convexity and the transverse concavity are highly variable. This variability exists in the same individual from the right to the left fossa.

The convex inferior surface of the eminentia articulates with the concave superior surface of the articular disk. The articulating surfaces are covered by a layer of fibrous tissue.

The bony roof of the mandibular fossa is very thin. This thinness seems to be indicative that this surface is not an articulating one.

THE HEAD OF THE MANDIBLE (CONDYLAR PROCESS) (Fig. 1-20B). The head of the mandible is composed of two sections, the capitulum or condyle and the neck. The condyle is the bulbous semicylindroid extremity with its long axis placed at right angles to the plane of the mandibular ramus and deviated from the frontal direction. The roughened lateral surface is inclined more anteriorly than the smooth medial surface. If the axes of the two condyles were extended medially and posteriorly, they would cross at or near the anterior circumference of the foramen magnum.

The smooth articulating surface of the condyle faces upward and forward. The posterior surface is fairly flat, but the anterior surface has an eminence near its midpoint that fits into a corresponding

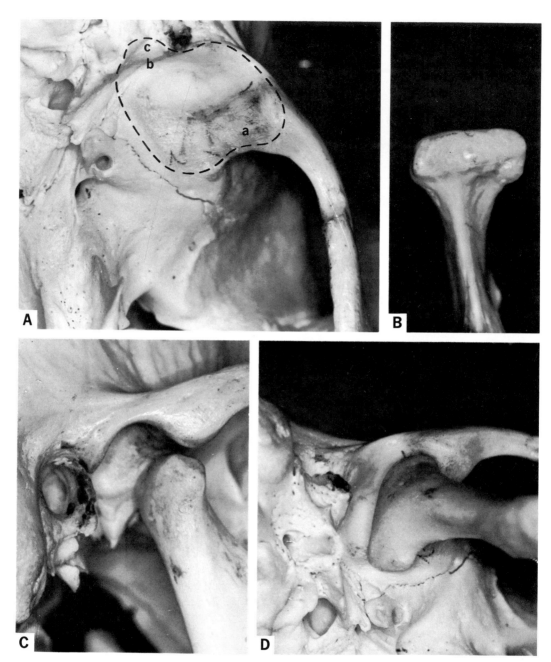

FIG. 1-20. *The osseous components of the temporomandibular joint involve the bones of the skull. The irregularities of the surface are obscured by the thick covering of fibrous tissue.* **A.** *The mandibular or glenoid fossa: articular eminence (a); petrotympanic fissure (b); posterior part (c).* **B.** *The head of the mandible.* **C.** *Lateral view of the fossa and condyle.* **D.** *Posterior view of the condyle elevated into the fossa to illustrate the similarity in contour of the fossa and the condyle.*

depression in the articular eminence. The condyle is a three-dimensional structure. It is strongly convex in an anteroposterior direction and slightly convex mediolaterally. The irregularities of the bony articulating surfaces are usually obscured and smoothed by the thick covering of fibrous tissue.

The convex superior surface articulates with the concave inferior surface of the articular disk.

Freese and Scheman, in the *Management of Temporomandibular Joint Problems,* state, "The exact correspondence of shape between the head of the mandible and the glenoid fossa is even more remarkable if we consider that between these two surfaces is interposed an articular disk. . . ."[13]

THE SOFT TISSUE COMPONENTS. The *articular disk* (Fig. 1-21*A*) is a flat, circular or approximately circular, dense, fibrous connective tissue plate. Islands

of cartilage, fibrocartilage, in the disk usually occur in the higher age groups. The disk varies in thickness; it is thickest posteriorly, thin at its center, and becomes somewhat thicker anteriorly. It is attached to the articular capsule and is directly fused in its anterior, medial, and lateral sections, whereas in the posterior section the disk and capsule are connected by a thick layer of loose connective tissue. The superior surface of the articular disk is concave as is the inferior surface (biconcave). Considerable significance is attached to the histology, attachments, and morphology of the articular disk. Blood vessels are absent in the fine central area of the articular disk, and this indicates that pressures exist in the joint. Avascular connective tissue is adapted to resist pressures. Since the disk is attached at its periphery to the capsule and the capsule envelops the joint, its presence divides the compartment into two spaces that contain the synovial

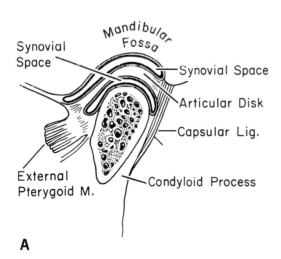

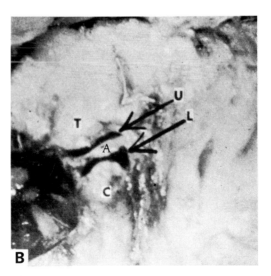

A   **B**

FIG. 1-21.   *The soft tissue components.* **A.** *A schematic illustration of the components of the temporomandibular joint and the insertion of the external pterygoid muscle.* **B.** *A partial dissection of the temporomandibular joint discloses the temporal bone (T), articular disk (A), condyle (C), upper compartment (U), and lower compartment (L). (From Freese and Scheman: Management of Temporomandibular Joint Problems. St. Louis, The C. V. Mosby Company, 1962.)*

fluid, the synovial spaces (Fig. 1-21B). The presence of the disk also allows two types of movement, diarthrodial (sliding) and ginglymus (hinge). The presence of the articular disk or meniscus also differentiates the temporomandibular joint from any other joint in the body, making it a bone-to-tissue (mandible to disk) and tissue-to-bone (disk to skull) articulation. The concavity of the disk on its superior and inferior surfaces should be indicative of where in the articulation the shape of the bony components will exert the most influence in mandibular movements. Convex surfaces fit into concave ones. Therefore, as the disk and the condyle approach the convex surfaces of the fossa, the two bony components become more closely approximated.

The *articular capsule* (Fig. 1-22) is a loose, thin sack of fibrous connective tissue that is attached to the border of the articulating surface of the temporal bone and to the neck of the condyloid process. It is attached to the skull as follows: to the posterior end of the zygomatic process, the anterior margin of the articular process, the medial edge of the mandibular fossa, and the posterior edge of the mandibular fossa anterior to the petrotympanic fissure. The lateral surface of the capsule is strengthened to a fairly distinct ligament, the tem-

poromandibular ligament. The attachment of the capsule between the skull and disk is very loose; however, the attachment between capsule, disk, and the neck of the condyloid process is tight. The capsule is especially tense between the disk and the two poles of the condyle.

The loose attachment between the capsule, skull, and disk allows the sliding diarthrodial movement in the upper compartment, whereas the tight attachment between disk, capsule, and condyloid process limits the movement to hinge or ginglymus in the lower compartment.

The *synovial membrane* is a connective tissue membrane which lines the fibrous articular capsule and covers the loose connective tissue between it and the posterior border of the disk. This membrane secretes the synovial fluid, a viscid, albuminous fluid which serves as a natural lubricant.

MANDIBULAR MOVEMENTS. The anatomical relation between the heads of the condyle and the articular capsule limits mandibular movements. This relation is described previously in the section on the articular capsule.

The sphenomandibular ligament arises from the angular spine of the sphenoid bone and inserts into the mandibular ligament, which is just superior to the mandibular foramen.

The stylomandibular ligament extends from the styloid process and stylohyoid ligament to the region of the mandibular angle.

The anatomical relation between the heads of the mandible and the dome-shaped concavities in the temporal bone with the interposed articular disk allows movements different in nature from the movements of any other joint in the body. The presence of the disk allows two types of movement, diarthrodial

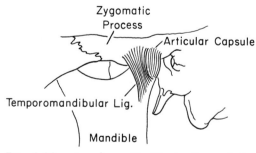

Zygomatic Process

Articular Capsule

Temporomandibular Lig.

Mandible

FIG. 1-22. *A schematic illustration of the thin, fibrous articular capsule of the mandibular joint. The lateral surface is strengthened to the temporomandibular ligament.*

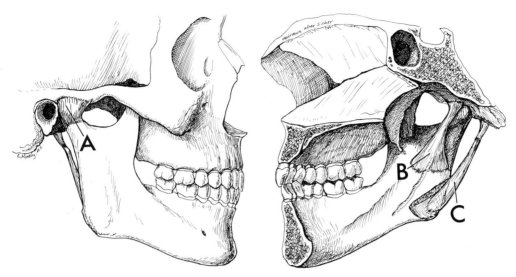

Fig. 1-23. *Lateral views of the temporomandibular joint showing the temporomandibular ligament* **(A),** *the sphenomandibular ligament* **(B),** *and the stylomandibular ligament* **(C).** *Only the temporomandibular ligament has a decisive influence in mandibular movements. (Redrawn after Sicher and DuBrul: Oral Anatomy. 6th ed. St. Louis, The C. V. Mosby Company, 1975.)*

(sliding) and ginglymus (hinge), thus the description, diarthrodial ginglymus joint. The movement in the upper compartment is chiefly a gliding motion in which the condyles and the articular disk move as a unit. This gliding movement is referred to as translation or a translatory movement; it is motion in which every point of the moving object has simultaneously the same velocity and direction of motion, distinguished from rotation. The pure hinge movement occurs between the articular disk and the condyles in the lower compartment. In most of the movements of the condyles, the glidings and the rotations cannot be isolated. The lateral rotations are slight movements and are made in the upper compartment. The lower compartment is not a ball and socket joint; it is a hinge. The shape of the condyle and the attachment of the articular capsule at the lateral and medial poles dictates this hinge movement.

Because of its peculiar form and manner of its attachments, the mandible is capable of, and subject to, a great variety of movements. So free and varied are these movements that they may appear to lack coordination. This is a deceptive appearance, for when movements that are made within the boundaries become uncoordinated beyond physiologic tolerances, pathologic conditions result. This has been repeatedly demonstrated by pathologic temporomandibular joints, pathologic wear of natural teeth, breakdown of the periodontium, and loss of osseous support to the teeth from malocclusion of the natural teeth. This has also been frequently seen with complete dentures, lesions of the oral mucosal covering of the residual ridges, the unseating of the dentures, and loss of osseous support resulting from the lack of harmony between the artificial substitutes and mandibular movements. Natural teeth, for all practical purposes, are fixed in bone, moving only within the limits of the periodontal attachments.

When the natural teeth are in contact and moving (gliding occlusion), they become a primary force in mandibular movements. Artificial teeth are attached to a movable denture base that is resting on displaceable tissue. The degree of displaceability varies in amount and direction. When the artificial teeth are in contact in dynamic gliding occlusion, they become a secondary force in mandibular movements.

The anatomy of the joint does allow some freedom of movement, but not random and freely swinging movements. The joint has a high degree of adjustability, but this adjustability varies greatly with different individuals, depending on the limits of physiologic tolerance in the individual joint. These movements also change in the same individual as a result of variance in muscle tonus. Movements recorded under stress conditions are not the same as those recorded under relaxed conditions. Movements noted on manual manipulation of the mandible are not necessarily the movements that will be initiated by the innate musculature. Movements in the same individual recorded during a period of lessened or increased muscle tonus will also vary. The joint movements are directed far less than any other joint by the articulating bones and by the articular ligaments, but to a greater degree by the play of muscles. The temporomandibular joint, its surroundings, and its controls are all living tissue capable of manifesting variabilities like all other similar living tissue, and these are the entities that make it difficult to understand the mechanics of temporomandibular articulation.

Movements of the mandible can be classified as masticatory and nonmasticatory. The masticatory procedures are the movements necessary in the introduction of food, the grasping, the crushing, the grinding, and finally, the swallowing of the triturated mass.

The nonmasticatory movements would then constitute all other normal movements, such as those used in speech and in wetting the lips, and also the habitual or abnormal movements such as bruxism, clenching, or tapping the teeth together.

In the mastication of food the movements are *"hingelike"* used in opening and closing the mouth for the introduction of food and to a lesser degree for the crushing of certain types of food, *protrusive* movement used in the grasping and incision of food, *right* and *left lateral* excursion for the reduction of fibrous as well as other types of bulky food. The combination of all these movements appears to be the most effective in the minute trituration of food.

Stuart states:

It seems obvious that jaw motions at condyle levels can be resolved into glidable rotating axes. Observers, viewing the action of the condyles during chewing, either by roentgenograms or by watching joints exposed to surgery, are impressed more by the gliding action than by the rotations. The only isolatable mandibular rotation movement capable of being seen is an opening and closing movement around the tranverse intercondylar axis when it is rearmost in the head.*

In addition to the movements that have been considered, there are two other movements that have a definite influence in prosthodontic procedures.

The *Bennett movement* is the bodily lateral movement of lateral shift of the mandible resulting from the movements of the condyles along the lateral inclines of the mandibular fossae in lateral jaw movements. Sicher describes this movement thusly:

*Stuart, C. E.: J. Prosth. Dent., 9:222, 1959.

In right lateral movement of the lower jaw the right condyle does, however, not rotate in situ as was formerly believed, but moves also slightly forward and outward.... The physiologic basis of Bennett's movement is the fact that a lateral shift of the mandible is possible only if the "resting" condyle is held in place by retrusive muscle fibers.... [The slide anteriorly and laterally is far enough to avoid any strain behind the rotating condyle.][41]

Stuart records the following pantographic findings:

The outward direction of a Bennett path may be combined simply with an upward, downward, forward or backward component. Its outward direction may be united with combinations of these, such as downward and backward, up and backward, down and forward, or up and forward. A Bennett movement may take place at the beginning of the lateral movement or it may be distributed throughout the lateral deflection. In other words, there is a definite timing in this side shift movement.*

Bennett movement, like all other movements from the centric occlusion position, is important if teeth contact or are in gliding occlusion as they move from and to centric occlusion or if clearance is provided to avoid contact.

Boswell described a phenomenon that can be interpreted as a unilateral vertical movement of the condyle in the glenoid fossa. This movement has not been reproduced in a mechanical substitute for the temporomandibular joint. Very little attention is paid to this movement, but if true, it has a very definite influence on jaw relation records. If a resistant object such as a stick is placed between the posterior teeth on one side and pressure is applied, the teeth can be made to almost contact on the opposite side. The interocclusal distance on the stick side will be more than on the non-stick side.

This phenomenon may also be the result of intruding the natural teeth or displacing the tissues under the denture bases.

When bilateral jaw relation records are being made, if the recording material is more resistant on the one side than the other, the contraction of the muscles can result in the jaws coming closer together on the least resistant side. Teeth arranged in this recorded jaw position will have a tendency to contact first on the more resistant side. The premature contact will depend upon several factors: the extent of displacement of the supporting soft tissue and the amount of intrusion of the condyle into the meniscus.

Boswell contended that the intrusion of the condyle into the meniscus was a result of the continued contracting of the muscles on the noncontacting side in an attempt to make the teeth contact. It appears that when recording media of unlike resistance are used, the muscles will cease to contract on the more resistant side and continue to contract on the least resistant side.[4a]

If the displacement of the soft tissue on the pressure side is greater than the intrusion of the condyle into the meniscus on the nonpressure side, the premature contact may be on the side of most pressure. This is not to be confused with bilateral differences in muscle contraction. Nor should it be overlooked that even though the bilateral pressure may be equal the displacement of the soft tissues may not be bilaterally the same. When McCollum was locating the terminal hinge axis at condyle level, this phenomenon was not demonstrated.

In considering mandibular movements and the temporomandibular joint it must be remembered that the movements within the joints are magnified when recording at distant points. The movement of the mandible at the point of the chin will be greater than at the posterior. Pantographic and strobe light studies are

* Stuart, C. E.: J. Prosth. Dent., 9:222, 1959.

magnified movements. This feature in no way invalidates their use, but they are not to be confused with the magnitude of movement in the joints.

In mastication the size and consistency of the bolus have a very definite influence on the direction and magnitude of movements.

The role of teeth in complete dentures must be considered as secondary in mandibular movements. When the teeth are in maximum occlusal contact in a static position, they could be responsible for a malposition of the condyles. If this is an uncomfortable position, the neuromuscular control will attempt to make correction. These corrections will be reflected in the denture-supporting structures more frequently than in the joint. If the teeth are not in harmony with mandibular movement when in gliding occlusion, the dictates at the joint level will predominate.

The joints are capable of more than one movement. It is possible that an individual could be trained to function in one or more of these movements.

Physiology

Definition: Physiology is the branch of biology dealing with the functions and vital processes of living organisms or their parts and organs.

The requirements of a successful complete denture are demanding: (1) compatibility with the surrounding oral environment, (2) restoration of masticatory efficiency within limits, (3) ability to function in harmony with the activity necessary in speech, respiration, and deglutition, (4) esthetic acceptability, (5) preservation of that which remains. To fulfill these requirements the prosthodontist needs to have a knowledge of the functions and vital processes of the body. Although a denture is not living tissue, it must function with and become a part of the body.

Since the Syllabus was first published, the study of and research in oral physiology has been pursued by physiologists who are dentally oriented. The findings and documentations of these students and researchers are revealing scientific evidence of factors which have been accepted on, more or less, an empirical basis. An example is that the soft tissues supporting the dentures not only are displaceable but also are compressible. These and other research findings have extensive practical application in dentistry, including complete denture prosthodontics.

It is not the purpose of this text to present in detail the subject of oral physiology; however, there are basic factors that the prosthodontist should know and understand. When the knowledge is applied, many of the Why's are understood. Many of the mechanical procedures, the How's, will be analyzed in a more objective manner. When one finds that a procedure used, taught, and passed down from generation to generation defies a basic fundamental principle in the functioning of the anatomical structure, he should question the validity of such a procedure. Persons who are trained in the technical procedures essential in complete denture prosthodontics can frequently satisfy the first four requirements for successful dentures; however, they rarely meet the fifth requirement.

PHYSIOLOGY OF BONE

Although considerable study has been devoted to the physiology of bone, the functions and vital processes of the osseous residual ridges supporting a denture need further study. Much of the knowledge pertaining to all skeletal bone is applicable, since the bone of the residual ridges is skeletal.

It is easy to understand why a study of the bone supporting dentures is extremely difficult: (1) vivisections only reveal the reaction of one section of bone to one denture, (2) bone responses in individuals vary in unaccountable ways, (3) roentgenographic studies are inconclusive as related to the stress-bearing potential of bone, (4) bone is one of the most unstable tissues in the body (Fig. 1-24).

ALVEOLAR PROCESS. The alveolar process appears to be the bony support most affected by dentures. The alveolar process supports the natural teeth and provides most of the vertical support for dentures. When the natural teeth are present, the roots occupy most of the space between the compact plates. This is particularly true in the anterior region in both arches. Healing of sockets after tooth extraction is similar to that for fractures: (1) primary clot formation in the socket, (2) organization of the clot by proliferating young connective tissue, (3) gradual replacement of the young connective tissues by coarse fibrillar bone, (4) reconstruction by resorptive activity on the one side and replacement of the immature bone by mature bone on the other, (5) epithelization and healing of the surface occurring simultaneously with the other reparative processes.

The reconstructive process leads generally to loss of bone in the area

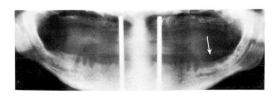

FIG. 1-24. *Roentgenogram of osseous residual ridge. The arrow points to bone loss. Was the loss a result of mental stress, pressure from a denture, systemic factors, or a combination of many factors?*

and to the formation of compact lamella at the surface of the scar. Histologic investigations have proved that the socket is filled with immature bone by the end of the second month. There is some quantitative loss when healing is uneventful; when the primary clot fails to form or is destroyed, the denuded bone necrotizes and is eliminated by resorption. This loss in quantity during normal healing after extraction is one of the reasons a waiting period of six weeks to two months is often advocated prior to the placement of dentures. To allow the immature bone to replace the young connective tissue is another reason.

BONE TISSUE. Bone tissue is in continuous flux throughout life. The regenerative reconstruction of bone is the result of the destruction of old bone, the action of the osteoclast, and the formation of new bone by the osteoblast. This regenerative reconstruction, although continuous throughout life, is not constant. During the period of bony growth the formation of bone outweighs resorption. In the adult, the two processes are more nearly balanced. In senility, resorption outweighs the formation. This regenerative reconstruction process accounts for the bony support reacting differently in different age groups. This is only one of the many reasons some dentures appear to be physiologically tolerated over a period of time and then seem to fail.

CHANGE IN FUNCTION. The reaction of bone to a change in function is subjected to the supreme test when the natural teeth are extracted and replaced with dentures. Wolff's law states that a change in form follows a change in function owing to alteration of the internal architecture and external conformation of the bone, in accordance with mathematical laws. Neufeld reported: "In some of the specimens studied, the trabecular pattern was arranged in such a way that it indicated that there was some adaptation of the structure of the bones to the presence of an appliance in the region near the superior surface of the alveolar process."[36] It seems possible that the trabecular pattern will arrange itself in such a manner that it will indicate resistance to the stress applied through such an appliance.

BLOOD SUPPLY. The blood supply to bone that supports dentures is derived principally from two sources. Smaller or larger arteries perforate the compact bone to supply the marrow or spongy bone. This internal supply arises from the interdental arteries. The arterioles and prearterioles derived from the periosteum supply the compact bone. The degree to which each of these contributes to the nourishment of bone is not known. It is known that the tooth sockets are filled with mature or compact bone. In many instances the alveolar process, because of shape and size, contains very little spongy bone. Atwood reported "a complete absence of periosteal bone over the residual ridge in all of the midsagittal specimens studied."[1] The type of bone in the healed alveolar process and the alteration of blood supply could account for some of the changes in the support. When pressure diminishes or destroys the blood supply of bone tissue or interferes with its venous drainage, resorption results.

REACTION TO PRESSURE. The reaction of bone to pressure has produced varied results; the variables in this type of study serve to indicate why the effects differ. Pressure of enough intensity applied to bone for a sufficient length of time is one of the main factors in bone resorption (Fig. 1-25). The gentle pressure exerted in orthodontic procedures, the steady pressure in the resorption of the

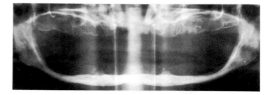

FIG. 1-25. *Roentgenogram of mandible which has been subjected to pressure from a mandibular denture for seventeen years.*

roots of deciduous teeth, and the pressure exerted by abnormally distended blood vessels are examples of this activity. The continuous presence of dentures is capable of exerting pressure of sufficient intensity to produce resorption. This is particularly true in the mandibular arch, since gravity exerts a steady pull on the denture. When pressure diminishes or destroys the blood supply of bone tissue or interferes with its venous drainage, resorption results. A denture is potentially capable of exerting steady pressure and also intermittent heavy pressure that can interrupt the blood supply. For this reason the dentures should be removed at least eight of every twenty-four hours.

When the natural teeth are present, the periodontal attachment provides tensile stimulation to the alveolar bone. With natural teeth, present or absent, the muscles and ligaments attached to the mandible exert the tensile stimulation to the body of the mandible. In certain individuals, muscle fibers of the mentalis may be attached to the slope of the alveolar ridge and therefore will provide stimulation to the bone. However, at times these fibers have a dislodging effect on the denture flanges when the lower lip is elevated.

Bone builds in response to stimulation, tensile in nature, like the pull of a ligament or muscle (Fig. 1-26). When the natural teeth are removed, no muscles or ligaments remain attached to the residual alveolar ridge. The force exerted by

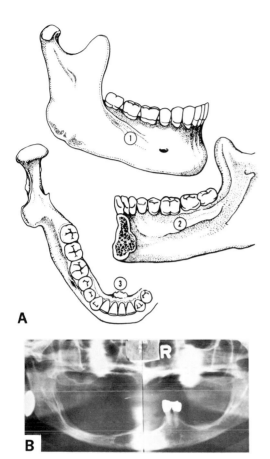

A

some stabilizing and others that cause shifting of the denture bases (Fig. 1-27). Weinmann and Sicher have reported, "Whether intermittent pressure is tolerated or even beneficial or whether it too leads to loss of bone depends entirely on its effects on the blood circulation, but it seems to be very difficult to assess these factors."[49]

METABOLIC CHANGES. Bone responds to all of the metabolic changes, dietary deficiencies, endocrine gland disturbances, and changes in function. These responses lead to periods of osteoporosis. Diseases of a debilitating nature, menopause, grand climacteric, and senility

B

FIG. 1-26. **A.** *Schematic illustration of areas of the mandible that are subjected to tensile stimulation: external oblique ridge (1), mylohyoid line (2), and genial tubercles (3).* **B.** *In the roentgenogram of a mandible note the alveolar ridge adjacent to the retained teeth and the absence of this ridge elsewhere.*

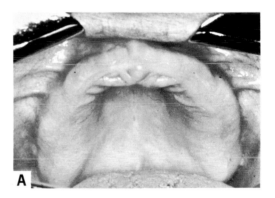

A

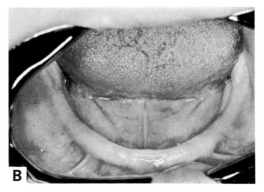

B

a denture cannot be classified as tensile in nature. Bone, such as the mandibular condyle, is resistant to pressure transmitted via avascular tissue since there can be no influence on circulation. Pressure to bone covered with periosteum disrupts circulation, and the bone is doomed to destruction. As the teeth contact, the force to the support increases and it is very questionable if this increase and decrease in force is physiologic. This force is directed in various directions and in varying magnitudes,

FIG. 1-27. *Intraoral photographs of residual ridges of a fifty-two-year-old male who has been completely edentulous for twelve years. The residual ridges have not been subjected to the pressure of dentures.* **A.** *Maxillary arch.* **B.** *Mandibular arch.*

are some of the conditions or periods in which there is a generalized loss of bone throughout the body.

With this knowledge of the physiology of bone, it is possible to institute procedures in the impression making, selection of teeth, arrangement of teeth, extension of the denture bases, and instructions to the patient that will assure a denture that should be more acceptable to the support: (1) recording the tissues in the impression at their rest position, (2) decreasing the number of teeth, (3) decreasing the size of the food table, (4) developing an occlusion that eliminates, as much as possible, horizontal forces and those that produce torque, (5) extending the denture bases for maximum coverage within tissue limits, (6) biting with the knife and fork, that is, placing small masses of food over the posterior teeth where the supporting bone is best suited to resist force, (7) removing the dentures for at least eight of every twenty-four hours for tissue rest.

PHYSIOLOGY OF MUSCLE

A muscle is made up of a large number of fibers bound together by areolar connective tissue into bundles, or fasciculi. The bundles are surrounded by connective tissue sheaths and grouped together into still larger bundles. The whole muscle is enveloped by a connective tissue sheath, the epimysium. The muscles receive an abundant blood supply; the blood vessels enter the muscle along the areolar tissue.

The human body is a very adjustable machine, capable of adapting to changes in environment. This mechanism is complex because it is composed of many organs, varying in their responses from day to day and to different situations. The nerve endings or sensory nerve terminals are the receptors. The *receptors* initiate the stimuli and the *effectors*

respond by acting. By means of the receptors the body is notified of the changes, and by the effectors it adjusts to these changes. The effectors of the body are the muscles and glands (Fig. 1-28).

The muscles that are intimately involved in complete denture service are defined as skeletal (from their site of origin or attachment), striated (from their morphology), and voluntary (controlled by the will). Skeletal muscle is controlled by the central nervous system and does not have automatic action. When a sensory nerve ending is stimulated, the afferent nerve carries the impulse to the central nervous system; it is relayed to the muscle by an efferent nerve, and contraction takes place. This is called reflex action, as opposed to voluntary action. The reflexes take place whether we are conscious of them or not, and we do not exercise any volitional control over them; that is, we cannot at will start or stop them.

In the ordinary sense of the term, we can voluntarily begin or stop the action of a skeletal muscle, although many skeletal muscles act when the individual is not conscious of the act. Individuals laugh, frown, scowl, and grin both consciously and subconsciously. Masticatory and nonmasticatory movements are of this same nature. A muscle can, under an individual's own volition, be activated. One muscle can be stopped and held in position, while another muscle can be activated. The mandible can be protruded and stopped before maximum protrusion. The external pterygoid can hold the meniscus and head of the mandible in this anteroposterior position, while the elevators and depressors can hinge the condyles on the meniscus. This control, by the will, of skeletal muscles accounts for the ability of an individual to function in a hinge movement under his own volition.

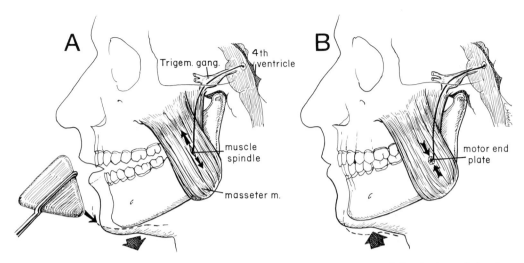

FIG. 1-28. *Schematic illustration of muscle response.* **A,** *opening and* **B,** *closing of the jaws. A sudden sharp blow on the chin point of the lower anterior teeth automatically stimulates a mandibular closure by a simple reflex. It is important to note that in recording procedures it is cogent not to stimulate the mandible in the chin region or the anterior tooth region because frequently a free slightly anterior closure is stimulated and not a posterior centric closure. Most anterior-free reflex closures are in a relatively protruded position; the posterior closures are more volitionally controlled and closer to the centric relation position. (Redrawn after Silverman: Oral Physiology. St. Louis, The C. V. Mosby Company, 1961.)*

Muscle is of primary interest because it exerts tension and performs mechanical work (Fig. 1-29). Resting muscle is soft and extensible; like most tissues it does not obey Hook's law, but becomes less extensible the greater the elongation. On stimulation there is a sudden and radical change in properties; it becomes hard, develops tension, resists stretching, and can shorten and lift a weight. The contraction takes place in the direction of the long axis of the muscle fibers, that is, in the direction from the insertion to the origin.

In the majority of skeletal muscles, the origins and insertions are in bone. However, many of the skeletal muscles involved in complete denture construction have a bony origin but insert into an aponeurosis, a raphe, or another muscle. The orbicularis oris has no bony origin or insertions, and its action is the contraction or closing of the oral orifice (sphincter). When the origins and insertions of a muscle are in bone, there is a limitation to the positions and action of the muscles. When an attachment is in an aponeurosis, a raphe, or a muscle, a more flexible relation exists.

The muscles of mastication have their origins and insertions in bone, with one exception. The uppermost fibers of the upper head of the external pterygoid insert into the mandibular articular capsule and thus indirectly into the anterior border of the articular disk. Part of the upper head and all of the inferior head insert to the anterior surface of the mandibular neck. This knowledge is utilized in making jaw relation records, particularly centric relation or centric position. Centric relation is a bone-to-bone relation controlled by the attached musculature, the tissue-lined bony fossae, the ligaments, and the neuromyons. It is a position that can be

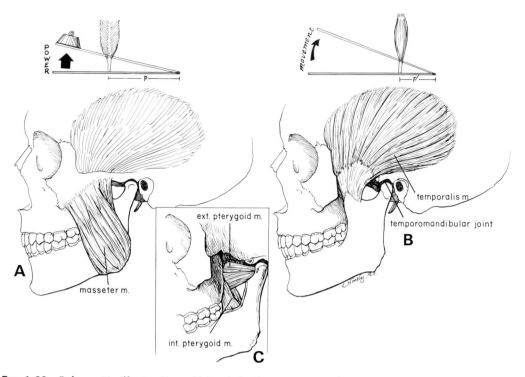

Fig. 1-29. *Schematic illustration of kinesiologic properties of muscle associated with the form and distribution of fibers in relation to connective tissue attachment.* **A** *shows the masseter, which has a long power arm (p) in comparison to that of the temporal muscle in* **B.** *The muscle moves a short distance and by virtue of its fiber form and distribution can create more energy in a given distance of movement.* **B** *represents the action of the temporal muscle, which has a short power arm (p') with action near the fulcrum. The muscle fibers are distributed in the direction of the movement, which results in quick movement and less energy.* **C.** *The external pterygoid is attached at the fulcrum. It is a small muscle with little total power and is associated primarily with movement. The internal pterygoid is a heavier, fleshier muscle further from the fulcrum and is thus similar to the masseter in its form and distribution. (Redrawn after Silverman: Oral Physiology. St. Louis, The C. V. Mosby Company, 1961.)*

recorded and repeated; in the absence of a pathologic condition, individuals can return to this position under their own volition; they can be guided to it and a record made can be repeated by others. This bone-to-bone relation can be a definite point of return, provided certain other factors are understood. The functions of muscle, tendons, ligaments, and connective tissue must be analyzed. Muscle and tendon elasticity, extensibility, stress and fatigue, and the plastic quality of bone are factors to be considered. When methods are considered for recording jaw relations, the neurologic control and the ease in which an imbalance can be induced by interfering nerve stimuli are all physiologic entities that must be correlated before any joint positions can be termed definite.

The muscles of facial expression, the muscles of the tongue, the suprahyoid muscles, the muscles of the soft palate, and the pharyngeal muscles do not have both origins and insertions in bone. These are the muscles primarily involved with the extent of the denture borders, the contour of the denture bases, and the positions of the teeth. The movable attachments of these muscles account for the various contours, borders, and positions of teeth that are seen in dentures. Impression techniques are influenced by these attachments. The muscles should not be stretched nor should they be left unsupported. The positions of the teeth, not the denture borders, support the muscles of expression. The available vestibular spaces should be utilized to their full extent but should not be over- or underfilled.

A muscle contraction is said to be *isometric* when the length of the muscle does not shorten during contraction. A muscle contraction is said to be *isotonic* when the muscle shortens, but the tension remains the same. In isometric contraction the muscle does no work, but the internal tension of the fibers has become greater. Muscles contract both isometrically and isotonically in the body; most contractions are actually a combination of the two. The contraction of the retractor and elevator muscles of the mandible during jaw closure is both isotonic and isometric—isotonic to move the mandible and isometric to brace the jaw when the teeth contact (Fig. 1-30).

Muscle tissue has two physical properties that must be considered, extensibility and elasticity. When a load is placed on a muscle, the muscle elongates, and within limits, the greater the load, the greater the stretch. When the load is released, the muscle shortens almost to its original length. Because a contracted muscle has greater elasticity than a resting muscle, an overloaded muscle may elongate when it contracts. These two properties limit or lessen the danger of rupturing when excessive strain is placed on a muscle. The property of elongation should be considered when jaw relations are recorded under manual

pressure, or when centric relation is recorded by the use of the Hickok strap. Fortunately, the same properties limit or lessen the danger of muscle rupture when such procedures are employed.

Skeletal muscle fibers vary greatly in size from one part of the body to another; the velocity of conduction is considerably less in some muscles and greater in other muscles. In most muscles, the fibers extend the entire length of the muscle, and usually each fiber is innervated by one or more neuromuscular junctions located somewhere on the middle third of the fiber. A stimulus is much more effective when applied to a neuromuscular junction than it is at other points of the fiber. The exact manner in which the action potential initiates this contraction has not as yet been discovered. The all-or-nothing law applies to muscle. A stimulus to a muscle fiber causes an action potential to travel over the entire fiber or fails to stimulate it at all, except at the local point of stimulus.

The all-or-nothing law should not be interpreted to mean that if a muscle contracts, it contracts with its maximum force. The force of contraction can vary: it can be weak or strong, depending on the presence of appropriate nutrients, or whether the fiber is already fatigued, or whether the muscle fiber is in a highly contractile state. The contraction of one fiber does not mean that all of the fibers in a muscle bundle are contracting. Some muscles contract very slowly and others very fast, depending on the physical and chemical characteristics of the individual muscles. Gradation of contraction refers to the different degrees of force that can be exerted by a muscle. A contraction of a postural muscle has slightly less gradation of contraction than that of the ocular or finger muscles. A muscle contraction is so well graded by the nervous control that almost any degree of con-

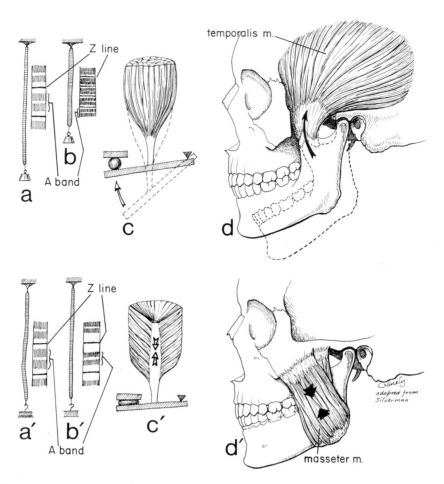

Fig. 1-30. *Two sequences to demonstrate muscle action in isometric and isotonic attraction. An isotonic contraction during which a muscle shortens its overall length is represented in* **a, b, c,** *and* **d.** *The temporalis muscle lies relatively close to the fulcrum at the condyle. It serves to accomplish work for closure and also to move the condyle so that another stronger muscle can perform greater work. The diverse muscle bundles distributed in the different directions indicate that the temporalis is essentially a placement or a movement muscle associated with the lever arm. Note in* **a** *and* **b** *that both light and dark striated components of the muscle fibers shorten;* **a** *represents the resting length, and* **b** *represents the shortened length.* **c** *demonstrates the effect of a shortening of both component bands. The effect of isometric contraction is shown in* **a′, b′, c′,** *and* **d′.** *The powerful masseter muscle is situated farther away from the fulcrum at the condyle than is the temporalis muscle. Its fibers are multipennate and contract in a plane oblique to the long axis of movement of the muscle organ.* **a′** *shows the muscle at rest, and* **b′** *shows the muscle in contraction but with the same overall length. The power has been generated by the shortening of the length of the dark striated bands and an elongation of the light bands. Such arrangement of the internal structure of the muscle allows power to be generated while the length remains constant. (Redrawn after Silverman: Oral Physiology. St. Louis, The C. V. Mosby Company, 1961.)*

traction can be called forth from a muscle. The gradation of contraction of almost any muscle of the body is almost lacking in limits. The phenomenon of muscle control is one of the reasons the reaction of the denture-supporting tissues in one individual varies from that of another; the degree of contraction is not the same.

Another interesting phenomenon of muscle is its power to undergo physical contracture. When a muscle length becomes shortened, as in the establishing of excessive interocclusal distance, the fibers of the elevator muscles actually shorten and re-establish new muscle lengths approximately equal to the maximum length of the lever system itself, thus re-establishing optimum force of contraction by a muscle. Constant overstretching of the depressor muscles, makes their normal contraction impossible and will cause these muscles to lose power, to weaken. Muscles do not act alone. When one muscle contracts, its antagonist must relax. When one muscle is shortened, its antagonist is stretched. When excessive interocclusal distance is established with dentures, the lessened force extended to the residual ridge is short-lived, but the depressor muscles are weakened.

When muscles are at rest, a certain amount of tonus usually remains. This residual degree of contraction in skeletal muscle is called *muscle tone*. Most skeletal muscle tone is caused by nerve impulses from the spinal cord. The nerve impulses are controlled by impulses from the brain and impulses that originate in the muscle spindles. The blocking of muscle spindle impulses causes loss of muscle tone, and the muscle becomes almost flaccid. The afferent impulses are necessary for the generating of tonus. They must originate in the muscles and tendons. The use of drugs to inhibit the nerve impulses is advocated in the mak-

ing of jaw relation records. The muscle relaxant drugs are not selective, and for this reason their use may be quite limited in recording jaw relations.

As the wear and tear of nerve tissue takes place, the power to innervate muscle diminishes. No matter how large an amount of carbohydrate or fat a diet may contain, a certain irreducible minimum of tissue wear and tear takes place; this can be restored only by eating protein. The majority of disorders involving muscle action is neurologic in origin; muscle without nerve innervation is useless. Lack of protein in the diet of the geriatric individual accounts for the loss of skeletal muscle tone, and this loss of tone is reflected in the muscles of mastication. This is why jaw relation records for some of these individuals are so hard to accomplish and repeat.

Prolonged and strong contraction of a muscle leads to fatigue. The nerve continues to function properly, the nerve impulses pass normally into the muscle fiber, and even normal potentials spread over the muscle fibers, but the contraction becomes weaker and weaker. If a muscle becomes fatigued to an extreme extent, it is likely to become continually contracted, remaining contracted for many minutes even without an action potential as a stimulus. If a muscle has become so fatigued that all the energy-giving compounds have been degraded, relaxation cannot be provided, and the muscle assumes a prolonged contracted state. When the fatigue is over, the muscle gradually relaxes. If an individual's mandible is protruded and allowed to remain until fatigue occurs, the antagonist action to the retractor and elevator muscles will be weakened. It would be possible to retrude and elevate the mandible to the centric position against very little or no opposing action from the external pterygoid. However, care must be exercised not to keep

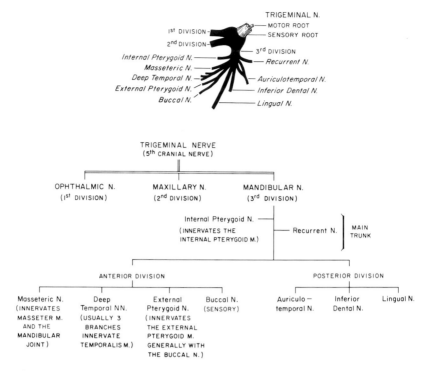

FIG. 1-31. *The fifth cranial nerve is responsible for the innervation of many of the structures involved in denture construction.*

the mandible in protrusion until extreme fatigue exists. This could defeat the purpose, at least for many minutes, as the external pterygoid could become continually contracted.

SOMATIC NERVOUS SYSTEM

The nervous and endocrine gland systems control the functions of the body. The two systems are complicated, and physiologists are the first to admit that there is a great deal to be investigated and learned about both systems. This is particularly significant as it applies to dentistry (Fig. 1-31).

The somatic senses refer to the nervous mechanism that collects sensory information from various areas of the body. This mechanism is differentiated from the special senses, such as those of sight, hearing, smell, and taste. It is concerned with physical states, including (1) the movement of the joints, (2) the positions of joints, (3) the tensions of muscles, (4) the tensions of tendons, and (5) the orientation of the body with respect to the pull of gravity or other acceleratory forces.

The somatic nervous system is composed of receptors, conductors, and effectors (Fig. 1-32). Guyton states that "receptors stimulate the nerve fibers in a different way from the stimulation that occurs following artificial stimulation."[15] We may expect that the result in the effector may also vary. This factor should be considered when mandibular movements are studied or when jaw closure is artificially elicited. The receptors of particular concern in complete denture prosthodontics are the mechanoreceptors and the receptors that detect pain.

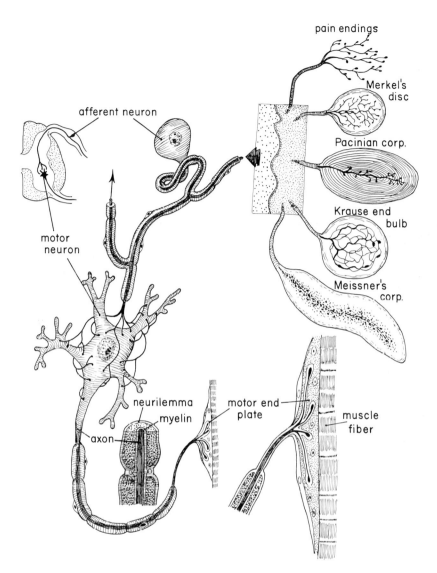

Fig. 1-32. *The nervous system is responsible for body protection. The pain endings, Merkel's disc, Pacinian corpuscle, Krause end bulb, and Meissner's corpuscle are examples of somatic sensory nerve endings that are mechanoreceptors. The afferent neurons conduct nervous impulses to a nerve center. The motor nucleus (not illustrated) in the central nervous system directs motor impulses to the motor neurons (efferent neurons) that conduct the impulses away from the center to the motor end plate upon the muscle fiber. The axon is the central core of the nerve cell and the essential conducting part. The neurilemma, a cellular sheath, encloses each nerve fiber and may be separated from it by a myelin sheath. (Redrawn after Silverman: Oral Physiology. St. Louis, The C. V. Mosby Company, 1961.)*

MECHANORECEPTORS. The receptors that detect stretch of the muscles and tendons, movements of the joints, and the stimuli of touch and pressure are the mechanoreceptors. Those that detect the stretch of the muscles are the muscle spindles, and those that detect stretch of the tendons are the Golgi tendon appa-

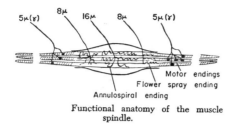

Functional anatomy of the muscle spindle.

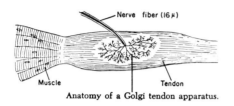

Anatomy of a Golgi tendon apparatus.

FIG. 1-33. *Schematic drawing of the anatomy of the muscle spindle (top) and the Golgi tendon apparatus (bottom). The muscle spindle can be stimulated by stretch of the entire muscle or contraction of the intrafusal fibers of the spindle. Note that the Golgi tendon apparatus is in the tendon, not at the junction of the muscle and the tendon. (From Guyton: Textbook of Medical Physiology, 4th ed. Philadelphia, W. B. Saunders Company, 1971.)*

ratuses (Fig. 1-33). The muscle spindle seems to insure that muscle tension will be proportional to stretch and to allow smooth coordination of phasic movement with posture.

Two types of receptors are located in the muscle spindle, the annulospiral and the flower spray endings. The Golgi tendon apparatus and the flower spray endings in the muscle spindle initiate an inhibitory reflex in the muscle that results in the relaxation of the muscle; the annulospiral endings reflexly excite the same muscle to oppose a change in length. Extreme loads can occur on tendons before the Golgi tendon apparatuses become maximally stimulated.

The *kinesthetic receptors*, which are proprioceptive end organs, detect movements at the joints. Physiologists appear to prefer that the term *proprioceptors* be limited to the receptors in and about the joints and that proprioception not be used when referring to the other receptors such as muscle spindles and Golgi tendon apparatuses. Mandibular movements and the effect of the movements are involved in practically all dental procedures, and the neurologic factors need to be investigated. Unfortunately, there has been little scientific research on the kinesthetic senses in and about the temporomandibular joints. In the absence of this information we can apply what is known about other joints and profit by it.

The *touch and pressure receptors* include (1) free nerve endings located in all tissues of the body, (2) Meissner's corpuscles located under the surface of the skin, (3) Pacinian corpuscles deep in the skin, and (4) other specialized end organs (Fig. 1-32). Some receptors adapt very rapidly; others can transmit impulses for prolonged periods of time. The Meissner's corpuscles are particularly abundant in the skin of the tips of the fingers. The sense of touch is advantageous to the prosthodontist in diagnosis and detecting abnormalities, but touch also elicits responses by the one who is being touched. What these responses will be cannot be foretold and may not be desired. The latter must be considered when recording maxillomandibular relations.

The deep sensibilities are the same as the sensibilities from the surface of the skin, except that they originate in the deep tissues and respond only crudely to mild tactile forces. An exception is the periosteum of bone. The end organs in the periosteum are especially sensitive to both light pressure and acceleratory effects. Bone reacts to pressure by resorbing. When force is applied to a denture, it is detected as pressure by the receptors in the periosteum. When the pressure is great enough to produce damage, the pressure receptors become involved, and the central nervous system is notified to alter the force. The availability of a protective mechanism is fortunate for the edentulous patient with dentures because excessive or constant pressure results in loss of the residual alveolar ridge. This same mechanism may be involved when the efficiency of artificial teeth is compared with the efficiency of natural teeth. In normal masticatory function, the patient may never generate the force to demonstrate the efficiency of the artificial teeth when comparing cusp and noncusp types of posterior teeth.

PAIN RECEPTORS. The recognition of pain by the pain receptors, which are free nerve endings found in all tissues of the body, is approximately even with different persons; however, the reaction may vary. Stoical persons react to pain less intensely than emotional persons. People of different nationalities differ in their emotional natures and react quite differently to pain stimuli. This difference may be the reason that some patients tolerate dentures even while the support is being destroyed. Psychic reactions to pain are subtle and include all the well-known reactions such as anguish, anxiety, crying, depression, nausea, and excessive muscle excitability. These reactions to pain are difficult to diagnose; when they are suspected in a denture patient, it may be necessary to have the patient consult a specialist in psychology and/or psychiatry.

Reflex motor reactions to pain are known as *withdrawal reflexes*. These reflexes remove a part of the body from the noxious stimulation. This protective mechanism does not function during sleep. This is one of the numerous reasons for removing dentures during sleeping hours.

CONDUCTORS. The type of nerve fibers that conducts the impulses and their organization determine the quality and efficiency of the reflex. Nerve fibers are myelinated or unmyelinated and may be large, intermediate, or small. The large myelinated fibers are the most rapid conductors of impulses. Saltatory conduction, which is of value because the conduction is faster and the system conserves energy, occurs in myelinated fibers (Fig. 1-34).

All sensory information in the somatic nervous system enters the spinal cord through the dorsal roots or goes directly to the brain stem. In the cord the fibers separate into the medial lemniscal system composed of large heavily myelinated fibers and the spinothalamic system composed mainly of small myelinated and some unmyelinated fibers. The small myelinated and unmyelinated fibers are slow conductors when compared to conduction of the fibers in the medial lemniscal system.

The somatic senses of primary concern to the prosthodontist are touch, kinesthetic sense, and pressure. These senses are conducted in the medial lemniscal system. Pain, heat or cold, crude touch, and crude pressure are conducted

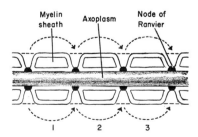

Fig. 1-34 *Saltatory conduction in a myelinated axon. (From Guyton: Textbook of Medical Physiology. 4th ed. Philadelphia, W. B. Saunders Company, 1971.)*

in the spinothalamic system. This rapid conduction may be the reason for the fast movements of the mandible that make intraoral checking of the contacting of teeth so difficult. The impulses from the annulospiral receptors of the muscle spindle and the Golgi tendon apparatus are conducted in the largest known sensory nerve fibers. Because the visual system detects images only by virtue of the many contrasts between the dark and light areas, movement in the semidark cavern of the mouth is not easily detected by sight. These factors are important when mechanical instruments are being used to study the contacts of teeth or when the jaws of the patient are being used as the articulator during the contacts.

Effectors (Fig. 1-35).   The effectors of the nervous system include skeletal and cardiac muscle, smooth muscle organs, some of the endocrine glands, and certain exocrine glands of the upper alimentary tract and skeletal muscles.

SALIVARY GLANDS AND SALIVA

The primary exocrine glands that secrete saliva are the parotid, submaxillary, and sublingual glands. In addition to these large glands, there are numerous small glands distributed throughout the oral cavity in the lips, tongue, and palate.

The secretions enter into the oral cavity by way of one or more common excretory ducts. The parotid gland empties through Stensen's duct, which has its orifice in the cheek above the molar teeth. The sublingual gland empties along the sublingual fold in the floor of the mouth and with the submaxillary gland in the sublingual caruncle situated to the lingual side of the mandible in the submandibular fovea. The accessory salivary glands empty through individual ducts at their respective locations. The small glands in the posterior two thirds of the palate are particularly significant in impression making and in the retention of the complete maxillary denture.

Saliva contains two types of secretions: (1) a serous secretion (thin, watery) containing the enzyme ptyalin for the digestion of starchy foods, and (2) a mucous secretion (viscid, sticky, or adhesive) for lubricating purposes.

The parotid glands secrete only serous type, and the molar (buccal) palatine and sublingual glands secrete only the mucous type. The submaxillary and sublingual glands secrete both the serous and mucous types, with the submaxillary secretion being more mucous, and the sublingual more serous. The quantity of daily secretion normally ranges between 1,000 and 1,500 milliliters with a pH of 6.0 to 7.0.

Although saliva contains an enzyme for digestive purposes, it is primarily a lubricating and protective agent. It not only lubricates the bolus of food but also coats the lining of the oral cavity to protect the lining mucosa. When the food particles are coated with mucus, they adhere to each other and slide along the epithelium with ease. Mucus is strongly resistant to digestion by the gastric juices and is capable of neutralizing small amounts of either acid or alkali. Saliva also lubricates the surfaces of a denture, thereby making the denture more compatible with the movements of the lips, tongue, and cheeks.

A knowledge of the nervous system regulating the salivary system is essential for evaluating prosthodontic problems and for educating patients in what to expect in this phase of denture use. The portion of the nervous system that controls the secretions of the body is the autonomic nervous system, a system that is not under voluntary control. The salivary glands are strongly stimulated by the *parasympathetic nervous system;*

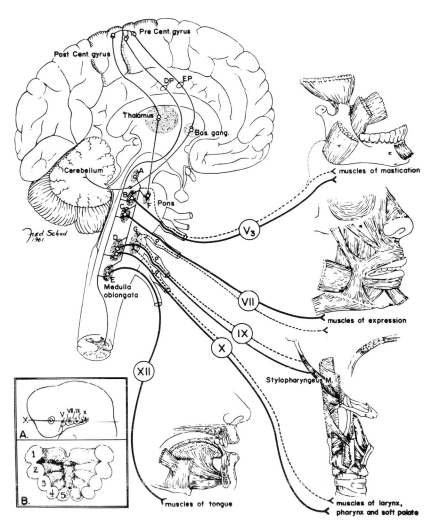

FIG. 1-35. *Innervation of the muscles of speech: mesencephalic nucleus (A); motor nucleus of mandibular nerve (B); motor nucleus of facial nerve (C); motor nucleus (ambiguus) of glossopharyngeal and vagus nerves (D); motor nucleus of the hypoglossal nerve, XII, medial to the motor nucleus of the vagus nerve, X (E); corticobulbar-corticospinal tract (DP); extra-pyramidal tract (EP); basal ganglia (Bas. gang.). Inset:* **A.** *Cross section of head of embryo showing indentations that represent the developing branchial arches on the lateral surface.* **B.** *Coronal section through the head of an embryo showing the relative positions of the branchial arches. (From Martone and Black: Physiology of speech. J. Prosth. Dent., 12:418, 1962.)*

the sympathetic system has little or no direct effect on salivation. The indirect effect, a reduction in the rate of secretion from sympathetic stimulation, is a result of the vasoconstriction of the blood vessels to the gland.

Stimulation of the submaxillary and sublingual glands is controlled principally by nerve impulses from the *superior salivary nuclei* and the parotid gland impulses from the *inferior salivary nuclei*. The parasympathetic fibers from the *seventh nerve* pass to the submaxillary glands, and fibers from the *ninth nerve* pass to the parotid glands. The excitation of the salivary nuclei, located near the junction of the pons and medulla, is both by taste and by tactile stimuli from the tongue and other areas of the oral cavity. The sight and/or smell of food can act as a stimulus, as can higher centers of the central nervous system. An example of this type of stimulation is the increase in salivation when a person eats food he particularly likes. When he eats a food he detests, salivation decreases appreciably.

Under physiologic conditions, salivation can be divided into three phases: (1) cephalic, (2) buccal, and (3) gastrointestinal. The *cephalic phase* of salivation occurs when one thinks about, smells, or sees food. The *buccal phase* is the response to the tactile and/or taste stimuli. The *gastrointestinal phase* results from the reflexes originating in the stomach or gastrointestinal tract and is thought to be particularly associated with foods which are irritating.

Physiologic factors that affect salivation include the following:

1. Agreeable taste stimuli result in profuse salivation, whereas distasteful stimuli can result in temporary cessation of salivation.

2. A smooth object inserted into the mouth will result in an increase in salivation, whereas a rough object will inhibit salivation. (The polished surfaces of a denture should be smooth.)

3. When a person is dehydrated, salivation decreases.

4. As one ages, the saliva becomes more ropy in consistency.

5. Emotions and other psychic effects excite the autonomic nervous system and in turn the functions of the body organs are altered.

Excitement, fright, or fear can almost stop gastrointestinal mobility and exocrine gland secretions. Anxiety, resentment, and prolonged worry can increase secretions and gastrointestinal mobility. The increased mobility can result in diarrhea, and the increase in gastric secretions in the development of a pathologic condition, peptic ulcers. When these gastrointestinal symptoms develop, the person also experiences an increase in salivation, at times profuse.

Some of the pathologic conditions that *decrease* salivation are (1) senile atrophy of the salivary glands, (2) irradiation therapy for head and neck tumors, and (3) diseases of the brain stem that directly depress salivary nuclei and block salivation. Other conditions include (4) some types of encephalitis, including poliomyelitis, (5) diabetes mellitus and/or insipidus, (6) diarrhea caused by bacteria or food, (7) elevated temperature from acute infectious diseases, and (8) vitamin deficiencies, particularly of vitamin A.

Pathologic conditions that may be accompanied by *increased* salivation are (1) digestive tract irritants and (2) painful afflictions of the oral cavity. These may be from vitamin deficiency or trauma from surgery, an ill-fitting denture, or inadequate interocclusal distance when artificial dentures are made.

Saliva is considered a major factor in evaluating the physical influences that contribute to denture retention. The physical forces in which saliva is involved are (1) adhesion, (2) cohesion, (3) capillarity, and (4) atmospheric pressure.

Adhesion is the binding force exerted by molecules of unlike substances in contact.

Cohesion is that force by which molecules of the same kind or the same body are held together.

Capillarity is a form of surface tension between the molecules of a liquid and those of a solid.

Thin, watery saliva of high surface

tension affords enough retention that patients do not have a problem with denture retention if all other retentive factors are acceptable. Patients who have ropy saliva do have problems with denture retention as do those who have profuse watery saliva.

The research report of Craig, Berry, and Peyton is significant to the dentists who provide complete denture treatment.[7c] They concluded "that capillary forces are the principal forces involved in denture retention." They found that increasing or reducing the surrounding pressure and temperature influences the retention of a denture because capillary force is affected. Discontinuity of the saliva film will reduce retention. This can be caused by reduction of outside pressure.

The practical applications of knowledge of the salivary glands and saliva in complete denture prosthodontics are many:

1. Excessive salivation, particularly by the submaxillary and sublingual glands, presents a problem in impression making. When this problem exists, atropine sulfate can be administered orally prior to the impression making.

2. Excessive secretions of mucus from the palatal glands may distort the impression material in the posterior two thirds of the palate. To counteract this problem (a) the palate may be massaged to encourage the glands to empty; (b) the mouth may be irrigated with an astringent mouthwash just prior to inserting impression material; or (c) the palate may be wiped with gauze.

3. When it is determined that saliva is a problem, the cause should be investigated. If necessary, therapy should be instituted to correct the problem.

4. When the cause is undetermined or there is no favorable response to therapy, the problem should be discussed with the patient prior to treatment.

When the patient understands the problem, his cooperation is usually assured. An example of this is the patient whose mucosa will not tolerate dentures because of xerostomia. It may be necessary to limit denture use to short periods and to restrict the diet to moist foods that are soft or liquid.

Summary

A summary of some of the practical applications of oral and general physiology in complete denture prosthodontics follows:

BONE

1. Alveolar residual ridge lost as a result of a pathologic condition, an accidental, or by surgical procedures does not undergo regenerative reconstruction. In short, that which is lost is no longer present nor will it be regenerated to provide denture support, stability, or retention.

2. When the natural teeth are removed or lost, the tensile stimulation provided by the periodontal attachments is lost. Bone builds in response to tensile stimulation, all other entities being favorable.

3. Bone resorbs in response to pressure, and complete dentures are capable of producing pressure sufficient to interfere with the blood supply. Gravity, when the teeth are not in contact, helps to release the pressure of the maxillary denture; however, gravity continues to exert a pulling force on the mandibular denture.

4. Under physiologic conditions it is questionable if the contact of teeth in dentures produce the extensive resorption seen in denture users. However, the contacting of the teeth in individuals with parafunction could contribute to excessive resorption. With dentures,

teeth contact in masticating approximately five minutes a day. The average time of tooth contact is three seconds; the total time in twenty-four hours is 17.5 minutes.

5. The use of weighted mandibular dentures would, because of the weight, increase the pressure on the blood vessels and the bone. It is possible that this disadvantage may be more damaging than has been reported or documented.

6. Osteoporosis, a disease in which the osteoblastic activity is lessened in the bone, occurs frequently in individuals who have complete dentures. The constantly changing bony base necessitates adjusting and altering the dentures; therefore, a definite recall system should be instituted.

7. Although the vertical stress produced by the contacting of artificial teeth in complete dentures is directed to the crest of the residual alveolar ridges in both arches, other areas can be used to help minimize this stress: the hard palate and the zygomatico-alveolar crest of the maxillary arch and the buccal shelf areas of the mandibular arch.

8. Although some prosthodontists may subscribe to a particular material for denture teeth, a certain occlusal form for the posterior teeth, and a definite arrangement of the denture teeth for individual situations, there are not sufficient scientific data that any of these result in *more* or *less* bone resorption. When the many variables are considered, this lack of data is understood.

MUSCLE

1. In that the muscles which move the mandible are under control of the will, i.e., the central nervous system, under physiologic conditions the muscles can be directed to move. At the first consultation appointment, patients can be given a training exercise that will prepare them for the time of jaw relation records. The exercise is accomplished at home, in a relaxed atmosphere, three times daily facing a large mirror. The mandible is relaxed and with the jaws separated slightly more than rest position, *not a wide separation*, the chin is brought forward (protruded) until it stops. From this position the jaw is carried backward (retruded) until the condyles are felt to stop (bump) in the fossae. This exercise is continued during the construction phase but make certain that the patient is fully conscious when the condyles stop in the fossae. At the time of recording the jaw relations the patient is first rehearsed and then with the recording records in place is directed to protrude, retrude to feel the condyle stop, and then close on the back teeth (recording media) until the anterior teeth touch (see Fig. 11-11).

2. With exercise, muscle alters its shape and size. This property of muscle provides a method for improving the shape and size of the tongues that are abnormal in size, position, and/or function.

3. When the artificial teeth are placed in positions that do not support the muscles of facial expression in the manner of the natural teeth or if for other reasons the muscles lose tonus, the facial expression changes. Another problem is the tendency to cheek biting when the denture teeth are placed in the positions formerly occupied by the natural posterior teeth. With patient training and a return of the tonus, the problem is relieved.

4. If a muscle contracts slowly or if contraction is rapid, the efficiency to do work is decreased. Maximum efficiency is developed when the velocity of contraction is about 30 per cent of maximum. If a muscle is in a highly contractile state, it may contract more strongly than normal. When a muscle contracts under physiologic conditions, the antag-

onist muscle relaxes. However, under abnormal conditions the antagonist muscle can become activated, and the result will be a change in the contracting muscle. If a muscle is already shortened before it is stimulated to contract, the force of contraction is less than normal. If it is stretched before contraction, the force will also be less than normal. These and other physiologic muscle actions are important in recording the jaw relations and also in educating patients in denture use.

5. The source of the energy for muscle contraction is adenosine triphosphate. Adenosine triphosphate is reformed rapidly, in milliseconds, and it is the source of energy for the contractile process. It is composed of the nitrogenous base adenine, the pentos sugar ribose, and three molecules of phosphoric acid. Cells can use carbohydrates, fats, and protein to synthesize large quantities of this source of energy. Muscle contraction will not occur without the energy from adenosine triphosphate; therefore, the dentist should be familiar with its source and the biochemistry involved in its metabolism.

SOMATIC NERVOUS SYSTEM

If one is to understand the contacting and noncontacting (separation) of the teeth, natural and/or artificial, he must know the basic fundamentals of the somatic nervous system. This does not mean or infer that members of the dental profession would not benefit from a knowledge of the intimate physiologic details of the system. However, when the practical application of the physiology of the somatic nervous system is considered, it is not necessary for dentists to know in detail the different brain centers through which nerve impulses are transmitted nor must they be expected to know all the nutritional factors involved in healthy nerve tissue. It is essential for

them to know the anatomy of the temporomandibular joints and the muscles and ligaments engaged in moving the mandible under physiologic conditions. When the normal physiology is understood, the abnormal or pathologic is more readily diagnosed and evaluated. The question is asked, what is normal? The term *normal* is applicable to an individual or to groups of individuals. Normal is defined as conforming to or consisting of a pattern, process, or standard regarded as usual or typical, regular or natural. *Pathologic* is defined as relating to, involving, concerned with, or caused by disease. *Physiologic* is defined as promoting or in accord with the proper functioning of an organism.

At times it is not difficult to differentiate whether the disease is the result of a normal or an abnormal function. A simple example is excessive wear to the enamel of the teeth of a person in the twenties who constantly eats gritty foods or citrus fruits. The loss of enamel is a pathologic situation but results from what one may expect to be a normal finding for the teeth of a person who eats gritty food or excessive citrus fruits.

Taste, sight, and hearing diminish for many as part of the aging process, estrogen production diminishes or ceases for females after menopause, the salivary glands may atrophy, and many prostate glands hypertrophy as the male ages. Are these conditions the results of normal or abnormal functions?

Osteoarthritic joints are diseased, but did the disease result because of abnormal function? An arthritic joint does not function in a normal manner, and this is of practical importance to the dentist who has a patient with arthritic temporomandibular joints or joint.

In edentulous situations the recording of jaw relations and the arrangement of the artificial teeth must be in harmony with the dysfunction. In the philosophy of "cuspid protected occlusion," does the mechanical contacting of the canines protect the remaining teeth? Do the canines wear excessively? Is the separation of the remaining teeth accomplished by the canines just missing? Are they being guided by the message sent to the central nervous system by the light touch receptors in the periodontal attachments surrounding the canines? A non-involved analysis of this phenomenon is as follows: When teeth contact, the central nervous system is notified by the touch, pressure, or pain somatic nerve receptors in and around the teeth, and at that instant the proprioceptors in and around the joint or joints responsible for the movement notify the central nervous system of the relation of the parts of the joint to each other. If either of these end factors is uncomfortable or is producing a pathologic situation, it is assumed that the central nervous system is notified. At this point the system becomes more complicated, and basic factors of the system must be evaluated. Also at this point subtle changes may first take place with no apparent corrective measure on the part of the system until damage of the degree of involving other receptors of pain, pressure, or touch occurs.

Proprioceptors provide information about the positions of the body in space at any given moment. However, the conscious component of the body in space is the input from the receptors in and around the joints *combined* with the information from the cutaneous and pressure receptors as well. The practical application of these factors to the dentist is that when the teeth are not in contact the mandible is at rest in space. The individual is not consciously aware of the relation of the mandible to the surrounding structures. However, the central nervous system is aware of the relation of the mandible and attached teeth to the maxillae, the tongue, lips, cheeks, and teeth

of the maxillary arch. This information is furnished by the receptors in and about the joint. When the mandible is elevated and retracted to make tooth contact, it will be directed in a manner to provide comfort, whenever possible, not only of the contacting of the teeth, but also of the relations of the condyles to their surrounding environment. When the teeth make contact, the mandible is no longer in space; therefore, the individual is aware or conscious of the contacting of the teeth. This awareness is particularly true if the contacts of the teeth or positions of the condyles in the fossae produce discomfort. Under physiologic conditions the central nervous system dictates that the jaw open to break the contact and further, when the jaw closes, it attempt to close to a comfortable relationship. Withdrawal reflexes can be produced by innocuous stimulaton; however, a strong flexor response for withdrawal is initiated only by stimuli that are noxious or potentially harmful to the person. These stimuli are called *nociceptive stimuli.* Pain in the periosteum initiates reflex contraction of nearby skeletal muscle. The reflex contraction is similar to the muscle spasms associated with injuries to bones, tendons, and joints. This phenomenon could well be a part of the problem with denture users whose dentures cause pain receptors in the periosteum to be stimulated. When a tendon or ligament attached to the periosteum is stretched to produce pain, the stretched muscle will be ordered to contract. This is important in all border positions of the mandible.

Conscious awareness of the positions of the various parts of the body in space depends upon impulses from sensory organs in and around joints. The organs involved are slowly adapting "spray endings" in the muscle spindle, Golgi tendon organ-like structures which are probably the pacinian corpuscles in the synovial membrane of the joints and ligaments. Although there is, according to researchers, a limited amount of information about the temporomandibular joint's receptor reflexes and few data involving the reflexes for the lateral pterygoid muscle, there is no reason to assume that receptors are not present, either in the joint or in any muscle involved in body equilibrium. Another researcher reports "the medial half of the anterior border of the meniscus is attached to the superior belly of the lateral pterygoid muscle. *Mahan* calls this the "foot portion." This portion contains many blood vessels and Golgi tendon organs. When the mandible retrudes, the meniscus is stretched at the "foot portion." This arrangement of receptors may account for the scarcity that has been demonstrated in the anterior belly of the digastric and the lateral pterygoid muscles.

REFERENCES

1. Atwood, D. A.: Some clinical factors related to rate of resorption of residual ridges. J. Prosth. Dent., *12*:441, 1962.
1a. ———: Reduction of residual ridges: A major oral disease entity. J. Prosth. Dent., *26*:266, 1971.
1b. ———: Clinical, cephalometric, and densitometric study of reduction of residual ridges. J. Prosth. Dent., *26*:280, 1971.
2. Barrett, S. G., and Haines, R. W.: Structure of the mouth in the mandibular molar region and its relation to the denture. J. Prosth. Dent., *12*:835, 1962.
2a. Baylink, D. J., Wergedal, J. E., Yamamoto, K., and Manzke, E.: Systematic factors in alveolar bone loss. J. Prosth. Dent., *31*:486, 1974.
3. Beaudreau, D. E., and Jerge, C. R.: An electrophysiological study of the gasserian ganglion (Abst.). International Ass. Dent. Res., *41*:105, 1963.
4. Block, L. S.: Muscular tension in denture construction. J. Prosth. Dent., *2*:198, 1952.
4a. Boswell, J. V.: J. Prosth. Dent., *1*:307, 1951.
5. Boucher, C. O.: Complete denture impressions based upon the anatomy of the mouth. J.A.D.A., *31*:1174, 1944.
6. Brill, N., Tryde, G., and Cantor, R.: The dynamic nature of the lower denture space. J. Prosth. Dent., *15*:401, 1965.
7. Campbell, R. L.: A comparative study of the resorption of the alveolar ridges in denture wearers and non-denture wearers. J.A.D.A., *60*:143, 1960.
7a. Cheraskin, E., and Ringsdorf, W. M. J.: Ecology of alveolar bone loss. Oral Surg., *30*:333, 1970.
7b. ———: Alveolar bone loss as a prognostic sign of diabetes in patients of the 60-plus age group. J. Amer. Geriat. Soc., *18*:416, 1970.
7c. Craig, R. G., Berry, G. C., and Peyton, M. A.: Physical factors related to denture retention. J. Prosth. Dent., *10*:459, 1960.
7d. Cutright, D. E., Brudvik, J. S., Gay, W. D., and Selting, W. J.: Tissue pressure under complete maxillary dentures. J. Prosth. Dent., *35*:160, 1976.
8. *Cunningham's Manual of Practical Anatomy*, Vol. 3, 12th ed., J. C. Brash, editor. London, Oxford University Press, 1958.
8a. DeMarco, T. J., and Paine, S.: Mandibular dimensional change. J. Prosth. Dent., *31*:482, 1974.
9. Edwards, L. F.: The edentulous mandible. J. Prosth. Dent., *4*:222, 1954.
10. ———: Some anatomic facts and fancies relative to the masticatory apparatus. J. Prosth. Dent., *5*:825, 1955.
11. ———, and Boucher, C. O.: Anatomy of the mouth in relation to complete dentures. J.A.D.A., *29*:331, 1942.
11a. El Mahdy, A. S.: Simulated functional studies of temporomandibular joints. J. Prosth. Dent., *26*:658, 1971.
12. Emig, G. E.: The physiology of the muscles of mastication. J. Prosth. Dent., *1*:700, 1951; Block, L. S.: Discussion of "The physiology of the muscles of mastication." J. Prosth. Dent., *1*:708, 1951.
12a. Fenton, A. H.: Bone restoration and prosthodontics. J. Prosth. Dent., *29*:477, 1973.

13. Freese, A. S., and Scheman, P.: *Management of Temporomandibular Joint Problems.* St. Louis, The C. V. Mosby Co., 1962.

14. *Gray's Anatomy of the Human Body,* 29th ed., C. M. Goss, editor. Philadelphia, Lea & Febiger, 1973.

14a. Guichet, N. F.: Biologic laws governing functions of muscles that move the mandible. Part I—Occlusal Programming. J. Prosth. Dent., *37*:648, 1977.

14b. ———: Biologic laws governing functions of muscles that move the mandible. Part II—Condylar position. J. Prosth. Dent., *38*:35, 1977.

14c. ———: Biologic laws governing functions of muscles that move the mandible. Part III—Speed of closure. J. Prosth. Dent., *38*:174, 1977.

14d. ———: Biologic laws governing functions of muscles that move the mandible. Part IV—Degree of jaw separation and potential for maximum jaw separation. J. Prosth. Dent., *38*:301, 1977.

15. Guyton, A. C.: *Textbook of Medical Physiology.* 4th Ed. Philadelphia, W. B. Saunders Company, 1971.

15a. Heartwell, C. M., Jr.: Complete denture failures related to improper interpretation and improper preparation of the anatomy of the mouth. Dent. Clin. N. Amer., *14*:379, 1970.

16. Hickey, J. C., Stacy, R. W., and Rinear, L. L.: Electromyographic studies of mandibular muscles in basic jaw movements. J. Prosth. Dent., *7*:565, 1957.

16a. Hirsch, B., Levin, B., and Tiber, N.: Effects of patient involvement and esthetic preference on denture acceptance. J. Prosth. Dent., *28*:127, 1972.

16b. Jacobs, R. M.: The effects of preprosthetic muscle exercise upon perioral tonus. J. Prosth. Dent., *18*:217, 1967.

16c. Jani, R. M., and Bhargava, K.: A histologic comparison of palatal mucosa before and after wearing complete dentures. J. Prosth. Dent., *36*:254, 1976.

16d. Jozefowicz, W.: The influence of wearing dentures on residual ridges: A comparative study. J. Prosth. Dent., *24*:243, 1970.

17. Jerge, C. R.: The neurologic mechanism underlying cyclic jaw movements. J. Prosth. Dent., *14*:667, 1964.

18. ———: The organization and function of the trigeminal mesencephalic nucleus. J. Neurophysiol., *26*:379, 1963.

19. Johnson, O. M.: The tori and masticatory stress. J. Prosth. Dent., *9*:975, 1959.

19a. Kapur, K. K., Collister, T., and Fischer, E. F.: Masticatory and gustatory reflex secretion rates and taste thresholds of denture wearers. J. Prosth. Dent., *18*:406, 1967.

20. Karies, A. K.: Palatal pressures of the tongue in phonetics and deglutition. J. Prosth. Dent., *7*:305, 1957.

21. Kamamura, Y., and Majima, T.: Temporomandibular joint sensory mechanisms controlling activities of the jaw muscles. J. Dent. Res., *43*:150, 1964.

21a. Kawazoe, Y., and Hamada, T.: The role of saliva in retention of maxillary complete dentures. J. Prosth Dent., *40*:131, 1978.

21b. Kelsey, C. C.: Alveolar bone resorption under complete denture. J. Prosth. Dent., *25*:152, 1971.

22. Kessler, B.: An analysis of the tongue factor and its functioning areas in dental prosthesis. J. Prosth. Dent., *5*:629, 1955.

22a. Klein, I. E.: The effect of thyrocalcitonin and growth hormones on bone metabolism. J. Prosth. Dent., *33*:365, 1975.

23. Kolb, H. R.: Variable denture-limiting structures of the edentulous mouth. Part I. Maxillary border areas. J. Prosth. Dent., *16*:194, 1966.

24. ———: Variable denture-limiting structures of the edentulous mouth. Part II. Mandibular border areas. J. Prosth. Dent., *16*:202, 1966.

25. Kraus, H.: Muscle function and the temporomandibular joint; Vaughan, H. C.: Discussion of "Muscle function and the temporomandibular joint"; Kraus, H.: Reply to the discussion of muscle function and the temporomandibular joint. J. Prosth. Dent., *13*:950, 956, 961, 1963.

25a. Kurth, L. E., and Feinstein, I. K.: The hinge axis of the mandible. J. Prosth. Dent., *1*:327, 1951.

26. Lawson, W. A.: Influence of the sublin-

gual fold on retention of complete lower dentures. J. Prosth. Dent., *11*:1038, 1961.

27. Lewinsky, W., and Stewart, D.: The innervation of the periodontal membrane of the cat, with some observations on the function of the end-organs found in that structure. J. Anat., *71*:232, 1937.

27a. Lye, T. L.: The significance of fovea palatini in complete denture prosthodontics. J. Prosth. Dent., *33*:504, 1975.

27b. Lyons, D. C.: The dry mouth adverse reaction syndrome in the geriatric patient. J. Oral Med., *27*:110, 1972.

27c. Maher, W. P., and Swindle, P. F.: Palatal vessels related to maxillary complete dentures. J. Prosth. Dent., *22*:143, 1969.

28. Maison, W. G.: Denture outline form. J.A.D.A., *59*:938, 1959.

28a. Manly, R. S., and Vinton, P.: Factors influencing denture function. J. Prosth. Dent., *1*:578, 1951.

28b. Margolese, M. S.: The role of endocrines in prosthodontics. J. Prosth. Dent., *23*:607, 1970.

29. Martone, A. L.: Anatomy of facial expression and its prosthodontic significance. J. Prosth. Dent., *12*:1020, 1962.

30. ———, and Black, J. W.: An approach to prosthodontics through speech science. Part V. Speech science research of prosthodontic significance. J. Prosth. Dent., *12*:629, 1962.

31. ———, and Edwards, L. F.: Anatomy of the mouth and related structures. Part I. The face. J. Prosth. Dent., *12*:1009, 1961.

32. ———: Anatomy of the mouth and related structures. Part II. Musculature of expression. J. Prosth. Dent., *12*:4, 1962.

33. ———: Anatomy of the mouth and related structures. Part III. Functional anatomic considerations. J. Prosth. Dent., *12*:206, 1962.

34. Millsap, C. H.: The posterior palatal seal area for complete dentures. Dent. Clin. N. Amer., November, 1964, p. 663.

34a. Nedelman, C., Gamer, S., and Bernick, S.: The alveolar ridge mucosa in denture and non-denture wearers. J. Prosth. Dent., *23*:268, 1970.

34b. Nedelman, C. I., and Bernick, S.: The significance of age changes in human alveolar mucosa and bone. J.

Prosth. Dent., *39*:495, 1978.

35. Nelson, A. A.: Significant factors involved in positional stability of the mandibular denture. Dent. Clin. N. Amer., November, 1964, p. 639.

36. Neufeld, J. O.: Dentures and their supporting oral tissues. Dent. Clin. N. Amer., November, 1964, p. 559.

37. Orban, B.: *Oral Histology and Embryology.* St. Louis, The C. V. Mosby Company, 1953.

37a. Parkinson, C. F.: Similarities in resorption patterns of maxillary and mandibular ridges. J. Prosth. Dent., *39*:598, 1978.

38. Pendleton, E. C.: The anatomy of the maxilla from the point of view of full denture prosthesis. J.A.D.A., *19*:543, 1932.

39. ———: The minute anatomy of the denture bearing area. J.A.D.A., *21*:488, 1934.

39a. Perry, C.: Neuromuscular control of mandibular movements. J. Prosth. Dent., *30*:714, 1973.

40. Pietrokovski, J., and Massler, M.: Alveolar ridge resorption following tooth extraction. J. Prosth. Dent., *17*:21, 1967.

40a. ———: Residual ridge remodeling of tooth extraction in monkeys. J. Prosth. Dent., *26*:119, 1971.

40b. Polter, R. B.: Evaluation of a delegated procedure: Posterior border of the maxillary denture. J.A.D.A., *81*:134, 1970.

40c. Porter, M. R.: The attachment of the lateral pterygoid muscle to the meniscus. J. Prosth. Dent., *24*:555, 1970.

40d. Ramfjord, S. P., and Blankenship, J. R.: Interarticular disc in wide mandibular opening in rhesus monkeys. J. Prosth. Dent., *26*:189, 1971.

40e. ———, and Endlow, R. D.: Anterior displacement of the mandible in adult rhesus monkeys: Long term observations. J. Prosth. Dent., *26*:511, 1971.

40f. Rayson, J. H., et al.: The value of subjective evaluation in clinical research. J. Prosth. Dent., *26*:111, 1971.

40g. Shannon, J. L.: The mentalis muscle in relation to edentulous mandibles. J. Prosth. Dent., *27*:477, 1972.

41. Shapiro, H. H.: Anatomic structures

which limit the borders of artificial dentures. New York Dent. J., *13*:136, 1947.

42. Sicher, H.: *Oral Anatomy.* St. Louis, The C. V. Mosby Company, 1952.

42a. Sicher, H., and DuBrul, E. L.: *Oral Anatomy,* 6th ed. The C. V. Mosby Company, St. Louis, 1975.

43. Silverman, S. I.: Denture prosthesis and the functional anatomy of the maxillofacial structures. J. Prosth. Dent., *6*:305, 1956.

43a. ———: Dimensions and displacement patterns of the posterior palatal seal. J. Prosth. Dent., *25*:470, 1971.

44. Sobolik, C. F.: Alveolar bone resorption. J. Prosth. Dent., *10*:612, 1960.

44a. Strohauer, R. A.: A comparison of articulator mountings made with centric relation and myocentric position records. J. Prosth. Dent., *28*:375, 1972.

45. Syrop, H. M.: Motion picture studies of the mechanism of mastication and swallowing. J.A.D.A., *46*:495, 1953.

45a. Tallgren, A.: The continuing reduction of the residual alveolar ridge in complete denture wearers: A mixed-longitudinal study covering 25 years. J. Prosth. Dent., *27*:120, 1972.

45b. Tardif, N.: An Electromyographic Study of the Behavior of the Masseter Muscle in Respect to the Utilization of Spiral-Spring Retention for Complete Dentures. M. S. Thesis, U. of Alberta, Canada, 1971.

45c. Trapozzano, U. R., and Lazzari, J. B.: The physiology of the terminal rotational position of the condyles in the temporomandibular joint. J. Prosth. Dent., *17*:122, 1967.

46. Turck, D.: A histologic comparison of the edentulous denture and non-denture bearing tissues. J. Prosth. Dent., *15*:419, 1965.

46a. Urinland, R. D., and Young, T. M.: Maxillary complete denture posterior palatal seal: variations in size, shape and location. J. Prosth. Dent., *29*:256, 1973.

47. Van Scotter, D. E., and Boucher, L. J.: The nature of supporting tissues for complete dentures. J. Prosth. Dent., *15*:285, 1965.

47a. Vaughan, H. C.: Need for changes in concepts relating to the temporomandibular joint and the mandibular articulation. J. Prosth. Dent., *17*:406, 1967.

47b. Vierheller, P. G., Speiser, W. H., and Al-Rahman, A. F.: Measuring mandibular vertical bone resorption by radiographic cephalometry. J. Prosth. Dent., *26*:33, 1971.

48. Weinmann, J. P.: Bone formation and bone resorption. Oral Surg., *8*:1070, 1955.

49. ———, and Sicher, H.: *Bone and Bones.* 2nd ed. St. Louis, The C. V. Mosby Company, 1955.

49a. Wical, K. E., and Swoope, C. C.: Studies of residual ridge resorption—Part I. J. Prosth. Dent., *32*:7, 1974.

49b. ———: Studies of residual ridge resorption—Part II. J. Prosth. Dent., *32*:13, 1974.

50. Woelfel, J. B., et al.: Electromyographic analysis of jaw movements. J. Prosth. Dent., *10*:688, 1960.

51. Wright, C. R.: Evaluation of the factors necessary to develop stability in mandibular dentures. J. Prosth. Dent., *16*:414, 1966.

52. ———, et al.: A study of the tongue and its relation to denture stability. J.A.D.A., *39*:269, 1949.

53. Yaeger, J. A.: Mandibular path in the grinding phase of mastication. J. Prosth. Dent., *39*:569, 1978.

Articulators

2

In the fabrication of indirect dental prostheses, a mechanical device is used to relate opposing models. Such a device is called an articulator. By definition, an articulator is "a mechanical device which represents the temporomandibular joints and jaw members to which maxillary and mandibular casts may be attached." A number of devices used by the profession do not satisfy this definition. Some do not make any type of hinge motion and others do not come close to duplicating excursive motion. Yet the profession refers to all these instruments as articulators.

Uses

The primary purposes of an articulator are (1) to hold opposing casts in a predetermined fixed relationship, (2) to open and close, and (3) to produce border and intra-border diagnostic sliding motions of the teeth similar to those in the mouth.

The uses of an articulator are (1) to diagnose dental occlusal conditions in both the natural and artificial dentitions, (2) to plan dental procedures that involve positions, contours, and relationships of both natural and artificial teeth as they relate to each other, (3) to aid in the fabrication of dental appliances and lost dental parts, and (4) to correct and modify completed restorations. Articu-lators can be helpful in the teaching and studying of occlusion and mandibular movements. To be of value, however, the elements should hold casts in the same relative position that occurs in the mouth and allow motion similar to that of the temporomandibular joints (TMJ's).

No matter how simple or complicated an articulator may be, if the operator does not use it properly or if it does not have the features for the basic purpose for which it is used, the results will be a disappointment. An articulator should have the following minimal requirements:

1. It should hold casts in the correct horizontal relationships.

2. It should hold casts in the correct vertical relationships.

3. It should provide a positive anterior vertical stop (incisal pin).

4. It should accept a face-bow transfer record.

5. It should open and close in a hinge movement.

6. It should allow protrusive and lateral jaw motion.

7. The moving parts should move freely and be accurately machined.

8. The non-moving parts should be of rigid construction.

Some of these additional features are desirable in an articulator:

1. Adjustable horizontal and lateral condylar guide elements.

2. The condylar elements as a part of the lower frame and the condylar guides as a part of the upper frame.

3. A mechanism to accept a third reference point from a face-bow transfer record.

4. A terminal hinge position locking device.

5. Removable mounting plates that can be repositioned accurately.

6. An adjustable incisal guide table.

7. Adjustable intercondylar width.

Limitations

An articulator is a mechanical instrument made of metal. Some articulators have parts made from a plastic material. The articulator is subject to human error in tooling and errors resulting from metal fatigue and wear. Even the best instrument is of little value if inaccurate casts or improper jaw relations are transferred to the articulator.

It is unlikely that any articulator will duplicate the condylar movements in the temporomandibular joints. The condylar elements and guidance surfaces should be thought of as cams that create equivalent-like motion in the area of the teeth. The movements simulated are empty-mouth sliding motions, not functional movements.

It might appear that since the articulator may not exactly reproduce border movements of the jaws or reproduce intraborder and functional movements either, the mouth would be the best place to complete the occlusion. Using the jaws as an articulator also has limitations. The intraoral analysis of occlusion has many limitations that are magnified when one studies occlusion in complete dentures. Some of the problems are: the adaptive capacity of the muscles as programmed by the somatic nervous system, the inability of humans to detect visually subtle changes in mo-

tion, the problem of making accurate marks in the presence of saliva, the inability to know exactly where the condyles are, the resiliency of the supporting structures, and the fact that dentures are movable.

The effectiveness of any articulator depends upon (1) how well the operator understands its construction and purpose, (2) how enthusiastic he is for the particular instrument, (3) how well the dentist understands the anatomy of the joints, their movements, and the neuromuscular system, (4) how much precision and accuracy are used in registering jaw relations, and (5) how sensitive the instrument is to these records.

Regardless of how simple or complex an articulator may appear, if the individual operator does not feel that it is capable of doing what he requires it to do or understands as its operation, he will be disappointed with the results. An articulator can do no more than what the operator does with it.

PRECISION, ACCURACY, AND
SENSITIVITY

No instrument is effective unless it will accurately adjust to the records. Errors in any of the maxillomandibular relation procedures are reproduced as errors in tooth relations.

The more stable the record bases, the more accurate will be the maxillomandibular relation records. Record bases or clutches attached to natural teeth are more stable than record bases resting on firm mucosal covering of an edentulous ridge. Record bases resting on a firm mucosal covering are more stable than those resting on pendulous or displaceable tissue.

The accuracy of recording methods and recording materials must be considered. Some dentists manually manipulate the patient's mandible to make maxillomandibular relation records; others allow the patient to make the movements voluntarily. Some dentists use graphic tracings, extraoral and intraoral; some use interocclusal records of wax, plaster, or compound to record maxillomandibular relations. One must analyze the procedures and the materials in these methods, remembering that the stability of the record bases and the resistance offered by the recording materials are of prime importance. Interference by the recording apparatus in maxillomandibular relation record procedures must be appreciated. The articulator cannot be blamed for errors; however, articulators that require intricate records for their adjustments may not be suitable for complete denture procedures. The manufacturer of the articulator provides instructions for setting and adjusting the parts and recommends records for which it can be used. As a rule, the best results are obtained when one follows these instructions.

Classification

Articulators have been classified as (1) arbitrary, (2) positional, (3) semiadjustable, and (4) fully adjustable. They have also been classified as (1) hinge joint, (2) average movement, and (3) fully adaptable.

These classifications may be confusing to the learner because they do not accurately describe the instruments now available. All articulators are fully adjustable and adaptable within the limits of the instrument. The hinge joint articulator, for example, is fully adjustable and adaptable to open and close in a hinge movement. It is questionable, however, if any articulator is fully adjustable and adaptable to all mandibular movements. *Semi,* a prefix meaning "half or partly," is not a scientific description of the articulators that are classified as semiadjustable.

Positioned instruments, or other mechanical instruments designed primarily for use in the construction of complete dentures, do not serve all of the primary purposes of an articulator. The limitations do not imply that they are not suitable for denture construction. The Stansbery Tripod is possibly the best known instrument of this class. A more descriptive classification of articulators for diagnosing dental problems and planning dental occlusion in natural and/or artificial dentitions follows:

CLASS I. Instruments that receive and reproduce pantograms or stereograms. These articulators can be adjusted to permit individual condylar movement in each of the three planes. They are capable of reproducing the timing of the Bennett shift on the balancing side and its direction on the working side. Timing can be considered another aspect of movement and is the reason this class of articulators has been called four-dimensional instruments. These instruments have variations; however, they all receive stereograms. Articulators of this They are designed to repeat the jaw motions at condyle levels in border positions. The jaw motion at condyle levels can be resolved into glidable rotating axes. The articulator should reproduce the glidings as faithfully as the rotations.

CLASS II. Instruments that will not receive stereograms. Articulators of this class are incapable of being set to the individual timing and direction of the Bennett movement unless the patient's movements accidentally coincide with the manufactured built-in settings. Most of these articulators are capable of being adjusted to protrusive jaw records. Some will accept lateral positional records. Several types of mini recording devices and pre-molded fossae are becoming popular for attaining better condylar guidance factors. This class is divided into four types:

Type 1 (Hinge). This type is capable of opening and closing in a hinge movement. A few instruments have limited nonadjustable excursive-like movements.

Type 2 (Arbitrary). This type is designed to adapt to specific theories of occlusion or are oriented to technique.

Type 3 (Average). This type is designed to simulate condylar pathways by averages or mechanical equivalents for selected aspects of mandibular motion. Adjustment of horizontal and lateral condylar guidance surfaces by means of positional jaw records or mini recordings is possible. Some types of face-bow can be used for the maxillary cast orientation.

Type 4 (Special). This type is designed and used primarily for complete denture construction.

Some examples of each class of articulator follows. Both historical and current models are included.

Class I
McCollum Gnathoscope
Granger Gnatholator
Ney Articulator
Cosmax
Stuart Gnathologic Computer
TMJ Stereographic
Denar D5A and SE
Aderer Simulator

Class II (Type 1)
The Barn Door Hinge
Gariot
Hageman Balancer
Gysi

Acme
Bonwill
Gysi Simplex and Adaptable
Stephens
Trubyte
The Centric Relator

Class II (Type 2)
Monson
Handy II
Galletti
The Gnathic Relator
The Correlator
Verticulator
Transograph

Class II (Type 3)
Hanau
Dentatus
House
Whip Mix
Denar Mark II
TMJ Mechanical Fossa
Panadent

Class II (Type 4)
Stansbery Tripod
Kile Dentograph
Irish Dupli-Functional

Articulators of Historic Interest

Gariot reputedly designed the hinge joint articulator about 1805 (Fig. 2-1). As originally designed it consisted of two metal frames to which the cast could be attached, a simple hinge to join them, and a set screw in the posterior of the instrument to hold the frames in a fixed vertical position.

The adaptable "barn door" hinge, (Fig. 2-2) with a vertical stop at the anterior end of the upper and lower members provides a more reliable instrument than some of the other hinge joint articulators.

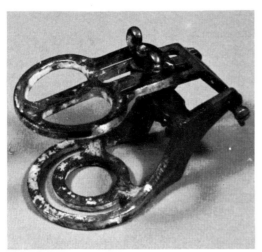

FIG. 2-1. *The Gariot hinge joint articulator. (From the collection of the Department of Prosthodontics, Virginia Commonwealth University, School of Dentistry.)*

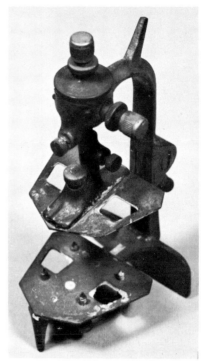

FIG. 2-3. *The Hageman Balancer. (From the collection of the Department of Prosthodontics, Virginia Commonwealth University, School of Dentistry.)*

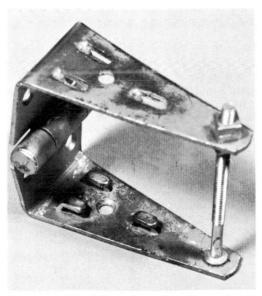

FIG. 2-2. *The fully adaptable "barn door" hinge. (A gift to the author from the Hanau Engineering Company, Buffalo, N. Y.)*

The Hageman Balancer (Fig. 2-3) opens and closes on a hinge. The design differed from most other articulators.

Other instruments with capabilities little removed from the adaptable "barn door" hinge are instruments designated as "mean value articulators." These instruments are capable of eccentric movement, but the condylar and incisal paths are not adjustable.

In 1858 Bonwill developed the first articulator with a serious effort to imitate the movements of the mandible in eccentric positions (Fig. 2-4).

The Acme (Fig. 2-5) is an elaboration of the Snow, which was designed in 1906. The Acme is available in three models to accommodate three ranges of intercondylar distance; the condylar

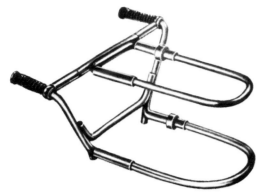

FIG. 2-4. *The Bonwill. (From Complete Denture Prosthodontics by J. J. Sharry. Copyright © 1962 by McGraw-Hill, Inc. Used by permission of McGraw-Hill Book Company.)*

paths are adjustable straight paths, the incisal guide pins rest on a changeable guide, and the Bennett movement is provided for, but is not limited or capable of limitation to the indications of a given patient. The Acme appears to be the forerunner of the Class II, Type 3 articulators.

The Gysi Simplex (Fig. 2-6A) was introduced in 1914 as a mean value articulator. The Gysi Adaptable articulator had been introduced in 1908 (Fig. 2-6B). It was an advanced instrument for the time, as it used extraoral graphic tracings and a particular condylar path plate. This instrument apparently was not accepted by the profession; therefore, the Gysi Simplex was introduced.

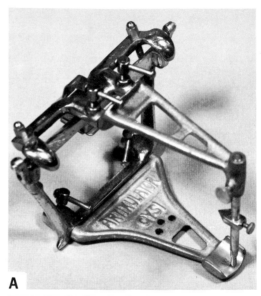

A

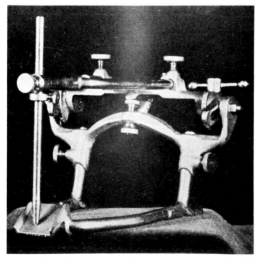

FIG. 2-5. *The Acme. (From Turner and Anthony: American Textbook of Prosthetic Dentistry. 6th ed. Philadelphia, Lea & Febiger, 1932.)*

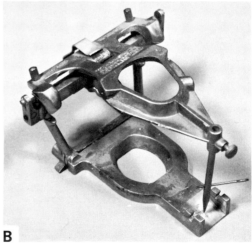

B

FIG. 2-6. A. *The Gysi Simplex.* **B.** *The Gysi Adaptable. (From the collection of the Department of Prosthodontics, Virginia Commonwealth University, School of Dentistry.)*

The arbitrary articulators were designed to meet the dictates of individual theories of mandibular movements and positions. These theories did not take into consideration individual variations. This type of articulator has limited use as a general rule.

In 1918 Monson presented the maxillomandibular instrument (Fig. 2-7), based upon the Spherical Theory. This concept is derived from an idea evolved by Von Spee that the lower teeth move over the surfaces of the upper teeth as over the external surfaces of a sphere with a radius of 4 inches. Movements reproduced in the Monson articulator are not in accord with the guidances afforded by the mandibular condyles in the lateral movements of the mandible.

The Bergström Articulator (Fig. 2-8) is an arcon instrument. This term appears to have been coined by Bergström to designate a mechanical feature. The term comes from the first two letters of *ARticulator* and the first three letters of *CONdyle*. The original Hanau H had many similar features.

The Precision Coordinator (Fig. 2-9), manufactured by the Precision Dental Mfg. Company, was a broken axis instrument. It also had a milling device built into its base.

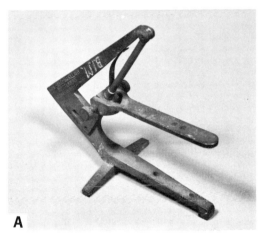

A

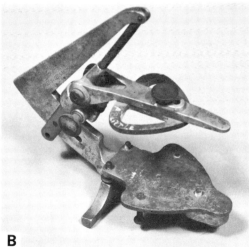

B

FIG. 2-7. *The maxillomandibular instrument by Monson.* **A.** *Without mounting plates.* **B.** *With mounting plates. (From the collection of the Department of Prosthodontics, Virginia Commonwealth University, School of Dentistry.)*

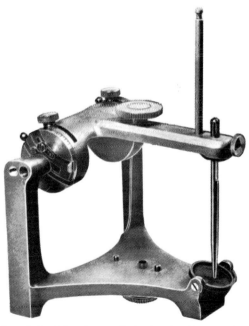

FIG. 2-8. *The "arcon" design by Bergström.* (From Complete Denture Prosthodontics by J. J. Sharry. Copyright © 1962 by McGraw-Hill, Inc. Used by permission of McGraw-Hill Book Company.)

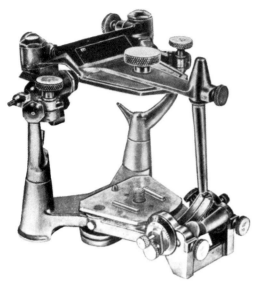

The Transograph presented in 1952 (Fig. 2-10) is a departure from the usual articulators. It is a split axis instrument designed to allow each condylar axis to function independently of the other. The designer does not accept that the condy-

lar axis is an imaginary line through the two mandibular condyles around which the mandible may rotate during a part of the opening movement.

In the Stansbery Tripod (Fig. 2-11) the maxillary cast is mounted in an arbitrary position. Later the instrument was modified to accept a face-bow transfer. The mandibular cast was mounted with a centric relation record of plaster. The record is made at the desired vertical dimension of occlusion and maintained at this position by a central bearing device. The eccentric records are made in plaster at a vertical dimension of occlusion equal to the height of the selected cusp with cusp-to-cusp contact. This vertical dimension is greater than that at centric occlusion. The turrets and slots are adjusted to these positional records, with the slots being adjusted to join the centric position with the eccentric positions by a straight path. Before teeth are arranged, the maxillary cast is raised 0.5 to 1.0 mm within the instrument to allow for milling after processing. A built-in

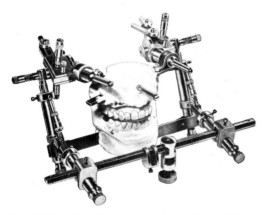

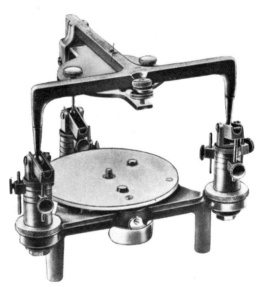

lathe attachment is used to mill the occlusion with abrasive paste to the desired dimension of occlusion. The milling device provides an elliptical horizontal freedom of the occlusion in the centric position.

Undoubtedly many acceptable dentures have been constructed with the Stansbery instrument and technique. Some of the limitations of the instrument are:

1. The teeth have to be arranged at the vertical dimension of occlusion for try-in, either on the tripod or another articulator, and then rearranged to accommodate the 0.5 to 1.0 mm opening.

2. No change in the vertical height of the cusps can be made during the construction without making new eccentric records.

3. Milling devices are not selective, and a desirable surface of tooth can be milled away.

4. Eccentric movements arc on a straight line.

5. No adjustments are possible for intercondylar distance.

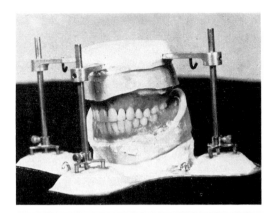

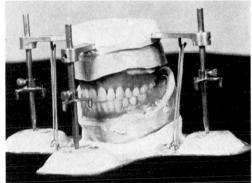

FIG. 2-12. *The Kile Dentograph. (From Kile, C. S.: The Kile Dentograph. J. Prosth. Dent., 5:169, 1955.)*

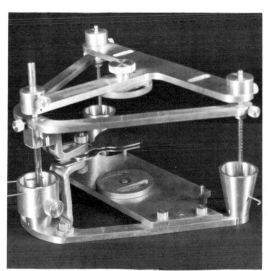

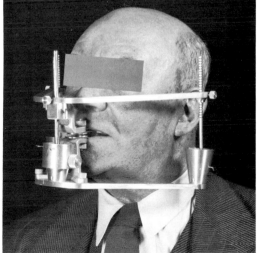

FIG. 2-13. *The Dupli-Functional by Irish. (Courtesy of the designer, E. F. Irish, D.D.S.)*

6. It will not accept a kinematic face-bow, although late models will accept arbitrary face-bow mountings.

7. It will not adjust for Bennett movement.

The Dentograph designed by Kile and presented in 1955 (Fig. 2-12) was designed primarily for use in complete denture construction. Kile states, "The Dentograph differs from all other articulating instruments in that it is custom built by and for each patient."[30] The vertical dimension of occlusion is established by the use of carborundum and plaster occlusion rims developed in a "generated path" by the Patterson method (pages 274–275).

The Dupli-Functional articulator (Fig. 2-13) was designed by Irish and presented in 1965. It was primarily for use in complete denture construction. It has two main purposes. First, it records each patient's mandibular movements and then, without further convertive procedures, serves as a three-dimensional tripod type of dental articulator upon which dentures may be constructed and their occlusion balanced.[28]

McCollum, a devoted student of gnathology, developed a mandibular movement recorder and an articulator (Gnathoscope) (Fig. 2-14) in 1939. The other instruments in this class are based in principle on this original work.

Granger's Gnatholator (Fig. 2-15) is slightly different from McCollum's Gnathoscope, but the principle is the same.

The Ney articulator (Fig. 2-16) was designed by Dr. A. J. DePietro. It can be set with a series of interocclusal stone records using a central bearing device and a gothic arch tracing. A pantogram can be used to set the articulator. Individual working side settings for the Bennett shift are not possible.

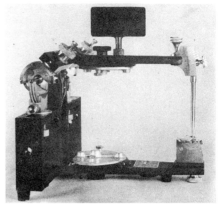

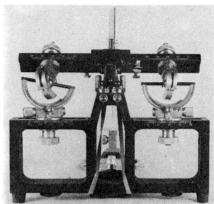

FIG. 2-14. *The McCollum Gnathoscope. (From McCollum, B. B., and Stuart, C. E.: A research report. S. Pasadena, California, Scientific Press, 1955.)*

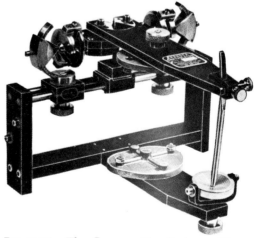

FIG. 2-15. *The Granger Gnatholator. (From Complete Denture Prosthodontics by J. J. Sharry. Copyright © 1962 by McGraw-Hill, Inc. Used by permission of McGraw-Hill Book Company.)*

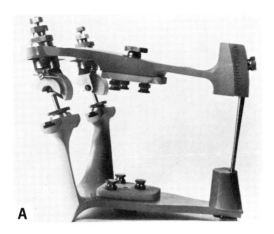

A

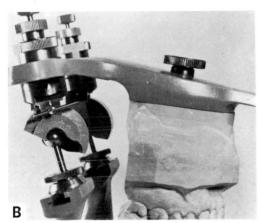

B

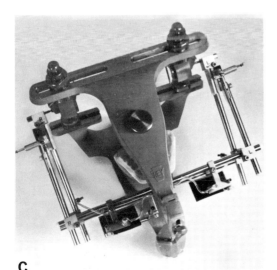

C

FIG. 2-16. *The Ney articulator.* **A.** *Side view.* **B.** *Contour of the eminentia inserts for condylar guidance.* **C.** *Pantograph attached.* *(Courtesy of the J. M. Ney Company.)*

Current Popular Articulators

STEPHENS CLASS II, TYPE 1 (Fig. 2-17). There are several models. The primary movement is a hinge opening and closing. These articulators will make a limited lateral movement. Some models have a set screw in the posterior of the instrument to hold the frames in a fixed vertical position. Others have an anterior pin to maintain vertical relation. This articulator is useful in the fabrication of small restorations and for prosthesis repairs.

GALETTI CLASS II, TYPE 2. In the Galetti articulator, each cast is held mechanically by two fixed posts and one adjustable post forming a tripod. The upper member can be adjusted by an extendable arm and a universal ball-and-socket joint to achieve the desired relationship of the upper and lower casts. Cast mounting is rapid. It has a fixed condylar path and a stop mechanism in the posterior region. It is useful to study static positional relationships of upper and lower casts.

TRUBYTE SIMPLEX CLASS II, TYPE I (Fig. 2-18). The new improved Simplex articulator uses average movements. The condylar guides are inclined 30 degrees with a Bennett movement of 7.5 degrees. The incisal guide table adjusts from 0 to 30 degrees. Model locking pins, rather than mounting plates, are used to attach casts. A mounting jig which doubles to level the occlusal plane is used for arbitrary mounting of the upper cast. As an alternate technique, a plane orientation jig positions the lower cast first and is used for positioning the Gothic arch transfer. It is useful with a special technique for complete denture construction.

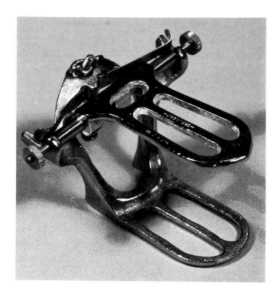

THE HOUSE ARTICULATOR (Fig. 2-19). This articulator was developed by M. M. House. It is adjusted with maxillo-mandibular relation records that use the Needles-House method (pages 274–275). The instrument has a milling device for occlusal adjustment after processing the dentures.

THE STUART ARTICULATOR, CLASS I (Fig. 2-20). The Stuart Gnathologic Computer was designed by C. E. Stuart. Stuart's contribution in the dental literature fur-

FIG. 2-17. *One model of the Stephens articulators.*

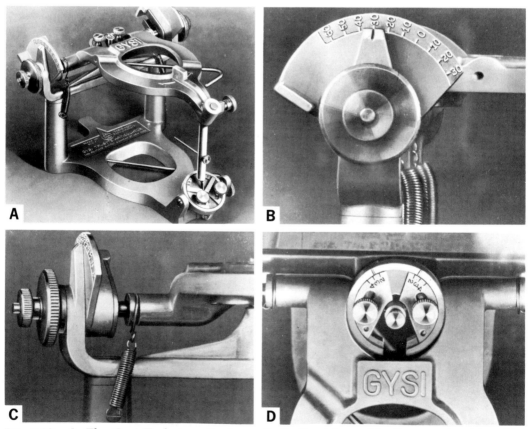

FIG. 2-18.   **A.** *The Gysi Trubyte articulator.* **B. C.** *Condylar guide.* **D.** *Incisal guide table.* (*Courtesy of the Dentists' Supply Company of New York.*)

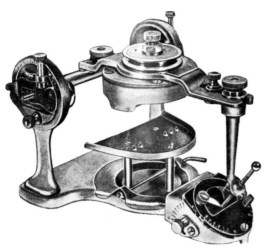

FIG. 2-19. *The House articulator. (From Complete Denture Prosthodontics by J. J. Sharry. Copyright © 1962 by McGraw-Hill, Inc. Used by permission of McGraw-Hill Book Company.)*

nished considerable information pertinent to the principles of gnathology and to the principles of an instrument that will receive and reproduce pantograms made in three planes. Not only does it record and repeat the positions in three planes and in the fourth dimension, that of time-sequence, it likewise records the amount and character of movement in one plane in relation to the other two planes.

The orientation of the maxillary cast is accomplished by using three known

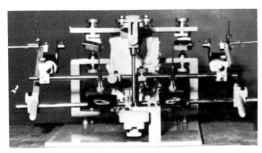

FIG. 2-20. *The Stuart Instrument. (From the collection of the Department of Prosthodontics, Virginia Commonwealth University, School of Dentistry.)*

points of reference. The skin locations of the hinge axis on the left and right sides of the face provide the two posterior reference points, and an anterior point is selected on the right side of the nose at a level near the lower orbit of the eye.

The axis of the articulator should be related to the teeth of the cast in the same way the patient's opening and closing axis is related to his teeth. Stuart states "If we wish to work on a laboratory instrument that is a mechanical and relational likeness of the mouth, we must have the dental casts open and close as they do in the mouth."* This can be interpreted that it is mandatory, in adjusting the instrument, to locate the terminal hinge axis. The instruments are fully capable of receiving casts from such positions and are not limited in this respect. However, the accuracy of the positions, as determined by the method used for hinge axis determination, is debatable with the edentulous patient.

Mandibular movements are recorded by magnetically controlled ballpoint styluses: two for the Gothic arch tracings, two for the vertical condylar glidings and two for the lateral condylar glidings (Fig. 2-21). The border positions and movements are reproduced because they are constant and dependable and can be repeated. After all records have been made, the axis-orbital relater is adjusted, and the recorder is locked together with quick-setting stone at centric relation. The four-dimensional records are transferred to the articulator. The articulator is then set to follow the tracings.

Once the articulator has been set, the maxillary cast is mounted to the maxillary frame using a hinge face-bow transfer record. The mandibular cast is mounted with a centric relation interocclusal record.[54]

Features of the Stuart instrument are:

*Stuart, C. E.: Conversation with the author.

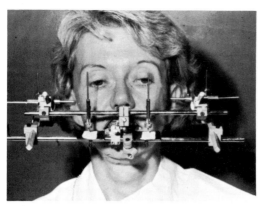

FIG. 2-21. *The mandibular movement recorder in position to write the effects of the movements. (Courtesy of J. M. Reynolds, Department of Restorative Dentistry, Medical College of Georgia.)*

1. The upper frame is of rigid construction and carries all of the cams that direct the gliding of the condyles and the fossae which carry the eminentiae.

2. The lower frame is of rigid construction and carries the condyles and simulates the mandible. The condylar spheres and guide controls duplicate the anatomic relationships of the jaws (a decided advantage for teaching).

3. The intercondylar distance is adjustable to each patient.

4. The fossa cups can be adjusted. Thus fossa likeness is cradled so that it can (a) be turned clockwise or counterclockwise horizontally, (b) be tilted down or up laterally to provide vertical adjustment or be maintained horizontally, and (c) be slanted anteriorly to give the eminentiae the desired inclination.

5. Eminentia blanks can be contoured and altered. If the protrusive line and lateral path differ, the plastic eminence can be altered to imitate the patient's.

6. The operating parts work freely and are devoid of set screws.

7. The nonoperating parts are rigid.

8. The surface of the condyle ball bears directly against the mechanical fossa and plastic eminentia.

9. Bennett timing is cut into the lateral wings.

THE SIMULATOR ARTICULATOR. An interesting feature of the Class I Simulator (Fig. 2-22) is the rotating condylar path. According to Granger, its developer, this feature makes the Simulator the only articulator that can be called an "anatomical articulator." In discussing the rotating condyle, he emphasizes several pertinent factors that are important in articulator evaluation: (1) they do not reproduce the anatomy of the temporomandibular joints; (2) they are mechanical equivalents; (3) the condyle paths either are fixed and rigid or are locked into position once the instrument has been adjusted to the pantogram; and (4) most articulators are adjusted to border movements, the paths being formed in plastic materials. On the Aderer Simulator, according to Granger, "the paths are not rigidly locked: they can rotate and move to reproduce all the paths of the condyles on the eminentia, border movements, and all their immediates."[16]

Although the Simulator articulator can be used in the procedures in complete denture construction, it is a sophisticated instrument and its capacity to simulate mandibular movements or condylar rotations requires accurate pantographs for its adjustments. To record the path of the condyles on the eminentia for the edentulous patient presents many problems that at this time do not appear to be satisfactorily surmounted. These problems are recognized and publicized by the Aderer Corporation, the manufacturers of the Simulator, in *A Practical Approach to the Instrumentation for the Treatment of Occlusion*.

The Simulator articulator was designed to be set with a conventional pantograph. A Minigraph (Fig. 2-23) has been developed. It can be applied when a full pantographic tracing would not be

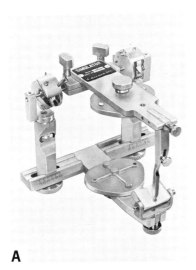

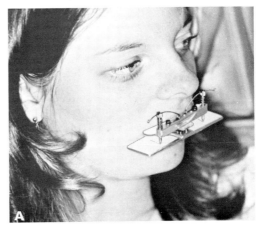

A

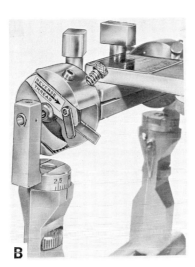

B

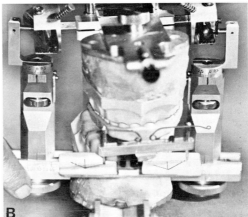

B

FIG. 2-23. **A.** *The minigraph showing a protrusive recording.* **B.** *The minigraph attached to the articulator. (Courtesy of J. Aderer, Inc., Long Island City, N. Y.)*

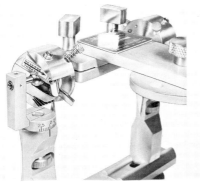

C

FIG. 2-22. **A.** *The Simulator articulator.* **B.** *Condyle path straight.* **C.** *Condyle path rotated. (Courtesy of J. Aderer, Inc.)*

feasible. It consists of only two anterior recording plates which are related to casts mounted to the hinge axis. Tracings of protrusive and both lateral movements are made.

An important aid to the Minigraph is a Mini-grip transfer vise.[62] It locks and holds the Minigraph for transfer back to the articulator. It is simpler and saves time by eliminating the need for stone cores, which would otherwise be necessary.

THE DENAR CLASS I (Fig. 2-24). The D5A articulator, a mandibular simulator of

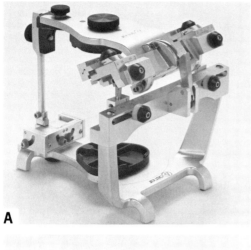

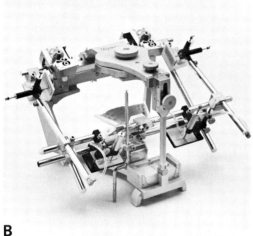

FIG. 2-24. **A.** *The Denar D5A Series articulator.* **B.** *Pantograph attached. (Courtesy of the Denar Corporation.)*

light weight and fairly rugged construction, is a precision-tooled instrument that should not be handled too roughly. It is a "mechanical equivalent of the lower half of the head. This articulator has total capacity to reproduce all mandibular movements of jaw positions recorded by any check-bite or chew-in technique or by the more sophisticated method employing a pantograph."[17]

The basic instrument is composed of a maxillary and a mandibular bow. The condylar elements are in the mandibular bow (arcon principle). When the side

shift adjustments are set at zero, the parts resist separation, but force will separate them. Force should therefore be avoided. The fossae are attached to the upper unit. The superior and medial fossa wall inserts are available in straight forms or in various anatomic curvatures and in either nylon or acrylic resin (Fig. 2-25). For the styli to follow the recorded tracing accurately when the instrument is adjusted to a pantographic tracing, the acrylic insert must be custom ground with a stone or bur having a diameter the size of the condylar element.

An adjustable metal incisal table and a custom incisal platform are available for the D5A. The foot of the incisal pin rests on an incisal pin stop, not on the adjustable lateral wings. Adjusting the foot of the incisal pin allows movement in the articulator to develop an area of occlusion in centric relation. The incisal platform can be used to hold self-curing acrylic resin in adjusting the horizontal and vertical overjet relation of the anterior teeth.

According to the *Manual for Occlusal Treatment*, the arbitrary hinge axis point can be used when the mandibular cast is related to the maxillary cast with a centric relation record.[17] When the record is made at an increased vertical dimension

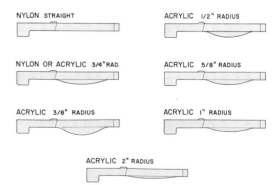

FIG. 2-25. *Inserts for superior and medial fossa walls of Denar D5A Series articulators. (Courtesy of the Denar Corporation.)*

of occlusion, the hinge axis is precisely located.

Anatomic landmarks are used with many articulators and techniques to establish the posterior and anterior reference points. The Denar Reference Plane Locator and Marker is useful for this purpose (Fig. 2-26). With it the anatomic points can be relocated accurately.

THE DENAR MARK II, CLASS II, TYPE 3. This system was developed primarily to satisfy the needs of undergraduate education. The articulator (Fig. 2-27) is a two-piece instrument incorporating a positive locking mechanism for the terminal hinge position. The horizontal condylar inclination can be adjusted from 0 to 60 degrees. It has an immediate Bennett shift adjustment of 0 to 4 mm plus a progressive Bennett shift adjustment of 0 to 15 degrees. The condylar elements are at a fixed intercondylar distance constructed to average anatomic dimensions. The posterior fossa wall is inclined posteriorly 25 degrees to allow for a backward movement of the rotating condyle as it moves outward during a Bennett shift.

The upper and lower members come apart and lock together in the open and closed positions. The articulator can be placed level in the upside down position for mounting casts without the need of a mounting stand.

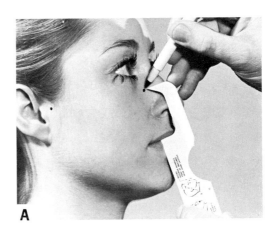

A

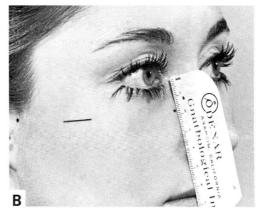

B

FIG. 2-26. *The Denar Reference Plane Locator and Marker.* **A.** *The anterior reference point is located by placing the notch of the Locator against the low lip line.* **B.** *The distance of the reference point from the inner canthus of the eye is recorded so that the anterior reference point may be relocated. The line represents the horizontal plane of reference that is marked on the face when the posterior reference point is located.* **C.** *The Locator is positioned forward from the middle of the upper margin of the external auditory meatus to the outer canthus of the eye to mark the posterior reference points. This measurement is needed when the mandibular cast is to be transferred to the articulator by a centric occlusion record. (Courtesy of the Denar Corporation.)*

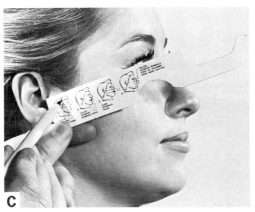

C

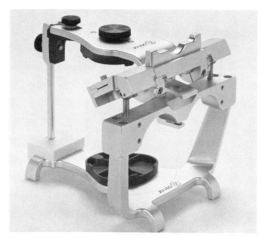

FIG. 2-27. *The Denar Mark II articulator.*

The standard face-bow (Fig. 2-28) has sidearms that are independently adjustable and have calibrated posterior reference pins. The transfer can be related to average anatomic axis reference points over the condyles or positioned in the external auditory meatus of the ears. Nylon earpieces are placed over the tips of the reference pins when used as an ear-bow.

When used as a face-bow, the posterior reference pins are attached into indexes on the lateral aspects of the condylar elements of the articulator when mounting the maxillary cast. It is attached into index holes on the lateral aspects of the fossae when used as an ear-bow.

There is also a slidematic face-bow (Fig. 2-29A). It features a unique slide gear mechanism which makes it easy and quick to assemble the bow on a patient. The posterior reference arms are designed to be used in the external auditory meatus of the ears similar to the Whip Mix bow. The sliding mechanism is calibrated to read off transcranial (intercondylar) distance in millimeters.

Once the face-bow record has been made on the patient, the sidearms are removed and set aside. A transfer jig (Fig. 2-29B) is attached to the toggle remaining on the face-bow fork. The transfer jig (Fig. 2-29C) is then inserted into the incisal guide table slot and attached to the lower member of the articulator. The face-bow fork is now properly related to the articulator for mounting of the maxillary cast.

The advantage of this face-bow is that the same bow can be used with additional transfer jigs for taking multiple face-bow records.

All Denar articulators can be calibrated to within (0.0001) one ten-thousandth of an inch of accuracy to each other. A special Denar Field Inspection Gage (Fig. 2-30) is used. Mounted casts can be transferred between calibrated articulators. With care, calibrated articulators will remain accurate for about ten mountings or remounts before recalibration is necessary.

THE TMJ ARTICULATOR (Fig. 2-31). This is a versatile instrument. Originally, it was primarily a Class I articulator. A method for recording mandibular movement by a four-dimensional stereograph modified from a technique by House is used to mold a set of individualized condylar fossae.

The recording is made intraorally on

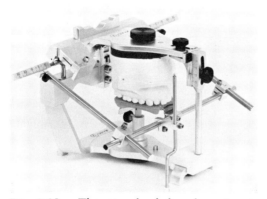

FIG. 2-28. *The standard face-bow is attached.*

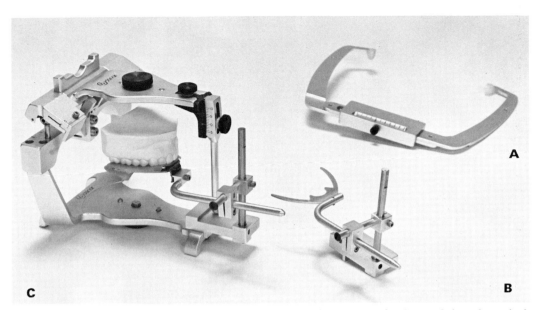

FIG. 2-29.   A. *The slidematic face-bow.* **B.** *The transfer jig.* **C.** *The jig and face-bow fork attached to the articulator.*

recording trays which fit over the teeth or edentulous arches. A central bearing pin and four special studs are placed in the general area of the canines and the 2nd molars. Four functional rhomboid recordings (Fig. 2-32) are generated in acrylic resin against an opposing platform holding the studs. The recordings are then transferred to the articulator using a hinge-axis face-bow. The trans-

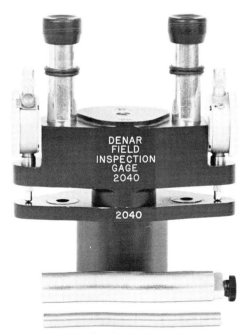

FIG. 2-30. *The field inspection gage.*

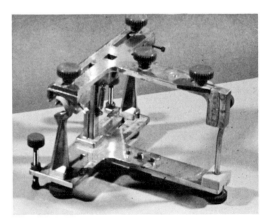

FIG. 2-31. *The TMJ articulator with molded fossae.*

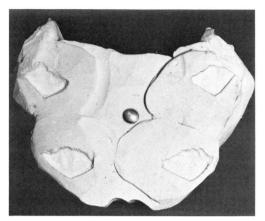

FIG. 2-32. *An intraoral functional stereographic recording. (Courtesy of Kenneth Swanson, Thousand Oaks, California.)*

fer is also used to set the intercondylar distance. Blank fossa boxes are filled with acrylic resin into which the curvature of the condylar pathways and the Bennett shift are molded as an analog of the recorded movements (Fig. 2-33).

A mechanical fossa (Fig. 2-34) accessory is available. It is used with the standard articulator and provides a simplified yet accurate method for determining rectilinear horizontal and lateral condylar guidance angles utilizing a check-bite setting technique. The mechanical fossa allows condylar inclina-

tion from 10 to 55 degrees and Bennett shift adjustment of 0 to 35 degrees. The superior wall of the TMJ has a 3-degree slant which produces a "Fisher angle" where the balancing pathway portion is steeper than the protrusive pathway. A double terminal hinge locking hook provides a method for securing the instrument in the terminal hinge position with no subluxation of the condylar elements. The locking device will permit a hinge opening of 115 degrees.

A series of premade fossae analogs are also available (Fig. 2-35). These are made with average curved protrusive paths varying in 5-degree differences and made in five different colors for easy identification. Early side-shift variations can be adjusted by sliding the box holder later-

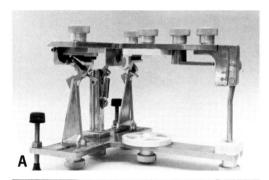

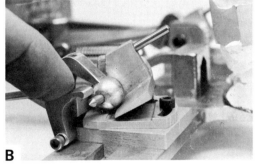

FIG. 2-34. **A.** *The TMJ articulator with mechanical fossae in place.* **B.** *The movable locking device (at end of finger) will allow the dentist to lock the instrument into terminal hinge position. (Courtesy of the TMJ Instrument Co.)*

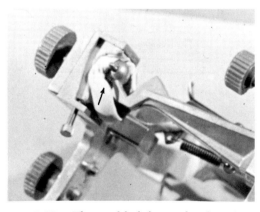

FIG. 2-33. *The molded fossa developed in acrylic resin from a stereographic recording.*

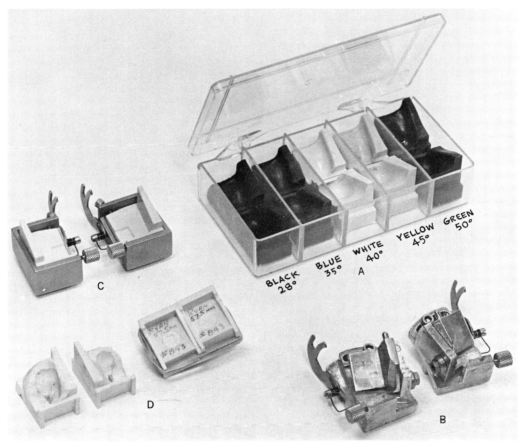

Fig. 2-35. A. *The series of premolded fossae.* **B.** *The mechanical fossae.* **C.** *Fossa blanks.* **D.** *A pair of molded fossae. Pertinent data can be marked on the back. (Courtesy of Kenneth Swanson, Thousand Oaks, California.)*

ally or medially on the articulator or by grinding a different Bennett control into the medial wall of the box. Data for a proper fossae selection can be made with check-bites, the TMJ Simplex MM Indicator, the Panadent Quick Analyzer, or the Denar Mini-Recorder.

The Simplex Mandibular Movement (MM) Indicator has been designed to quickly indicate the movement paths of the condyles. Rapid and accurate settings can be made for the TMJ or any other adjustable articulator by using these accessories. The curvature and inclination of the protrusive and/or lateral pathway of the condyles can be

speedily plotted. Also, the early and total Bennett shift can be closely determined. From the Indicator, the specific premade analog fossae can be determined which should be inserted in the articulator in order to most accurately follow the individual movement pathways of the condyles.

The following claims are stressed by the manufacturer:

1. The instrument will arc open to 115 degrees at which point it will counterbalance for stability.

2. It will sit on the laboratory bench inverted, as well as upright, without the use of special jigs.

3. Visibility is completely unobstructed.

4. There is a positive centering guide.

5. It can be locked in terminal hinge position.

6. The newly designed hinge axis styli will accept most face-bows in use today, including ear-bows.

7. There is sufficient space between the upper and lower members that casts for any technique can be attached easily.

The articulator and its accessories can meet a variety of needs. It can meet the needs of a Class II, Type III articulator using only the mechanical fossae. The standard premade fossae analogs and the simplex MM Indicator increase its capabilities. The custom molded fossae from intraoral stereographic recordings further increase its usefulness without any major additional cost. It can satisfy the instrument needs for teaching occlusion, occlusal analysis, the fabrication of simple and complex fixed and removable prosthodontic restorations, and complete denture construction.

HANAU ARTICULATORS. Until recently, the Hanau Model H (Fig. 2-36) was possibly the best known and most widely used of the Class II, Type 3, articulators for complete dentures. Other instruments that are adjustable to more than one jaw movement are of similar construction. For these reasons the Model H will be discussed in some depth.

When Hanau introduced the Model H articulator, he presented the *Intraoral Technique for Hanau Articulator Model H*. In this publication he acknowledged that some of the outstanding prosthodontists of his time—Drs. E. J. Farmer, Felix A. French, Robert Gillis, Victor Sears, R. O. Schlosser, and W. H. Wright—assisted in arranging and revising the technical procedures. Since these prosthodontists did not and do not subscribe to the same concepts of occlusion, it can be assumed that the Hanau articu-

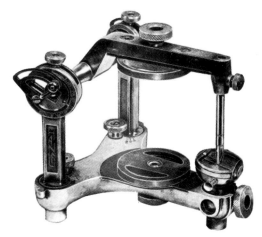

FIG. 2-36. *The Hanau Model H. The original articulators did not have the universal incisal guide table. (From the collection of the Department of Prosthodontics, Virginia Commonwealth University, School of Dentistry.)*

lator can be used to develop different concepts.

According to the literature, Hanau did not intend the Model H to be an anatomic articulator. He designed it for complete denture construction and outlined a specific technique for its use. From his research Hanau concluded that "the articulator jaw members should produce movements equivalent to those of the mandible to the maxillae" and that "the movements of the jaw members of the articulator have a definite relation to the anatomical movements, and that both are by no means the same, but must be equivalent, in order to compensate for the effect of the resilient supporting tissues upon which prosthetic dentures function in the mouth."[24]

In the Model H the maxillary cast is mounted with a face-bow transfer. Since the instrument is not designed to receive a kinematic face-bow, the average points of location for the hinge axis are used.

The mandibular cast is mounted by any acceptable centric relation record made at the desired vertical dimension of occlusion. Hanau admired the Gothic arch tracing (graphic method). However, he observed:

The arrow point tracing is a basic contribution to denture prosthesis, as important as the face bow. It constitutes a link in a chain of operations, but does not give results per se. It, therefore, should not be underestimated, nor in enthusiasm be overrated. . .

The protrusive relation record is required to adjust the horizontal condylar indication, so that the instrument jaw members perform movements which are equivalent, but not identical to the relative movements of the mandible to the maxillae.[24]

Hanau held the opinion "that the setting of a lateral indication by an anatomical record does not offer any particular advantages to start with." His experience was that "the required overprotrusion on the working side in lateral cannot and need not be predetermined, but, that it is to be established on the finished case in the mouth, by records, observation, and interpretation of symptoms on the ridges."[24]

Dentures built on the Model H articulate in the mouth with a component of overprotrusion within a range mentioned. That means they have a tendency to find premature contact of the distal inclines of the lower cusps with the mesial inclines of the upper cusps, if they would have to articulate in what is considered theoretical anatomic articulation. Hanau defined anatomic articulation as "the articulation of natural teeth in the mouth." He recommended the following formula to arrive at acceptable lateral inclinations:

$$L = \frac{H}{8} + 12$$

where L = lateral condylar inclination in degrees and H = horizontal condylar inclination in degrees as established by a protrusive record.

This technique ordinarily does not employ lateral relation rest records taken in the mouth for articulator adjustments, yet a lateral relation rest record is sometimes obtained and its use indicated because the patient fails to give a true protrusive relation record. In such a case, the lateral relation rest record is used to adjust the articulator's horizontal condyle inclination on the balancing side only. Lateral relation records made in the articulator are frequently verified in the mouth.[24]

The balancing condylar movement is downward, forward, and medially. The intercondylar rod passing through the condylar element on the working side produces upward, backward, and lateral movement. If the Bennett movement is in any other direction or component of directions, the Model H will not accurately receive the record.

The Model H meets all minimum requirements of an articulator and, in addition, allows movements in lateral and protrusive directions. It will receive an arbitrary face-bow transfer, and the case can be remounted to correct for processing errors within a limited range without new eccentric records. The standard incisal guide table consists of a spherical element having specially formed guiding surfaces, adjustable in three dimensions. The incisal guide pin is notched, the notch being used as a third point of reference for mounting the maxillary cast.

Limitations of Hanau Articulators

1. Only an arbitrary face-bow transfer of the maxillary cast is allowed.

2. Intercondylar distance is not adjustable.

3. It will not receive all lateral records, that is, will not adjust to all Bennett movements.

4. The condylar elements are in the upper member; this position is confusing as related to the skull.

5. An arbitrary reference point (notch

on the incisal pin) is used as the third point of reference for maxillary cast mounting.

6. The condylar elements are ball-and-axle construction. In this type of construction, four clearances must be provided in tooling. Tooling of this nature is subject to error.

7. The condylar elements travel in a straight line.

8. The condylar elements do not remain constant in all eccentric movements. The condylar balls can move on the axle.

Weinberg conducted a mathematical study on the Hanau Model H of the effects of various adjustments to the development of occlusion. In this study the use of average location of the hinge axis, arbitrary location of the anterior point of orientation, and the straight condylar path produced the greatest amount of error. He concluded: "because of the relative mobility of denture bases, the Hanau Model H articulator and others of this type are adequate. However, fixed restorations (in natural teeth) require a higher degree of accuracy in lateral excursions than complete dentures."[68] Weinberg's work seems to verify the claims of Hanau.

The current Model H is designated the 96H2. It maintains all the features of the original Model H. In addition, auditory pins have been added to the terminal hinge condylar locking mechanism (Fig. 2-37). They insert into the earpieces and secure the ear-bow (Fig. 2-38) to the articulator when it is used. The condylar elements are fixed at the 110 mm width. The horizontal condylar adjustments range from 0 to 75 degrees and the lateral adjustment from 0 to 30 degrees. A 145 series exists with the same features, but the space between the upper and lower members is 3/4" less (Fig. 2-39).

A newer model 158 is now available (Fig. 2-40). It has the same inside dimen-

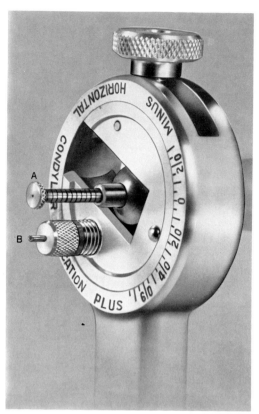

FIG. 2-37. *Extendable shaft for kinematic face-bow transfer* **(A)**. *Pin on locking bolt for relating ear-bow* **(B)**.

sions and condylar features as the H-2 but has arcon type movements. It does not need a mounting stand. A special face-bow (Fig. 2-41) is available for this articulator. It may be used either as a face-bow or ear-bow with provisions for proper mounting on the articulator for either position.

There are four models in the University series of articulators. The 130-21 model is an arcon articulator intended for occlusal reconstruction (Fig. 2-42). It has intercondylar width adjustment from 94 to 150 mm. A split vertical and lateral compound axis permit adjustments from −30 to +30 degrees in both planes. The lateral condylar angle is adjustable from 0 to 40 degrees. The upper

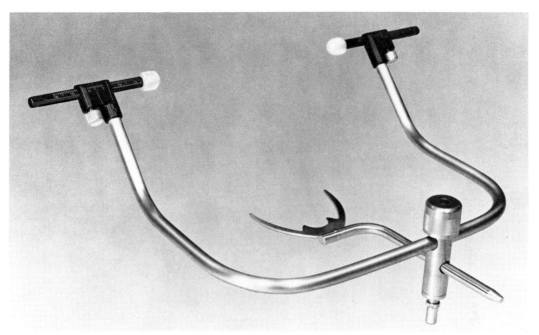

FIG. 2-38. *This face-bow can be used in the regular manner or as an ear-bow.*

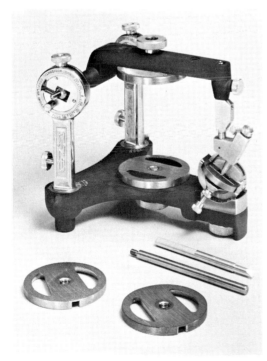

FIG. 2-39. *The Hanau Model 145-2. (Courtesy of the Hanau Engineering Company, Buffalo, N. Y.)*

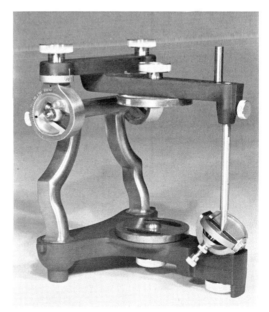

FIG. 2-40. *The Hanau 158 series.*

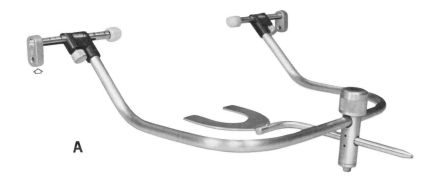

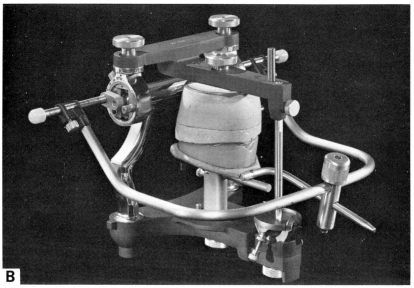

FIG. 2-41. **A.** *Adaptor (arrow) for using ear-bow with model 158.* **B.** *Adaptor and face-bow attached to the articulator.*

member may be separated from the lower member by loosening a retention lock. The 130-22 model is a nonarcon articulator used primarily for restoration of natural teeth. It has variable intercondylar width settings of 94 to 150 mm. The upper and lower members can also be separated.

The 130-28 model is an arcon checkbite articulator. (Fig. 2-43). It is suggested for standard fixed and removable partial prosthodontic cases. It has intercondylar width adjustment capability of 94 to 150 mm. Condlyar inclination adjustments of 0 to 60 degrees and lateral ad-

justment of 0 to 40 degrees. The 130-30 model is the same with the addition of a special retrusive-protrusive condylar adjustment.

All of the Hanau articulators described are axle and slot type instruments. This type of condylar mechanism is not well suited as a diagnostic instrument for natural dentitions or for many fixed prosthodontic situations. A model 154 may be better suited for such cases.

DENTATUS. Another adjustable articulator is the Dentatus, Class II, Type 3, a shaft-type instrument (Fig. 2-44). The

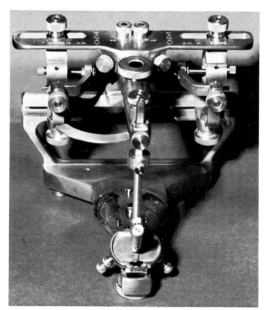

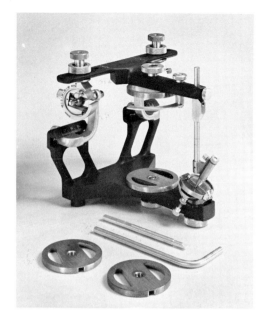

FIG. 2-42. *The University Model 130-21.* (*Courtesy of the Hanau Engineering Company, Buffalo, N. Y.*)

FIG. 2-43. *Hanau model 130-28.*

condylar elements are attached to the upper members, and the condylar path is straight. The Bennett angle is calibrated to 40 degrees. The intercondylar distance is fixed. This articulator will receive a hinge axis face-bow.

PANADENT. The Panadent articulator, Class II, Type 3 (Fig. 2-45) is the latest approach to dental instrumentation. It may be the way articulators will go in the future.

The Panadent system is the result of recent research in the area of mandibular motion. Research has shown that condylar movement patterns are similar in many respects. It is suggested that it is possible to classify individual condylar movements into groups based upon their amount of immediate Bennett shift.

The articulator is of rigid design. It uses $\frac{1}{4}''$ condylar elements instead of the usual $\frac{1}{2}''$ size. A series of statistically selected three-dimensional analogs of condylar axis motion are used. The ana-

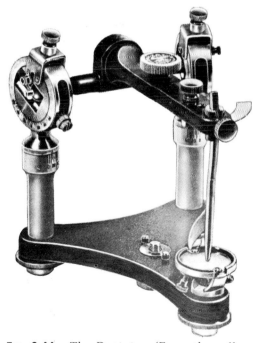

FIG. 2-44. *The Dentatus.* (*From the collection of the Department of Prosthodontics, Virginia Commonwealth University, School of Dentistry.*)

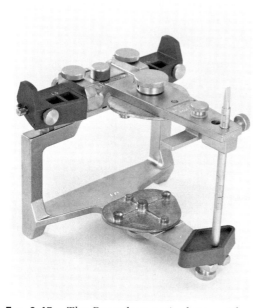

FIG. 2-45. *The Panadent articulator with a 1.5 mm immediate side shift premolded fossae. (Courtesy of Panadent Corp., Colton, California.)*

1. A series of preformed statistically molded three-dimensional motion analogs guide the actual pathways of the condylar elements.

2. Five wall analog guides for each condylar element for producing the rhombus geometric and total envelope of motion.

3. Lateral guide walls in the motion analogs for better working side control.

4. All major parameters of condylar movement control including curved surfaces for protrusive, balancing, and Bennett pathways.

5. An upper frame that can be locked to the lower frame for precise centric axis motion during mounting and remounting.

6. Accurate fixed condylar elements.

7. Designed for use with most commonly used face-bows.

log fossae feature curvilinear protrusive and balancing pathways with the medial wall angulation of 6 degrees. There are five pairs (Fig. 2-46) in the set with immediate Bennett shift of 0.5, 1.0, 1.5, 2.0, and 2.5 mm.

The articulator is designed to be set with an extraoral quick analyzer (Fig. 2-47), although it can be set with checkbites. The analyzer is used to plot the condylar pathways and register immediate Bennett shift. The appropriate analogs are then selected and inserted in the articulator. The analog fossae are then rotated to duplicate the slope of the protrusive pathways. The analogs can be mixed so that each side may have different amounts of Bennett shift.

The articulator can be used with any of the available face-bows (Fig. 2-48).

The analog fossae can be fitted to the Whip Mix articulator (Fig. 2-49). The following claims are stressed by the manufacturer:

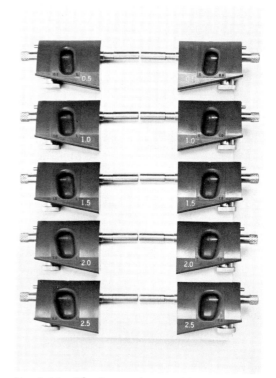

FIG. 2-46. *The 5 sets of premolded Panadent fossae.*

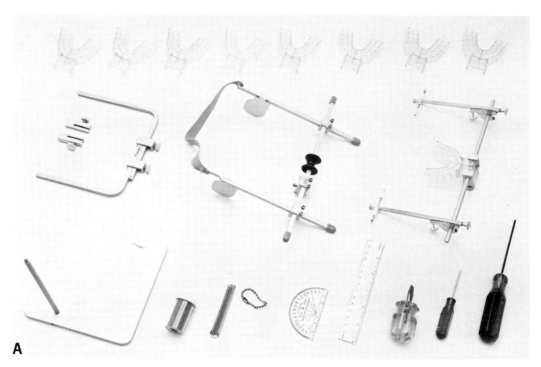

A

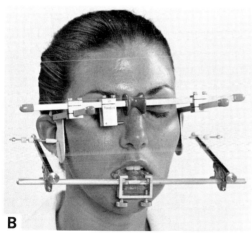

B

FIG. 2-47. **A.** *The Panadent quick analyzer kit.* **B.** *The analyzer positioned on a patient ready to record condylar vertical paths and the amount of side shift.*

8. The articulator can be set with conventional check bites.

WHIP MIX ARTICULATORS. The Whip-Mix Articulator (Fig. 2-50) is designed for complete denture construction, as an accessory instrument for quick diagnosis of the occlusion of natural teeth, routine restorative and fixed prosthodontic pro-

cedures and for educational purposes (Fig. 2-51). It is a Class II, Type 3, instrument but does not have shaft-and-ball construction. In addition to the advantages of many instruments of this type, it offers additional features.

1. The condylar elements are on the mandibular (lower) member. When the student of occlusion advances and decides to progress to a gnathologic type of instrument, his thinking as to the movements of instrument and jaw will not have to be reversed.

2. The intercondylar distance is adjustable to three positions. The narrowest distance is 96 mm, the intermediate distance is 110 mm, and the widest distance is 124 mm. This is similar in concept to the use of an average hinge axis location. Slight errors of intercondylar

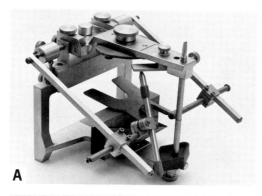

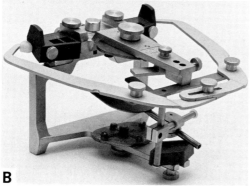

FIG. 2-48. **A.** *The Panadent face-bow attached to the articulator.* **B.** *The modified articulator with face-bow attached.*

distance have the least affect on working and balancing cusp path directions. Condylar spacers are either removed or replaced as the condylar elements are changed for different intercondylar settings. Care should be exercised to always return each spacer to the same position. When changing spacers, make sure the condylar housing is positioned in tight opposition to the side of the upper member of the articulator.

3. The distance between the condylar elements remains constant in all eccentric movements. The condylar elements are not on an axle.

4. The distance between the hinge axis and the mandibular anterior teeth remains constant in all eccentric positions. This is the same as the anatomic arrangement in the skull.

5. The instrument is equipped with two incisal guide tables, one of metal and the other of plastic. The plastic provides for the construction of an individual incisal guidance table for each patient. This is an aid in arranging teeth, but as with other instruments, once the teeth are contoured and harmonized with the condylar path, the teeth should act as the incisal guides.

6. The axis-orbital plane is the undersurface of the maxillary arm. The maxillary arm is rigid and constant to the assembly of the entire instrument. It would be almost impossible to make an error in the orientation of the maxillary cast.

7. All condylar guidance is derived

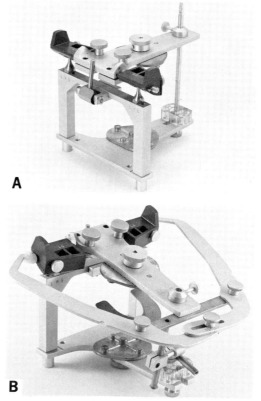

FIG. 2-49. **A.** *Whip Mix articulator modified to use the Panadent premolded fossae.* **B.** *The modified articulator with face-bow attached.*

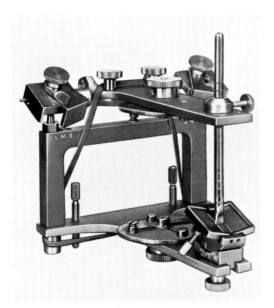

FIG. 2-50. *The Whip Mix 8500 articulator. (Courtesy of the Whip Mix Company, Avery-Louisville, Kentucky.)*

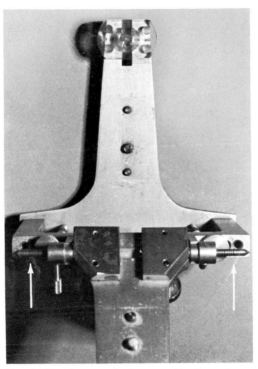

FIG. 2-52. *Arrows designate attachments on the Whip Mix to receive a kinematic face-bow (Courtesy of the Whip Mix Company, Avery-Louisville, Kentucky.)*

from the upper part of the articulator and remains constant to the upper teeth as in the human skull.

8. The condylar housing allows a horizontal condylar inclination of 0 to 65 degrees and a Bennett shift lateral adjustment of 0 to 45 degrees. Special condylar housing units allow for immediate Bennett shift, but are not recommended, since the articulator does not

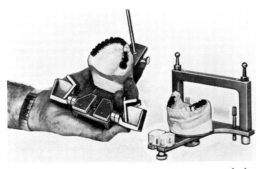

FIG. 2-51. *The simplicity of design and the arcon principle make the Whip Mix a useful teaching instrument. (Courtesy of the Whip Mix Company, Avery-Louisville, Kentucky.)*

have a positive midsagittal locking device.

9. The instrument will receive a true hinge axis registration (Fig. 2-52). A series 8800 articulator is now available (Fig. 2-53). It has $\frac{1}{2}''$ more space between the upper and lower members. The additional space is an advantage for complete denture fabrication. In addition, there is a spring locking mechanism in terminal hinge position.

10. The Whip Mix Quick-Mount Face-bow has made organized cast mounting much easier. The face-bow permits a convenient quick and surprisingly accurate method of securing on average axis location. It employs special designed ear plugs that are placed in the external auditory meatus of the ears (Fig. 2 54A). The anterior support is attained by posi-

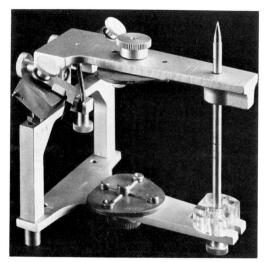

FIG. 2-53. *The Whip-Mix 8800 articulator.*

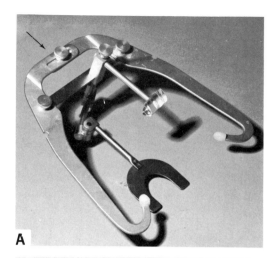

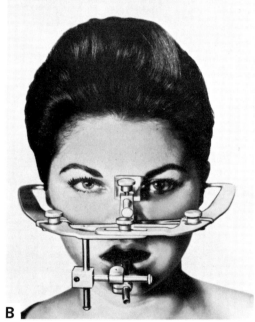

FIG. 2-54. A. *The quick mount Whip Mix face-bow with nasion relator. Arrow designates scale for determining intercondylar distance adjustment.* **B.** *The face-bow assembled on a patient.*

tioning a curved plastic block into the deepest part of the nasion. The plane of reference is automatically created 25 mm below the nasion and through the centers of the left and right external auditory canals. The facebow also has a three-sectional scale (Fig. 2-54B) that measures the transcranial width corresponding to the three (S, M, L) settings of intercondylar distance for the condylar elements of the articulator. The articulator has lugs on the latter walls of the condylar housing. Corresponding holes in the earpieces of the face-bow make for easy transfer of the face-bow to the articulator. The lugs on the articulator are correctly positioned when the horizontal condylar inclination is set at 30 degrees.

Evaluation

In recent years investigators have carried out scientific research to evaluate the capabilities of many of the articulators to determine the advantages and disadvantages of the features that are built into the instruments. The findings of these investigators are significant, and some are useful in the selection of an articulator.

THE FACE-BOW

The movements of the teeth are the result of the rotations and slidings made by the condyles. The better the casts on an articulator duplicate the distances to the condylar rotational centers, the less the potential for articulator-produced errors of motion. A face-bow record is used to transfer these relationships.

A face-bow will record the location of the maxillary teeth (or arch) to the opening-closing axis of mandible in centric relation (terminal hinge position). When an anterior reference point is used, the teeth are also recorded to a fixed plane in space as determined by the three reference points.

The face-bow is an integral part in the procedures in analyzing and studying the occlusion of natural teeth. Its use is also an integral part in procedures in developing the occlusion for complete dentures. Deviations from the relationships of the condylar rotational centers to the maxillae to the rotational centers on an articulator produce some differences in occlusion on the instrument from that in the mouth.

A correct centric occlusion can be developed on an articulator without a face-bow transfer record provided it is developed at the exact vertical dimension used to mount the casts. Any increase or decrease of the vertical dimension will cause a difference between the centric occlusion on the articulator and that in the mouth when the dentures are inserted.

When a face-bow transfer is made, the two posterior points of reference are the left side and right side facial locations of the terminal hinge axis. The axis may be found kinematically using a hinge-axis locator or it can be estimated (arbitrary axis) using anatomic landmarks. Some techniques use measurements from anatomic landmarks on the lateral aspects of the face and others relate the axis to the external auditory meatus of the ears.

The anterior reference point varies. Some use the infraorbital notch or a point related to this anatomic landmark. Others choose a point related to some other specific landmark. For instance, the Whip Mix uses a point 25 mm below the deepest part of the nasion. Regardless of where the third point is positioned, it is selected to approximate a near horizontal plane and can be relocated accurately.

When a third reference point is not used, the face-bow transfer record is positioned on the articulator so that the plane of occlusion is horizontal or the maxillary central incisors are positioned in the middle between the upper and lower members of the articulator.

The true transverse hinge axis should be located where stereographic recordings are to be used. When one pantographs in three dimensions simultaneously, one must duplicate one axis. When other forms of articulation are used (Class II types) the arbitrary axis may be satisfactory.

After a mathematical evaluation of face-bow transfers, Weinberg came to the following conclusions:

A reasonable error in the transverse hinge axis location (within ±5 mm) results in negligible anteroposterior mandibular displacement (in the magnitude of 0.2 mm) when a 3-mm centric relation record is removed and the articulator is closed. This anteroposterior displacement can be limited further by a thinner interocclusal centric relation record.

When the centric relation record is obtained without a change in vertical dimension, there is no anteroposterior mandibular displacement at all. The face-bow mounting in this instance is mainly concerned with the accurate transfer of the condylar inclination. A marked change in vertical dimension because of a thick centric relation record causes gross anteroposterior mandibular displacement that requires more extensive intraoral adjustment.

Marked deviations from the transverse hinge axis of the patient, resulting from arbitrary mounting, can cause anteroposterior mandibular displacement even with small vertical dimension changes. Eccentric records with an arbitrary mounting are practically valueless.

When an anterior point of reference is used for cast mounting, the occlusal plane is orientated. Elevation of the occlusal plane decreases the condylar readings; lowering the occlusal plane increases them. With any of the commonly used anterior points of orientation, the degree of variation produced is in the magnitude of 0.2 mm at the second molar balancing cusp and less anteriorly.

The working cusp inclines are not measurably affected by changes in the condylar readings. In normal use, the working condyle movement on the Hanau type of articulator is constant regardless of the condylar readings. It consists of rotation with lateral Bennett movement of zero degrees.

The small degree of error at the balancing cusp inclines is well within the accuracy of the cast construction, centric relation record, and the instrument itself. However, completely arbitrary maxillary cast mounting can produce not only significant anteroposterior mandibular displacement but also serious cuspid inclination disharmonies.[68]

CONDYLE PATH

The study of skulls and the observations of pantograms reveal a condyle path for most individuals as concavities and convexities. The majority of the articulators of Class II have a straight condyle path. Granger states that the average condylar path follows a curvature of approximately a ¾″ radius. Weinberg showed that the maximum difference between a straight condylar path and one with a ½″ radius is 0.4 mm. A maximum condylar error of 0.4 mm produces an 0.2 mm error at the second molar. This calculation is based on a 3-mm cusp height and a constant incisal guidance (Table 2-1).

The arcon principle, in which the condyles in the lower member with the condylar slots are fixed to the upper member, has been investigated, and the

findings of Beck and Morrison, Weinberg, and Villa follow.

Beck and Morrison concluded:

By fixing the condylar guide to the upper member of the arcon articulator, and the shaft axis to the lower member, a constant relationship exists between the occlusal plane and the arcon guides of the instrument at any position of the upper member, making the reproduction of mandibular movement more accurate.[3]

Weinberg concluded:

Both the arcon and condylar instruments produce the same motion because condylar guidance is the result of the interaction of a condylar ball on an inclined plane. One without the other is ineffective. Reversing the relationship does not change the guidance produced. The only change is in the numbers used to record the inclination. Mathematical evidence supports the view that neither instrument has any specific advantage over the other.[66]

Villa's findings are summarized as follows:

The most important requirement in the reproduction of the protrusive movement on the articulator is to establish the inclination and curvature of the condylar path and its relation to the incisal path and the upper cast. The relationship between these three factors should not be altered at any time. This means that the condylar guide, the upper cast, and the incisal guide must be fixed to the upper member of the articulator because such is the condition in nature.[63]

In 1958 Beck conducted further investigation in the arcon concept of articulators. He compared the clinical results of dentures which were constructed in duplicate for six patients. The articulators used were the Bergström and Hanau Model H because of the similarity of the dimensions of the instruments. Beck's conclusions follow:

TABLE 2-1. *Summary of Mathematical Study of the Hanau H Articulator**

	Approximate Error at the Second Molar Balancing Cusp Height (mm)	Approximate Error at the Second Molar Working Cusp Height (mm)
1. Average anatomic location of the hinge axis	0.2	0.2
2. Arbitrary location of the anterior point of orientation	0.2	No error
3. Straight condylar path	0.2	0.2
4. No Fischer angle	0.1	No error
5. No individual working condylar motion	No error	0.8
Maximum total error	0.7	1.2

* Weinberg, L. A.: An evaluation of basic articulators and their concepts. Part II. J. Prosth. Dent., *13*:659, 1963.

No conclusive results could be recorded from duplicate dentures which were constructed on the Arcon and the Model H. However, the study is limited in scope and further investigation is advisable. No definite superiority could be noted in the clinical evaluation of complete dentures constructed on the arcon (Bergström) over the condylar type of instrument (Hanau Model H).

LATERAL MAXILLOMANDIBULAR RELATIONS

The ability of an articulator to accept lateral maxillomandibular relation records is particularly desirable when balanced occlusion in complete dentures is required. Most rectilinear, Class II, Type 3, articulators produce the working movement by combining the balancing condylar movement with a camlike fulcrum on the working side. Since the working condylar element remains against the posterior wall it acts as a fulcrum. The lateral Bennett Shift of the instrument is produced by the freedom of lateral movement of the working condylar element. The amount of lateral shift is controlled by the medial movement (Bennett Angle) of the balancing condylar mechanism. An adjustable intercondylar distance provides an adjustable fulcrum rather than a fixed fulcrum on the working side. This permits some degree of adjustability on the working side but not complete three dimensional guidance. Therefore, this type of articulator will accept some but not all check records. The Whip-Mix and Denar Mark II may accept more lateral records than the Hanau series, since they don't have an axle. The Class I instrument would, of course, take any lateral positional records.

MANDIBULAR AND ARTICULATOR MOVEMENTS

A comparison of the findings of investigators reveals lack of agreement. This is expected and should not contribute confusion to the person who is willing to take the time to evaluate the methods used and the concepts and philosophies of the investigators and to compare the findings with those of others. The investigations of Shanahan and Leff in mandibular and articulator movements resolved into the following conclusions:

1. The normal opening and closing movements of the mandible do not coincide with the opening and closing movements of a hinge-axis articulator.[47]

2. Photographs of projected tracings of movements of the mandible provide knowledge of the movements of the mandible during mastication and during lateral protrusive excursions. However, projected tracings do not necessarily reveal the true nature of the movements of the mandible.

Mandibular tracings indicate that there is considerable difference in the quality of these two groups of movements. Horizontal, lateral, and protrusive excursions are slow and hesitant, whereas the vertical masticatory cycles are smooth and rhythmic. The mandible shifts its position to accommodate the changes in muscular function at both ends of the cycles.

Masticatory cycles do not coincide with opening and closing arcs of hinge axis articulators. Also natural protrusive movements do not coincide with straight line protrusive movements of an adjustable articulator.[48]

3. A study of the tracings of the natural opening, closing, and masticating movements of the mandible does not show the presence of a mandibular axis in the region of the condyles. An artificial mandibular axis can be produced during the opening and closing movements by forcing the chin backward. However, an artificially produced mandibular axis, jaw position, or jaw movement is not a normal physiologic movement.

There is no evidence of rotation about a mandibular axis in the region of the condyles with concomitant anterior translation in these studies of the opening, closing, and masticating movements.[49]

4. A geometric study of the opening and closing cyclic movements of the mandible showed the untenability of the concept that the mandible rotates about a translating axis. The meaning of this concept or belief is simply that the mandible does not change its size or shape during the movements.[50]

5. The theory that the mandible rotates about vertical axes in the region of the condyles during lateral movements has been investigated and found untenable.

The use of a central bearing point produces unnatural influences upon the lateral movements of the mandible. The direction and the character of the movements made with a central bearing point in the mouth are entirely different from those movements made under normal conditions, such as lateral movements made with the teeth in contact. The sagittal axes could not be related to the opening and closing, the lateral, or rocking movements of the mandible.[51]

The conclusions reached by Shanahan and Leff are generally true. The mandible in normal functional movements slides and rotates and creates what is called compound movement. There is both an instaneous axis of motion and an axis of rotation in compound motion. The problem in analyzing compound motion is that the instaneous axis is the only one detectable. Motion must be reduced to a simple form to resolve motion and locate the axis of rotation.

Clayton,[9a] Messerman,[37] and Lundeen have shown that masticatory function does occur along border positions and that the condyles do return to the centric relation position. Normally both condyles are not in the centric relation terminal position at the same time. Either one condyle or the other seats itself briefly in the terminal position during part of the closing chewing stroke.

Lundeen and Wirth found that on fifty condylar tracings, a point corresponding to 5 mm of protrusive movement, the angle formed with the axis-orbital plane ranges from 25 to 75 degrees, with a medium of approximately 40 degrees.[33] For lateral movement, a point corresponding to 5 mm of balancing condyle movement forms an angle with the axis orbital plane of between 25 and 75 degrees. The medium angle was between 45 and 50 degrees. They also found that the Bennett movement of the balancing condyle was composed of two identifiable portions. There is an early Bennett shift up to about 3.0 mm with a median of about 1.0 mm. The remainder of the pathway showed arcs of circles which were nearly parallel to each other. Very few subjects had pure immediate shift. All of the shift occurred within the first few degrees of rotation. The remainder of the movement made an angle of about 6 to 7.5 degrees.

Selection

Operators do not always use instruments to their full capabilities, but this is not always necessary with an articulator. However, one can use too complex an instrument for a simple case or too simple an articulator for a complex case. Key factors in determining articulator needs are the amount and timing of the Bennett shift, the type of anterior guidance, and the angle of the first millimeter or so of the condylar path. The toughest cases to treat are those with a lot of early Bennett shift, no anterior guidance (or flat anterior guidance), and flat, early

condylar movement. The posterior tooth forms, concepts of occlusion, the extent of the restoration, and the type of support, whether tooth or tissue, have a bearing. The articulator must be within the understanding and capabilities of the operator. An instrument will perform no better than the ability of the operator to use it.

When the information in this chapter is reviewed and analyzed, the following factors are pertinent to the selection of an articulator:

1. No mechanical instrument will produce the movements of the condyles in the temporomandibular fossae for all individuals. Instruments of metal cannot be expected to reproduce all the movements of living tissues in normal and pathologic situations. The goal of articulation is to simulate tooth movements along border pathways in whatever plane is important.

2. The accuracy of an articulator in reproducing mandibular movements is in direct relation to the records made of mandibular movements; therefore, an articulator that will reproduce the movements recorded by natural teeth is not necessarily the instrument of choice with the edentulous patient.

3. Clinical evaluation of articulators, particularly in complete denture construction, has so many variables that each dentist must be honest with himself in appraising results. An honest appraisal is not based on the patient's tolerance but on the physiologic acceptance of the supporting tissues.

4. It is essential that the concepts and philosophies of designers of articulators and the conductors of investigations are known and correlated with the features in the articulator and the underlying motivations in the investigating procedures.

5. A pantograph usually is not indicated for complete denture procedures.

An acceptable registration is possible only if the patient has exceptionally stable residual alveolar ridges. When the bases are not stabilized, the lack of accuracy for the edentulous mouth offsets any advantages. A good interocclusal record is better than a poor pantograph. In addition, a pantogram is hardly worthwhile with articulators that cannot be set to follow the tracings.

6. An immediate side shift of the mandible without rotation is an anatomic and technical impossibility. Individually controlled side shift must be molded for each patient. This is usually a curved path and is not made by changing the angle of a metal or plastic fossa.

7. The single, most important requirement of an articulator is to maintain centric relation. Next in importance is maintenance of the vertical dimension of occlusion once it has been established.

8. No incisal guide can reproduce the arrangement of the anterior teeth. One way to reproduce incisal guidance is to mold a shape that corresponds to the existing or proposed arrangement of the anterior teeth.

9. Sophisticated instruments require sophisticated methods to record mandibular movements. The use of auxiliary personnel in laboratory procedures is becoming more prevalent and necessary to meet dental needs. Their level of skill in using articulators is an important factor in selection.

10. The sophisticated instruments have been too expensive for students.

When an articulator is used in the reconstruction procedures involving natural teeth, the articulator of preference is one that will accept pantograms in three planes, a four-dimensional instrument.

When an articulator is selected for complete denture construction, the type will depend on (a) the type of occlusion to be developed and (b) the kind of jaw relation records that will be made to adjust the articulator.

REFERENCES

1. Bailey, Rush L.: Recording edentulous jaw relationships. Dent. Clin. North Am., 21:271; 1977.
2. Beck, H. O.: A clinical evaluation of the arcon concept of articulation. J. Prosth. Dent., 9:409, 1959.
3. ———: Selection of an articulator and jaw registrations. J. Prosth. Dent., 10:878, 1960.
4. ———, and Knapp, F. J.: Reliability of fully adjustable articulators using a computerized analysis. J. Prosth. Dent., 35:630, 1976.
5. ———, and Morrison, W. E.: Investigation of an arcon articulator. J. Prosth. Dent., 6:359, 1956.
6. Bell, L. J., and Matich, J. A.: Study of acceptability of lateral records by the whip-mix articulator. J. Prosth. Dent., 38:22, 1977.
7. Bellanti, N. D.: The significance of articulator capabilities. J. Prosth. Dent., 29:269, 1973.
8. Boucher, L. J., et al: Occlusal articulation. Dent. Clin. North Am., 23:155, 1979.
9. Bowman, J. F.: Selection of an articulator for undergraduate teaching of removable partial prosthodontics. Presented at the Ass. of Den. Schools Meeting, Toronto, Canada, 1965.
9a. Clayton, J. A., et al: Graphic recording of mandibular movements: J. Prosthet. Dent., 25:287, 1971.
10. Cortino, R. M., and Stallard, H.: Instruments essential for obtaining data needed in making a functional diagnosis of the human tooth. J. Prosth. Dent., 1:66, 1957.
11. Coye, R. B.: Study of variability of setting fully adjustable gnathologic articulator to a pantographic tracing. J. Prosth. Dent., 37:460, 1977.
12. Dean, H. D., Jr.: Articulator, academics, and attitudes. J. Prosth. Dent., 31:88, 1974.
13. Finger, I. M., and Tanaka, H.: New semi-

adjustable articulator—Part III. J. Prosth. Dent., *37*:310, 1977.

14. Gibbs, C. H., and Perda, H. J.: New articulator emphasizing centric occlusion and the anterior determinants. J. Prosth. Dent., *37*:382, 1977.

15. Gillis, R. R.: Articulator development and the importance of observing the condyle paths in full denture prosthesis. J.A.D.A., *13*:3, 1926.

16. Granger, E. A.: *The Function of the Rotating Condyle Path of the Aderer Simulator.* Long Island City, N. Y., J. Aderer, Inc.

17. Guichet, N. F.: *Procedures for Occlusal Treatment. A Teaching Atlas.* Anaheim, California, Denar Corporation, 1969.

18. ———: Applied gnathology: Why and how. Dent. Clin. North Am., *13*:687, 1969.

19. Gysi, A.: Some reasons for the necessity of using adaptable articulators. Dent. Dig., *37*:224, 1931.

20. Hall, R. E.: The problem of the articulator. J.A.D.A., *21*:446, 1934.

21. Hanau Engineering Company: *University Series Articulator Technique.* Buffalo, N. Y., 1963.

22. Hanau, R. L.: Dental engineering. Reprinted from J. Nat. Dent. Ass., July, 1922.

23. ———: The relation between mechanical and anatomical articulation. J.A.D.A., *10*:776, 1923.

24. ———: *Full Denture Prosthesis—Intraoral Technique for Hanau Articulator Model-H.* 4th Ed. Buffalo, N. Y., 1930.

25. Harper, R. N.: Survey of opinions on adaptable articulator technique. Reprint Dental Items of Interest, Sept., 1930.

26. Hickey, J. C., Lundeen, H. C., and Bohannon, H. M.: A new articulator for use in teaching and general dentistry. J. Prosth. Dent., *18*:435, 1967.

27. Hobo, S., Shillingburg, H. T., and Whitsett, L. D.: Articulator selection for restorative dentistry. J. Prosth. Dent., *36*:35, 1976.

28. Irish, E. F.: The dupli-functional articulator. J. Prosth. Dent., *4*:642, 1965.

29. Javid, N. S.: Comparative study of sagittal and lateral condylar paths in different articulators. J. Prosth. Dent., *31*:130, 1974.

30. Kile, C. S.: The Kile Dentograph. J. Prosth. Dent., *5*:169, 1955.

31. Lauciello, F. R., and Appelbaum, M.: Anatomic comparison to arbitrary reference notch on Hanau articulators. J. Prosth. Dent., *40*:676, 1978.

32. Lee, R. L.: Jaw movements engraved in solid plastic for articulator control. J. Prosth. Dent., *22*:209, 1969.

33. Lundeen, H. C., and Wirth, C. G.: Condylar movement patterns engraved in plastic blocks. J. Prosth. Dent., *30*:866, 1973.

34. ———, et al.: An evaluation of mandibular border movements. Their accuracy and significance. J. Prosth. Dent., *40*:442, 1978.

34a. ———: Personal communication.

35. McCoy, R. B., et al.: A method of transferring mandibular movement to computer storage. J. Prosth. Dent., *33*:510, 1976.

36. Messerman, T.: A means of studying mandibular movements. J. Prosth. Dent., *17*:36, 1956. Rosenblatt, J.: Discussion of "A means of studying mandibular movements." J. Prosth. Dent., *17*:44, 1967.

37. ———, et al.: Investigation of functional mandibular movements. Dent. Clin. North Am., *13*:629, 1969.

38. Mitchell, D. L., and Wilkie, N. D.: Articulators through the years—Part I. J. Prosth. Dent., *39*:324, 1978.

39. ———, and Wilkie, N. D.: Articulators through the years—Part II. J. Prosth. Dent., *39*:451, 1978.

40. Mjor, P. S.: The effect of the end controlling guidances of the articulator on cusp inclination. J. Prosth. Dent., *6*:1055, 1965.

41. Mohamed, S. E., Schmidt, J. R., and Harrison, J. D.: Articulators in dental education and practice. J. Prosth. Dent., *36*:319, 1976.

42. Needles, J. W.: Mandibular movements and articulator design. J.A.D.A., *10*:927, 1923.

43. Paraskis, C. S.: Criteria for selecting an articulator to occlude and articulate teeth for full denture construction. Dent. Clin. North Am., November, 1964, p. 629.

44. Philips, G. P.: Use of the occlusoscope. J.A.D.A., *26*:1332, 1939.

45. Schweitzer, J. M.: The transograph and transographic articulator. J. Prosth. Dent., *7*:595, 1957.

46. Sears, V. H.: Requirements of articulators in dentistry. Dent. Items Int., *48:*685, 1926.

47. Shanahan, T. E. J., and Leff, A.: Mandibular and articulator movements. J. Prosth. Dent., *9:*941, 1959.

48. ———: Mandibular and articulator movements. Part II. Illusion of mandibular tracings. J. Prosth. Dent., *12:*82, 1962.

49. ———: Mandibular and articulator movements. Part III. The mandibular axis dilemma. J. Prosth. Dent., *12:*292, 1962.

50. ———: Mandibular and articulator movements. Part IV. Mandibular three dimensional movements. J. Prosth. Dent., *12:*684, 1962.

51. ———: Mandibular and articulator movements. Part V. Vertical and sagittal axes myths. J. Prosth. Dent., *13:*872, 1963.

52. Smith, B. J.: Adjustment of lateral condylar guidances of Dentatus AR series of articulators. J. Prosth. Dent., *34:*208, 1975.

53. Stansbery, C. J.: Functional position check bite technic. J.A.D.A., *16:*421, 1929.

54. Stuart, C. E.: The growth of accuracy in measuring functional dimensions and relations. Read before the Academy of Denture Prosthetics, Detroit, Mich., May 8, 1958.

55. ———: Condylar determinants to be found in the patient and put in the controls of an articulator if cusps are to be prepared on teeth correctly. Presented during midwinter meeting of the Chicago Dental Society, February, 1962.

56. Swanson, Kenneth H.: Complete dentures using the TMJ articulator. J. Prosth. Dent., *41:*497, 1979.

57. Tanaka, H., and Beu, R. A.: A new semi-adjustable articulator. Part I—Concept behind the new articulator. J. Prosth. Dent., *33:*10, 1975.

58. ———, and Beu, R. A.: A new semi-adjustable articulator—Part II. J. Prosth. Dent., *33:*158, 1975.

59. ———, and Finger, J. M.: A new semi-adjustable articulator—Part IV. J. Prosth. Dent., *40:*288, 1978.

60. Thomas, C. J.: A classification of articulators. J. Prosth. Dent., *30:*11, 1973.

61. *T.M.J. Newsletter. 1:*1, 1971.

62. Tradowsky, M.: Articulator adjustments using the transfer vise. J. Prosth. Dent., *39:*47, 1978.

63. Villa, A. H.: Requirements of articulators for protrusive movements. J. Prosth. Dent., *9:*215, 1959.

64. ———: Requirements of articulators for lateral movements. J. Prosth. Dent., *9:*422, 1959.

65. ———: Requirements in articulators: Contraindicated features. J. Prosth. Dent., *9:*619, 1959.

66. Weinberg, L. A.: Arcon principle in the condylar mechanism of adjustable articulators. J. Prosth. Dent., *13:*263, 1963.

67. ———: An evaluation of basic articulators and their concepts. Part I. Basic concepts. J. Prosth. Dent., *13:*622, 1963.

68. ———: An evaluation of basic articulators and their concepts. Part II. Arbitrary, positional, semiadjustable articulators. J. Prosth. Dent., *13:*645, 1963.

69. ———: An evaluation of basic articulators and their concepts. Part III. Fully adjustable articulators. J. Prosth. Dent., *13:*873, 1963.

70. ———: An evaluation of basic articulators and their concepts. Part IV. Fully adjustable articulators. J. Prosth. Dent., *13:*1038, 1963.

71. Winstanley, R. B.: Observations on the use of the Denar pantograph and articulator. J. Prosth. Dent., *38;*660, 1977.

Educating the Patient

3

A willingness to instruct the patient in the care and use of his dentures and an understanding of his desires are essential to assure a successful prognosis. An informed patient will realize when his denture requires attention and will seek treatment before an ill-fitting denture damages the oral tissues (Fig. 3-1).

Skill in mechanics is only one facet of denture service. The dentist must also know anatomy, physiology, and psychology so that he can correctly evaluate

normal and abnormal situations. Only with this knowledge can he be sincere and convincing in his statements to the patient. Patients are reluctant to carry out instructions when they doubt the dentist's sincerity. In many situations firmness is required; in others sympathy. A dentist is at a decided disadvantage if he presents a patient a treatment plan without being convinced that the treatment is based on sound scientific factors.

What patients relate about denture

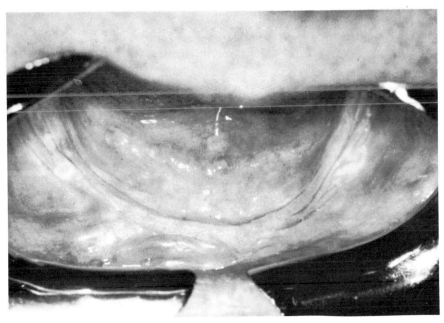

FIG. 3-1. *Illustration of loss of residual ridge and damage to soft tissues resulting from constant pressure of ill-fitting dentures. If the patient had been properly instructed in denture care, such deterioration may have been avoided.*

91

use is not always scientific. What can be physiologically tolerated and what some patients tolerate can be quite different. One of the primary objectives of dentures is to preserve the supporting tissues within physiologic limitations. The preservation of the supporting tissues is essential to continuous successful use of dentures, and today's increasing life expectancy makes this requirement more important than ever. Therefore, the patient should be educated to understand his responsibility in denture service.

Understanding the Patient

The dentist must know human psychology because the ability to understand the patient's mental processes is frequently the difference between the acceptance and the rejection of dentures. First of all, the dentist should find out why the patient wants dentures. Is the patient interested only in cosmetic factors or does he expect the dentures to restore the masticatory function of the natural teeth? Did the patient decide by himself to seek dental care or did the members of his family exert pressure? Is he prepared to devote the time necessary for the procedures and to accept the inconvenience and the responsibility of denture care?

The patient who seeks dentures as a result of pressure by others is rarely a successful denture patient unless he is educated during the treatment. The dentist must explain the nature of the procedures and must prepare the patient for this new experience.

Another patient who does not seek care in the broad terms of health maintenance but is concerned only with the contour of a tooth, wrinkles in the lip, or white straight teeth lacks motivation in the essentials. Before treatment the dentist must discuss the specific require-

ments and evaluate them with the patient.

Since the loss of the natural teeth is a traumatic experience, it should not be treated in a light manner by either the patient or the dentist. The loss of the natural teeth presents problems, but dentures alone are not a panacea for dental problems. The success of the treatment will depend upon the willingness of the patient to accept his responsibility in the treatment, the use and care of the dentures, and the postinsertion procedures.

Instructing the Patient

Scientific terminology can be confusing to a layman. However, it is not advisable to oversimplify the instructions. Oversimplification may offend some patients. Acceptable terminology seems to stimulate patients to seek more information by asking questions.

Physiology that the dentist can discuss with his patient involves bone, muscles, and the nervous system (pages 24–41). The limitations they impose should be discussed with the patient. Mechanical factors likewise must be considered, but they should be correlated with the biologic entities.

Patients do not always remember verbal instructions; therefore, instructions should be given verbally *and* in writing during the consultation interview in a relatively painless situation. To reinforce this information, request the patient to read and become familiar with the instructions. Review this information with the patient at appropriate stages in the procedures. Charts and slides are additional methods of instructing the patient (Fig. 3-2).

It is not possible to prepare instructions that cover all situations. However, the following questions and answers serve as a basis for patient education.

The Care of your dentures

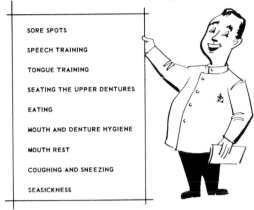

SORE SPOTS

SPEECH TRAINING

TONGUE TRAINING

SEATING THE UPPER DENTURES

EATING

MOUTH AND DENTURE HYGIENE

MOUTH REST

COUGHING AND SNEEZING

SEASICKNESS

**U. S. NAVAL DENTAL CLINIC
NAVAL BASE
NORFOLK, VIRGINIA**

FIG. 3-2. *Example of a visual aid for education in the care of dentures from a booklet of instructions in the use and care of dentures. (Courtesy of Dental Division, Bureau of Medicine and Surgery, U. S. Navy.)*

WHY REPLACE TEETH

It is necessary to have artificial replacements for the natural teeth because the body cannot function properly if some of the important organs involved in speech, swallowing, and mastication are lost. Most people desire to be accepted in society and to associate with others in ease and comfort. This is not always possible when missing teeth cause poor speech and appearance.

A change in facial expression occurs when teeth are not replaced. The lips and cheeks are supported by teeth. When the lips and cheeks are unsupported, the muscles do not function properly and become weak. As a result, the skin wrinkles, the lips and cheeks sag, and one looks older. (Fig. 3-3.)

The tissues of the mouth should be kept in the healthiest possible condition at all times. Within limits this is possible with dentures, but they are not the same as the natural teeth. The factors that contributed to the loss of the natural teeth may be an adverse influence to the successful use of dentures. Dentures may aid in keeping the tissues of the mouth in a healthy condition if the patient follows instructions in the use and care of the dentures.

The loss of teeth affects speech. In most situations this difficulty is overcome in a relatively short time if the teeth are replaced.

WHAT TO EXPECT FROM DENTURES

The majority of patients do not know what to expect from dentures. Unfortunately, well-wishing friends may tell the patient, "My dentures are as good as or better than my natural teeth, and I've never had a minute's trouble." Although this is possible, it is usually not true. As a result, a disappointed patient must learn for himself what he may realistically expect.

Patients rarely expect to see with an artificial eye or to have natural use of an artificial hand or leg, yet they frequently expect the artificial teeth to duplicate the natural teeth in form and function. Dentists have contributed to this mistaken belief. The dentist should neither oversimplify nor overcomplicate the procedures. He should be frank and honest in evaluating the situation and instructing the patient.

Dentures are artificial substitutes and have limitations. It is perfectly normal to feel awkward with new dentures. The appearance has undergone a slight change; speech may seem altered and a feeling of mouth fullness may be

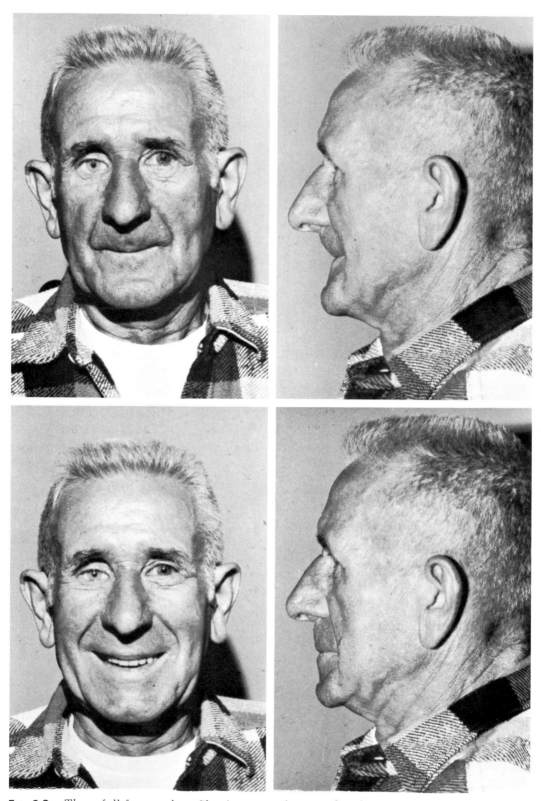

FIG. 3-3. These full face and profile views are photographs of an edentulous patient before and after the insertion of dentures. Appearance is important to both sexes. Even the artificial eye appears more natural when the facial contours are restored. The patient is aware of an acceptable facial expression and is pleased.

present. Time, patience, and cooperation in following instructions will bring about a relaxation of the muscles of the lips, tongue, and cheeks. Eventually the slight change in appearance becomes a pleasant change; speech will be normal, and eating will be less difficult.

Artificial teeth are placed in positions that will provide compatibility with the surrounding environment in speech, swallowing, and masticating. In most situations this is the position formerly occupied by the natural teeth. Malrelations of the mandible to the maxillae are not corrected by removing the natural teeth, and the artificial teeth are not, as a rule, tolerated if they are placed in an attempt to correct the malrelation. Patients frequently request that the teeth be placed in positions that are not compatible with function. They must be educated to accept the positions that are considered more desirable to meet all of the requirements for successful denture service. Patients must understand that to change the positions of the teeth to meet their requirements may necessitate placing the teeth in an unacceptable position for total function. To meet their desires may require a compromise in another area.

Force directed at right angles to the support is more stabilizing than that directed at an inclined plane. The buccal shelf areas in the mandibular arches and the crests and slopes of the residual ridges in the maxillary arch are considered the primary stress-bearing areas for denture support. In these areas the artificial teeth can be positioned so that vertical forces of occlusion, when the mandible is in terminal hinge position, will be more at right angles to the support than in other arch areas. Another reason that these areas are considered primarily stress bearing is the configuration of the bone and the character of the overlying soft tissues. The buccal shelves are usually broad expanses of dense basal bone. The residual ridges in the first molar area in the maxillary arches are usually broad, and between the cortical plates the cancellous bone is usually plentiful. The overlying soft tissue has a tightly attached submucosa that contributes to uniform tissue resiliency. The contour of the zygomaticoalveolar crest in the molar areas of the maxillary arches affords stability. Although the overlying soft tissue is not considered desirable to resist pressure, the area can be used to aid in stability.

The bone in the anterior arches is not structured to withstand stress. The cortical plates of bone are thin, and the cancellous bone is usually sparse. When forces of occlusion occur in the anterior arch, the forces are directed at inclined planes. The rotational centers of the mandible are located so that a long lever is created between the centers of rotation and the area of tooth contact. Damage usually results when a denture base is unseated from the basal seat.

Skeletal muscle is adaptable. The adaptability of the muscle in the lips, tongue, and cheeks helps to stabilize dentures. Patients can be advised of this and taught muscle exercises that can be beneficial. This is particularly applicable in situations of lack of supporting structures.

An excessive flow of saliva frequently accompanies the insertion of new dentures. This is a reaction to a new stimulus.

The dentures will feel tighter and looser throughout the day. This will vary with the amount of blood in the tissues.

Frequently a burning sensation on the palate and tongue may occur at the time of denture insertion. This may not result from denture insertion but from an endocrine gland disturbance.

Soreness of the gums frequently

develops with dentures. This can occur as a result of pressing the soft tissues between the bone of the jaws and the hard denture base, or the teeth may not be contacting evenly.

The dentures, particularly the lower, may dislodge during speech and eating. The upper denture is easier to become accustomed to than the lower denture for two reasons. The supporting area of the upper jaw is much larger than the lower and is relatively still; the lower jaw is constantly moving in speech, swallowing, and eating. The mandibular denture is proximate to the most active muscle in the body, the tongue. In its activity the tongue frequently unseats the denture, which in turn traumatizes the mucosa and increases pressure on the supporting bone.

In time all dentures do not fit as well as they did at first. The dentures themselves do not change appreciably, but the supporting tissues change constantly. This is a *normal* occurrence and is due to a loss of bone and a shrinkage of the soft tissues supporting the denture. The greatest change usually takes place in the first six to eight months after denture insertion.

HOW TO USE DENTURES

If the patient experiences difficulty in pronouncing words clearly, instruct him to practice reading aloud. Words that give him trouble should be repeated often. The patient should practice pronouncing words with similar sounds. For example, if it is difficult to say *late*, have him practice pronouncing *pate*, *Kate*, *mate*, and *late*. If this drill reveals that the *l* sound is the source of the difficulty, have him practice *light*, *loose*, *lane*, and *late*.

Training the tongue aids in stabilizing the dentures. When the mouth is opened, the tip of the tongue should be moved forward until it rests against the inside of the denture flange and the lower front teeth. This action helps to seat the lower denture. Once the habit is formed, it becomes automatic. If the upper denture feels loosened from its seat, closing the mouth and then swallowing will elevate the tongue to the palate and reseat the denture.

Eating with ease and efficiency requires time, patience, and training. The most efficient artificial teeth are only about one third as efficient as the natural teeth. Eating habits must be changed to compensate for this difference. The type of food eaten and the nourishment received from the food affects the success or failure in the use of dentures. Hard foods that require considerable force to masticate or sticky foods, such as caramels, pineapple upside-down cake, peanut butter, and boiled rice, should be avoided. Most breads become glutinous when chewed. Few denture wearers can chew gum without tissue damage. Foods requiring minimum force in chewing, such as well-cooked cereals, boiled eggs, and very tender or ground meats, should be selected.

Food should be cut into small portions, placed on the back teeth, and chewed slowly on both sides of the mouth at once. Biting with the front teeth, even if possible, should be avoided. If this practice is continued, the support will be lost, and the dentures will become loose. Biting on the front teeth is comparable to taking a seat on one end of a seesaw with no one on the other end. The denture flange will hit against the anterior bone and the soft tissue. The tissues will be damaged by the unstabilizing force, and the dentures will require frequent remaking or rebasing. (The younger the patient the more important the instruction about biting becomes, as his life expectancy is longer.)

The acts of coughing and sneezing

often dislodge the dentures and result in an embarrassing situation. Embarrassment can be avoided by covering the mouth with a handkerchief.

Many dentures are lost during the nausea accompanying seasickness, car sickness, or air sickness. When vomiting seems imminent, the dentures should be removed and kept in water until the patient recovers.

HOW TO CARE FOR DENTURES

Good oral hygiene and denture hygiene are essential. It is extremely important that dentures be kept clean, not only for sanitary reasons but also because debris under dentures produces pressure that will result in bone loss. Bone loss results in loose dentures. The dentures should never be cleaned or immersed in boiling water, for it is possible to distort the denture base.* Another precaution is to hold the dentures over a container of water while cleaning them. If the denture slips, the water will cushion the fall. Dentures should be cleaned after each meal, preferably with a brush and a dentrifice made especially for the purpose, not with an abrasive powder. When the lower denture is cleaned, it should not be held in the palm of the hand. If the denture slips, it may snap into two pieces when it is clutched. Instruct the patient to grasp the denture between the thumb and the forefinger. If dentures develop an odor, they should be immersed in an oxidizing solution (Clorox, one teaspoonful to a half pint of water) for about a half hour.

The dentures should be removed for at least eight of each twenty-four hours to allow the tissues to rest. There are many scientific reasons for this rest. Chinese women demonstrated by bind-

*Woefel, J. B., and Paffenbarger, G. C.: Method of evaluating the clinical effect of warping a denture. J.A.D.A., 59:250, 1959.

ing their feet that constant pressure makes the bones "shrink." Dentures may produce similar deterioration of the oral tissues on which they rest. A denture is capable of exerting both steady pressure and intermittent heavy pressure that can interrupt the blood supply to the supporting tissues. This is particularly true in the mandibular arch. When the mandible is in rest position, gravity exerts a pull on the mandibular denture. The pull of gravity on the maxillary denture could aid in releasing some of the pressure of the maxillary denture, and this may be a factor in the varying rates of resorption when comparing the two arches.

When the soft tissues are damaged by constant pressure, the dentures become loose. Unfortunately for the patient, injury to the tissue is not usually accompanied by pain until the damage is extensive. The supporting tissues therefore require rest from the force of the denture. The blood should be allowed to circulate freely through the vascular tissue because the bone receives part of its supply from this tissue.

The eight-hour rest period is best managed during the sleeping hours. In the waking hours the somatic nervous system acts as a protective mechanism. Through this system the central nervous system is advised when a denture is accurately seated in a position that is acceptable to the surrounding environment. When a hard object encountered in mastication or functional tooth contacts causes pain, the jaw reflexly opens. This nociceptive or withdrawal reflex that protects the oral tissues from excessive pressure during working hours does not function during sleep. The denture can become unseated or the wearer may swallow and make tooth contact. The resulting force can be damaging to the tissues. The absence of the reflex phenomenon during sleep is one reason for leaving the denture out of the mouth during sleeping hours.

During the rest period the dentures should be kept in water or in a diluted mouth antiseptic.

When soreness develops and is continuous, the patient should return for an examination. He should *not* attempt to adjust dentures with sandpaper or files and should not depend upon liners, pads, or adhesives. It is accepted that when the interocclusal distance is encroached upon beyond acceptable limits that the soft tissues will be damaged and the bone will resorb until an acceptable distance is created. It is also accepted that disharmony between the contacting of the teeth and mandibular movements is potentially damaging. When denture adhesives, pads, suction cups, or soft liners are inserted in the tissue side of the dentures, control over interocclusal distance and occlusal balance is lost. The immediate relief to the patient may appear promising, but the end result may be devastating. Casts cannot be poured to correct the occlusion or to reestablish the vertical dimension of occlusion. When soreness persists, the problem should be evaluated by the dentist.

The patient should likewise return to the dentist when the dentures become loose. Regular postinsertion appointments must be kept. The use of self-applied denture liners or denture adhesives is potentially damaging. Such measures often provide temporary relief but can result in changes that are not compatible with successful continued use of dentures.

IMMEDIATE DENTURES

When the dentures are inserted at the same sitting at which the last remaining natural teeth are extracted, the patient must take additional precautions and procedures. The period of denture adjustment is more critical than it is when healing has taken place. As the tissues heal, there is tissue loss, and the foundation for the denture base changes. It is important that the dentures be altered to accommodate to this change. If adjustments are not made, uncomfortable sore spots may develop, or the dentures may become ill-fitting and loose. Immediate dentures will need a remake or a rebase within the first eight months.

The patient should be instructed to take the following precautions:

1. Exercise care in eating until the tissues have an opportunity to heal.

2. Keep all recall appointments.

Oral and written instructions are given to aid the patient in having a pleasant and successful experience with dentures. No two people have the same foundation for dentures. Therefore, some patients take longer than others to adjust to dentures. Advice from other patients is cheap and given in good faith. However, the dentist is the only one specially trained to help with denture problems. When a dentist accepts the responsibility of rendering denture service, he must also accept the responsibility of educating the patient in the use and maintenance of dentures.

REFERENCES

1. Atwood, D. A.: Some clinical factors related to rate of resorption of residual ridges. J. Prosth. Dent., *12*:441, 1962.

1a. Baseheart, J. R.: Nonverbal communication in dentist-patient relationships. J. Prosth. Dent., *34*:4, 1975.

1b. Bell, D. H., Jr.: Prosthodontic failures related to improper patient education and lack of patient acceptance. Dent. Clin. N. Amer., *16*:109, 1972.

2. Bills, E. D.: Council to the aging dental patient. J. Prosth. Dent., *9*:881, 1959.

3. Bliss, C. H.: Psychologic factors involved in presenting denture service. J. Prosth. Dent., *1*:49, 1951.

4. Brill, N., Tryde, G., Schübeler, S.: The role of learning in denture retention. J. Prosth. Dent., *10*:468,1960.
5. Collett, H. A.: Background for psychologic conditioning of the denture patient. J. Prosth. Dent., *11*:608, 1961.
6. ———: Motivation: A factor in denture treatment. J. Prosth. Dent., *17*:5, 1967.
6a. Grieder, A.: Psychologic aspects of prosthodontics. J. Prosth. Dent., *30*:736, 1973.
6b. Guckes, A. D., Smith, D. E., and Swoope, C. C.: Counseling and related factors influencing satisfaction with dentures. J. Prosth. Dent., *39*:259, 1978.
7. Hooper, B. L.: Instructions for edentulous patients. J.A.D.A., *19*:205, 1932.
8. Kapur, K. K., and Soman, S. D.: Masticatory performance and efficiency in denture wearers. J. Prosth. Dent., *14*:687, 1964.
9. Koper, A.: Why dentures fail. Dent. Clin. N. Amer., November, 1964, p. 721.
10. LaVere, A. M.: Denture education for edentulous patients. J. Prosth. Dent., *16*:1013, 1966.
10a. Levin, B., and Landesman, H. M.: Practical questionnaire for predicting denture success or failure. J. Prosth. Dent., *35*:124, 1976.
11. Maison, W. G.: Instructions to denture patients. J. Prosth. Dent., *9*:835, 1959.
12. Manly, R. S., et al.: Oral sensory thresholds of persons with natural and artificial dentitions. J. Dent. Res., *31*:305, 1952.
13. Mann, A. W.: Diet and nutrition in the edentulous patients. Dent. Clin. N. Amer., March, 1957, p. 285.
14. Means, C. R.: The home reliner materials. The significance of the problem. J. Prosth. Dent., *14*:1086, 1964.
14a. Nassif, J., Blumenfeld, W. L., and Tarsitano, J. T.: Dialogue—a treatment modality. J. Prosth. Dent., *33*:696, 1975.
14b. ———: A self-administered questionnaire—An aid in managing complete denture patients. J. Prosth. Dent., *40*:363, 1978.
15. Naylor, J. C.: What a patient should know about complete dentures. J. Prosth. Dent., *9*:832, 1959.
16. Östlund, S. G.: Saliva and denture retention. J. Prosth. Dent., *10*:658, 1960.
17. Perry, C.: Nutrition for senescent denture patients. J. Prosth. Dent., *11*:73, 1951.
17a. Pilling, L. F.: Emotional aspects of prosthodontic patients. J. Prosth. Dent., *30*:514, 1973.
18. Rothman, R.: Phonetic considerations in denture prosthesis. J. Prosth. Dent., *11*:214, 1961.
19. Schabel, R. W.: Patient education with prosthodontic acrylic resin models. J. Prosth. Dent., *17*:104, 1967.
19a. Silverman, S., Silverman, S. I., Silverman, B., and Garfinkel, L.: Self-image and its relation to denture acceptance. J. Prosth. Dent., *35*:131, 1976.
19b. Smith, M.: Measurement of personality traits and their relation to patient satisfaction with complete dentures. J. Prosth. Dent., *35*:492, 1976.
20. Southwood, L.: Educating patients who request contraindicated dentures. J. Prosth. Dent., *15*:272, 1965.
21. *The Standard Edition of the Complete Psychological Works of Sigmund Freud.* Vol. VII. Trans. from the German under the general editorship of James Strachey in col. with Ann Freud assisted by Alix Strachey and Alan Tyson. London, Hogarth Press, 1953–66.
22. Stephens, A. P., Cox, C. M., and Sharry, J. J.: Diurnal variation in palatal tissue thickness. J. Prosth. Dent., *16*:661, 1966.
23. Strain, J. C.: Influence of complete dentures upon taste perception. J. Prosth. Dent., *2*:60, 1952.
23a. Straus, R., Sandifer, J. C., Hall, D. S., and Haley, J. V.: Behavior factors and denture status. J. Prosth. Dent., *37*:264, 1977.
24. Wannemacker, E.: Should dentures be worn at night? D. Abst., *3*:158, 1958.
25. Wright, C. R., et al.: Study of the tongue and its relation to denture stability. J.A.D.A., *39*:269, 1949.

Diagnosis

4

Definition: Diagnosis is (1) the act or process of deciding the nature of a diseased condition by examination, (2) a careful investigation of the facts to determine the nature of a thing, or (3) the determination of the nature, location, and causes of disease.

These definitions do not define the full extent of the investigation that should be considered before formulating a treatment plan for complete dentures. All the pathologic, nonpathologic, normal, and abnormal conditions must be evaluated and corrected. The following diagnostic considerations pertain to the completely edentulous patient or to one whose natural teeth have been condemned by other diagnostic procedures.

Diagnosis in complete dentures is a continuing process and is not accomplished in a short time. In many patients the most pertinent findings elude the operator until the planned treatment nears completion. The dentist should be the first to recognize the problem and be ready to change the treatment plan to meet the new findings. This should pose no embarrassment if the dentist properly instructs the patient before treatment. Treatment does not terminate with the construction and delivery of complete dentures, and the patient should be so advised.

Treatment planning is a consideration of all of the diagnostic findings, systemic and local, which influence the surgical preparations of the mouth, impression making, maxillomandibular relation records, occlusion to be developed, form and material in the teeth, the denture base material, and instructions in the use and care of dentures.

The factors in these findings will be governed by (1) the patient's mental attitude, (2) the patient's systemic status, (3) past dental history, and (4) local oral conditions. Thorough investigation of these factors before the discussion of treatment procedures with the patient often means the difference between success and failure in the service rendered.

Mental Attitude

House classified patients as philosophical, exacting, indifferent, and hysterical.* As these four classifications are analyzed, the patients who are well motivated, disturbed, frustrated, or anxious, those who have the power to adjust and the will to learn, and those whose minds determine the character of the disease (psychosomatic) can be so designated. The gradations in these characteristics must be evaluated carefully.

*Lecture by M. M. House

PHILOSOPHICAL PATIENT

The best mental attitude for denture acceptance is the philosophical type. This patient is rational, sensible, calm, and composed in difficult situations. His motivation is generalized, as he desires dentures for the maintenance of health and appearance and feels that having teeth replaced is a normal, acceptable procedure. The philosophical patient overcomes conflicts and organizes his time and habits in an orderly manner; he eliminates frustrations and learns to adjust rapidly.

EXACTING PATIENT

The exacting type may have all of the good attributes of the philosophical patient; however, he may require extreme care, effort, and patience on the part of the dentist. This patient is methodical, precise, and accurate and at times makes severe demands. He likes each step in the procedure explained in detail. If the exacting patient is intelligent and understanding, he can be the best type; however, if he lacks intelligence and understanding, extra hours spent, prior to treatment, in patient education until an understanding is reached is the best treatment plan.

INDIFFERENT PATIENT

The indifferent type of patient presents a questionable or unfavorable prognosis. This patient evidences little if any concern; he is apathetic and uninterested and lacks motivation. The indifferent patient pays no attention to instructions, will not cooperate, and is prone to blame the dentist for poor dental health. Unfortunately, many young patients are this type.

An education program in dental conditions and dental treatment is the recommended treatment plan before denture construction. If interest cannot be stimulated, it is best to refuse this patient in hope that interest can be stimulated by someone else. In many instances this lack of interest is the reason the patient is edentulous.

HYSTERICAL PATIENT

The hysterical type is emotionally unstable, excitable, excessively apprehensive, and hypertensive. The prognosis is often unfavorable, and additional professional help (psychiatric) is required prior to and during treatment. This patient *must* be made aware that his problem is primarily systemic and that many of his symptoms are not the result of dentures.

Systemic Status

No prosthodontic procedures should be planned until the systemic status of the patient is evaluated. This may seem rather involved to the person who considers dentistry as related to digital dexterity. This is not involved to the person who realizes that dentistry is part of a health service and that oral health is closely associated with the general health of the patient. Except in cases of accidents, individuals who are losing or have lost their natural teeth are manifesting a pathologic condition. This loss may be as a result of systemic factors or may be associated with unfavorable systemic conditions. The dentist is not always in a position to appraise these factors and should request other professional assistance.

The dentist not only must be aware of the systemic factors but must also consider them in the treatment plan. Some systemic diseases have a direct relation to denture success even though no local manifestations are apparent. Many systemic diseases have local manifestations with no apparent systemic symptoms and others have both local and systemic reactions.

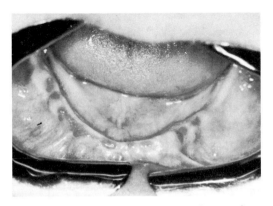

FIG. 4-1. *This intraoral view shows the poor healing following the extraction of the mandibular teeth of a patient with diabetes. The areas of granulation tissue have not resolved, and the residual alveolar ridge is severely resorbed.*

DEBILITATING DISEASES

Patients with diseases *debilitating* in nature should be under medical control. Diabetes (Fig. 4-1), tuberculosis, and blood dyscrasias are examples. These patients require extra instructions in oral hygiene, eating habits, and tissue rest. It is advisable to consult the physician and determine the health status before denture construction. Since the supporting bone may be affected by the disease, frequent recall appointments should be arranged to keep the denture bases adapted and the occlusion corrected.

DISEASES OF THE JOINT

Diseases involving the joint (Fig. 4-2), particularly osteoarthritis, present a different problem. It is estimated that 37 out of every 100 adults have this breakdown of the cartilage and other tissues that make the joints move properly. People under the age of 45 are affected at the rate of two men for every woman. From 55 to 65 more women are affected than men, and after 65 the ratio is about equal.

The weight-bearing joints, such as the knees, spine, and hips, are prone to become involved. Frequently affected are the terminal joints of the fingers and the joints at the base of the thumb and of the big toe. Less frequently involved are the second row of joints in the fingers and the temporomandibular joints.

Heberden's nodes are bony enlargements of the terminal joints of the fingers (Fig. 4-3). This primary osteoarthritis, which is more prevalent in women than

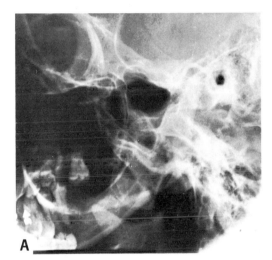

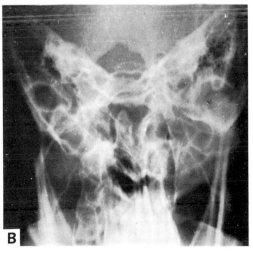

FIG. 4-2. *Arthritic involvement of the temporomandibular joint.* **A.** *The left joint appears normal.* **B.** *The right joint is involved.*

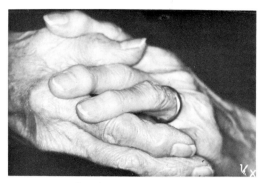

FIG. 4-3. *Heberden's nodes. The joints of the fingers are stiff and sometimes painful when moved.*

in men, sometimes occurs as early as age 40 and has a tendency to run in families. When the terminal joints of the fingers are arthritic, it is difficult for the patient to insert and clean dentures.

Osteoarthritis of the temporomandibular joint presents a problem in complete denture construction, for mandibular movements are painful. In extreme conditions surgery may be indicated, and the oral surgeon should be consulted. Special impression trays are often necessary because of limited access from reduced ability to open the jaws. Jaw relation records are difficult to record and repeat, and occlusal correction must be made often because of subsequent changes in the joint.

CARDIOVASCULAR DISEASES

Consultation with the patient's cardiologist is indicated for a patient with a *cardiovascular* disease. Denture procedures of any nature may be contraindicated. Short appointments with premedication may be required.

DISEASES OF THE SKIN

Dermatologic diseases, such as pemphigus, often have oral manifestations. The oral mucosa of the patient with pemphigus becomes extremely painful.

Medical treatment may or may not give comfort. The constant use of dentures is contraindicated, and their use is primarily for mental comfort (Fig. 4-4).

NEUROLOGIC DISORDERS

Bell's palsy and Parkinson's disease are indicative of *neurologic* involvement. Patients with these diseases can be treated, but it is essential that they understand their problems. Denture retention, maxillomandibular relation records, and supporting the musculature are some of the added denture problems.

ORAL MALIGNANCIES

Most oral *malignancies* are detected by the dentist (Fig. 4-5). Oral lesions that cannot be readily diagnosed should be further studied by biopsy. Eradication of the lesion by surgery or by radiation therapy is the primary important factor. Subsequent prosthodontic treatment is best handled by the maxillofacial prosthodontist. Accurate casts made before surgery or radiation are helpful when this prosthodontic treatment is undertaken (Fig. 4-6).

The radiation therapist and maxillofacial prosthodontist have not determined how long a time should elapse after *radiation therapy* prior to subject-

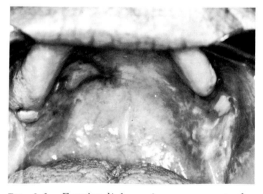

FIG. 4-4. *Erosive lichen planus prevents the satisfactory use of dentures for this 66-year-old male.*

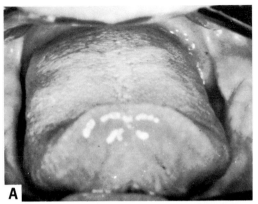

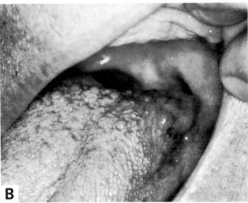

Fig. 4-5. *Areas of the tongue most frequently involved with malignancy.* **A.** *The inferior surface of the apex of the tongue.* **B.** *The lateral margins. These areas are easy to examine visually.*

ing the tissues to the stresses of a denture. The tumor prognosis, the amount of radiation, the tone and the appearance of the tissues govern the time factor. The radiation therapist should be consulted, and no denture should be constructed unless approved by him. Where prognosis is unfavorable, dentures may be constructed to bolster the patient's morale. If prognosis is favorable but the tissues still have a bronze color and lack tonus, denture construction should be delayed. When dentures are constructed, the tissues should be watched carefully for any signs of radiation necrosis (Fig. 4-7). The dentures should be used on a

limited time basis, depending upon the reactions of the tissues.

CLIMACTERIC

Climacteric is one of the periods in the life of both the male and the female when an important change in bodily function occurs. In the female, this period is termed *menopause*. The glandular functional changes that occur have varying effects on different individuals. A majority undergo bone changes, a generalized osteoporosis. The mental disturbances vary from mild irritability to complete nervous breakdown. Hot flashes, burning palate, burning tongue, the tendency to gag, inability to adjust, and vague areas of pain are some of the symptoms experienced by these patients. They should receive every consideration possible. Medication helps some patients; psychiatric treatment helps others. The use of tranquilizers as medication should be carefully evaluated, as the side effects and habit-forming potential may contraindicate their use. Before dentures are constructed, the patient *must* be made aware of these conditions and their possible effect during the period of adjustment to dentures. (See Fig. 21-14, page 436.)

Local Factors

Unfortunately local factors are the only ones considered by many dentists. However, it is not enough to make a cursory examination and note the presence or absence of teeth. If teeth are present, every effort should be expended to retain them. The diagnostic procedures for the partially edentulous mouth are not the same as the procedures for the completely edentulous mouth.

If all avenues for the retention of natural teeth have been exhausted and it is determined that the teeth must be

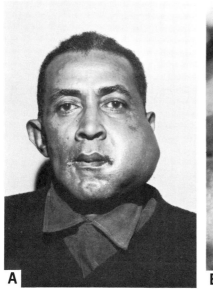
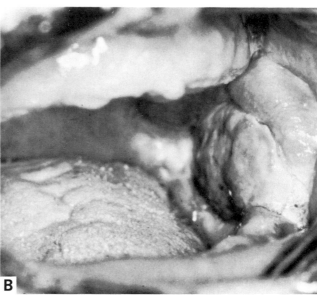

FIG. 4-6. *The pathologic report of a biopsy of this mass revealed a rhabdomyosarcoma. Impressions and cast can be made at this time, regardless of the necessity for their use at a later date.* **A.** *The swelling still permits access through the lips to make intraoral impressions of* **B.**

removed, the question of immediate dentures must be considered. The diagnostic evaluations for immediate dentures vary from those for dentures that will be inserted later. Many of the existing conditions have the same influence in the treatment plan, but many differ. They are considered in the chapter on immediate dentures.

An appreciation of the influences of local factors is based on the anatomy and physiology of the supporting tissues, the functions of the muscles of mandibular movements, and the temporomandibular joint. When this knowledge is applied in evaluating the local factors, the type of impression to be made, the material to be used in making the impression, the method to be used in making maxillomandibular relation records, the form of posterior teeth, and the occlusion to be developed can be determined.

Local factors that are considered to afford the ideal environment for complete dentures are (Fig. 4-8):

1. Broad square ridges devoid of undercuts and bony abnormalities;

2. Definite cuspid eminences and alveolar tubercles; a broad palate with uniform depth of vault in the maxillary arch;

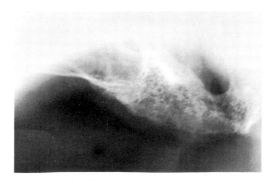

FIG. 4-7. *Radiation necrosis may not occur immediately after radiation therapy. This area of necrosis is demonstrated five years post radiation treatment.*

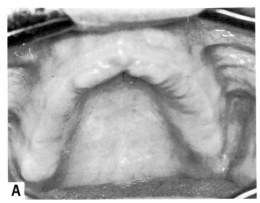

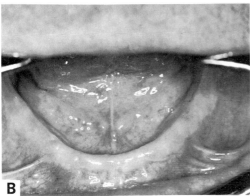

FIG. 4-8. **A.** *Nearly ideal maxillary arch and mucosa. The cuspid eminences and labial cortical plate have either undergone resorption or have been removed with surgical procedures.* **B.** *The ideal mandibular arch and mucosal covering.*

3. Broad buccal shelf and firm retromolar papillae in the mandibular arch;

4. A definite vestibular fornix, devoid of muscle attachments;

5. Frenum attachments high in the maxillary and low in the mandibular arches;

6. A clearly defined and well-developed lingual sulcus;

7. A lateral throat form that allows suitable extension into the retromylohyoid space;

8. A firm mucosal covering over the denture-bearing area;

9. Mucous membrane in the vestibular fornix and floor of the mouth which is loosely and movably attached for denture seal;

10. A gradually sloping palate with a passive reflection at the junction of the hard and soft palate;

11. A tongue normal in size, position, and function;

12. A normally related maxillae to mandible;

13. Good muscle tonus and coordination in mandibular movements;

14. Adequate inter-ridge space for the favorable placement of teeth;

15. Saliva of suitable viscosity and quantity;

16. Hard and soft tissues devoid of any signs of pathology.

Unfortunately deviations from these ideal conditions are more often the rule than the exception (Fig. 4-9). Any deviation should be noted in the diagnosis so that appropriate procedures can be incorporated in the treatment plan. In the majority of patients foreign bodies are removed, undesirable undercuts are eliminated or altered, and areas of exostosis (palatal tori and mandibular tori) are surgically removed.

A complete roentgenographic study furnishes information as to the presence of foreign bodies, exostosis, pathologic areas, and generalized osteoporosis in the bony support (Fig. 4-10A). The vertical contour is best studied with the Panorex (Fig. 4-10E); the horizontal contour, with an occlusal view (Fig. 4-10C). A lateral jaw view is usually sufficient for the temporomandibular joint study unless pathologic symptoms exist (Fig. 4-10B). It is questionable whether roentgenographic study furnishes pertinent information regarding the stress-bearing potential of bone. Research, either laboratory or clinical, has not demonstrated this potential when the dense appearing bone is compared to the less dense or numerous large nutrient canals are present or absent.

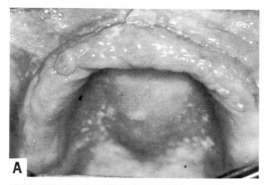

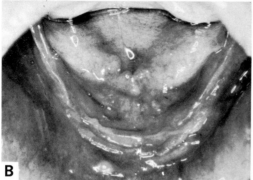

FIG. 4-9.   *Deviations from ideal environment for dentures.* **A.** *The mucosa over the palate and the anterior residual ridges is abused.* **B.** *The mucosa over the mandibular residual ridge is pendulous and contains bands of fibrous tissue.*

The maxillomandibular relation, the size of the residual ridges, the amount of interarch space, the patient reaction to impression making, the stability of the record bases, and the neuromuscular coordination can be evaluated by making diagnostic casts, recording maxillomandibular relations, and accurately mounting the casts on an articulator. No other method is an accurate procedure (Fig. 4-11).

If Freud's concept in psychoanalysis is accepted, at the time of local factor evaluation, it can be determined if the patient will accept or reject dentures. The patient may reject even the placing of fingers in the oral cavity. He may also reject the placing of dentures even

to the extent of gagging at the thought of dentures or becoming nauseated.

The color, tone, texture, and presence or absence of lesions are indices of health or disease in the soft tissues. The skin, the lips, the intraoral mucosa, the tongue, the tissue attachments, and the palate should be examined both digitally and visually. All lesions of the soft tissues should be investigated. Pale color may be indicative of anemia or hyperemia of acute infection.

The lips vary in size: some are thin and tight; others, full and relaxed. The thin, tight, short lips make impressions difficult, as the insertion and removal of the impression trays may cause discomfort. This type of lip also presents an esthetic problem, as these patients often reveal the entire edentulous maxillary residual ridge when speaking or smiling.

If the mucous membrane of the denture-bearing areas is flabby, pendulous (Fig. 4-9B), or thin, stability and retention are difficult to secure. This type of mucosa does not offer a stable base for record bases; therefore, maxillomandibular relation records must be verified repeatedly. If the mucosa is hard and unyielding, retention is difficult to secure.

Hypertrophied tissue often requires surgical removal. Soft and hard tissues that are abused from the use of other prosthesis should be allowed to recover before prosthodontic treatment, the best procedure being to *remove* the source. (See Chapter 20.) Knife-edge ridges, high V-shaped vaults, and the absence of the alveolar ridge present problems in stability, retention, and soreness that can result in hyperemia of the palatal mucosa and loss of the residual bone (Fig. 4-12). When the residual ridge is absent, there is no resistance to horizontal forces, and the posterior tooth form must be adapted accordingly. The knife-edge ridge, which includes the mylohyoid and external oblique ridges, is a constant

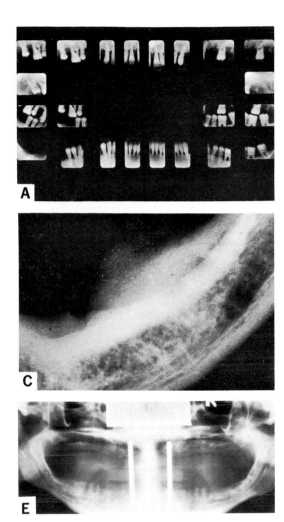

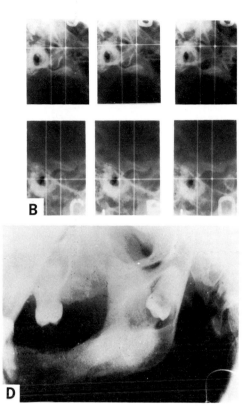

FIG. 4-10. *Studies of the denture-bearing area.* **A.** *Periapical views.* **B.** *A series of roentgenograms of the temporomandibular joints.* **C.** *The contour of the mandibular torus.* **D.** *An unsuspected dentigerous cyst.* **E.** *The Panorex screening method.*

source of discomfort to most patients. Tissue attachments, frenums, if attached low or high enough to cause interference (Fig. 4-13), are best removed surgically.

When the origins of the genioglossus and geniohyoid (Fig. 4-14) and the insertions of the superior constrictor and origin of the mylohyoid muscles interfere with denture stability and retention, they can be repositioned surgically or accommodated in the impression procedure.

The size, position, and functions of the tongue influence denture acceptance (Fig. 4-15). The muscle of the tongue, like other muscles of the body, will adapt to a new environment and alter form.

Only after carefully evaluating all of the diagnostic factors can the dentist intelligently discuss with the patient the treatment plan, the probable prognosis, and the time and expense involved. It is only through a clear understanding that patients are in a position to assume their part of the responsibility in the treatment. A clear understanding entails an honest evaluation of all the diagnostic factors. Patients should recognize that dentures are artificial substitutes and have limitations.

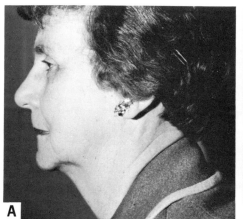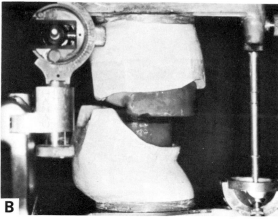

FIG. 4-11. *One would not suspect this retruded relation of the mandible to the maxillae when viewing the patient.* **A.** *The patient automatically compensates for the retruded position of the mandible.* **B.** *Articulated casts provide an accurate method for the appraisal of maxillomandibular relations.*

The Geriatric Patient

Definitions: Gerontology is the scientific study of the process and phenomena of aging; *senility* is old age accompanied by infirmity. In 1959 the Gerodontological Society further defined gerontology as "the branch of knowledge which is concerned with situations and changes inherent in increments of time, with particular reference to postmaturational stages." Gerodontology, or gerodontics, is the branch of dentistry that deals with the oral health problems of older people.

The geriatric person is one who has reached the age when important changes in bodily functions occur. His health and well-being pose a major challenge to society and particularly to the persons who are responsible for his care.

The number of persons in the United States who are past 65 years of age has increased from three million in 1900 to twenty million in 1971, of whom 4 per cent were in nursing or rest homes. The increase in life expectancy is the result of (1) improved hygiene, (2) prevention and control of infections in childhood, (3) development of new drugs, and (4) better dietary habits.

One of the problems of aging is that some of the bodily functions do not maintain their efficiency. Fortunately, not all of these functions change simultaneously. The cells, tissues, and organs do not age at the same rate. To obtain successful results with complete dentures in the postmaturation group of patients, the dentist must understand these bodily changes. He must, if possible, anticipate the time at which they will occur and recognize the symptoms in the diagnostic phase of his procedures. He must know (1) why the changes occur, (2) how the changes are related to the physiologic and psychologic status of the patient, and (3) what influence the changes will have on the prosthodontic procedures.

The prosthodontist must realize that treatment of the aging can be difficult. When the dentist does not have the time, patience, or knowledge to treat the geriatric patient, he should refer the patient to a dentist who has these qualifications. The prosthetic dental problems of the

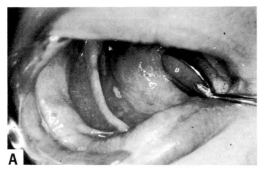

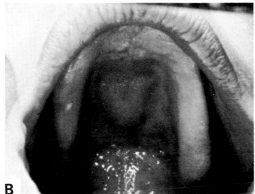

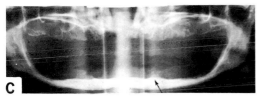

FIG. 4-12. *Some sources of problems with denture stability and retention.* **A.** *Knife-edge ridge which is more prevalent in the mandibular than in the maxillary arch.* **B.** *High vault. The soft tissue covering of the residual bone contains bands of fibrous tissue and is pendulous.* **C.** *The most superior bony area, the genial tubercles (designated by arrow).*

geriatric should *not* be arbitrarily placed in the untreatable category.

YOUR OFFICE. Dentists who treat geriatric patients should consider the changes of age when they plan their offices and select their auxiliary personnel. Accidents account for many deaths in the aging, and safety must be considered in office planning. The reception

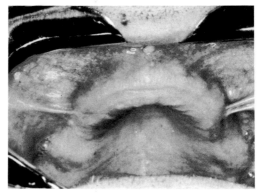

FIG. 4-13. *Buccal frenum attachments that should be corrected by surgical procedures.*

room should be well lighted; the furniture should be sturdy to offer support; the seats should be easy to get in and out of. The floor covering should not impede walking; neither should it present unsure footing. The walking space should not have obstacles such as scatter rugs, low tables, or stools. The decor should be cheerful, not gaudy or somber. Reading material should be constructive, not trite or obscene.

In addition to a safe, pleasant waiting or reception room the operatory must also meet certain requirements. The

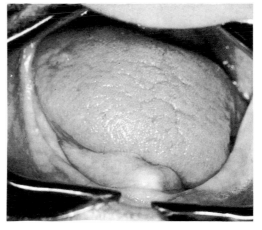

FIG. 4-14. *The genial tubercles on this patient's mandible are not good support for a denture.*

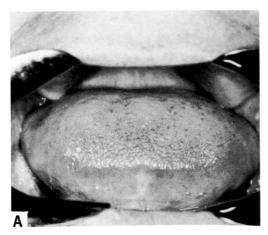

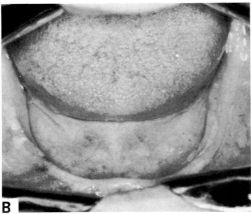

FIG. 4-15. **A.** *An abnormally large tongue. The extracted natural teeth were not replaced with artificial substitutes, and the tongue was used to crush food against the palate, with the result that the tongue gained in bulk.* **B.** *A poorly positioned tongue. The apex of this relaxed tongue is retracted and rests in the middle third of the anterior lingual vestibule. In the edentulous mouth the apex of a relaxed tongue should rest against the lingual surface of the anterior residual ridge.*

dental chair should not be a contoured type. It should have a cup-type headrest that will be comfortable and offer positive head support. The armrest should be movable to allow easy entrance and exit. The footrest should be adjustable to give positive support to the feet.

A mobile dental unit is best. The cuspidor should be mobile and adjustable. An evacuator is desirable.

It has been suggested that teenage girls and boys be used as receptionists. The teenager usually has no dislike for old age, a philosophy which may not be shared by the dentist. The teenager is more likely to fascinate the geriatric patient who may not care for an older receptionist. Most old people respond to youth in a more pleasant manner.

It has been found that many old people are made uncooperative by being cuddled and treated like a child or as "Mother" or "Dad." The dentist should not cajole, be humorous, or talk down to old people. To be overly sympathetic may make them unfriendly rather than win their friendship and cooperation. This does not mean that the dentist must show a lack of sympathy or be unfriendly. To be abrupt in speech or discourteous in manner is as distasteful as being overly solicitous or too talkative. Even the person who is growing old gracefully is conscious of the changes that are taking place; he does not have to be reminded by the dentist's actions.

COMMUNICATION. Communication between persons of all ages presents problems. Since many older patients have a partial or a total loss of hearing, communications with them is more difficult. Losing patience with these people leads to frustration and confusion. An understanding of what the dentist plans to do and why he is doing it is essential prior to treatment. The average English-speaking person has a vocabulary of two thousand words, which have ten thousand definitions. These meanings vary from speaker to speaker, from place to place, and from time to time. The aging person has probably been exposed to more of the definitions than the young, and he remembers things in the past.

With most geriatric patients it is advisable to hold a consultation prior to the chairside diagnostic procedures. It is helpful to record the proceedings on tape for review prior to making the treatment plan. Tape recording the treatment plan and financial arrangements is also desirable.

During the consultation it is advisable to allow the patient to talk freely about his problems, general health, dental health, socioeconomic status, and family *with the agreement* that once treatment begins relaxation on his part is vital. He does not need to review the information already discussed.

When the patient begins to repeat himself, the time has come to end the interview. If other specific information is desired, this may be obtained from members of the family or the physician. When it is determined that the patient has cardiovascular, pulmonary, metabolic, skeletal, oncologic, or psychologic problems, consultations should be held with the patient's physician(s), or the patient should be referred to his physician for a thorough investigation of the systemic status.

CLASSIFICATION. The changes in the geriatric patient can be classified as (1) physiologic, (2) psychologic, and (3) pathologic. In the use of any classification there must be flexibility. Not all patients can be classified in the strictest sense. One must analyze the aging process and describe the effects of the changes on the patient to understand this classification better.

Aging persons usually fit into one of three groups: (1) those who are well preserved physically and emotionally, (2) those who are really aged and chronically ill (senile), and (3) those who fall between the two extremes. Another way of grouping the aging is by their psychologic reactions to the aging process. One group are *realists;* another have an attitude of *resentment;* an in-between group are *resigned* to their position.

It is not difficult to recognize the aging person who is a realist, for he is growing old gracefully. The realists are the *philosophical* and *exacting* types (page 102). They are vigorous, alert, active, and usually economically secure, and their advice is respected at home and in the community. They do show some regressive changes but accept these as normal. Their alertness to the changes and their realism in accepting them allow them to enjoy their old age. They follow instructions, take pride in their appearance, practice good oral hygiene, seek dental care, and accept a proper diet. The treatment plan for these patients is based on the diagnostic findings described on pages 102–105.

The *resenters* are also easily recognized, for they are the *indifferent* and *hysterical* types (page 102). They are chronically ill emotionally and physically. They do not accept or adapt to tissue and organ changes, even though the changes are mild. They resent and resist aging and consequently become psychologically involved. Their advice loses its soundness; therefore, it is not respected and they become indignant. They will not listen to advice, rarely follow instructions, become negligent in body care as well as in oral hygiene, and rarely *seek* dental care. The psychologic change is one of involution, a reversal of development that is referred to as second childhood. They often crave attention and feel neglected and unloved. These are the people who accuse others of "stealing" their belongings and money. They become "security addicts," frequently placing several locks on the same door in the home. Learning about these acts may be the first clue the dentist receives during diagnosis as to the patient's response to the aging process.

Dental treatment for the resentful group is difficult from a physiologic, psychologic, and technical aspect. Frequently the treatment must be merely palliative, for these patients are subject to heart disease, cerebrovascular problems, nutritional disorders, and debilitating diseases. Forgetfulness leads to broken appointments. Treatment by one dentist may be confused with that performed by another. They cannot remember fees and misquote figures. They may want to talk and reminisce; they may describe soreness where no evident symptoms exist. To get attention they lose or destroy their dentures. Male patients will sandpaper, file, or mechanically alter their dentures. Women, as well as men, will try all of the advertized do-it-yourself reliners, denture adhesives, and even cloth and cotton to alter the tissue surface of the denture.

Although the resenters rarely seek dental care on their own initiative, concerned members of the family frequently seek treatment for them. Definitive procedures may not be advisable in all situations, as some of these patients do not want treatment. When these conditions are explained to the concerned family, they usually appreciate the advice and will not develop a "guilt" complex as they see their edentulous parent.

Many of the resentful geriatric patients make up the 4 per cent who are in nursing or rest homes. Directors of these homes frequently seek advice from the dentist. Members of the family or directors of the home should not be told that the patient's complaints are imaginary (all in the mind) or that the individual is "just getting old." When this type of answer is related to the patient, it can only make a difficult situation more severe.

Evaluation of the in-between group, the *resigned,* may be a problem because they vary in their emotional and systemic status, and the treatment plan may be definitive or palliative in nature. For example, it may be advisable to rebase or reline the existing dentures (page 412) rather than construct new dentures. The passive submission of this group does not always lead to successful prosthodontic results and is frustrating, not only to those responsible for their care but also to the dentist.

Certain signs discernible to the knowledgeable observer are clues to the identification of the resigned and resentful patients. An expression of *indifference,* for example, may reflect lack of concern, or it may relate to a state of depression, sorrow, or despair.

An expression of *hostility* may indicate that the patient does not desire treatment but is being coerced by members of his family. It may also indicate that he resents his oral condition and defies the dentist to correct the problem. The dental problem may be his "crutch" for attention which he is not about to give up. It may also be a reflection of his feeling toward members of the health professions in general.

The expression of *fear* may reflect an uneasy feeling that something may happen contrary to his desire. It could mean that he dreads the procedures because of previous experience or is concerned that the examination will reveal a condition he has been concealing.

The expressions of *anxiety* and fear are sometimes hard to separate. Anxiety may indicate a disturbance of the mind because of unpleasant experiences, or it may be an expression of eagerness to proceed and get the experience over. In psychiatry, anxiety is defined as a tense emotional state characterized by fear and apprehension regarding what is to happen.

PHYSIOLOGIC CHANGES

The physiologic changes of aging do not necessarily mean that a pathologic condition is not present. However, the condition is considered benign in comparison to the pathologic processes of the chronically ill group. The more prevalent physiologic changes are loss or graying of the hair and diminution of the senses of sight, hearing, and taste.

Loss of teeth, difficulty in hearing, and diminishing vision can be offset by artificial aids such as complete dentures, hearing aids, and eyeglasses. In many instances those who will not wear a hearing aid or glasses will reject dentures.

THE SENSES. The average person at age 60 needs twice the illumination for reading as one 25 years of age. Persons 80 to 85 years of age need over three times as much illumination as a person 25 to 30. The dread of glaucoma and/or surgery for cataracts often makes the geriatric patient secretive about his loss of sight, and the family may not be aware of the change. When an aging person relates this phenomenon of diminishing vision, he should be referred to an eye specialist. It is the prerogative of the dentist to inform the patient that the change *can occur* in the *absence* of glaucoma or cataract and that an eye examination should be sought. Thus both anxiety and accidents may be avoided.

About 55 out of every 1,000 persons 65 to 74 years of age are functionally deaf. This condition is said to be irreversible.

Young adults have approximately 245 taste buds on each papilla of the tongue, but by the age of 75 to 80 years the number has declined by 64 per cent. The loss of taste buds results in a decrease in perception of all four taste attributes—salt, sweet, bitter, and sour.

LOSS OF TEETH. The loss of teeth has been and still is a problem for the aging. Sixty per cent of men and 70 per cent of women over 65 years of age are edentulous. The loss of teeth and the loss of

some taste sense frequently leads to malnutrition.

SKIN. As one ages, the skin becomes thin, wrinkled, dry, and freckled. The wrinkled skin of the face, particularly around the mouth, may be cause for great mental anguish for some aging persons (Fig. 4-16A). It is far better to discuss this normal phenomenon of aging during the diagnostic interview rather than later in the prosthodontic procedures. To eliminate wrinkles, the patient frequently requests the dentist to place the artificial teeth in undesirable relations to the support, to overextend or overcontour the borders, or to decrease the interocclusal distance.

An accumulation of melanin, the brownish-black pigment in the skin (Fig. 4-16B) and hair, occurs as the skin becomes thinner. This normal phenomenon occurs particularly on the dorsa of the hands and is of concern to anyone with carcinophobia unless he understands the process.

ORAL MUCOSA. The oral mucosa undergoes changes similar to those in the skin; it becomes thin, is easily abraded, and frequently reacts unfavorably to the pressure of dentures (Fig. 4-16C).

SALIVA. The saliva decreases in quantity and changes in quality. Lack of lubrication or viscous or ropy saliva decreases the retention of the dentures and increases frictional trauma to the thin mucosa.

NEUROMYAL CHANGES. A generalized "slowing down" of normal activity means that housework and yardwork seem to take longer, and the body tires more easily. Muscle activity lacks coordination, and the muscles lose tonus. The cheeks sag, and the mandible, when at rest, appears to drop slightly more in a protruded position. These changes are

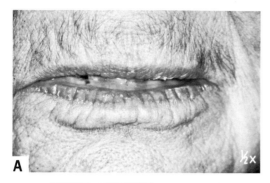

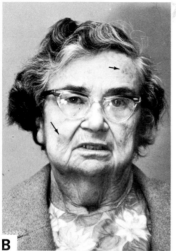

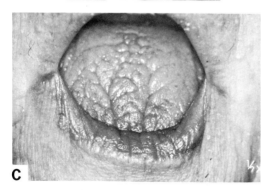

FIG. 4-16. *Signs of aging in the skin.* **A.** *Loss of muscle tonus and wrinkling of the skin around the mouth.* **B.** *Arrows point to accumulations of melanin.* **C.** *Thin, wrinkled oral mucosa of the lips, tongue, and cheeks. Although this patient uses a complete maxillary and a removable mandibular partial denture, they are not used continuously for long periods of time.*

understandable when one knows that fibrous tissue replaces some of the muscle fibers. The conduction of nerve impulses diminishes only slightly—approximately 15 per cent between the ages of 30 and 90. During this same period the excretory capacity of the kidneys decreases approximately 50 percent, an excellent example of differences in the aging process. The decrease in nerve conduction, loss of muscle tonus, "slowing down" of muscle activity, lack of moisture in the skin, and lack of muscle coordination all influence the recording of maxillomandibular relations.

SEXUAL DRIVE. The change in sexual drive varies with individuals and sex. Women may become frigid. The drive of males diminishes, but men frequently do not want to admit this. The effect, when the change is not accepted gracefully, is usually a psychologic change, one of frustration.

GENERALIZED OSTEOPOROSIS. The most common systemic bone condition occurring in both sexes is osteoporosis. It is likely to appear earlier in women than in men. Back pain, loss of body height and face height, stooping, and some types of deformity are some of the symptoms. In the advanced disease spontaneous fractures occur. The atrophy of bone is particularly noticeable in the residual alveolar ridge (page 25), more so when the ridge is subjected to the continuous pressure of dentures.

MEMORY. A decrease in mental capacity to remember recent events, new names, and new places occurs, but recall of past events and places seems less impaired. During conversation the geriatric person may distress or bore his listener by repeating the same incidents many times. However, correction does not help the situation.

CIRCULATION, ALIMENTATION, AND ELIMI-
NATION. The flow of blood and lymph
slows down as one ages. The gastric
juices become less acidic, and the digestive processes slow down. Elimination of
waste products may become irregular.
These slowing processes tend to make
the elderly practice self-medication,
using cathartics so indiscriminately as to
produce dietary problems. Vitamins A
and D are not utilized when mineral oil
is present in the digestive tract. Harsh
laxatives force food through the digestive tract before nutrients can be ingested.

NUTRITION AND DIET

Nutrition and diet are important factors with all edentulous patients, but
particularly with the geriatric. Their diet
often presents a challenge, not only to
the dentist but also to those who are
responsible for their care. Many geriatric
patients live alone and do not have the
energy or the desire to prepare well-
balanced meals for themselves. Many
are undergoing a decline in their mental
faculties, and time means nothing to
them. As a result, they may eat only one
meal a day, and symptoms of dietary
deficiencies may develop (Fig. 4-17).

As the aging process advances, people
become less active. Since muscle activity
is limited, caloric requirement is lower.
The time for more proteins and fewer
carbohydrates and starches has come,
but many revert to childhood habits, frequently consuming excess carbohydrates. They seem to crave sweets and
starches and may rebel against milk,
cheese, and eggs. Vitamin therapy, so
essential as a diet supplement for them,
may be looked upon as medicine that
they often refuse to take. The cooperation of the family is frequently the only
solution to treating these patients.

Decline in sensibility to taste can result in appetite loss. Loss of appetite can
result in malnutrition that contributes to
chronic physical disorders, deteriorating
in nature.

Obesity can result from an excessive
intake of refined carbohydrates. This excessive intake may be caused by emotional disturbances, metabolic disorders,
and/or atrophy of the taste buds for
sweets. The relation of obesity to cardiac
problems is well documented. The use
of drugs to decrease appetite is not without danger. The action of these drugs on
the central nervous system causes ner-
vousness and also elevates blood pressure.

In starvation diets the stores of the
water-soluble vitamins of the B group
and vitamin C do not last long. Dieting
as treatment for obesity may have side
effects as a result of vitamin deficiency.
Patients who are successfully using
complete dentures may suddenly find
that the dentures are no longer comfortable because the supporting tissues
change with the weight loss.

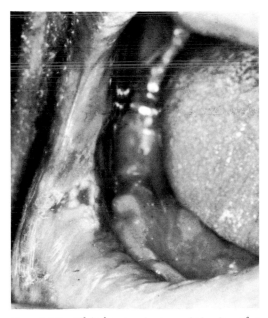

FIG. 4-17. *This benign lesion of the lip of a
74-year-old male is attributed to dietary
deficiency.*

Patients who will not discipline themselves in diet control may not be very cooperative in carrying out the instructions given for the care and use of dentures (Chapter 3).

PSYCHOLOGIC CHANGES

The dentist must understand how to deal with the psychologic problems, as well as the dental problems of his patients. The psychologic reaction to any or all of the biologic changes can be favorable or unfavorable and frequently determines into which group the patient will fall—the well-preserved, the chronically ill, or the in-between group. Even when the changes are benign, the psychic reactions to them may have such adverse effects on the well-being of some persons that they do not grow old gracefully. The knowledgeable dentist is frequently in a position to allay their anxiety or suppress their fears and thereby avert a psychologic problem. This is *not* to be interpreted that the dentist should substitute for a psychiatrist, but rather that he should counsel the patient and members of his family and, when necessary, refer them for psychiatric consultation.

A dentist should know what behavior or personality changes occur with aging and recognize them during his clinical examination of the patient. He will then be in a position to give special attention when needed, to recognize the individual problem, and to understand the reaction. This knowledge does *not* place him in the position to treat the psychologically involved patient unless he is also a specialist in psychology who has had training in understanding, predicting, and trying to change human behavior. It is the responsibility of every member of the health team, of which the dentist is an important member, to educate aging persons in what changes may be expected.

The psychologic problems influencing the behavior of the aging can be divided into (1) reactions to physiologic changes and (2) reactions to social changes, changes in environment, and changes in mental capacity.

REACTIONS TO PHYSIOLOGIC CHANGES. The changes influencing one's appearance seem to affect women more than men. This may *not* actually be so. Women frequently voice their concern over the loss of hair and face height, wrinkling of the skin, changes in tooth appearance, and the loss of the natural teeth. A man may not vocally register his concern; however, his reaction may be more dramatic but concealed. In replacing the lost natural teeth with artificial ones the dentist must be aware of this concern for appearance and strive to meet the esthetic requirements of all patients (page 327). Pride is a proper sense of personal dignity and worth—honorable self-respect. Vanity suggests undue admiration for oneself and an excessive desire to be admired by others for one's achievements and appearance. Providing dentures for the patient who has a justified belief in his appearance and a proper sense of personal dignity is a pleasure. It may be a very unpleasant experience with someone who has developed a vain personality.

Meeting esthetic requirements is sometimes impossible, for some patients will not accept normal changes in appearance. They will insist that the artificial teeth be placed and contoured to recreate their youthful appearance. When this is not done, they will reject the dentures. Patients in their late forties and early fifties who insist that their natural teeth be removed because their position, the relationship of the jaws, or the signs of age are distasteful to them or relate that they had the teeth removed because they could not stand their looks frequently react in an unfavorable manner to dentures. It is difficult to create beauty where beauty did not exist and have harmony with the surrounding environment. Malrelated jaws are not corrected by extracting the natural teeth and replacing them with artificial teeth. Trying to compensate for malrelated jaws when placing artificial teeth can be disastrous. Not only may the support for the dentures be destroyed, but also the teeth may be placed in positions that are out of harmony with mandibular movements and the functions of the lips, tongue, and cheeks. The gain in appearance is usually overshadowed by the difficulties, whereupon the patient becomes emotionally upset.

Women during and after menopause, particularly those who have been admired for their beauty, may be quite demanding about the cosmetic arrangement of their artificial teeth. These women may blame the loss of their natural teeth on dentists and readily condemn all dentists for their "enormous fees." If they will not consent to a psychologic evaluation and treatment, their dental problems may remain unsolved.

The loss of or decline of the senses of vision, hearing, and taste have psychologic implications. The loss of sight complicates a person's activities. The learning processes are slowed, and distinguishing objects rapidly is not possible; therefore accidents occur. Hearing loss can result in growing isolation. Isolation can result in profound personality changes that may be resentful in nature. The loss of teeth coupled with loss of the sense of taste and often a consequent appetite loss can contribute to deteriorating mental, as well as physical, disorders.

The loss of sex drive, skin changes, generalized slowing of manual activity, and changes in other bodily functions and bodily appearance sometimes cause personality changes. The type of change is unpredictable and varies from extroversion to withdrawal and can be unfavorable for those who are involved in their health care.

REACTIONS TO SOCIAL CHANGES. As a person ages, changes over which he has no control take place in his social life. In many instances, these changes occur in a relatively short period. Death claims relatives, friends, and neighbors; relatives and friends retire from business or professions and move to other localities. When one changes his residence, it is not always easy to make new friends. Severance of social ties leads to isolation, particularly for those who were habitually unsociable or who no longer derive pleasure from activities enjoyed in former years. Isolation can lead to resentfulness and unreasonable demands on the time of others. The aged who resent being sent to rest or nursing homes frequently draw into their shells and isolate themselves from their neighbors.

Many older workers do not wish to retire. Retirement can lead to anxiety over loss of income and fear that they will have to depend upon someone else for support. For an able-bodied person idleness can result in a guilt complex and a loss of self-esteem. The feeling of worthlessness, of loss of identity, and of being rejected or forsaken can lead to a lack of desire to live.

It is generally assumed by both young and old that loss of mental powers accompanies old age and that the problem is uncorrectable. Physiologic and biologic aging is a contributing factor to the slowing down of mental activity; however, many other contributing factors, such as anxiety, fear, malnutrition, isolation, chronic illness, and boredom, can be controlled, and the aged can be rehabilitated.

Healthy people who have a high level of intelligence and a good education, who practice continuous self-learning, and who keep up with current events show less deficit in memory than do those in poor health. People in poor health frequently "give up" and live in the past. Concern over bodily symptoms is frequently concentrated on the mouth, and minor problems become major ones.

During the diagnostic procedures it is therefore important for the prosthodontist to be alert for clues that will reveal the patient's psychologic responses to aging. If the problems are severe, the patient may have to be referred for psychiatric counseling before any attempt is made to fit him with complete dentures.

PATHOLOGIC CHANGES

Acute inflammatory infections are less frequent after maturity, but chronic disorders are a menace to good health. The pathologic disorders or changes most frequently encountered are (1) metabolic, (2) skeletal, (3) muscular, (4) circulatory, (5) neoplastic, and (6) psychologic. To evaluate and treat the total patient the dentist must know the basic factors that are involved in the processes and be in a position to discuss intelligently the conditions with the patient, to refer him for consultation to specialists, and to review the findings with the consultant.

Not all pathologic changes produce a state of senility, nor can the dentist classify the changes as benign. One such condition, infrequently encountered but devastating when present, is pain when wearing dentures. Repeated examinations reveal that *all* of the factors which usually provide denture success have been met—the oral mucosa evidences no hyperkeratosis, no hyperemia, and no ulcerations; the patient is not taking medication; his diet is well balanced; and in general he appears and feels well. The exception to this feeling of being well is *pain* when using the dentures.

The pain may be caused by the following:

1. Osteoporosis, bone sore mouth discussed on page 400.

2. A diminished blood supply and, as a result of this lack of blood the abused area does not become hyperemic; therefore the sign of irritation is absent.

3. Metabolic, e.g., thiamine deficiency. This deficiency allows an accumulation of pyruvic acid in the tissues. The principal clinical manifestation is peripheral neuritis.

4. A lack of estrogen resulting in tissue tone loss. This problem is not to be confused with psychogenic facial pain, for neither the type of pain nor the individual are characteristic.

The principal causes of disability in persons 65 years of age and older are heart disease, hypertensive vascular disease, tuberculosis, diseases of the bones and joints (other than tuberculosis and arthritis), accidents, nephritis, diabetes, cancer, and eye disease. The commonest causes of death after the age of 65 are cerebral hemorrhage, heart disease, cancer, general arteriosclerosis, and accidents. Many of the accidents result from pathologic changes that are not benign in nature. They produce a state of mental and physical infirmity characterized by weakness, a lack of mental stability or firmness of purpose, and illness (senility) ending in death. It is important to realize that when a person has pathologic changes of this magnitude the treatment plan may be only palliative in nature, i.e., it may ease the symptoms without eliminating the problems.

Signs and symptoms of psychologic, physiologic, and pathologic changes can be observed and recorded during the initial interview prior to the consultation interview and intra-oral examination. There is no justification for subjecting a geriatric patient to extensive examinations and diagnostic procedures if the examiner is reasonably certain that the psychologic or physical condition of the patient is such that treatment will be very limited. When any of the signs and symptoms of disease are observed in the face, complexion, posture, voice, or walking or breathing pattern of an aging patient, a more thorough investigation of the systemic status should be instituted prior to detailed dental diagnostic procedures. Signs and symptoms are *not* conclusive evidence of disease; therefore, the dentist should not attempt a diagnosis at this time. Neither should he alarm the patient or the family. A calm, honest appraisal of the situation is indicated. The concerned persons will appreciate the consideration, the thoroughness of the procedure, and the honest effort not to involve them in unnecessary expense.

FACIAL EXPRESSION. An absence of facial expression may indicate a loss of muscle tonus, but, of far more importance, it may exist because of tic douloureaux. The patient consciously holds his facial muscles in an immobile position for fear of "triggering" the excruciating pain. A masklike expression may also be the result of numerous plastic surgery procedures, and the chronologic age given by the patient may be far from correct. The esthetic requirements of this patient may be impossible to fulfill. A masklike expression may have more serious significance, for it occurs as a result of disorders of the central nervous system such as paralysis agitans and of endocrine gland disease such as hypothyroidism.

COMPLEXION. Pallor may be indicative of anemia, hypothyroidism, or degenerative lesions of the renal tubules (nephrosis). A pale complexion may also result from a debilitating systemic disease such as tuberculosis. It may be due to lack of nourishment.

A ruddy complexion may be a sign of polycythemia (increase in red blood cells) or of a neoplasm. Redness has also been noted in some chronic alcoholics, particularly on (or in) the skin of the nose.

Bronzed skin occurs in Addison's disease. However, bronzed areas of the skin of the head and neck may signify that the patient is receiving or has received radiation therapy.

A diffuse bluish-purple color may indicate vitamin B_2 deficiency. This should not be confused with the cyanotic complexion. The color changes of cyanosis, which is associated with diseases of the heart and lungs, vary from bluish-purple to red-purple in fair-skinned persons.

The lemon-yellow complexion of jaundice is associated with gall bladder, liver, or bile duct disorders.

An increase in pigmentation is sometimes caused by adrenal gland insufficiency.

A complexion marred by ulcerated lesions may be due to basal cell or squamous cell carcinoma.

When the complexion of the aging woman is marred by the growth of hair, one may suspect Cushing's syndrome or postmenopausal syndrome (Fig. 4-16A). It can also be a normal phenomenon.

POSTURE AND WALKING PATTERN. Stooped shoulders may indicate changes in the spine. The majority of patients who are stooped also tend to protrude the mandible. However, the protruded mandible may indicate temporomandibular joint discomfort.

Tremor of the head accompanies Parkinson's disease. It occurs also as a habit spasm but recently has been observed in patients who have been taking tranquilizing drugs.

When a patient drags one leg as he

walks (hemiplegic), one should suspect a cerebrovascular problem that has caused a stroke.

Involuntary *hurried* walking (festinating) occurs in certain nervous disorders such as Parkinson's disease.

Slapping the sole of the foot occurs in tabes dorsalis and may also occur following spinal cord injury.

Dropping the toe when walking may be the result of poliomyelitis.

Staggering can result from excessive intake of alcohol, excessive medication with muscle relaxant drugs, hyperventilation, or from damage to the brain or spinal cord.

THE VOICE. *Hypernasality* of the voice may be caused by a paralysis of the musculature of the soft palate and/or lateral and posterior wall of the throat or by a perforation of the palate.

Hoarseness can be caused by a paralysis of one or both vocal cords. It can also result from laryngitis, polyps, or ulcerations. However, in the aging the cause may be excessive smoking or a tumor of the vocal cords. Elderly women may develop a masculine-sounding voice as part of the menopausal syndrome.

BREATHING PATTERN. Wheezing is most commonly present in bronchial asthma and emphysema. It may also occur in bronchial infection and heart failure.

Shortness of breath (dyspnea) is not limited to lung disease, for it frequently occurs with heart failure. Shortness of breath may be more profound when one is reclining (orthopnea).

Shallow breathing at a rapid rate indicates advanced pulmonary fibrosis.

Erratic breathing, continuous *hyperventilation,* or *periodic* breathing should alert one to the possibility of serious pulmonary, renal, or cardiac problems. Heavy sighing or hyperventilation may indicate an emotionally disturbed person.

The patient who sits on the edge of the chair and appears reluctant to sit back may have difficulty breathing when in a supine position (orthopnea).

LOCAL FACTORS. In addition to the local factors that were described on pages 105–110, other signs and symptoms of physiologic or pathologic change are equally important in diagnosis.

1. Halitosis can result from (a) poor oral hygiene, including a lack of care of dentures; (b) soft tissue lesions with necrosis, ulceration, or hemorrhage; (c) an unhealed surgical site; (d) heavy smoking; (e) a diet of highly flavored foods or beverages; (f) respiratory disease; (g) a gastrointestinal problem; (h) the acetone breath of the diabetic; or (i) the ammoniacal odor associated with uremia.

2. Crinkly, sparse, coarse hair and slow speech and perception may indicate a low basal metabolic rate.

3. An enlarged head may relate to Paget's disease (osteitis deformans). This disease usually begins during or after middle age. In the roentgenogram the bone has a "cottonball" appearance.

4. Enlargement of the finger joints may be visible evidence of osteoarthritis (Fig. 4-3). Spindle fingers denote rheumatoid arthritis. Swollen hands and/or swollen feet may indicate heart failure or kidney disease.

5. Obesity is more noticeable as the patient is seated and may present dental procedure problems in addition to psychic or systemic involvement.

6. Dry skin and dry lips may be indicative of xerostomia (Fig. 4-16C). The facial skin of the aging usually becomes more wrinkled, darker, and drier. The loss of moisture, fat, and tonus of the skin is indicative of the condition of the oral mucosa. Cancer of the lip is the most common malignant neoplasm of the mouth. It is usually found on the lower lip of males.

7. Mouth breathing may be due to a

loss of fat and elasticity and to drying of the nasal mucosa. Breathing through the nostrils may be painful because of sensitive tissue lining the airways. Mouth breathing may also be due to nasal congestion, passages closed with polyps, or a deviated septum. Mouth breathing dries the oral mucosa. Difficulty in breathing through the nose may present problems in some types of impression making.

8. In addition to temporomandibular joint discomfort, a protruded mandible may be (a) a compensating posture to help balance a body that is stooped, (b) a sign of oral aggression against treatment, or (c) a malrelation of the jaws.

9. Congenital syphilis may be suspected when a patient has narrow pupils that respond to light with accommodation.

10. Wide pupils of the eyes are indicative of glaucoma.

11. If the eye lens is cloudy or appears to have a film over a portion of it, the patient may have glaucoma.

12. Unilateral protrusion of the eyeball is usually due to a local lesion. One should suspect a tumor.

13. Distension of the veins of the neck while a person is sitting in a semi-reclined position may indicate heart failure, pericarditis, or obstruction of the superior vena cava.

14. Vigorous pulsating of the arteries of the neck may indicate aortic insufficiency, arteriosclerosis, or aneurysm.

15. When the thyroid gland or the lymph nodes of the neck are palpated and found to be enlarged, one should suspect a goiter, an infection, or a neoplasm, respectively.

PAIN. Not all of the signs and symptoms of pathologic conditions are visible. Pain is one of these, and a recognition of its relationship to systemic disease is essential to an understanding of the total patient and his problems.

In *renal* disease, the pain of kidney origin is dull and located in the back or in one or both flanks. The pain usually involves the groin and scrotum and is accentuated during urination.

The pain of *kidney stones* resembles the acute abdominal pain experienced with colic and spreads from the kidney area to the scrotum.

In the United States the incidence of *cancer of the prostate* in men over 75 is more than 500 per 100,000. The pain is intense and is referred to the bladder, urethra, rectum, perineum, sacrum, gluteal region, and the legs.

Gallbladder pain is usually localized in the upper right quadrant.

Bowel obstruction is accompanied by pain in the area of obstruction.

Chest pain may have its origin in the heart, pleural cavity, or mediastinum. Severe retrosternal pain is present when there is an accumulation of air in the mediastinum after pneumothorax.

Glossodynia, pain in the tongue, usually occurs with women in the post-menopausal years, infrequently with the male.

Paroxysmal pain, lasting several seconds to several minutes, burning and stabbing in nature, and localized to the posterior pharynx, back of the tongue, middle ear, and region of the tonsils is termed *glossopharyngeal neuralgia.* It occurs primarily with males of middle age and can be triggered by talking, swallowing, protruding the tongue, or touching the tonsil or pharynx.

The pain of *tic douloureux* (trigeminal neuralgia) is burning and comes quickly. It is one of the worst pains experienced by humans and may be located in one or more branches of the trigeminal nerve. The pain is of short duration, lasting only seconds or minutes.

Pain located over the maxillary sinus may indicate carcinoma of the antrum. Neoplasms of the nasopharynx are associated with persistent facial pain. *Psy-*

chogenic facial pain is frequently described as burning, fleeting, pulling, draining, gripping, or boring. It is usually described as being in an area rather than in a specific location and is frequently experienced by postmenopausal or menopausal females.

INTRAORAL CHANGES

Since many of the physiologic and pathologic changes of the aging are reflected in the oral mucosa, the dentist should be able to recognize those that are frequently encountered. The changes from the normal that he does not recognize should be thoroughly investigated.

1. In the majority of edentulous patients 65 years of age and older there is a marked resorption of the residual alveolar ridge. The overlying mucosa shows signs of use and age, particularly if the mucosa has supported dentures (Fig. 4-14).

2. In the presence of ill-fitting dentures one will find inflammatory hyperplasia (Fig. 4-9). Palatal inflammatory hyperplasia (Fig. 4-12B) is also associated with ill-fitting dentures. In many instances it is associated with improper palatal relief in the maxillary denture base. Failure to remove the denture for tissue rest and to clean the soft tissue of the palate produces palatal inflammatory hyperplasia.

3. White lesions of the buccal mucosa include lichen planus, leukoplakia, or fungus plaque (moniliasis). However, if the lesion feels hard and is deeply fissured, one must suspect squamous cell carcinoma. White lesions or keratotic patches on the lateral margin of the tongue or in the floor of the mouth in the anterior segment on either side of the midline near the orifices of the salivary glands are frequently squamous cell carcinoma.

4. A painless, nonulcerated, poorly defined firm mass covered by normal pink mucosa may be a fibrosarcoma. A pink or light red, well-circumscribed mass of firm consistency located in the hard or soft palate may be a mixed tumor.

5. A unilateral swelling in the hard palate, in the second bicuspid, and/or molar area may indicate a neoplasm of the maxillary antrum.

6. When the tongue has a distinct purple discoloration and atrophy of the superficial papilla and appears shiny and smooth, riboflavin deficiency should be suspected.

7. Mucositis may be an indication of vitamin B_{12} deficiency. If the saliva is thick and ropy and the mucosa is inflamed, the patient may be receiving or has received radiation therapy.

8. Generalized cyanosis of the oral mucosa of the elderly suggests either heart or lung disease or polycythemia.

9. The thinning of the mucosa of the geriatric patient allows Fordyce's spots to become more apparent. The appearance of this developmental disturbance sometimes upsets the person who has carcinophobia.

10. Red petechial areas of the buccal mucosa may indicate a blood abnormality, a thinning or fragility of the blood vessel walls, or a disturbance in the blood-forming organs.

11. Nicotine stomatitis refers to lesions that occur in the palatal mucosa, usually of pipe smokers. The lesion is usually extensive, showing flat or compressed smooth gray patches. Gray nodules or projections appear throughout the patches. Pale red depressed lines may course throughout the area. Hypertrophied and inflamed mucous glands frequently appear.

12. Hyperplastic filiform papillae make the dorsal surface of the tongue immediately anterior to the circumvallate papillae appear hairy (hairy tongue). Tobacco and food stain the papillae, and

the area becomes dark. Fungus and yeast organisms are commonly detected in hairy tongue.

13. Macroglossia (acquired) usually results from relaxation of the tongue musculature. This occurs in disturbance of the endocrine glands as in hyperpituitarism; however, the extraction of the mandibular posterior teeth allows the musculature to relax and is probably the most prevalent etiologic factor.

14. Varicosity of the veins of the ventral surface of the tongue may indicate a cardiovascular or pulmonary problem. When the varicose veins extend to the lateral surfaces of the tongue, the posterior lingual flanges of the mandibular denture may present a problem to the patient.

15. As the serous glands decrease in activity, the saliva becomes more mucous and ropy. When the salivary glands atrophy, the reduction of salivary flow results in a dry mouth (xerostomia).

Diagnostic Procedures

Past dental history furnishes valuable information as to the mental attitude of the patient toward dentistry and the dentist. The patient may reveal instances of traumatic experiences dating to his first visit to the dentist. Traumatic experiences have very lasting effects and make patients tense in the dental chair. Experiences with previous prosthodontic restorations are important in determining patient tolerance, tissue tolerance, and esthetic acceptability. What the patient expects from dentures is divulged. Patient education in dental health is revealed as they discuss their dental treatment. Unfortunately, very few patients are instructed in the use and care of their dentures. The majority of patients state they were instructed to "go wear the dentures." Any existing prosthesis should be examined thoroughly in an objective manner. To condemn a prosthesis on the complaint of the patient is often incorrect diagnosis.

During the consultation and medical history taking, two very important factors are revealed: (1) the patient's behavior pattern, personality, temperament, and ability to communicate (hearing is essential to communication) and (2) the medications he is taking, including nonprescribed proprietary drugs.

MEDICATION

The value of knowing what medication a patient is taking is twofold: (1) it can be an indication of systemic problems and (2) the dental treatment can be influenced by the effects of the drug. The dental treatment may include the prescribing of drugs, and these must be compatible with those already being taken. Drugs can act as synergists, and the combined effect may not be desired or promote good health. Drugs can also be antagonists, one drug counteracting or neutralizing the effect of another. Therefore, the dentist should be aware of any synergistic actions of drugs he may prescribe with those the patient is already taking. Patients can also be sensitive to drugs. Sensitivity is determined by questioning the patient and those who are responsible for his care.

It is equally important to understand the side effects of the drugs the patient is taking. Salicylates like aspirin, which is widely used in the treatment of osteoarthritis, can act as anticoagulants, upset digestion, produce gastric pain for patients with peptic ulcers, and cause ringing in the ears. Certain tranquilizing drugs produce tremors similar to those of Parkinson's disease in 15 per cent of those who take them. One of the side effects of a drug that is recommended for these tremors is xerostomia. Phenothiazines may have a hypertensive effect on older people, and drugs that reduce blood pressure reduce salivary gland function. These few examples illustrate the importance of a thorough investigation in this area during the diagnostic procedures.

When prescribing drugs for an aging person one should furnish completely understandable written information to the patient.

Following are the common drugs and their effects that can influence the successful treatment of a patient prosthodontically:

I. Xerostomia (dry mouth)
   A. Antihistamines—Benadryl
   B. Probanthine, atropine, belladonna —decrease in GI secretions and motility to control conditions of stress and tension; used by ulcer patients
   C. Many antihypertensives
   D. Nitroglycerin—for angina pectoris
   E. Most antipsychotic drugs—phenothiazines (Thorazine, Compazine, thioxanthines, and butyrophenones)
   F. Antiparkinsonian agents—Artane, Akineton, Norflex, Parsidol
   G. Antiarrhythmic agents—quinidine, procainamide, disopyramide
   H. Tricyclic antidepressants—imipramine (Tofranil)
   I. Antianxiety agents—diazepan (Valium)
   J. Amphetamines—used in the control of obesity and as a central nervous system stimulant
   K. Antisialogogues—drugs purposely used to dry up the mouth, e.g., atropine
   L. Decongestants—Contac and others
II. Changes in the Oral Flora
   A. Antibiotics—especially the broad spectrum type
III. Possible Mucosal Changes
   A. Dilantin
   B. Adrenal corticosteroids—may cause an atrophy of skin and mucosa
IV. Sialorrhea—Salivation
   A. Cholinesterase inhibitors—for treat-

ment of myasthenia gravis which has a syndrome of fatigue and exhaustion of the muscular system marked by a progressive paralysis of muscles without sensory disturbance or atrophy (cholinesterase, an esterase present in all body tissues, hydrolyzes acetylcholine into choline and acetic acid), e.g., Prostigmine
   B. Adrenergic-stimulating drugs, e.g., epinephrine—cause mucous salivary flow
   C. Sialogogue—name given to a drug such as pilocarpine purposely used to increase salivation, as it stimulates the chorda tympanic nerve causing a copious flow of saliva
   D. Other drugs which may cause excessive flow of saliva are:
      1. Iodides—rarely used therapeutically; previously used for thyroid disorders and stomatitis; currently used mostly as an expectorant
      2. Mercurial salts—used as diuretic to keep down edema, e.g., Neohydrin, Thiomerin
      3. Ammonium salts—ammonium chloride, nitrate—rarely used except in combination with diuretic or as an expectorant
      4. Foreign bodies in the mouth (dentures, gum, etc.).
V. Dysphagia—difficulty in swallowing; gagging; could cause difficulty during the making of an impression
   A. Phenothiazine derivatives (Thorazine, Sparine, Prolixin, Mellaril)
   B. Belladonna derivatives—Belladonna tincture, atropine
   C. All agents that produce xerostomia—could lead to dysphagia
VI. Postural or Orthostatic Hypotension—fainting on standing up or changing position
   A. Glyceryl Trinitrite—anti-anginal
   B. Sedative and centrally acting skeletal muscle relaxants (especially in the aged), e.g., Valium, Equanil
   C. Phenothiazine derivatives (Thorazine, Sparine, Compazine, thio-

xanthines, and butyrophenones).

D. Antihypertensives (e.g., reserpine), and including diuretics
E. Narcotic analgesics—morphine
F. Tricyclic antidepressants—imipramine and others

VII. Bronchial Spasm and At-rest Bradycardia (abnormal slowness of heart beat) and Dyspnea (labored breathing)—could cause difficulties in managing the patient during the construction procedure
A. Inderal—blocking agent used to prevent arrhythmia in heart patient

VIII. Hypoglycemic Shock—concentration of glucose in the blood below the normal limit
A. Insulin

IX. Behavioral Changes or Confusion—patient acceptance of dentures could be affected by these drugs
A. Adrenal corticosteroids—for arthritis, allergies
B. Anti-parkinsonism agent—e.g., Artane, Akineton, Norflex
C. Some antihistamines—varies by patient
D. Digitalis and related cardiac glycosides—e.g., digoxin, digitoxin
E. Tricyclic antidepressants—e.g., Elavil, Tofranil
F. Darvon

X. Nausea and Vomiting
A. Aspirin—in small doses can cause nausea and vomiting
   1. In large doses for rheumatic condition—can cause dizziness and confusion
   2. Good drug, but one of the most abused drugs—greatest cause of accidental poisoning with infants
B. Any analgesic, but especially Darvon
C. Digitalis or other cardiac glycosides—when used over a long period of time

XI. Anticoagulants
A. Used for stroke and CV patients, e.g., heparin (usually used in hospitals only), dicumarol, Coumadin
B. The dentist should not perform any treatment that involves bleeding without consulting a physician about a prothrombin time test. Drug should *not* be withdrawn, but dosage adjusted, if necessary.

XII. Drug Induction of Parkinson-like Syndrome and other Bizarre Muscle Movements, including Facial Muscles
A. Phenothiazines, thioxanthines, and butyrophenones
B. Tricyclic antidepressants

FIRST APPOINTMENT

During the first appointment the procedures are as follows:

1. Seat the patient in the dental chair and record all local factors on a chart (Fig. 4-18).

2. Make preliminary impressions of the edentulous ridges and adjacent areas.

3. Pour the impressions with stone to make study casts.

4. Accurately mount the casts on the articulator.

5. Take roentgenograms.

6. If the patient has complete dentures, examine the border extensions, stability, retention, esthetics, the vertical dimension of occlusion, interocclusal distance, phonetics, and occlusion. In some instances this may include mounting the dentures for occlusal study.

7. Record the reactions of the patient to oral procedures.

8. Record the information voluntarily related by the patient, particularly that pertaining to previous dental experiences and dentist-patient relations.

9. Advise the patient that at the next appointment a treatment plan can be discussed more intelligently after the first appointment procedures have been studied and correlated.

SECOND APPOINTMENT

During the second appointment the procedures are as follows:

Diagnostic Data For Complete Dentures

Consultation Interview

Patient:
Address:
Age: Sex
Referred by:

Date:
Telephone: Business_____
            Home   _____
Occupation

Systemic Status:
Have you ever had any of the following?

Rheumatic Fever	Yes	No	Tuberculosis	Yes	No	Diabetes	Yes	No
Arthritis	Yes	No	Epilepsy	Yes	No	Anemia	Yes	No
Jaundice	Yes	No	Fainting Spells	Yes	No	X-ray Treatment	Yes	No
Heart Disease	Yes	No	Syphilis	Yes	No	Radium Treatments	Yes	No

(If so, where and when)

Have you ever been troubled with:

High Blood Pressure	Yes	No	Prolonged Bleeding	Yes	No
Low Blood Pressure	Yes	No	Reactions to Medicine or		
Shortness of Breath	Yes	No	Anesthetics (Novocain)	Yes	No
Swollen Ankles	Yes	No	Sweating at Night	Yes	No
Pain Over the Heart	Yes	No	Loss of Voice	Yes	No
Pain Under Breast Bone	Yes	No	Sinus Involvement	Yes	No
Persistent Cough	Yes	No	Asthma or Allergies	Yes	No
Skin Condition or Rash	Yes	No	Excessive Thirst	Yes	No
Burning Tongue	Yes	No	Any Bladder or Kidney		
			Involvement	Yes	No

Have you ever had any childhood or other diseases of lasting effect? Yes   No
Have you ever had any serious digestive disorders? Yes   No   If so, please
describe them _____.
Have you ever been treated for any mental or nervous condition? Yes   No
Do you tire easily? Yes   No
Do you have any trouble sleeping flat, or must you prop up with several pillows?
No trouble   Prop Up
How long since your physician gave you a complete physical "check-up"?_____
Physician's name _____ Address _____ Phone _____
May we have your permission to consult with him? Yes   No
Are you taking any medicine now? If so, can you tell us what it is? _____
If under the care of a physician for pregnancy, what is your expected date of
delivery? _____
Have you ever had penicillin? Yes   No   If so, did you have any bad effects?
Yes   No
Physician's report:

Dental History:
Date of Extractions: _____ Maxillary _____ Mandibular _____
Reasons for the loss of teeth_____ Periodontal_____Caries_____Other____
Dental Experiences prior to the loss of the natural teeth:
  (Patient's Words)

Number and Type of Previous Dentures:

Removable Partial: Maxillary _____ Mandibular _____

Complete dentures: Maxillary _____ Mandibular _____

Experiences with previous dentures: (Patient's Words)

Mental Attitude:
  Philosophical_____ Exacting_____ Hysterical_____ Indifferent_____
What the patient expects:
  1 Understands limitations____ 2 Function_____ 3 Esthetics_____ 4 Utopia_____
Coordination In:
A Speech_____ Walking_____ Thinking _____

FIG. 4-18. *Example of a diagnostic chart. Diagnostic data recorded on charts is not always definitive.*

Examination:

    Roentgenographic Findings:

    Muscle Coordination of Mandibular Movements:
      1. Normal_____   2. Fair_____   3. Uncoordinated_____

Residual ridge contour:	Maxillary_____	Mandibular
Smooth	_____	_____
Irregular	_____	_____
Full	_____	_____
Knife edge	_____	_____
Flat	_____	_____

Mucosa:	Maxillary_____	Mandibular
Normal resiliency	_____	_____
Hard unyielding	_____	_____
Displaceable	_____	_____
Spongy	_____	_____
Hyperemic	_____	_____
Hypertrophy	_____	_____

Tongue:	Size	Normal_____	Abnormal_____
	Position	Normal_____	Abnormal_____
	Function	Normal_____	Abnormal_____

Hard Palate: High Vault _____   Medium Vault _____   Flat _____
Soft Palate: Class 1 _____   Class 2 _____   Class 3 _____
                Active _____   Passive _____
Lateral Throat Form: Class 1 _____   Class 2 _____   Class 3 _____
Alveolar Tubercle: Normal _____   Bulbous_____ Pendulous_____ Undercut____
Frenum Attachments: Normal _____ High to crest _____ Broad - Single _____

Tori: Palatinus _____   Mandibularis _____

Intermaxillary Space.   Favorable _____   Limited _____   Excessive _____

Antero-Posterior Jaw Relations: 1. Even _____   2. Mandible Protruded _____
                                               Maxillae Protruded _____

Arch Size:	Maxillary	Mandibular
Average	_____	_____
Small	_____	_____
Large	_____	_____

Surgical Procedures Necessary:
    Teeth for extraction R. 8-7-6-5-4-3-2-1   1-2-3-4-5-6-7-8 L.
                          R. 8-7-6-5-4-3-2-1   1-2-3-4-5-6-7-8 L.

Roots: _____   Unerupted Teeth: _____
      Alveoplasty: Area _____
      Exostosis: Area _____
      Soft tissue: Area _____

Prognosis   Favorable _____   Unfavorable _____

B

FIG. 4-18 (*cont.*)

1. Conduct the consultation interview in a private reception room in pleasant surroundings, devoid of any dental equipment.

2. Make every effort to encourage the patient to relax and relate his problems. Leading questions are sometimes necessary, but once started most patients will talk freely, and they should be allowed this privilege with few interruptions. This conversation affords the dentist an excellent opportunity to begin evaluating the mental attitude of the patient.

3. After the patient has related his problems, information regarding general health should be obtained. The use of a prepared questionnaire is most helpful (Fig. 4-18). It is often more relaxing to the patient for him to fill in the form. Invariably he will discuss his health as he asks for assistance in answering the questions.

4. Record past dental history in the same manner; however, more general information often results from having the patient relate his dental experiences. Certain pertinent information is divulged, such as when and why the teeth were removed, whether partial or complete dentures were ever used, how many complete dentures have been made, whether immediate dentures were made, and what is wrong with present dentures. The discussion of past dental history leads to the subject of the use and care of dentures.

5. Begin educating the patient in his responsibilities in the treatment (Chapter 3). If the patient evidences indifference or an uncooperative attitude at this time, the prognosis presents unfavorable aspects, and the subject should be pursued again after all the factors have been evaluated. Some personality clashes become evident when attempting to educate a patient. If they are still evident when the discussion is continued, it is far better to let the patient seek treatment elsewhere.

When all the diagnostic information has been evaluated, the dentist is in a position to plan the treatment and present it to the patient as part of health care. For the chronically ill patient treatment may be merely palliative (Fig. 4-19). The completely edentulous person who has poor tissue tone, a loss or absence of alveolar residual ridge, and other unfavorable local factors (page 105 presents a challenge; however, it is one which should be approached with caution. It is often advisable to construct well-adapted denture bases of polished, processed acrylic resin and see if the tissues will tolerate their presence. The artificial teeth may be added later.

Proceed with caution with the patient who has complete dentures and who has received treatment elsewhere. When possible, it is better to construct new dentures and not try to alter the existing ones. For the chronically ill it may be best to rebase or reline the existing dentures; however, problems do arise from this type of treatment.

When new dentures are constructed, it is *mandatory* that the patient leave the former dentures with the dentist until the new dentures have been evaluated and accepted or rejected. It is surprising what problems can be encountered unless this is done. This understanding should be reached before treatment is begun.

Finally, the patient is advised about the time required for the procedure, the expense, and the probable prognosis. He is again told of the limitations of dentures, the problems to be expected, and the need for cooperation in following instructions. These instructions in the use and care of dentures should be given to the patient in writing (Chapter 3) and discussed with him again before and after the dentures have been placed.

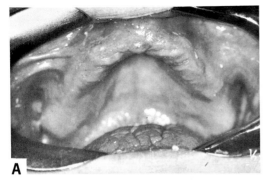

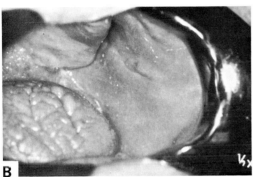

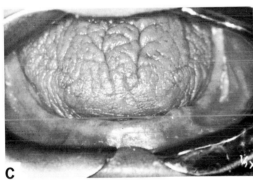

FIG. 4-19. *Oral soft tissues of a chronically ill patient.* **A.** *Mucosa covering the residual alveolar ridge, the palate, and the vestibular fornix is devoid of moisture.* **B.** *The dry mucosa lining the cheek will adhere to the denture surface. This is irritating and painful.* **C.** *The tongue is dry, and although there is little loss of residual ridge, dentures are not tolerated.*

REFERENCES

1. Appleby, R. C., and Ludwig, T. F.: Patient evaluation for complete denture therapy. J. Prosth. Dent., 24:11, 1970.

2. Applegate, O. C.: Conditions which may influence the choice of partial or complete denture service. J. Prosth. Dent., 7:182, 1957.

3. Barbenel, J. C.: Physical retention of complete dentures. J. Prosth. Dent., 26:592, 1971.

3a. Barker, B. F., Moffit, M. W., and Johnson, J. K.: Sjörgren's syndrome: Diagnosis and dental treatment. J. Prosth. Dent., 39:536, 1978.

4. Barone, J. V.: Diagnosis and prognosis in complete denture prosthesis. J. Prosth. Dent., 14:207, 1964.

4a. ———: Nutrition—Phase one of the edentulous patient. J. Prosth. Dent., 40:122, 1978.

5. Bernier, J. L.: Tumors of the lips. Dent. Clin. N. Amer., November, 1957, p. 637.

6. ———: Clinical features of early malignant growths of the oral cavity. Dent. Clin. N. Am., July, 1958, p. 235.

7. Bhaskur, S. N.: Oral pathology in the dental office: Survey of 20,575 biopsy specimens. J.A.D.A., 76:761, 1968.

8. Blackwood, H. J. J.: Adaptive changes in the mandibular joints with function. Dent. Clin. N. Am., November, 1966, p. 559.

9. Bolender, C. L., Swoope, C. C., and Smith, D. E.: The Cornell Medical Index as a prognostic aid for complete dentures. J. Prosth. Dent., 22:20, 1967.

10. Bortel, R. H.: Problems of old age in dental prosthetic and restorative procedures. J. Prosth. Dent., 26:250, 1971.

10a. Bottomley, W. K., and Terezhalmy, G. T.: Management of patients with myasthenia gravis who require maxillary dentures. J. Prosth. Dent., 38:609, 1977.

11. Brewer, A. A.: Treating complete denture patients. J. Prosth. Dent., 14:1015, 1964; Schweitzer, J. M.: Discussions of "Treating complete denture patients." J. Prosth. Dent., 14:1031, 1964.

12. Brill, N., Tryde, G., and Schubeler, S.: The role of learning in denture retention. J. Prosth. Dent., 10:468, 1960.

13. Bruno, S. A.: Neuromuscular disturbances causing temporomandibular dysfunction and pain. J. Prosth. Dent., 26:387, 1971.

14. Buckley, G. A.: Diagnostic factors in the

choice of impression materials and methods. J. Prosth. Dent., 5:149, 1955.

15. Budtz-Jorgensen, E.: Delayed hypersensitivity to Candida albicans in man. Demonstrated in vitro: the capillary tube migration test. Acta Allerg. (Kobenhavn), 27:41, 1972.

16. ———: Denture stomatitis. IV. An experimental model in monkeys. Acta Odont. Scand., 29:513, 1971.

17. Cheraskin, E.: The systemic influences. In *Complete Denture Prosthodontics*, 2nd ed., J. J. Sharry, editor. New York, McGraw-Hill Book Co., Inc., 1968.

18. ——— and Ringsdorf, W. M.: A fortunate erratum. J. Oral Med., 26:75, 1971.

19. Colby, R. A.: Odontogenic tumors. Dent. Clin. N. Amer., November, 1957, p. 709.

20. ——— et al.: *Color Atlas of Oral Pathology*, 3rd ed. Philadelphia, J. B. Lippincott Co., 1971.

21. Collett, H. A.: Influence of dentist-patient relationship on attitudes and adjustment to dental treatment. J.A.D.A., 79:879, 1969.

22. Crandell, C. W.: Roentgenographic examination of edentulous jaws. J. Prosth. Dent., 9:552, 1959.

23. DeVan, M. M.: Methods of procedure in a diagnostic service to the edentulous patient. J.A.D.A., 29:1981, 1942.

24. ———: Physical, biological and psychological factors to be considered in the construction of dentures. J.A.D.A., 42:290, 1951.

25. ———: Procedures preceding the prosthodontic prescription. J. Prosth. Dent., 13:1006, 1963.

26. Dreizen, S., Stone, R. E., and Spies, T. D.: Oral manifestations of nutritional disorders. Dent. Clin. N. Am., July, 1958, p. 429.

27. Dresen, O. M.: Relief and postdam areas of denture base. J. Wis. Dent. Soc. 24:97, 1948.

27a. Emory, L.: The face in patient evaluation and diagnosis. J. Prosth. Dent., 35:247, 1976.

27b. Ettinger, R. L.: Etiology of inflammatory papillary hyperplasia. J. Prosth. Dent., 34:254, 1975.

28. Friedman, A. P.: Differential diagnosis of facial pain. Dent. Clin. N. Am., November, 1966, p. 545.

29. Gochin, R. J.: Tumors of the buccal and labial mucosa. Dent. Clin. N. Am. November, 1957, p. 661.

30. Gordon, D. F.: Are new dentures necessary? J. Prosth. Dent., 23:512, 1970.

30a. Grieder, A.: Psychologic aspects of prosthodontics. J. Prosth. Dent., 30:736, 1973.

31. Halperin, V.: Tumors of the palate. Dent. Clin. N. Am., November, 1957, p. 667.

31a. Hartsook, E. I.: Food selection, dietary adequacy and related dental problems of patients with dental prostheses. J. Prosth. Dent., 32:32, 1974.

32. Heartwell, C. M., Jr.: Psychologic considerations in complete denture prosthodontics. J. Prosth. Dent., 24:5, 1970.

33. Hygel, I. M.: Geriatrics and dental service. J. Prosth. Dent., 1:295, 1951.

34. Jankelson, B.: Communication with the completely edentulous patient. Dent. Clin. N. Amer., 14:427, 1970.

35. Jensen, M. B.: Overgeneralization in geriatrics. J. Amer. Soc. Geriat. Dent., 2:2, 1967.

36. ———: *Measuring Attitudes toward Old People*. Veterans Administration Center, Prescott, Arizona (mimeographed) 1966.

36a. Joglekar, A. P.: Biologic approach to complete dentures. J. Prosth. Dent., 30:700, 1973.

36b. Jones, P. M.: Complete dentures and the associated soft tissues. J. Prosth. Dent., 36:136, 1976.

37. Kaaber, S.: Studies on the permeability of human oral mucosa. I. Gravimetric determination of biologic fluids at microgram levels. Acta Odont. Scand., 29:653, 1971.

38. ———: Studies on the permeability of human oral mucosa. II. The permeability of dry palatal mucosa to water, sodium, and potassium. Acta Odont. Scand., 29:663, 1971.

39. ———: Studies on the permeability of human oral mucosa. III. The permeability of dry palatal mucosa to water, so-

dium, and potassium. Acta Odont. Scand., *29*:683, 1971.

40. Kelly, H. T.: Psychosomatic aspects of prosthodontics. J. Prosth. Dent., *5*:609, 1955.

41. Kingery, R. H.: Examination and diagnosis preliminary to full denture construction. J.A.D.A., *23*:1707, 1936.

42. Kirschner, H., and Osterlok, G.: Clinical photography in the dental practice. Quintessence International, *3*:71, 1972.

43. Kleemeier, R. W.: Behavior and organization of the bodily and external environment. In *Handbook of Aging and the Individual: Biological and Psychological Aspects.* Chicago, The University of Chicago Press, 1959.

44. Klein, I. E., Blatterfein, L., and Miglino, J. C.: Comparison of the fidelity of radiographs of mandibular condyles made by different techniques. J. Prosth. Dent., *24*:419, 1970.

45. Koper, A.: The initial interview with complete denture patients: Its structure and strategy. J. Prosth. Dent., *23*:590, 1970.

45a. ———: Human factors in prosthodontic treatment. J. Prosth. Dent., *30*:678, 1973.

46. Kraus, H.: Muscle function of the temporomandibular joint. Dent. Clin. N. Amer., *10*:553, 1966.

47. Krogh-Poulson, W. C., and Olsson, A.: Occlusal disharmonies and dysfunction of the stomatognathic system. Dent. Clin. N. Amer., November, 1966, p. 627.

47a. Kydd, W. L., Daly, C. H., and Nansen, D.: Variation in response to mechanical stress of human soft tissues as related to age. J. Prosth. Dent., *32*:493, 1974.

48. Lamont-Hauers, R. W.: Arthritis of the temporomandibular joint. Dent. Clin. N. Amer., November, 1966, p. 621.

49. Landa, J. S.: Diagnosis of the edentulous mouth and the probable prognosis of its rehabilitation. Dent. Clin. N. Amer., March, 1957, p. 187.

50. ———: The total personality in the dentist-patient relationship. New York J. Dent., *29*:80, 1959.

51. Lew, I., and Jury, K. W. M.: The subperiosteal implant and the geriatric patient. J. Amer. Soc. Geriat. Dent., *6*:3, 1971.

51a. Loiselle, R. J.: Practical approach to denture fabrication. J. Prosth. Dent., *30*:490, 1973.

52. Lovestedt, S. A.: Oral roentgenographic manifestations of systemic disease. Dent. Clin. N. Amer., July, 1958, p. 413.

53. Lyons, H.: The professional gentleman: His responsibilities. J. Am. Coll. Dent., *33*:127, 1966.

54. Mann, A. W.: Diet and nutrition in the edentulous patient. Dent. Clin. N. Am., March, 1957, p. 285.

55. ———, Spies, T. D., and Springer, M.: The oral manifestations of vitamin B complex deficiencies. J. Dent. Res., *20*:269, 1941.

56. Martone, A. L.: Clinical applications of concepts of functional anatomy and speech science to complete denture prosthodontics. VI. The diagnostic phase. J. Prosth. Dent., *12*:817, 1962.

56a. Massler, M.: Geriatric dentistry: The problem. J. Prosth. Dent., *40*:324, 1978.

57. Mehringer, E. J.: The saliva as it is related to the wearing of dentures. J. Prosth. Dent., *4*:312, 1954.

58. Miller, A. A.: Psychological considerations in dentistry. J.A.D.A., *81*:941, 1970.

58a. Miller, E. L.: Types of inflammation caused by oral prostheses. J. Prosth. Dent., *30*:380, 1973.

58b. ———: Clinical management of denture-induced inflammations. J. Prosth. Dent., *38*:362, 1977.

59. Miller, S. C.: *Oral Diagnosis and Treatment,* 3rd ed. New York, McGraw-Hill, Inc., 1957.

60. Moore, C.: Cigarette smoking and cancer of the mouth, pharynx, and larynx: A continuing study. J.A.M.A., *218*:553, 1971.

61. Moulton, R. E.: Emotional factors in nonorganic temporomandibular joint pain. Dent. Clin. N. Am., November, 1966, p. 609.

61a. Nater, J. P., Groenman, N. H., Wakkers-Garritsen, B. G., and Timmer, L. H.: Etiologic factors in denture sore mouth syndrome. J. Prosth. Dent., *40*:367, 1978.

62. National Institutes of Health: *Parkin-*

son's *Disease, Hope through Research.*
Bethesda, Maryland, National Institute
of Neurological Diseases and Stroke.

63. Neufeld, J. O.: Dentures and their supporting oral tissues. Dent. Clin. N. Am., November, 1964, p. 559.

64. Niiranen, J. V.: Diagnosis for complete dentures. J. Prosth. Dent., 4:726, 1954.

65. Nokamoto, R. Y.: Bony defects on the crest of the residual alveolar ridge. J. Prosth. Dent., 19:111, 1968.

66. Ortman, H. R.: Factors of bone resorption of the residual ridge. J. Prosth. Dent. 12:429, 1962.

67. Östlund, S. G.: Saliva and denture retention. J. Prosth. Dent., 10:658, 1960.

68. Payne, S. H.: Diagnostic factors which influence the choice of posterior occlusion. Dent. Clin. N. Am., March, 1957, p. 203.

68a. ———: Preventive prosthodontics. J. Prosth. Dent., 30:491, 1973.

68b. Perrelet, L. A., Bernhard, M., and Spirgi, M.: Panoramic radiography in examination of edentulous patients. J. Prosth. Dent., 37:494, 1977.

69. Perry, C.: Examination, diagnosis, and treatment planning. J. Prosth. Dent., 10:1004, 1960.

70. Pickett, H. G., Appleby, R. C., and Osborn, M. O.: Changes in the denture supporting tissues associated with the aging process. J. Prosth. Dent., 27:257, 1972.

70a. Pilling, L. F.: Emotional aspects of prosthodontic patients. J. Prosth. Dent., 30:514, 1973.

71. Plainfield, S.: Psychological consideration in prosthetic dentistry. Dent. Clin. N. Am., November, 1962, p. 669.

72. Pruden, W. H.: The role of study cast in diagnosis and treatment planning. J. Prosth. Dent., 10:707, 1960.

73. Ramsey, W. D.: The relation of emotional factors to prosthodontic service. J. Prosth. Dent., 23:4, 1970.

74. ———: The role of nutrition in conditions of edentulous patients. J. Prosth. Dent., 23:130, 1970.

75. *Research on First-admission Geriatric State Mental Hospital Patients.* Age,

disability and rehabilitation. Iowa City, Iowa, The Institute of Gerontology, University of Iowa, 1963.

75a. Roberts, A. L.: Prosthodontic approach to edentulous patients. J. Prosth. Dent., 30:493, 1973.

76. Robinson, H. B. G.: Neoplasms and "precancerous" lesions of the oral regions. Dent. Clin. N. Am., November, 1957, p. 621.

77. Ryan, E. J.: The dental problems of senescence. J. Prosth. Dent., 1:64, 1951.

78. Sarnat, B. G.: Developmental facial abnormalities and the temporomandibular joint. Dent. Clin. N. Am., November, 1966, p. 587.

79. Schuyler, C. H.: Elements of diagnosis leading to full or partial dentures. J.A.D.A., 41:302, 1950.

80. Schwartz, L., and Chayes, C. M.: The examination of the patient with facial pain and/or mandibular dysfunction. Dent. Clin. N. Am., November, 1966, p. 537.

81. Seifert, I.: Evaluation of psychologic factors in geriatric denture patients. J. Prosth. Dent., 12:516, 1962.

82. Shafer, W. G.: Benign tumors and cysts of the jawbones. Dent. Clin. N. Am., November, 1957, p. 693.

83. Sherwood, E. D.: Geriatrics: An emerging challenge for the health profession. The American Society for Geriatric Dentistry, January, 1971.

84. Sinick, D.: Psychologic factors in dental treatment. J. Prosth. Dent., 14:506, 1964.

85. Stahl, S. S., Wilson, J. M., and Miller, S. C.: Influence of systemic diseases on alveolar bone. J.A.D.A., 45:277, 1952.

86. Sussman, M. B., and Burchinal, L. G.: Intergenerational family continuity and economic activity. In *The Older Person in the Family: Challenges and Conflicts,* H. L. Jacobs, ed. Iowa City, Iowa, The Insititute of Gerontology, University of Iowa, 1965.

87. Swoope, C. C.: Identification and management of emotional patients. J. Prosth. Dent., 27:434, 1972.

87a. ———: Predicting denture success. J. Prosth. Dent., 30:860, 1973.

87b. ——— and Hartsook, E.: Nutrition analysis of prosthodontic patients. J. Prosth. Dent., *38:*208, 1977.

88. Tiecke, R. W.: Tumors of the tongue and the floor of the mouth. Dent. Clin. N. Am., November, 1957, p. 647.

89. Thomas, C. C.: Cutaneous disease of interest to the dentist. Dent. Clin. N. Am., July, 1958, p. 371.

89a. Tolentino, A. T.: Prosthetic management of patients with pemphigus vulgaris. J. Prosth. Dent., *38:*254, 1977.

90. Toto, P. D.: Tumors of the gingiva. Dent. Clin. N. Am., November, 1957, p. 679.

91. Ucellani, E. L.: Evaluating mucous membrane. J. Prosth. Dent., *15:*295, 1965.

92. Updegrave, W. J.: Interpretation of temporomandibular joint radiographs. Dent. Clin. N. Am., November, 1966, p. 567.

93. Vinton, P. W.: The geriatric complete denture patient. Dent. Clin. N. Am., November, 1964, p. 759.

94. Vosburg, F.: Psychoneurosis in oral diagnosis and treatment planning. J. Prosth. Dent., *26:*329, 1971.

95. Waldron, C. A.: The differential diagnosis of radiolucent areas in the jaws. Dent. Clin. N. Am., July, 1964, p. 299.

96. Weikstein, M. S.: Basic psychology and dental practice. Dent. Clin. N. Am., *14:*379, 1970.

97. ———: Practical application of basic psychiatry to dentistry. Dent. Clin. N. Am., *14:*397, 1970.

98. Weinberg, L. A.: An evaluation of duplicability of temporomandibular joint radiographs. J. Prosth. Dent., *24:*512, 1970.

99. Weinshell, E.: Psychiatric considerations of the forty-year-old denture patient. Dental Abstracts, *9:*20, 1964.

100. Weiss, A. D.: Sensory functions. In *Handbook of Aging and the Individual: Biological and Psychological Aspects.* Chicago, University of Chicago Press, 1959.

101. Wright, C. R., et al.: A study of the tongue and its relation to denture stability. J.A.D.A., *39:*269, 1949.

102. Young, H. A.: Diagnostic survey of edentulous patients. J. Prosth. Dent., *5:*5, 1955.

102a. Zakhari, K. N., and McMurry, W. S.: Denture stomatitis and methods influencing its cure. J. Prosth. Dent., *37:*133, 1977.

103. Zucker, A. H.: A psychiatric appraisal of tongue symptoms. J.A.D.A., *85:*649, 1972.

Surgical Preparation for Complete Dentures

5

The objective of this chapter is to develop an understanding of the surgical preparation of the mouth within boundaries of acceptable basic surgical techniques. The results of the surgical procedures are residual ridges and a mucosal covering free of disease and of sufficient quantity and quality to give adequate stability and retention to dentures. The prognosis for successful complete denture service is often in direct proportion to the proper preparation of the support. In the surgical preparation of the mouth for complete dentures it is necessary to have a mental picture of the ideal. A square arch with parallel walls is the ideal form for stability and retention. (Fig. 5-1).

Since the oral cavities of patients vary markedly, preparation for complete dentures sometimes becomes complicated. The preparation often requires the attention of one with special surgical interest and training. These procedures should be performed by a surgeon thoroughly familiar with the requirements for good stability and retention of a denture. Results that are surgically acceptable are not always the best suited prosthodontically. The team approach is advocated for those patients whose surgical and prosthodontic treatment is performed by different operators.

Preoperative Examination

The examination of a patient requiring surgical preparation prior to denture construction necessitates additional evaluation in the diagnostic procedures. The medical status is more carefully reviewed. The past and present therapies, the patient's idiosyncrasies, and allergic responses to medication are recorded. Care must be used to establish and rule out hemorrhagic tendencies. Additional roentgenographic study is often required. In many of these patients the success or failure depends upon patient cooperation. The *mental attitude* of the patient must be evaluated to determine whether he will accept treatment. Most of these patients are aged; it is not enough that their families desire this treatment. The patient himself must understand the extensiveness of the procedures, particularly the postoperative prosthodontic observations and adjustments. (It is well to confirm such instructions in writing.) The patient's mental attitude must be such that he not only desires the treatment but is willing to carry out the instructions in the use and care of the dentures. Patients who claim that the oral condition is a result of negligence on the part of all the dentists who have treated them should

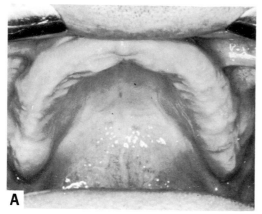

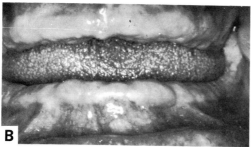

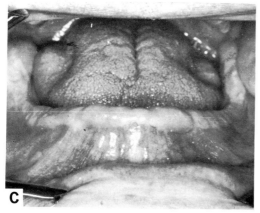

FIG. 5-1. A. *An ideal edentulous maxillary arch. Note the fullness of the residual ridge, the preservation of the cuspid eminences, the absence of undercuts in the alveolar tubercle areas, and the positions of the frenum attachments.* **B.** *These edentulous arches are ideal in shape and relation.* **C.** *An ideal edentulous mandibular arch. Note the contour of the residual ridge, the absence of undercut areas, the preservation of the integrity of the tissues in the retromolar pad and masseter groove areas, and the attachment of the frenums.*

not be accepted for treatment. Failure to participate in the discussions about treatment may indicate an indifferent attitude, which makes for an unfavorable patient. What the patient expects from dentures should be discussed; if he expects performance like the natural teeth, education is indicated. A complete understanding and acceptance of the limitations of denture performance must be accomplished before treatment. Explanations before treatment are diagnoses; those after treatment are excuses.

The patient's *physical status* should be carefully evaluated to determine any medical limitations and to establish the surgical risk. The surgical procedures may be compromised by the physical limitations of the patient. A thorough knowledge of the physical condition of a patient reduces the surgical and postoperative problems. Many systemic conditions contraindicate the use of dentures; others make for unfavorable prognosis; and still others must be controlled before denture construction.

There should be no medical or physical findings that contraindicate a planned surgical procedure. This conclusion can be reached only by a thorough physical examination. Extensive surgical procedures often require hospitalization, affording the opportunity for a more thorough evaluation of the patient's physical condition. The patient should be free of any active disease or should be in a controlled state under medical surveillance.

The medical history should be carefully reviewed, drug idiosyncrasies should be recorded, and care should be taken to delete these drugs from the treatment plan. The nature of these surgical procedures requires an investigation of the bleeding and clotting time; any discrepancies should be controlled prior to surgery. Physical standards to tolerate a general anesthetic should be met. Due to the postoperative debilitating effects of diet deficiencies, the nutritional needs should be controlled and continued postoperatively as long as necessary.

The surgical evaluation and preparation should take into account the mental preparation of the patient to reduce the emotional and physiologic shock of the surgical procedures. The patient should fully understand the reasons for the procedures, the tissue responses expected, the postoperative difficulties, and the anticipated prognosis. A good working rapport allows the patient to be an active responsible participant.

Retained Dentition

CLINICALLY EVIDENT TEETH

In the extraction of clinically evident teeth the instrumentation and detach-

ment should preserve as much of the bony and soft tissue as needed to result in a suitably contoured ridge for denture support.

ROOT TIPS

Root tips must be evaluated individually (Fig. 5-2). Those with roentgenographic evidence of pathologic change should be removed. Root tips that are covered by a millimeter of sound bone and show no roentgenographic evidence of pathologic change, especially if they have withstood denture trauma in the past, can be justifiably left in the mandible. The mandible is more highly calcified than the maxillae and the likelihood of the root tips moving or becoming a pathologic problem under a denture is slight. In the maxillary alveolar process this is not an ironclad finding because of the porosity of the bone. Large maxil-

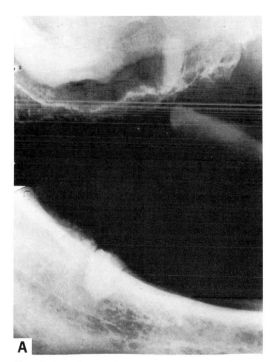

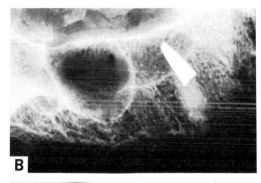

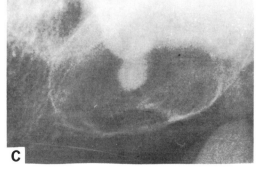

FIG. 5-2. *A roentgenographic study frequently reveals root tips.* **A.** *These roots should be removed.* **B.** *and* **C.** *These roots and the elevator tip need not be removed, but the patient should be advised of their presence.*

lary root tips that are not involving the sinus or those that can be removed without leaving a surgical defect should be prophylactically removed.

If any root tips remain, the patient should be advised of their presence, and a record of their location should be placed in the patient's chart.

UNERUPTED TEETH

Unerupted teeth in an edentulous arch or in a condemned dentition should be evaluated with several thoughts in mind: (1) evidence of associated pathologic activity, (2) the location of the unerupted tooth, (3) the age of the patient, and (4) the history of whether or not the tooth has been symptomatic. In the very elderly, any impacted tooth that is surrounded by normal bone and shows no alteration in follicular activity should

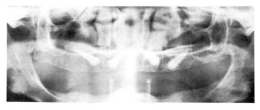

FIG. 5-3. *These unerupted cuspids are present in a maxillary arch that has supported a denture for over twenty years. The treatment plan should not include removing these teeth.*

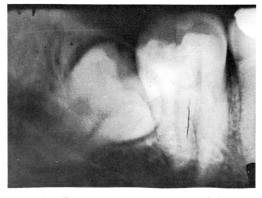

FIG. 5-4. *Roentgenogram of an ameloblastic transformation.*

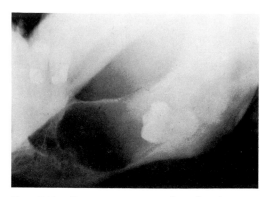

FIG. 5-5. *Roentgenogram of a dentigerous cyst. Ameloblastic transformation can lead to this cystic area.*

not be removed under a denture (Fig. 5-3).

The majority of embedded or impacted teeth usually should be removed at the time the other teeth are being removed and the mouth is being prepared for dentures. Operators of special skill and experience can remove most impacted or embedded teeth without surgically creating a large defect.

There are reasons for the removal of impacted teeth before construction of the dentures. A relatively high percentage show ameloblastic transformation (Fig. 5-4) in their early stages of development. If eruption is delayed or arrested, this transformation may result in the formation of a dentigerous cyst (Fig. 5-5). This cyst can become so large as to jeopardize the continuity of the mandible or weaken it to the extent that a pathologic fracture results. Such cysts can further differentiate into ameloblastic tumors that may require resection of the jaws before they are surgically controlled.

If an embedded or an impacted tooth is left and is covered with a denture, it should be recorded, and the patient should be made aware of its presence. Roentgenograms should be taken at reasonable intervals to be sure that no adverse results occur.

Nonpathologic Bony Conditions

ALVEOLECTOMY

The definition of an alveolectomy as it is considered here is "the surgical removal of part of the alveolar process of the upper or lower jaw." An alveolectomy is necessary in instances of alveolar fracture and where uneven interseptal or interproximal spines exist (Fig. 5-6). Opposing undercuts present obstacles to the path of insertion and removal of the denture. These undercuts should be altered or removed (Fig. 5-7). Bilateral alteration or removal is not always neces-

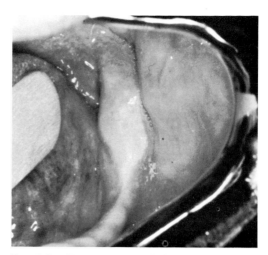

FIG. 5-8. *Examination of the lingual aspect at the posterior termination of the mylohyoid line of this patient reveals a bony tubercle, referred to as a lingual tuberosity.*

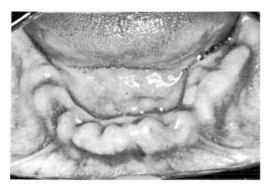

FIG. 5-6. *An edentulous mandibular residual ridge that is not considered desirable for denture insertion and removal. Note the undercut and irregular areas. To insert and remove a denture over the bony irregularities will lead to discomfort and bone destruction.*

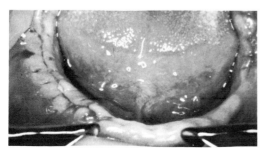

FIG. 5-7. *This edentulous mandibular residual ridge has been prepared to reduce or eliminate the undesirable undercuts.*

sary. It is important to realize that the removal of bone should be done with prudence and care because once the bone tissue is removed, it cannot be reinserted.

Although the operator can anticipate the need for alveolectomies at the time of extraction, it is not always possible to determine the extent. In patients with advanced periodontal pathosis it is best to remove the teeth and limit the alveolectomy to fractures or uneven spines, with further evaluation after both the hard and soft tissues have healed. Often areas that at the time of extraction do not appear to need contouring exhibit this need after some healing has ensued. It is best to evaluate the ridges and soft tissue response about three weeks after extractions.

In the mandibular arch an area that often requires an alveolectomy is the lingual aspect at the posterior termination of the mylohyoid line (Fig. 5-8). The denture flange should extend below this area, but not beneath it. If it extends under it, the bone will be denuded, resulting in necrosis and sequestration.

The removal of these bony projections should be bilateral.

In the atrophied mandible the alveolar process, because of the lateral resorption, presents a very thin bony ridge called "knife-edge ridge" (Fig. 5-9A and B). The overlying soft tissue is often rolled or pendulous with a fibrous base and is mobile to pressure (Fig. 5-9C). The patient complains of pain during tooth contact. In the severe instances, two things should be accomplished surgically. The knife-edged bone should be made blunt to decrease the irritability to denture pressure. The soft tissue should be stabilized by excising the roll of fibrous tissue. The surgical area should not be subjected to the trauma of a denture until it is healed. If a surgical splint is used, it should not be opposed by a functional denture.

In the maxillary arch an area that frequently requires an alveolectomy is the alveolar tubercle (Fig. 5-10). The tubercles often present opposing undercuts that present a problem in impression making and, if reproduced, interfere with the insertion and removal of the denture. If no undercuts are present in the anterior section of the arch, it is not always necessary to remove the undercuts from both tubercles. The alveolar tubercles frequently approximate the retromolar papillae and pad area to the extent that adequate denture coverage is not possible. If the bony

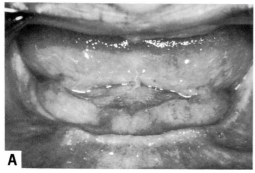

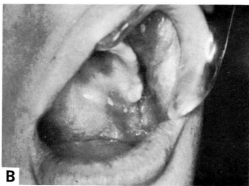

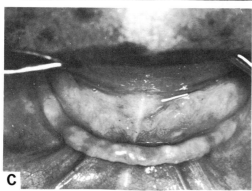

FIG. 5-9. *Studies of atrophied arches.* **A.** *The knife-edge ridge is frequently found in the mandibular arch.* **B.** *The knife-edge ridge is less frequently found in the maxillary arch.* **C.** *Pendulous or rolled soft tissues can be pinched between the denture base and bone with resulting discomfort and tissue damage.*

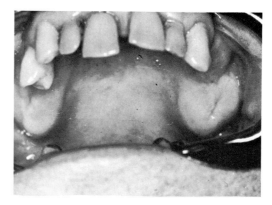

FIG. 5-10. *A maxillary arch with alveolar tubercles that can pose a problem in insertion and removal of the denture or a problem of adequate space between the tubercle and the retromolar papilla and pad.*

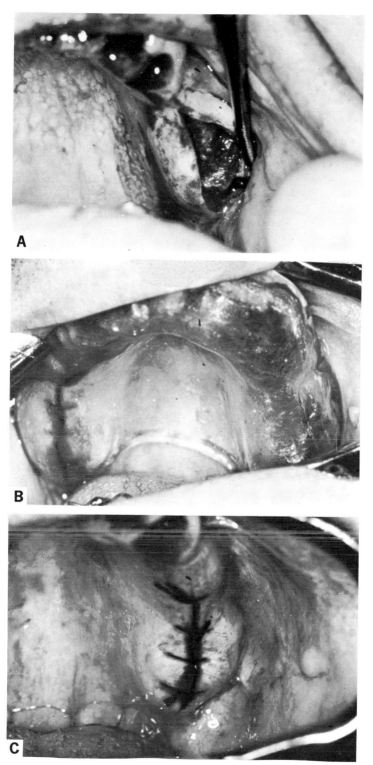

FIG. 5-11. *The surgical and prosthodontic procedures to prepare a maxillary arch for the insertion of an immediate complete maxillary denture when the bony undercuts in the anterior segments oppose bony undercuts in the alveolar tubercle areas.* **A.** *The maxillary anterior teeth are extracted, and the bony undercut areas are reduced in the alveolar tubercle areas.* **B.** *The preformed clear acrylic resin splint, provided by the prosthodontist, is used prior to the final suturing procedures.* **C.** *The left alveolar tubercle surgical site is sutured prior to denture insertion.*

tissue of the tubercle is involved and of sufficient vertical height to allow reductions, it should be reduced (Fig. 5-11). (Soft tissue involvement is discussed later.)

The surgical technique of alveolectomies requires an adequate mucoperiosteal flap to allow the removal of the bone with a minimum of trauma to the soft tissue. The alveolar process should be smoothed with a rongeur, file, and rotary bone bur. The wound should be cleansed of all debris and the mucoperiosteal flap repositioned in its anatomic position. A surgical splint will exert a positive upward force to hold the soft tissue in place and enhance healing.

TORI

Although tori and generalized bony exostoses are classified as tumors, they probably represent bony hyperostosis and are so common that they will be discussed with the nonpathologic bony conditions.

TORUS PALATINUS.   The torus palatinus is located at the junction of the palatine process of the maxillary bones in the midline of the palate. The torus may be smooth or pedunculated and covered with a mucosa that varies in quality and quantity.

Small tori that do not act as fulcrum points under a denture may not require removal. The torus, even when small, will act as a fulcrum under a denture if the mucosal covering of the crest and slopes of the ridges are displaceable to a greater extent than the mucosal covering of the torus. In these instances, the denture base over the area must be relieved to compensate for this difference or the torus should be surgically removed.

When a torus is large or grossly undercut, it should be surgically removed (Fig. 5-12). The surgical technique re-

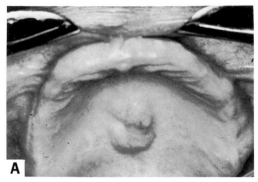

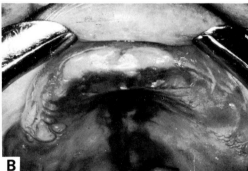

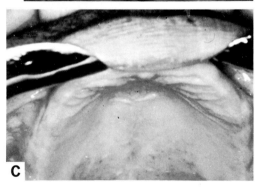

FIG. 5-12.   *Procedure in preparing a maxillary arch with a large torus. The use of a surgical splint is advocated when the maxillary torus is removed.* **A.** *Preoperative.* **B.** *Splint in place.* **C.** *Sixth day postoperative.*

quires careful reflection of a midline mucoperiosteal flap laterally because this mucosa is often very thin, tears readily, and has a poor blood supply. The poor healing qualities of this tissue necessitate the mechanical support and protection of a surgical splint. The splint should be constructed before surgery and should fit accurately and be extended and contoured like a finished denture. The splint acts as a bandage, a training device, and later as the individualized impression tray.

TORUS MANDIBULARIS.   This bony growth is found on the lingual cortical surface of the mandible; it is usually of bilateral growth and is located in the bicuspid area (Fig. 5-13). The tori vary in size and shape. The mucosal covering is usually thin. The tori should be removed prior to denture construction, as a relief in the denture base rarely suffices for comfort. As a rule the patient will not tolerate the denture. The reflection of the mucoperiosteal flap should be adequate in size, and care should be exercised not to traumatize the flap. The torus is removed with rotary bone burs or chisels. A smooth bony base, devoid of undercuts, should result. A surgical splint is not usually necessary because the mucoperiosteal covering can be readapted; it is vascular and heals rapidly. Usually denture construction procedures are not delayed more than five or six days. With a careful suturing technique and digital pressure approximately fifteen or twenty minutes after the procedure, the mucoperiosteal flap repositions itself very quickly. The normal position and weight of the tongue help to maintain the tissue in its anatomical position.

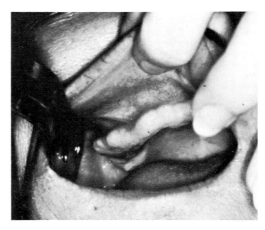

FIG. 5-14. *Areas of exostosis on this patient's maxillae present objectionable undercuts and multiple undesirable fulcrum points under a denture.*

GENERALIZED EXOSTOSIS

Exostoses are bony nodules located on the alveolar process of the mandible and the maxillae. The buccal aspect in the molar region of the mandible and the buccal aspect from the bicuspids posteriorly to the alveolar tubercle in the maxillae are the more frequent locations (Fig. 5-14). These exostoses usually present undercuts to the path of insertion and removal of the denture and should be removed by alveolectomy techniques. In the majority of these operations, no surgical splints are required, as the thickness of the mucosal covering permits adequate stabilization by suturing.

Soft Tissue

ALVEOLAR TUBERCLE AREA

Frequently the alveolar tubercle area that approximates the retromolar papilla or pad is composed primarily of fibrous connective tissue. Many tubercle areas that do not approximate the retromolar papilla or pad are pendulous. The pendulous area does not offer a stable base

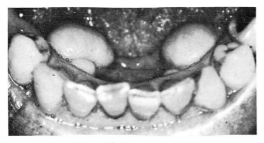

FIG. 5-13. *Mandibular tori such as these rarely support a denture comfortably.*

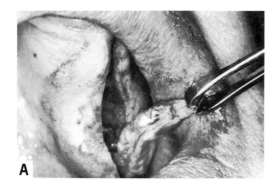

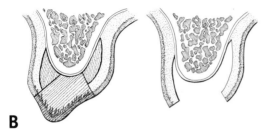

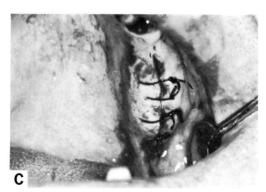

FRENUMS

The maxillary and mandibular *labial* and *buccal* frenums can present undesirable situations if they are attached too near the crest of the residual alveolar ridge. If the labial frenum has been irritated by a pre-existing denture and has become hyperplastic, it interferes with the border extension and presents an unstable base for a denture.

A frenectomy accomplishes two important results: (1) the procedure allows border extension, and (2) it releases a mobile band of tissue that is in contact with the denture. A frenectomy is the treatment of choice rather than a "Z-plasty" or frenotomy because not only is the release of the tension on the frenum important, but also the detachment of the frenum from the attached gingiva is necessary (Fig. 5-16). A surgical splint

FIG. 5-15. **A.** *Removal of soft tissue in the alveolar tubercle area.* **B.** *Diagram of the surgical procedure: wedge incision, left; undermining the mucosa, leaving the periosteum attached to the alveolar bone, right.* **C.** *The lateral and medial mucosal segments are fixed with sutures. A surgical splint is not necessary.*

for a denture. In both of these conditions, the fibrous or pendulous tissue should be removed by a series of wedging incisions (Fig. 5-15A, and B). Suturing is usually adequate to hold the tissues in close approximation for healing (Fig. 5-15C).

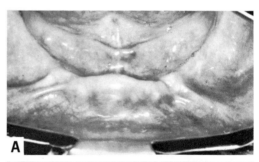

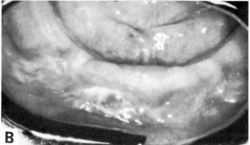

FIG. 5-16. **A.** *Preoperative view of a mandibular edentulous residual ridge that presents a fulcrum point in the midline and buccal frenum attachments that are undesirable for denture stability.* **B.** *The midline fulcrum point and the frenums have been removed by surgical procedures.*

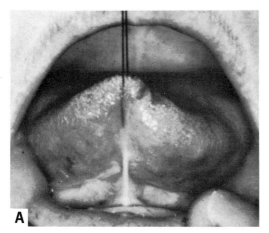

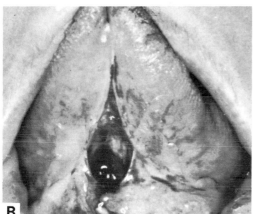

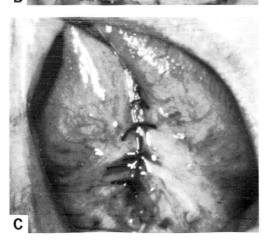

FIG. 5-17. *A frenectomy is the treatment of choice for the lingual frenum that is attached in an unfavorable position. **A.** The tongue is elevated with a suture. **B.** The frenum is removed. **C.** The surgical site is sutured.*

is not needed with the frenectomy unless a sulcus extension is performed. The frenectomy should be anticipated prior to denture insertion, and the denture flange should be contoured to occupy the space that is created.

LINGUAL FRENUM

The *lingual frenum* should always be carefully evaluated because in some instances of excessive alveolar resorption the genioglossus muscle could be mistaken for a high frenum attachment. If the attachment results in a partial ankyloglossia, a simple release (frenotomy) is sufficient surgery (Fig. 5-17). However, a wide band attachment that is strong and resistant to displacement when the tongue is elevated will necessitate an alveolar detachment as an additional dissection.

Individual isolated muscle origins that interfere with border extension, provided they are not extensive, can often be handled with single transverse excisions and suturing the detached muscle at a more desirable vestibular level. The released tissue should be sutured through the firm attached tissue at the base of the incision to assure firm immobilization (Fig. 5-18).

Benign Pathologic Soft Tissue

LIPS

The lips of denture patients should be devoid of fissures, ulceration, or masses before denture procedures. The extension of the lips during the fabricating procedure and while using dentures indicates the need for the removal of all pathologic tissues prior to denture construction. Any unhealed soft tissue ulceration that remains two weeks after a mechanical etiology should be biopsied for diagnosis (Fig. 5-19). The most common pathology of the lips includes

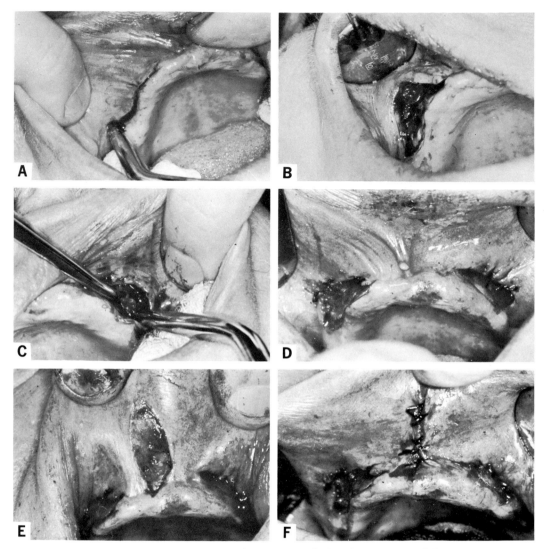

FIG. 5-18.   *Correction to provide a satisfactory vestibular fornix for stability and retention of the maxillary denture.* **A.** *Single transverse incision.* **B.** *Muscle attachment exposed.* **C.** *Muscle detached from the periosteum.* **D.** *The muscle sutured at the desired position.* **E.** *Labial frenum removed.* **F.** *Sutures in place.*

papilloma, mucocele, scar tissue, hyper-keratosis, lichen planus, epidermoid carcinoma, hemangioma, irritation fibroma, recurrent aphthous ulcer, and recurrent herpes labialis.

HYPERPLASIA OF ORAL MUCOSA

Inflammatory fibrous hyperplasia of the alveolar mucosa (epulis fissuratum) is usually a result of denture irritation and frequently is seen about the anterior vestibule when the patient has natural mandibular anterior teeth opposing a complete maxillary denture (Fig. 5-20). It is also seen in this same area when patients have received an immediate complete maxillary denture and have used it until the resorption results in labial flange irritation.

Inflammatory hyperplasia of the

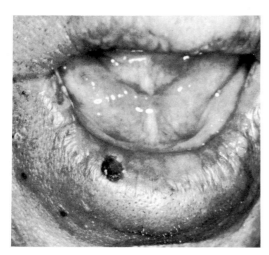

FIG. 5-19. *Soft tissue ulceration. The patient stated that the sore resulted from a cigarette wrapper sticking to his lip ten days before. The surgical biopsy revealed a malignant tumor.*

palatal mucosa (papillomatosis) is frequently observed under ill-fitting maxillary dentures, especially those having an unnecessary relief chamber (Fig. 5-21).

These two hyperplastic reactions of the oral mucosa are usually painless and often well advanced before professional treatment is sought. The treatment consists of (1) the removal of the irritant for tissue recovery, and (2) surgical removal by excision or cautery.

The use of an accurate fitting nonfunctional surgical splint is indicated when the inflammatory fibrous hyperplasia is excised. The splint serves to stabilize the tissue during the healing stage and to mold the vestibular fornix. The removable surgical splint is not necessary after excision of hyperplastic palatal mucosa if cauterization is used. Often the irritation, even of a well-constructed removable prosthesis, offsets the advantage of covering the surgical site.

HYPERKERATOSIS WITHOUT DYSKERATOSIS

The only true means to differentiate between hyperkeratosis and dyskeratosis

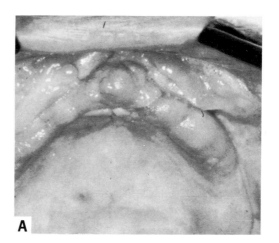

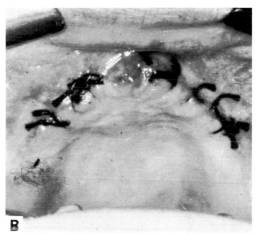

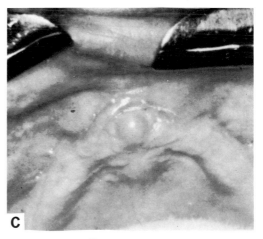

FIG. 5-20. *Inflammatory hyperplasia in the maxillary labial vestibule. Biting with the anterior teeth can produce this reaction.* **A.** *Preoperative.* **B.** *Surgical procedures.* **C.** *Postoperative.*

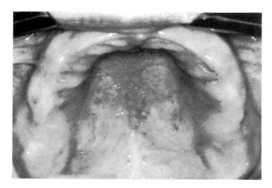

Fig. 5-21. *The papillomatous type of hyperplasia is not easily eradicated without surgical procedures. The pathologic change is not reversible.*

is by surgical biopsy and histologic examination. Areas of hyperkeratosis associated in or near the weight-bearing area of the denture should be removed if they are small enough to be excised as an excision biopsy. Large or small diffused areas should be microscopically diagnosed and should be removed if associated with the peripheral extension or the denture-bearing area. In most instances removal can be satisfactorily handled by a stripping technique with a low intensity electrocautery wire. The areas that are not surgically treated should be noted and monitored frequently by the dentist, and any clinical change in the appearance would indicate another biopsy of the lesion.

LICHEN PLANUS

Lichen planus is a white plaque-like lesion closely resembling hyperplasia of the oral mucosa (Fig. 5-22). The buccal mucosa is the most common site in the mouth, and it is thought to be caused by debilitating disorders and anxiety. It is important to differentiate between this lesion and dyskeratosis and this is best done by a biopsy. Once the diagnosis of lichen planus has been made, it is not necessary to treat this patient further surgically but rather to try to improve the oral hygiene and treat the patient

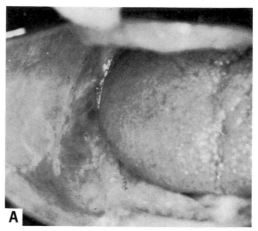

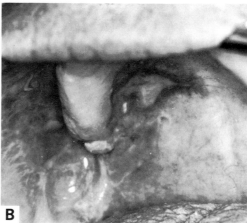

Fig. 5-22. *Lichen planus.* **A.** *This type presents no problem in denture use.* **B.** *This erosive type prevents the use of dentures for this patient.*

symptomatically. Dentures are not contraindicated for these patients, but patients affected with the erosive form of this disease may have difficulty with dentures. Dentures help improve general health, as the ability to masticate is improved.

MUCOCELES AND RETENTION CYSTS

Mucoceles and retention cysts are the result of the mucous retention phenomenon. Mucoceles are described as diffuse or well-circumscribed mucous pools in the connective tissue stroma without an epithelial lining. Retention cysts are mucous pools that are lined by epithelium, e.g., intraductal. They are often soft and fluctuant but may be firm. They are usually not fixed and are painless (Fig. 5-23). They are often traumatically ruptured and usually recur. Surgical excision is indicated for the removal of these cysts, with exception of the large retention cysts located in the floor of the mouth and more often called *ranulas*. Because of the size and depth of a ranula, complete removal by excision is often impossible, and in these patients a marsupialization is indicated. Often the original examination of an edentulous patient with marked alveolar resorption reveals that the structures of the floor of the mouth actually fold over the alveolar process, giving the impression of a ranula. Digital examination will help in differentiating between the two conditions.

DERMOID CYST

The dermoid cyst is also located in the floor of the mouth and often is confused with a ranula. It is usually in the mid-

line, however, and the ranulas are usually located laterally in the submental space. This cyst usually has a much firmer wall and is more easily enucleated surgically than a ranula, and excision is the treatment of choice. A dermoid cyst seldom recurs if excision is complete.

PAPILLOMAS AND FIBROMAS

Papillomas and fibromas are rather common benign neoplasms of the oral mucosa (Fig. 5-24). The *papilloma* is

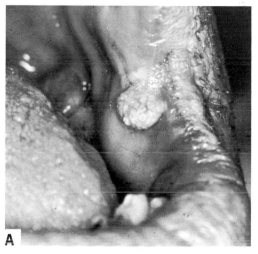

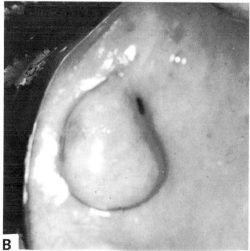

FIG. 5-24. **A.** *A papilloma. Notice the cauliflower-like surface.* **B.** *A fibroma that should be excised.*

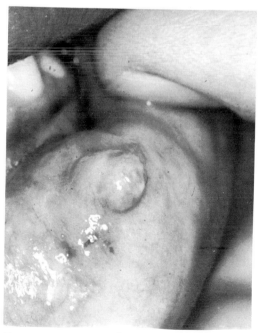

FIG. 5-23. *A retention cyst that should be surgically removed.*

usually pedunculated, and its surface may be described as cauliflower-like. A *fibroma* is usually pedunculated too, but its surface is smooth and appears to be normal mucosa. The papilloma is of surface epithelial origin. The fibroma is comprised of connective tissue. Both of these tumors should be excised before denture construction.

Bony Pathology (Nonmalignant)

BONY CYST

Any cystlike lesion should be surgically explored, and a pathologic diagnosis made (Fig. 5-25). The traumatic bone cyst often seen in the body of the mandible in the bicuspid and molar area is painless and usually discovered by roentgenography. A surgical approach to the area should be made, designing the approach so that the surgical defect is minimal. On opening into the area, one usually finds a void in the portion of the bone with no epithelial lining. In this instance, the wound should be debrided and closed, and prosthodontic treatment continued.

CYSTS OF ODONTOGENIC ORIGIN

Cysts of odontogenic origin are more commonly seen in the mandible than in the maxillae (Fig. 5-26); however, they do appear in both jaws. A dentigerous cyst or a follicular cyst associated with impacted or embedded teeth may grow rather large, causing marked bone destruction and jeopardizing the denture base. These cystic growths are best surgically managed by enucleation. Occasionally the marsupialization technique is indicated first to reduce the pressure of the cyst, to allow shrinkage and bone fill-in, and to prevent a surgical fracture; then as shrinkage allows, enucleation is performed at a later date. Large infected dentigerous cysts should be enucleated. The resulting wound is then saucerized, packed, and permitted to heal by secondary intention. As granulation progresses, the dressings are necessarily reduced in size. Because of the propensity for these cysts to undergo ameloblastic transformation, they should all be examined histologically.

The apical and lateral periodontal cyst and residual cyst are likewise handled surgically whenever possible, depending upon their size and location. The construction of dentures should be

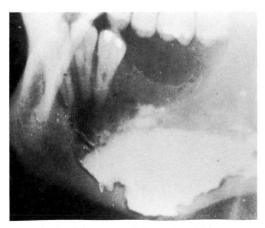

FIG. 5-25. *A bony cyst that should be investigated by surgical means.*

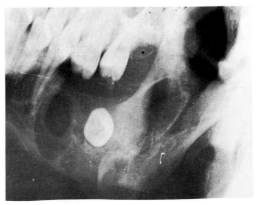

FIG. 5-26. *Roentgenogram of cysts of odontogenic origin in the mandible.*

delayed until the overlying mucous membrane is well epithelialized.

A follicular cyst may show ameloblastic change in the cyst lining; and if this becomes far advanced before the diagnosis and treatment, usually a large block of bone has to be dissected to control or eradicate this tumor. An ameloblastoma is not an encapsulated tumor; it is locally infiltrative and therefore has to be treated more radically with a larger bone dissection. An exception to this rule is the adenoameloblastoma, which is usually well encapsulated and appears cystic on a roentgenogram.

CYSTS OF
NONODONTOGENIC ORIGIN

Cysts of nonodontogenic origin result from proliferation of embryonic material at fusion sites of the jaw (Fig. 5-27). These developmental cysts are the nasolabial cysts, median palatal cysts, incisal canal cysts, and globulomaxillary cysts. These cysts should also be surgically managed, enucleated prior to construction of the denture, as they are slow growing and may perforate into the oral cavity and become contaminated and infected. They grow at the expense of the bony structures that are the base of the denture, and the earlier they are surgically controlled, the less bone loss and hence a better denture base.

MISCELLANEOUS LESIONS

Other radiolucent lesions noted in the mandible ought to be surgically explored, diagnosed, and treated as indicated. The most common of these are the central giant-cell tumors, the early cementomas, and the isolated eosinophilic granulomas.

NONODONTOGENIC
BENIGN LESIONS

The myxoma, osteoma, osteoblastoma, ossifying fibroma, aneurysmal bone cyst, fibrous dysplasia, and rarely the chondroma are nonodontogenic lesions that may be found in the jaws. They require surgical treatment and management before denture construction (Fig. 5-28). In handling these benign lesions, the operator should attempt to leave a residual ridge that will be satisfactory for a denture support. These lesions should be treated conservatively (e.g., currettage) whenever possible; however the definitive surgical care is dictated by the nature and extent of the clinical problem.

ODONTOGENIC TUMORS
OF THE JAWS

Odontogenic tumors of the jaws are classified by Thoma and Goldman* as ectodermal—the ameloblastomas—mesenchymal—the odontogenic myxoma and fibroma and the cementoma—and mixed—the ameloblastofibroma and odontoma. These lesions are essentially treated surgically and rather conserva-

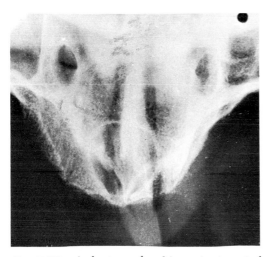

FIG. 5-27. *A denture should not be inserted until this incisal canal cyst is eradicated.*

*Thoma, K. H., and Goldman, H. M.: Odontogenic tumors; classification based on observations of epithelial, mesenchymal, and mixed varieties. Amer. J. Path., 22:433, 1946.

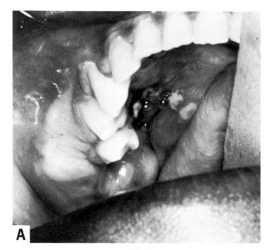

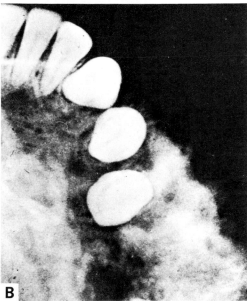

FIG. 5-28. *Benign bony lesions like this fibrous dysplasia should be treated prior to denture construction.* **A.** *Intraoral view.* **B.** *Roentgenogram of the area.*

tively with the exception of the ameloblastoma, which has the ability to grow rather rapidly. Marked bone destruction often requires a bony resection for surgical control as indicated in our earlier discussion. All of these tumors cannot be diagnosed by roentgenography alone, inasmuch as they may often be multilocular and mimic each other.

They require a pathologic diagnosis by biopsy techniques. A maxillofacial prosthodontist should be consulted when surgical procedures will be extensive.

Other Osteolytic Lesions

GAUCHER'S DISEASE; NIEMANN-PICK DISEASE

Acute cases of Gaucher's disease and Niemann-Pick disease, which are disturbances of the lipid metabolism, may result in osteolytic lesions of the jaws. However, inasmuch as these patients seldom reach maturity, it is unusual to see a patient with this disease becoming a prosthetic problem. Diagnosis is made by a microscopic examination of the tissue.

PAGET'S DISEASE (OSTEITIS DEFORMANS)

Since Paget's disease is most common after the age of 40, prosthetic patients may manifest symptoms of this disease. It has been noted by many dentists that this disease has a predilection for the maxillae. The X-ray findings will vary, depending upon whether the disease is in an osteolytic or osteoblastic stage. Both stages may appear simultaneously, producing the classic "cotton wool" appearance radiographically. This disease is diagnosed by characteristic blood chemistry changes, such as an increase in the alkaline phosphatase level, and microscopic alterations in the bone pattern. When the maxillae are involved, the teeth become loose and spaced wider apart. There is no known medical treatment, but a number of the cases develop into osteogenic sarcoma. These patients become candidates for dentures early in life, and their jaws grossly expand, necessitating the remaking of dentures to compensate for this growth. This should be explained to the patient prior to treatment.

HYPERPARATHYROIDISM

Osteitis fibrosa cystica, now more often called hyperparathyroidism, also must be differentiated from other osteoporotic lesions of the jaws. It is identified by making a diagnosis of hyperparathyroidism with its characteristic blood and urine chemistry changes. The increased presence of the parathyroid hormone causes an increase in the blood calcium and a lowering of the blood phosphorus levels. This is accompanied by an increase in both the calcium and phosphorus found in the urine. The loss of these minerals results in an increased bone resorption. As this disease progresses, lesions develop that are designated as "brown tumors" of hyperparathyroidism. Brown tumors histologically are indistinguishable from the central or peripheral giant cell granuloma of the jaws.

HYPERTHYROIDISM

Hyperthyroidism is characterized by an excess secretion of thyroxin with most of its symptoms originating from an increased metabolism. This is manifested by the patients showing an increased basal metabolic rate, being nervous, having loss of weight, and showing marked perspiration. In advanced cases there is evidence of alveolar atrophy.

FIBROUS DYSPLASIA

Fibrous dysplasia is of unknown etiology. The jaws may be enlarged and the teeth are malpositioned. Generally there are no changes in the serum calcium and phosphorus. On roentgenographic examination the affected bone will show a mottled, ground glass appearance. Depending on age, surgical correction may be the treatment of choice.

OTHER DISEASES

Some other diseases of systemic origin that cause a change in the roentgenograms of the jaws should be noted and then referred for treatment. The prosthodontist should be aware of his responsibility in this field. Among these diseases are condensing osteitis, Albers-Schönberg disease, the rather often seen osteomyelitis, and the seldom seen actinomycosis.

Procedures for Specialists

Certain surgical procedures in preparing the mouth for complete dentures should be delegated to practitioners of special interest and training in oral surgery and prosthodontics. Areas for special concern are the residual alveolar ridges of the mandibular and maxillary arches.

RESIDUAL ALVEOLAR RIDGE

Not all patients who present for treatment with extensive loss or absence of the residual alveolar ridge or ridges should be condemned to an existence without dentures. This condition, which is becoming more evident as life expectancy increases, is more frequently encountered in the mandibular arch than in the maxillary. With the loss of alveolar ridge the origins of some of the muscles attached to the mandible and maxillae become intimately involved with the denture borders. The bony landmarks also present limiting problems to adequate denture border extensions.

The surgical and prosthetic evaluation, splint design, and treatment are executed as a combined effort by the prosthodontist and the oral surgeon. The desirable result is a base that will offer stability and retention. Stability is the more important. Excessive retention often permits patients with dentures to perform functions that could be most damaging to the supporting tissues; therefore, excessive vertical height is not desired. Factors furnishing the maximum stability are broad support, frenum attachments that do not encroach on the crest or slope of the support, a definite vestibular fornix devoid of muscle attachments, and a mucous membrane covering of equal resiliency. Prior to discussing with the patient plans for surgery or prosthodontic treatment, the prosthodontist and the oral surgeon should conduct a joint evaluation and correlate the findings.

The *dental history* is of considerable concern, as the etiology of the excessive loss of residual ridge may be determined. An examination of any existing prosthesis may furnish an index to patient tolerance and/or physiologic tolerance of the support. Past dental history, as related by the patient, is a good method for determining the type of patient— philosophical, exacting, indifferent, or hysterical. Indifferent and hysterical patients should not be accepted for treatment. If the patient has been edentulous for a period of years, without prosthetic restorations, the prognosis is unfavorable.

The *local findings* should be evaluated by a complete roentgenographic study, accurately articulated study casts, and a visual and digital examination of the soft and hard tissues. The Panorex is an excellent screening device and will furnish information regarding the vertical height of the existing bony support, the position of the mandibular canal, the mental foramina, and the general contour of the bone (Fig. 5-29).

The accurately articulated study casts are necessary not only in the analysis of maxillomandibular relationships and interocclusal distance but also in the fabrication of the surgical splints. Occlusion rims properly contoured and adjusted on the articulated cast are most helpful in predetermining the esthetic results.

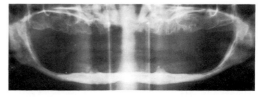

FIG. 5-29. *A Panorex screening to evaluate the bony topography of a patient with atrophied jaws. Note the loss of vertical residual alveolar ridge and the contour of basal bone in the buccal shelf areas.*

Palpation and visual examination of the soft tissues determine the resistance, positions, and extent of the attachments. In the mandibular arch, the muscles of particular concern are the mentalis, quadratus labii inferioris, depressor anguli oris, genioglossus, geniohyoid, mylohyoid, and buccinator; in the maxillary, the buccinator, levator anguli oris, and quadratus labii superioris.

The contour, position, and character of the genial tubercles, the mylohyoid line, and the external oblique line are palpated. Undercut areas are noted, particularly those distolingual to the mandibular bicuspids. The tissue covering in the maxillary anterior region may be hypertrophied, pendulous, and excessively displaceable. The fibrous bands, if present in this displaceable tissue, can be palpated, and they act as irritants under a denture.

Surgical splints are used in the treatment of these patients to mold soft tissues, to hold the attachments in their new positions, and to protect the underlying de-epithelized surfaces. The extension of the splints is preplanned and designed by the oral surgeon and the prosthodontist (Fig. 5-30).

The tonus of the tissues determines the material of choice in the impression making for the splint. If the attached tissues lack tonus and are easily displaced, adequate extension for the splint can be produced with an impression

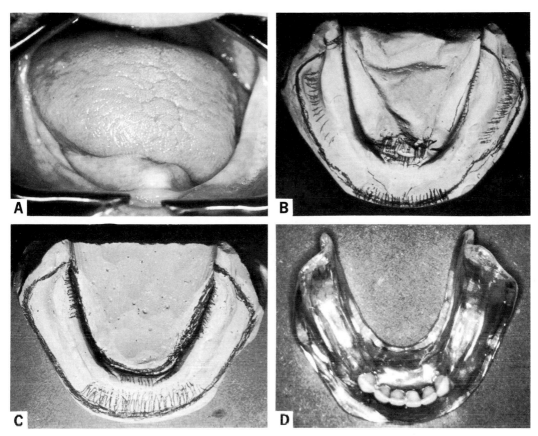

FIG. 5-30. **A.** *Intraoral photographs are valuable in designing surgical splints.* **B.** *The cast is outlined for altering.* **C.** *The altered cast.* **D.** *The surgical splint.*

compound in a slightly overextended impression tray. The impression should extend to the desired border positions. In areas where displacement is not desired, some of the impression compound should be removed, and a refined impression of a free flowing material should be used.

If the attached tissues are not displaceable and overextended, the impression is made with either a reversible or irreversible hydrocolloid. Stone casts are made and altered to the desired border positions.

The material of choice, clear methyl methacrylate resin, is processed. The splint should be accurately adapted for stability. The tissue surfaces should be smooth; the borders should be rounded and polished. The posterior segments should be designed for controlled pressure, contacting evenly in centric occlusion on polished flat occlusal ramps. These ramps should not be designed for mastication, and the patient should be so instructed. Anterior teeth may be placed in the splint for esthetic reasons. If circumferential wire pins or screws are used for the mechanical fixation, holes are placed through the ramp at the base.

MANDIBULAR ARCH

There are four areas in the mandibular arch of special concern. These areas are (1) the labial vestibule, (2) the posterior lingual sulcus, (3) the distobuccal flange, and (4) the anterior lingual flange.

LABIAL VESTIBULE.   The anterior sulcus extension begins from slightly anterior to the mental foramen to the same relative position on the opposite side of the arch. The origins of the mentalis, quadratus labii inferioris, and depressor anguli oris are usually involved. Of the several techniques in this extension, the following are used:

1. The *anterior sulcus slide* is per-

formed by making a horizontal incision along the flexible line of the mucosa at the junction of the attached and unattached gingiva (Fig. 5-31A,B).

Care should be exercised not to expose the periosteum. With sharp dissection the muscle attachments are severed, and the dissection carried to the depth of the predetermined peripheral extension (Fig. 5-31C). The epithelized mucosa on the anterior aspect of the incision is undermined, reinserted, and sutured at the depth of the new sulcus (Fig. 5-31D).

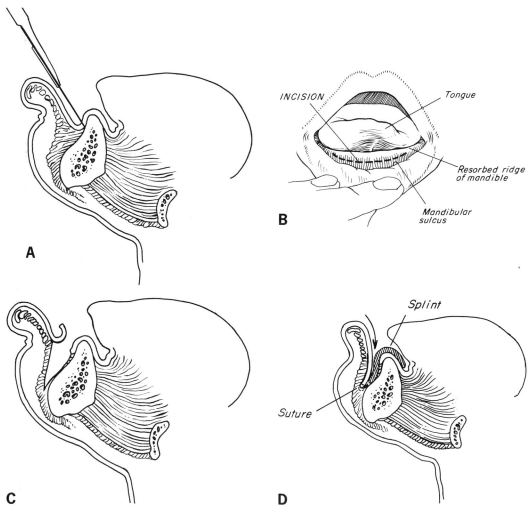

FIG. 5-31.   *Diagrams of a mandibular anterior sulcus slide. Initial incision:* **A,** *midsagittal section;* **B,** *anteroposterior view.* **C.** *Inferior extent of the incision (midsagittal section).* **D.** *Suturing and splint insertion (midsagittal section).*

A surgical splint is inserted and stabilized bilaterally with circumferential wiring in the bicuspid area or with metal screws in the molar area. The methods of mechanically fixing a surgical splint are circumferential wiring, pins, or metal screws. The method used is determined by the thickness and contour of the bone and varies with each patient.

2. The *reverse anterior sulcus slide* is indicated in patients requiring any bone surgery in the area. The incision is made to the lip side of the sulcus (Fig. 5-32A). Care is exercised to preserve the anterior extension of the mental nerve. The extent of the incision is from the cuspid to cuspid area and a thick mucosal flap is reflected posteriorly. After the osseous surgery is completed, the muscle attachments are severed, and the flaps are repositioned in a sliding technique (Fig. 5-32B). The de-epithelized surface is on the lip side. The reverse anterior sulcus slide technique does not require a surgical splint if care is taken in approximating and collapsing the mucoperiosteal flap. This flap should be sutured into the depth of the sulcus extension. If the flap requires further immobilization, small tack stitches are indicated midway between the alveolar crest and the sulcus extension (Fig. 5-32C).

The *mucosal graft* is an autogenous graft from the buccal vestibule extended to the area requiring sulcus extension. The technique involves the sulcus slide and the placing of the graft. The oversized mucosal graft is thinned by "defatting" the underside prior to insertion. The graft edges are fixed into the recipient edges with deep sutures. The advantage of this technique is that the denuded area is immediately covered by epithelized tissue. The disadvantages are that it creates two surgical sites, grafts break down, and it prohibits the use of a molding splint. The pressure of a splint may cause a delay in the proliferation of the blood supply to the graft.

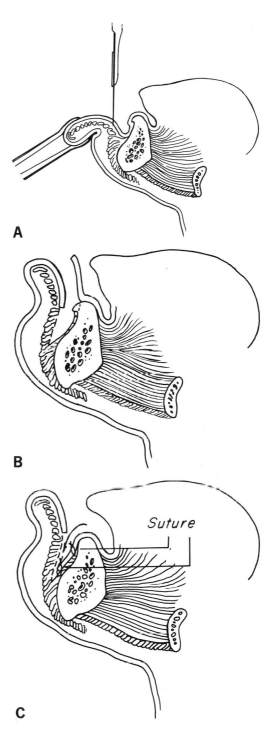

FIG. 5-32. *Diagrams of a mandibular reverse anterior sulcus slide (midsagittal section).* **A.** *Initial section.* **B.** *Inferior extent of the incision and alveoplasty.* **C.** *Location of sutures.*

POSTERIOR LINGUAL SULCUS. The *posterior lingual sulcus extension* is performed by making an anteroposterior midline incision following the residual ridge (Fig. 5-33A). The incision begins distal to the retromolar pad and extends approximately to the mental foramen (Fig. 5-33B). The mucosa and mucoperiosteal flap are reflected lingually until the attachment of the mylohyoid muscle is exposed. The overlying mucosa is stripped to approximately one-half centimeter lingually; this allows full mobility of the overlying mucosa (Fig. 5-33C). With sharp dissection the mylohyoid muscle is detached from its distal origin, extending to the bicuspid area. Inferior to the muscle is a layer of fatty tissue; this is a definite surgical landmark. The posterior extension and inferior extension depend upon the limitations imposed by the other anatomical entities in the area. If the mylohyoid and/or the external oblique lines are objectionable in contour or sharpness, they should be rounded with a rotary bone bur and hand files. Finally, the mucosa is sutured into position along the original incision line.

A peripherally extended surgical splint is then placed with mechanical fixation (Fig. 5-34). A roentgenograph can be made to evaluate a splint for position when the splint material is radiopaque acrylic resin.

DISTOBUCCAL FLANGE.   One of the most neglected areas in the mandible is the *lateral posterior vestibule.* If the buccal shelf is not covered with a prosthesis, or if marked alveolar resorption exists in the absence of the prosthesis, the buccinator muscle collapses. Failure to utilize this area properly in the presence of a prosthesis often results in inversion of the residual ridge with the forming of a trough. The external oblique line becomes prominent, or in some instances the entire buccal cortical aspect is lost

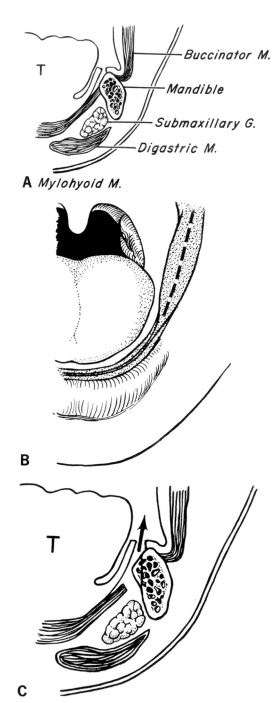

FIG. 5-33. *Diagrams of a posterior lingual sulcus extension (T = tongue). Initial incision:* **A,** *frontal section;* **B,** *anteroposterior view.* **C.** *Mylohyoid muscle detached and bone contoured (arrow = direction of removal of sharp mylohyoid bony ridge).*

as denture support. At times the buccinator muscle is found overlying the mylohyoid line. This area can be made readily available for denture support by the *buccinator muscle push-back technique.*

An anteroposterior midline incision following the crest of the residual ridge is made from the retromolar pad to the

cuspid area. A lateral oblique line incision from the most posterior point of the midline incision is carried laterally and superiorly for approximately a centimeter to give further relief and to allow a mucosal anterior advancement to give more depth to the buccinator vestibule when the splint is inserted (Fig. 5-35). A full thickness of periosteal flap is reflected laterally, care being exercised to preserve the mental nerve. The mucoperiosteal flap is reflected to or near the lateral inferior border of the mandible (Fig. 5-36A). If the external oblique line

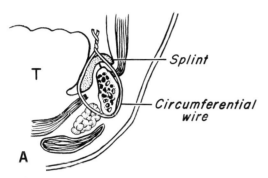

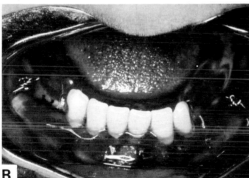

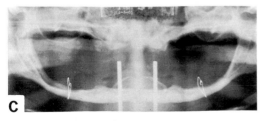

FIG. 5-34. *A mandibular splint for a posterior lingual sulcus extension.* **A.** *Diagram of a circumferential wire* to retain the splint.* **B.** *Photograph of a splint in position.* **C.** *A roentgenograph of a splint that is not radiopaque.*

* Mersilene suture has replaced the wire for splint fixation.

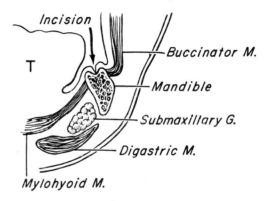

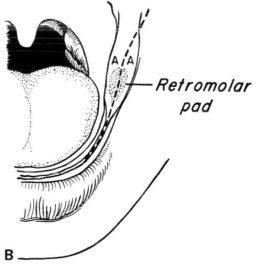

FIG. 5-35. *Diagrams of the initial incision for a distobuccal vestibular extension.* **A.** *Frontal section* (T = tongue). **B.** *Anteroposterior view.*

presents problems in contouring or sharpness, it should be altered with rotary bone burs and hand files. The mucosa is undermined along the lateral edge of the initial incision and the mucosa is advanced anteriorly and sutured (Fig. 5-36B). This relieves the tension of the incision and allows the flange of the splint to be inserted over the external oblique line thereby creating the buccal sulcus (Fig. 5-36C). In this technique a surgical splint must be used and the lateral aspect should be extended over this buccal shelf. This splint should be mechanically fixed.

ANTERIOR LINGUAL FLANGE.   The *anterior lingual sulcus* extension involves the genioglossus and geniohyoid muscles and the genial tubercles. If this tubercle is

prominent and becomes a fulcrum for denture displacement or if the genioglossus muscle is prominent and there is no lingual sulcus, one should carefully evaluate whether this procedure would be helpful. The loss of a genial sulcus may allow excessive anterior displacement of the denture during tongue and masticatory movements. A midline incision is made just lingual to the height of the ridge (Fig. 5-37), and the mucoperiosteal flap is reflected lingually and posteriorly. The genial tubercle is exposed, and the dissection is carried laterally on either side to its inferior length. With blunt dissection the attachments of the genioglossus muscle are separated from the more deeply attached fibers of the geniohyoid muscle. Anatomically this may be one group of muscle

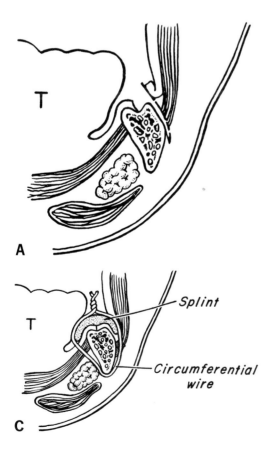

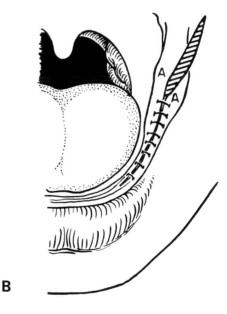

FIG. 5-36.   *Diagrams of distobuccal vestibular extension (T = tongue). **A.** Mucosal reflection and muscle detachment (frontal section). **B.** Mucosal anterior advancement and suturing (anteroposterior view). **C.** Circumferential wire to retain splint in position (frontal section).*

attachments. The genioglossus is tagged with a heavy silk suture under tension and is then detached from the genial tubercle. Then it is carried to the belly of the geniohyoid and sutured into the muscle (Fig. 5-37B). This allows a physiologic contraction of the muscle that has been severed. If indicated, the genial tubercle is removed with rotary burs and hand files. The wound is debrided and closed at its original incision site. A surgical splint is placed and mechanically fixed and circumferential wires are passed around the mandible bilaterally in the bicuspid area (Fig. 5-37C).

MAXILLARY ARCH

There are two areas in the maxillary arch of special concern. These areas are the (1) buccinator sulcus and (2) the labial vestibule.

BUCCINATOR SULCUS. The buccinator sulcus in the maxillary arch can be extended; however, the maxillary sulcus requires less surgical management than the mandibular, as the palate greatly enhances retention of a denture. A relief incision runs parallel to the maxillary crest just above the mucoflexure line (Fig. 5-38A). The surgical splint is extended into the area (Fig. 5-38B). The nature of this extension often requires splint alteration for more accurate peripheral extension at the time of surgery.

LABIAL VESTIBULE. Severe resorption of residual alveolar process without concomitant atrophy of overlying soft tissues results in extremely mobile ridges. Although this condition can be seen in any location, it occurs most often in the

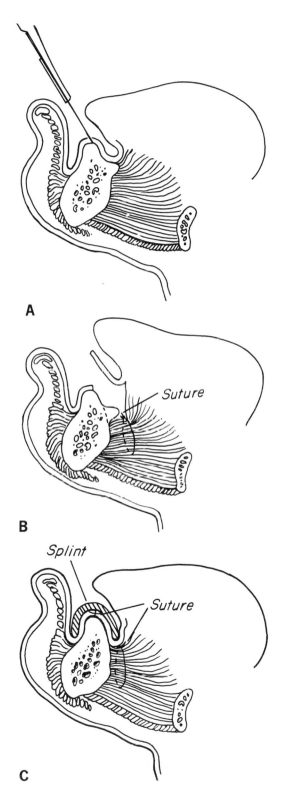

A

B

C

Suture

Splint

Suture

FIG. 5-37. *Diagrams of anterior lingual sulcus extension (midsagittal section).* **A.** *Initial incision.* **B.** *Detachment and reinsertion of the genioglossus muscle and removal of genial tubercle.* **C.** *Splint insertion.*

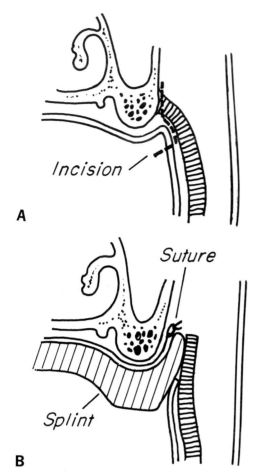

A

B

FIG. 5-38. *Diagrams of a maxillary buccal vestibular extension (frontal section).* **A.** *Initial incision.* **B.** *Suturing and splint insertion.*

maxillary anterior region. It is frequently observed when natural mandibular anterior teeth function against maxillary complete dentures which have inadequate posterior occlusion (combination syndrome). Laskin has advocated a sclerosing procedure for such situations,[18a] and Starshak has described a surgical procedure to firm the denture seating area.[30a] However, injection of sclerosing agents precludes wearing of dentures for four to six weeks and sometimes results in soft tissue necrosis of varying severity. Starshak's surgical approach, which is similar to that for surgical reduction of

hyperplastic gingiva of the maxillary posterior ridge, has the disadvantages of tending to reduce vestibular depth and decreasing the ridge surface area covered by keratinized epithelium.

Keagle has devised a surgical procedure which firms the hypermobile soft tissue and preserves the keratinized epithelium without shortening the vestibule. (Fig. 5-39).[13a] A facial incision (Fig. 5-40) is made at the mucogingival junction perpendicular to the tissue surface (Fig. 5-41, incision A). It is carried to the periosteum if the mucogingival junction is lateral to the alveolar crest or to a depth equal to half the thickness of the soft tissue if the mucogingival junction is occlusal to the alveolar crest. The direction of the incision is then changed so that the hypermobile tissue

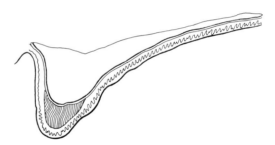

FIG. 5-39. *Cross-sectional diagram of hypermobile maxillary anterior ridge. Shaded area depicts excess connective tissue to be excised. This tissue is generally inflamed, collagen-poor, and spongy.*

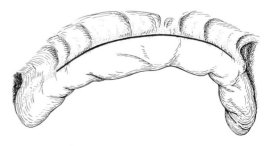

FIG. 5-40. *Incision at mucogingival junction.*

will be dissected supraperiosteally or bisected supracrestally (Fig. 5-41, incision B) stopping 2 to 2.5 mm short of the soft tissue crest.

While holding the keratinized mucosa with Jerald or Adson forceps, the superfluous, spongy connective tissue is then removed from the inner side of the flap (Fig. 5-41, incision C) between the first (a) and second (b) incisions, taking care to leave the tissue a uniform 2 to 2.5 mm thick.

Tension is then placed on the keratinized tissue to pull it over the alveolar ridge toward the vestibular fornix (Figs. 5-42 and 5-43). It may be necessary at this point to remove a wedge of superfluous spongy connective tissue from the palatal (lingual) aspect of the ridge. This is accomplished by sharp dissection, and the excess tissue is discarded (Fig. 5-42, incisions C and D). This step is not always required.

While holding the mobilized, thinned, keratinized mucosa firmly against the alveolar crest, an incision is made at its border into the alveolar mucosa (Fig. 5-43, incision F). This mucosa is then sharply dissected from the alveolar ridge periosteum in a coronal direction (Fig. 5-43, incision G). The mobilized ridge mucosa is then sutured snugly to the periosteum using interrupted mattress sutures (Fig. 5-44). Conventional interrupted sutures tend to be easily pulled through the fragile periosteum underly-

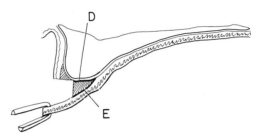

FIG. 5-42. *Excess spongy connective tissue is removed from the palatal (lingual) side of the ridge crest by sharp dissection and discarded (Incisions **D** and **E**).*

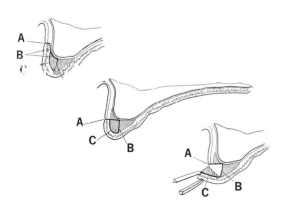

FIG. 5-41. *Initial incision (**A**) is extended to center of supracrestal soft tissue (to periosteum if mucogingival junction is facial to alveolar process). The line of incision is then changed 90 degrees and directed toward the ridge crest. (**B**) It is terminated about 2.5 mm from the crest surface. Incision **C** is made to remove superfluous spongy tissue from the inner aspect of the keratinized mucosa.*

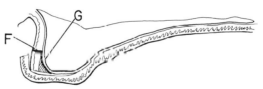

FIG. 5-43. *While extending and holding the mobilized, thinned keratinized mucosa firmly against the ridge an incision (**F**) is made at its border into the alveolar mucosa which is then sharply dissected from the underlying periosteum in a coronal direction (Incision **G**).*

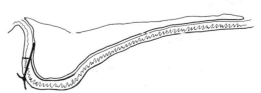

FIG. 5-44. *Cross-sectional view of gingivoperiosteal mattress suture.*

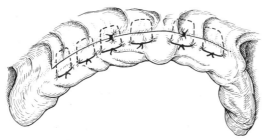

Fig. 5-45. *Facial view of gingivoperiosteal mattress sutures and gingivomucosal sutures which may be required for good coaptation of the gingiva to the mucosa.*

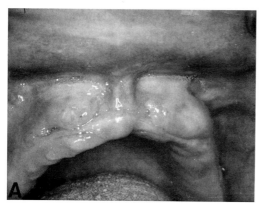

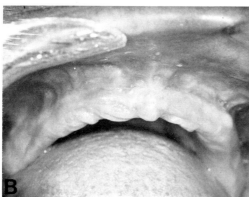

Fig. 5-46. *Pre- and postsurgical (**A** and **B**) views of a maxillary anterior ridge treated as described. In addition to treatment of the hypermobile ridge, pendulous hyperplastic tissue (epulis fissuratum) was removed from the alveolar mucosa on both sides of the midline.*

ing the alveolar mucosa and to become embedded and difficult to remove. Once the keratinized mucosa has been immobilized, the cut margin of the alveolar mucosa can be sutured to it if necessary (Fig. 5-45).

The patient's denture is then relined with a tissue conditioning material which will serve as a dressing during healing. The material should be changed at one- to two-week intervals for four to six postoperative weeks before attempting new denture impressions (Fig. 5-46). Another surgical technique involves stripping the hypertrophied mucosa and suturing the vestibule at the height of its extension (Fig. 5-47).

If the extension and excision of the hypertrophied mucosa are performed at the same operation, the use of a surgical splint is mandatory. The lack of muscle tension at the site and the ability to obtain good retention with a maxillary splint often eliminates the necessity for mechanical fixation. If fixation is neces-

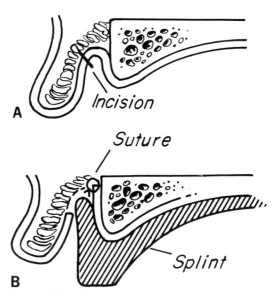

Fig. 5-47. *Diagrams of a maxillary labial vestibular extension (frontal section). **A.** Initial incision. **B.** Suturing and splint insertion.*

sary, pins can be placed in the lateral aspects of the buccal flanges. The exposed pins should be covered with autopolymer resin to protect the cheeks. Another method of fixation employs a nasal alveolar spine wire in conjunction with a midpalatal screw. The splint is used in its fixed position for approximately ten days.

Malrelated Jaws

Malrelated jaws are not corrected by the removal of teeth. Disharmonies of tooth relations and occlusal contacts that result from skeletal disharmonies in the natural dentition are an index to the problems in tooth arrangement that will be present when the patient receives complete dentures. Malrelated jaws should be analyzed early in the diagnostic procedures, and surgical correction should be performed prior to removal of the teeth. The teeth act as landmarks during the orientation of the jaws and also act as stabilizers while the jaw is healing. It is possible to correct these malrelations surgically in the absence of teeth, but the construction of splints and the immobilization of these splints prolong the treatment plan.

Congenital Deformities

Congenital deformities that affect construction of complete dentures are usually of the cleft lip and cleft palate type. In most instances surgical procedures are undertaken early in life. Every effort should be made to keep the natural teeth to use for retention. When dentures are indicated, additional surgery is often indicated to prepare the support for their retention and stability. The use of special materials in impression making, denture construction, and speech bulb fabrication must be considered. These patients can be helped by the surgeon and the prosthodontist.

Postoperative Procedures

After extensive surgical techniques, care should be exercised to maintain and support the patient. This requires dietary control and often intravenous fluid therapy to keep intake up to minimal daily requirements. Occasionally, electrolytic imbalances have to be corrected. Appropriate analgesics and sedatives should be prescribed. Oral hygiene should be maintained by irrigations with saline solution and dilute hydrogen peroxide.

In the more extensive procedures of muscle repositioning, sulcus extensions, and tissue removal, antibiotic therapy should be used to control secondary infection and enhance healing.

Immobilized splints are maintained in place from two to three weeks, depending upon the procedures performed and the ability of the patient to tolerate the splint. Muscle repositioning should be maintained from two and one-half to three weeks. Sulcus extensions do not require more than ten days.

During the postoperative healing period, rigid discipline is needed, both by the clinician and by the patient. This insures that minimal trauma is being transmitted through the fixed appliances to the healing surgical sites. Regulation of the patient's physical activity, dietary intake, and psychologic status requires constant monitoring. This is an uncomfortable time for the patient, and he requires encouragement and surveillance. In the more extensive cases requiring hospitalization, postoperative care should be carried on in the hospital until the patients are able to care for themselves. Heavy manual work is contraindicated. The occlusal stresses should be checked for excessive trauma on the splints, and the prosthodontist becomes more active in the care of the patient. After splints and sutures have been removed, the patient is seen jointly by the prosthodontist and the oral surgeon until the epithelization has been completed. During the period from mobilization to epithelization, the patient should be wearing some type of physiologic splint.

Prosthodontic Treatment

At the time of surgery the role of the prosthodontist is that of consultant and associate to the oral surgeon. If alterations of the surgical splints are necessary, the prosthodontist should make them.

If the borders need to be extended, additional material should be added accurately, then smoothed, and polished. The material should be stable. Autopolymerizing methyl methacrylate is the material of choice. The method of application is the "sprinkle on" technique which lessens the quantity of free monomer. After polymerization any excess monomer is eliminated by placing the splint in hot water in a pressure cooker at twenty-four pounds of pressure for fifteen minutes. Alterations requiring grinding should be smoothed and polished.

The postoperative prosthodontic treatment period begins with the removal of the mechanical fixation devices. This treatment period is designed to promote a molding and conditioning of the soft tissues as well as to allow the alteration in the trabeculation of bone to resist the new forces. The healing period varies with individuals but usually involves six to eight weeks. The surgical splint with the occluding ramps is used for the surgically treated arch.

A new denture is made for the opposing arch using noncusp teeth at the desired occlusal plane. The tissue side of the splint is ground out and is resurfaced with an autopolymerizing soft liner.

The liner should be stable and easily cleaned, should allow a cast to be poured without distortion, and should remain pliable. The denture and splint should be accurately mounted on an articulator, and the maxillary posterior teeth must contact equally with the occlusal ramps. This contacting should be with the jaws in centric relation at the desired vertical dimension of occlusion. The anterior teeth should not contact in the centric occlusal position. Since the patient should not perform extensive masticatory functions, the occlusal ramps are used to discourage the eating of other than soft foods. The patient is instructed to incise with knife and fork and to place the food in the posterior part of the oral cavity. He is instructed to remove the prosthesis for at least eight of the twenty-four hours, preferably at night.

When healing and molding of the soft tissue are adequate, as determined by the tonus and color of the mucosa, noncusp teeth are used to replace the acrylic resin ramps. The occlusion is refined by remounting precedures. The patient is thoroughly instructed in the use and care of the dentures. These instructions are given in writing as well as verbally. Emphasis is placed on tissue rest at night, small pieces of food, use of the knife and fork for incising, and oral hygiene. The patient is placed on a definite recall system for observation (Fig. 5-48).

Again, varying with individuals, new dentures may be constructed approximately six to eight months after surgery. The same type of posterior occlusion is reestablished. If additional weight is needed for stability, the mandibular denture is constructed with a full cast base weighing approximately 26 dwt. The weight will vary to meet the specific situation. Gold is the metal preferred for the cast base denture.

It must be recognized that there are

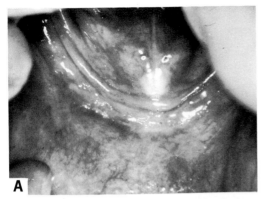

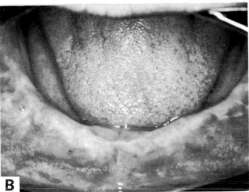

FIG. 5-48. **A.** *This preoperative photograph of an atrophied edentulous mandible reveals no vertical residual alveolar ridge. The vestibular mucosa and muscles attach near and on the crest of the denture supporting area, and the mucosa that covers the posterior supporting areas is pendulous.* **B.** *This postoperative photograph discloses a mandibular basal seat that is favorable for denture stability.*

other surgical and prosthodontic approaches to the management of patients who have extensive loss or an absence of the residual ridge or ridges.

Cobalt chromium alloys are used in mesh form and inserted subperiosteally. The male members are a part of the implanted mesh and the female attachments are in the denture.

Cobalt chromium buttons that are fabricated in the denture may be used for the maxillary arch in selected conditions.

Attracting magnets may be inserted subperiosteally with the other section of the magnet being fabricated in the denture base.

Opposing magnets may be fabricated in the dentures. This approach requires no particular surgical procedure.

In recent years there has been extensive clinical research in augmentation to increase basal bone in a vertical and horizontal direction for denture base stability. In general, autogenous bone has been the preference of most clinicians. There are numerous techniques and modifications. The actual bony augmentation is an insertion subperiosteally of either rib, split rib, iliac bulk bone, or particularized bone. These procedures are generally followed by a vestibuloplasty using a split-skin technique. However, occasionally techniques such as interpositional grafting negates the need for secondary soft tissue skin graft to obtain a vestibular fornix. This can be done either in the maxillae or the mandible. A midsagittal mandibular split Visor technique has a distinct advantage of allowing a pedicle medial cortical segment to be advanced superiorly in the mandible and then recontoured in bulk by particularized bone grafting. This technique shows a considerable amount of promise because of maintaining vascular supply to the segment. As previously described in this text, the vestibular fornix extension or vestibuloplasty based on re-epithelization is a predictable procedure when you have knowledgable prosthetic support and good stent construction. The vestibular fornix extension obtained by split-skin graft can often be done without a stent when the potential height of the mandible is 10 mm or greater. This allows healing without insertion of a stent; however, it does mean that the patient has to be without a prosthesis for a while.

Obwegeser describes in detail the

procedure done for stent construction.[11] This procedure works well when no bone surgery is indicated for recontouring or when the patient will accept hospitalization and skin grafting.

Long-term studies with augmentation techniques of the mandible show a high percentage of vertical height loss of the graft material. There is, however, clinical evidence of mass change, particularly in the buccal lingual dimension which allows an increase in basal support for the lower prosthesis. This clinical impression is supported by the findings of Davis et al.[7b] At this time there are a number of preprosthetic clinical research projects going on, and it is expected that some qualifications of these techniques will be indicated for treatment of the severely atrophied mandible or maxilla, to obtain predictable results.

Processed medicinal Silastic (silicone rubber), a Dow Corning Company product, has been implanted subperiosteally to add supporting area for a denture. Hypertrophied and pendulous tissue has been injected with medicinal Silastic to firm the tissue for better support of the denture. The implantation and injection of medicinal Silastic are in the research stage and their value has not been determined.

Any efforts based on sound anatomic, physiologic, histologic, surgical, and prosthodontic procedures that will help these patients should be encouraged.

REFERENCES

1. Baker, R., and Connole, P.: Preprosthetic augmentation grafting—autogenous bone. J. Oral Surg., *35*:541, 1977.
1a. Bauman, R.: Inflammatory papillary hyperplasia and homecare instructions to denture patients. J. Prosth. Dent., *37*:608, 1977.
1b. Bear, S. E.: Surgical correction of oral anomalies as related to dental prosthesis. Dent. Clin. N. Amer. July, 1967, p. 337.
1c. Bell, W. H.: Current concepts of bone grafting. J. Oral Surg., *26*:118, 1968.
2. Behrman, S. L.: Surgical preparation of edentulous ridges for complete dentures. J. Prosth. Dent., *11*:405, 1961.
3. Boyer, H. E., and DeJean, E. K.: Principles of management of oral surgery patients. Dent. Clin. N. Amer., July, 1964, p. 349.
4. Boyer, M. J., and Salb, H. S.: Surgical preparation of the oral cavity for prosthetic restorations. J. New Jersey Dent. Soc., *27*:14, 1955.
4a. Boyne, P. J.: Transplantation, implantation, and grafts. Dent. Clin. N. Amer., *15*:433, 1971.
5. Cardwell, J. B.: Lingual ridge extension. J. Oral Surg., *13*:287, 1955.
6. Clark, H. B., Jr.: Deepening of labial sulcus by mucosal flap advancement. Report of Case. J. Oral Surg., *11*:165, 1953.
7. Craddock, F. W.: Surgical preparation of mouth for dentures, Part I. New Zeal. Dent. J., *42*:165, 1946.
7a. Davis, W. H., et al.: Transoral bone graft for atrophy of the mandible. J. Oral Surg., *28*:760, 1970.
7b. ———, et al.: Long-term ridge augmentation with rib graft. J. Maxillofac. Surg., *3*:103, 1975.
8. DeVan, M. M.: Role of oral surgeon in prosthodontics. Oral Surg., *22*:458, 1966.
9. Dinon, L. R., and Strang, J. E.: The dental patient with heart disease. Dent. Clin. N. Amer., July, 1958, p. 335.
9a. Donoff, R. B.: Biological basis for vestibuloplasty procedures. J. Oral Surg., *34*:890, 1976.
9b. Ettinger, R. L.: Etiology of inflammatory papillary hyperplasia. J. Prosth. Dent., *34*:254, 1975.
9c. Friedlander, A. H., and Renner, R. P.: Selective resection of circumoral musculature for enhancement of mandibular denture stability. J. Prosth. Dent., *37*:602, 1977.
10. Gazabatt, C. A., ParaNany, H., and Meissner, E. V.: A comparison of bone resorption following intraseptal alveolectomy and labial alveolectomy. J. Prosth. Dent., *15*:435, 1965.

10a. Harle, F.: Visor osteotomy to increase the absolute height of the atrophied mandible. A preliminary report. J. Maxillofac. Surg., 3:257, 1975.

11. Heartwell, C. M., Jr., and Peters, P. B.: Surgical and prosthodontic management of atrophied edentulous jaws. Part I. The evaluation of edentulous jaws. Part II. The surgical and prosthodontic treatment. J. Prosth. Dent., 16:613, 1966.

12. Jordan, L. G.: Cooperation of oral surgeon and prosthodontist in rendering artificial denture service. J. Prosth. Dent., 2:55, 1952.

13. Kazanjian, V. H.: Surgery as an aid to more efficient service with prosthodontic dentures. J.A.D.A., 22:566, 1935.

13a. Keagle, J. G.: Personal communication. Medical College of Georgia, School of Dentistry, 1979.

14. Kelly, E. K.: The prosthodontist, the oral surgeon, and the denture supporting tissues. J. Prosth. Dent., 16:464, 1966.

14a. Kelly, J. F., and Friedlaender, G. E.: Preprosthetic bone graft augmentation with allogeneic bone: a preliminary report. J. Oral Surg., 35:268, 1977.

14b. Kent, J. N., et al.: Pilot studies of a porous implant in dentistry and oral surgery. J. Oral Surg., 30:608, 1972.

15. Kjell, W.: Ridge extension: A modified operative technic. J. Oral Surg., 21:54, 1963.

16. Koslin, A. J.: Fixation technic for sulcus deepening. J. Oral Surg., 21:60, 1963.

17. Kruger, G. O.: Ridge extension: Review of indications and technics. J. Oral Surg., 16:91, 1958.

18. Lambson, G. O.: Papillary hyperplasia of the palate. J. Prosth. Dent., 16:636, 1966.

18a. Laskin, D. M.: A sclerosing procedure for hypermobile edentulous ridges. J. Prosth. Dent., 23:274, 1970.

19. Lee, J. H., and Downton, D.: Frenoplasty. J. Prosth. Dent., 8:19, 1958.

20. Lewis, E. T.: Repositioning of the sublingual fold for complete dentures. J. Prosth. Dent., 8:22, 1958.

20a. MacIntosh, R., and Obwegeser, H.: Preprosthetic surgery: a scheme for its effective employment. J. Oral Surg., 25:397, 1967.

21. Meyer, R. A.: Management of denture patients with sharp residual ridges. J. Prosth. Dent., 16:431, 1966.

21a. Michael, C. G., and Barsoum, W. M.: Comparing ridge resorption with various surgical techniques in immediate dentures. J. Prosth. Dent., 35:142, 1976.

21b. Miller, E. L.: Sometimes overlooked: preprosthetic surgery. J. Prosth. Dent., 36:484, 1976.

22. Morris, J. H.: Anatomic considerations pertinent to general practice oral surgery. Dent. Clin. N. Amer., July, 1964, p. 383.

22a. Obwegeser, H.: Surgical preparation of the maxilla for prosthesis. J. Oral Surg., 22:127, 1964.

23. Orlean, S. L., and Mallon, C. F.: Vestibuloplasty and prosthodontic transfers in the rehabilitation of edentulous patients. Case Reports. J. Prosth. Dent., 13:240, 1963.

23a. Peterson, L., and Slade, E.: Mandibular ridge augmentation by a modified visor osteotomy: Preliminary report. J. Oral Surg., 35:999, 1977.

24. Pressman, R. S.: Prophylaxis of transient bacteremias. Dent. Clin. N. Amer., July, 1958, p. 351.

24a. Roberts, B. J.: Mylohyoid ridge reductions as an aid to success in complete lower dentures. J. Prosth. Dent., 37:486, 1977.

25. Schmitz, J. F.: A clinical study of inflammatory hyperplasia. J. Prosth. Dent., 14:1034, 1964.

26. Schuchardt, K.: Die epidermistransplantation un der munduohoffastic, deutashe zahn - Mund -. u. Keifer, 7:364, 1952.

27. Shea, C. R., and Wolford, D. R.: Removal of genial tubercle for prosthesis. Oral Surg., 8:1044, 1955.

28. Simpson, H. E.: Experimental investigation into the healing of extraction wounds in macacus rhesus monkeys. J. Oral Surg., 18:391, 1960.

29. ———: Healing of surgical extraction wounds in macacus rhesus monkeys. J. Oral. Surg., 19:3; 227, 1961.

30. Sindoni, A., Jr.: The diabetic dental patient. Dent. Clin. N. Amer., July, 1958. p. 459.

30a. Starshak, T. J.: *Preprosthetic Oral Sur-*

gery. St. Louis, The C.V. Mosby Company, 1971, pp. 138–141.

30b. Steinhauser, E.: Free transplantation of oral mucosa for improvement of denture retention. J. Oral Surg., *27:*955, 1969.

30c. ———: Ergebonisse der Vestibulumplastik mit freier Hauttransplantation am Ober-und Unterkiefer. Fortschr. Kiefer Geischtschir., *10:*19, 1965.

30d. ———: Vestibuloplasty—skin grafts. J. Oral Surg., *29:777,* 1971.

30e. ——— and Obwegeser, H. L.: Second International Conference on Oral Surgery—1965. Copenhagen, Munksgaard, 1967, pp. 203–208.

30f. Terry, B. C., Albright, J. E., and Baker, R. D.: Alveolar ridge augmentation in the edentulous maxilla with use of autogenous ribs. J. Oral Surg., *32:*429, 1974.

31. Trauner, R.: Alveoplasty with ridge extensions on the lingual side of the lower jaw to solve the problems of a lower dental prosthesis. J. Oral Surg., *5:*40, 1952.

32. Walker, R. V.: Surgical procedures in the correction of prognathia: Prepared by invitation for the sixty-first annual meeting of the American Ass. of Orthodontists. Dallas, Texas, May, 1965.

33. Walsh, J. P.: Surgical preparation of the mouth for the reception of dentures. New Zeal. Dent. Survey, *23:*461, 1947.

34. Weiss, L. R.: Intraoral skin graft as aid to denture construction. J.A.D.A., *34:*389, 1947.

34a. Wilkie, N. D.: The role of the prosthodontist in preprosthetic surgery. J. Prosth. Dent., *33:*386, 1975.

35. Wyatt, J. L., Jr., and Welhorn, J. F.: Prosthetic management of mandibular prognathism. J. Prosth. Dent., *15:*174, 1965.

36. Yrastorza, J. A.: Surgical problems in edentulous jaws associated with denture construction. J. Oral Surg., *21:*203, 1963.

Complete Denture Impressions

6

An impression is the negative form of the teeth and/or other tissues of the oral cavity, made in a plastic material which becomes relatively hard or set while in contact with these tissues. One makes an impression in order to produce a positive form or cast of the recorded tissues.

A *complete denture impression* is a negative registration of the entire denture bearing, stabilizing, and border seal areas present in the edentulous mouth.

A *preliminary impression* is an impression made for the purpose of diagnosis or for the construction of a tray.

A *final impression* is an impression for making the master casts. The master casts are used in constructing the dentures.

We do not "take," but we "make" an impression. To make a box to fit within another box, we must record the limits of the first box by measuring with ruler and calipers. The bottom, sides, corners, and ends are the guides or limits. To make an impression we measure with our eyes and fingers the anatomic limits in the oral cavity. The impression material is shaped and molded into a negative likeness of the supporting area, a cast is made from this impression, and the denture base is constructed on the cast. As a result, the denture base fits the supporting tissues within the oral cavity. A knowledge of the origins of the

muscles of facial expression and of the anatomic landmarks is essential. If one knows the oral anatomy, both gross and histologic, he can readily decide how to make the impression, what material to use, and how to position the tissues when the impressions are made.

Muscles of Facial Expression

When the residual ridges are considered adequate in width and height to give stability and retention to a denture base, the *origins* (Fig. 6-1) of the

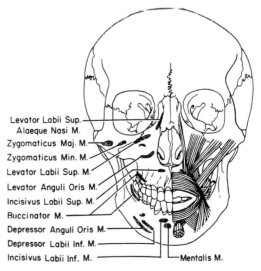

Levator Labii Sup. Alaeque Nasi M.
Zygomaticus Maj. M.
Zygomaticus Min. M.
Levator Labii Sup. M.
Levator Anguli Oris M.
Incisivus Labii Sup. M.
Buccinator M.
Depressor Anguli Oris M.
Depressor Labii Inf. M.
Incisivus Labii Inf. M.
Mentalis M.

FIG. 6-1. *Origins of the muscles of facial expression.*

muscles of facial expression rarely present a problem in border extensions. When the residual ridges are lost, the *origins* become more intimately involved in the positions of the borders. The *insertion* of the muscles of facial expression distal to the corners of the mouth at the modiolus (Fig. 6-2A) and the position and action of the orbicularis oris have a definite influence in impression making. These muscles can be relaxed with

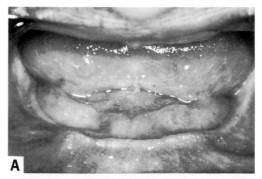

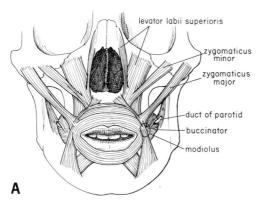

levator labii superioris
zygomaticus minor
zygomaticus major
duct of parotid
buccinator
modiolus

A

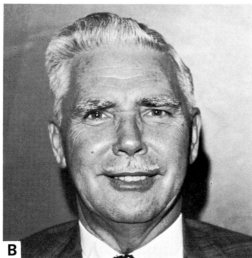

B

FIG. 6-2. A. *Intersection of the muscles at the corners of the mouth is the modiolus. The orbicularis does not arise from or insert into bone.* **B.** *This patient can be trained to relax the muscles of facial expression. Relaxation of the lips and the muscles at the corners of the mouth makes it easier to insert and remove impression trays and material.*

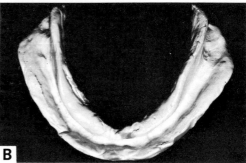

FIG. 6-3. A. *The masseter groove area. The action of the masseter muscle reflects the buccinator muscle in a superior and medial direction.* **B.** *An impression of the masseter groove area. Notice that the impression material is reflected in the directions of the action of the muscles.*

the jaws open, and this relaxation is desirable when introducing the impression tray or impression material. The patient should be trained to open the jaws and relax the lips and cheeks to avoid interference from a pair of tense lips (Fig. 6-2B). When the lips are tense, a stretching action often results in lacerations at the corners of the mouth and/or distorted impression material. The buccinator muscle joins the superior constrictor at the pterygomandibular raphe distal to the retromolar pad area. It is buccal to this area that the action of the masseter muscle pushes the buccinator muscle toward the retromolar pad. The impression will be reflected superiorly and medially forming a groove called the masseter groove (Fig. 6-3). If the distobuccal flange of the mandibular denture base is not contoured to allow freedom for this action, the denture will be displaced.

Anatomic Landmarks

Mouths vary; that is, the same anatomic landmarks do not appear prominently when impressions of one mouth are compared with those of another.

Therefore, each patient must be studied individually because each patient is different. A knowledge of oral anatomy will help the operator provide enough landmarks to act as positive guides to the limits of the impressions.

THE MAXILLARY ARCH (Fig. 6-4A)

1. The labial frenum may be single or multiple; it appears as a fold of mucous membrane extending from the mucous lining of the mucous membrane of the lips to or toward the crest of the residual

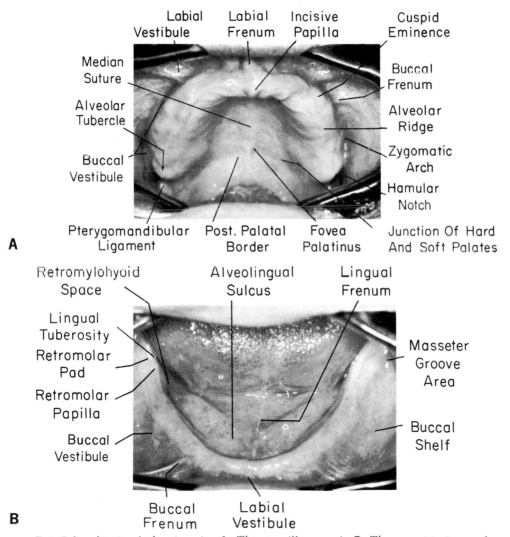

FIG. 6-4. *Anatomic landmarks.* **A.** *The maxillary arch.* **B.** *The mandibular arch.*

ridge on the labial surface. The frenum may be narrow or broad. It contains no muscle fibers of significance; therefore, it can be surgically excised if it attaches too near the crest of the alveolar ridge. It inserts in a vertical direction.

2. The labial vestibule or labial flange area extends on both sides from the labial frenum to the buccal frenum. The reflection of the mucous membrane superiorly determines the height. The area of mucous membrane reflection contains no muscle.

3. The buccal frenum, a fold or folds of mucous membrane, varies in size and position and extends from the buccal mucous membrane reflection area to or toward the slope or crest of the residual ridge. This frenum, like the labial one, contains no muscle fibers of any significance. Its reflection is in an anteroposterior direction.

4. The buccal vestibule area, or the buccal mucous membrane reflection area, is the space distal to the buccal frenum. It is bound externally by the cheek and internally by the residual ridge. At the distal end of the residual ridge is the alveolar tubercle. In the area of the buccal flange of the denture base where it rounds the distobuccal area of the tubercle sometimes a small muscle attachment is found. When the vestibular space that is distal and lateral to the alveolar tubercles is properly filled with the denture flange, the stability and retention of the maxillary denture is greatly enhanced.

5. The hamular notch is distal to the alveolar tubercle. This narrow cleft extends from the tubercle to the pterygoid hamulus. The pterygomandibular ligament attaches to the hamulus. The narrow cleft of loose connective tissue is approximately 2 mm in extent anteroposteriorly.

6. The distal palatal termination of the denture base is termed the *posterior*

palatal seal area. It is distal to the junction of the hard and soft palate. This is not a straight line from hamular notch to hamular notch but follows the contour of the distal border of the palatal bone. The vibrating line is the area at the junction of the hard and soft palates where movement is seen as the patient says "Ahhhh" in a moderate manner. Movement may be active or passive. This junction is more definitely demonstrated if the patient's nostrils are closed, and he is asked to exhale through his nose. The soft palate will flex at the junction. From this vibrating line is determined the posterior extension of the posterior palatal seal.

7. The fovea palatina, usually two in number, are found one on each side of the midline and slightly posterior to the junction of the hard and soft palates.

8. The median palatal suture is the area extending from the incisive papilla to the distal end of the hard palate. The mucosa over this area is usually tightly attached and thin, the underlying bony union being very dense and often raised. It is here that the palatal torus, if present, is located.

9. Rugae are raised areas of dense connective tissue radiating from the median suture in the anterior one third of the palate. This area is a secondary bearing area, as it resists anterior displacement of the denture.

10. The incisive papilla is a pad of fibrous connective tissue overlying the orifice of the nasopalatine canal. In the dentulous mouth it is located between the two central incisors on the palatal side. In the edentulous mouth it may lie on or labial to the crest of the residual ridge.

THE MANDIBULAR ARCH (Fig. 6-4B)

1. The labial frenum, like the maxillary one, is a fold of mucous membrane. It is not usually as pronounced as the

frenum in the maxillary arch but is histologically and functionally similar.

2. The labial flange space extending from the labial frenum to the buccal frenum is limited inferiorly by the mucous membrane reflection, internally by the residual ridge, and labially by the lip.

3. The buccal frenum is a fold or folds of mucous membrane extending from the buccal mucous membrane reflection to or toward the slope or crest of the residual ridge in the region just distal to the cuspid eminence. This membrane may be single or double, broad U-shaped, or sharp V-shaped. The reflection is in an anteroposterior direction.

4. The buccal shelf area is bordered externally by the external oblique line and internally by the slope of the residual ridge. The bone in this area is very dense and the trabeculation is arranged almost at right angles to the path of jaw closure. Forces of occlusion can be directed more nearly at right angles to the buccal shelf than at any other area of support.

5. The external oblique line is a ridge of dense bone extending from just above the mental foramen superiorly and distally, becoming continuous with the anterior border of the ramus.

6. The retromolar pad is a pear-shaped area of glandular tissue, loose areolar connective tissue, the lower margin of the pterygomandibular raphe, fibers of the buccinator muscle, and fibers from the temporal tendon. The retromolar papilla is a small pear-shaped area just anterior to the retromolar pad. It is dense, fibrous connective tissue.

7. When the tip of the tongue is elevated, a fold of mucous membrane can be observed. This, the lingual frenum, overlies the genioglossus muscle which takes origin from the superior genial spine on the mandible.

8. The fold of mucous membrane from the tongue to the residual ridge is the sublingual fold.

9. The mylohyoid muscle forms the muscular floor of the mouth. It arises from the mylohyoid ridge of the mandible. This ridge is near the inferior border of the mandible in the incisal region but becomes progressively higher on the body of the mandible until it terminates just distal to a slight prominence, the lingual tuberosity.

10. The retromylohyoid space lies at the distal end of the alveolingual sulcus. It is bounded medially by the anterior tonsillar pillar, posteriorly by the retromylohyoid curtain—which is formed posteriorly by the superior constrictor muscle, laterally by the mandible and pterygomandibular raphe, anteriorly by the lingual tuberosity, and inferiorly by the mylohyoid muscle.

INTERPRETING ANATOMIC LANDMARKS

MAXILLARY LANDMARKS (Fig. 6-5A)

1. Frenum attachments (a) appear as notches.

2. Mucous membrane reflections (b) in the labial and buccal vestibule are responsible for the impression being turned out toward the lips and cheeks. The reflections are smooth.

3. The residual ridge forms the alveolar groove (c).

4. The alveolar tubercle produces a depression (d) at the distal ends of the alveolar groove.

5. If an extreme opening is allowed in making the impression, the pterygomandibular ligament will form an anteroposterior notch (e) distal to the alveolar tubercles.

6. If the patient is allowed to open wide, protrude, and go into lateral movements, the distobuccal flange in the distobuccal vestibule will be contoured by the anterior border of the coronoid process (f).

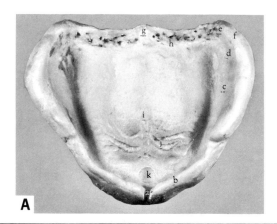

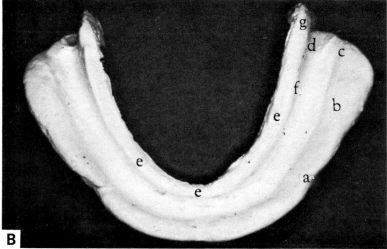

FIG. 6-5. *Final impressions.* **A.** *The maxillary final impression: frenum notch* (**a**); *mucous membrane reflection* (**b**); *alveolar groove* (**c**); *alveolar tubercle depression* (**d**); *notch for pterygomandibular ligament reflection* (**e**); *distobuccal flange contour* (**f**); *fovea palatinus* (**g**); *junction of hard and soft palates* (**h**); *midpalatal suture* (**i**); *rugae* (**j**); *incisive papilla* (**k**). *(Courtesy of A. L. Martone, Medical Towers, Norfolk, Virginia.)* **B.** *The mandibular final impression: notch for buccal frenum reflection* (**a**); *buccal shelf area* (**b**); *reflection of masseter groove area* (**c**); *depression of the retromolar pad* (**d**); *sublingual fold reflection* (**e**); *area of mylohyoid muscle* (**f**); *eminence in retromylohyoid space* (**g**).

7. The fovea palatina (g) usually form two small raised dots in the impression.

8. At the junction of the hard and soft palates the impression usually appears smooth (h). However, in this area the impression will show the influence of very active palatal glands. The surface will not be smooth but irregular and the glandular secretions will adhere to the impression material.

9. The median suture forms an ir-regular groove anteroposteriorly in or near the middle of the vault (i).

10. The rugae appear as small grooves radiating laterally from a central groove much like branches from a tree (j).

11. The incisive papilla appears as a small round depression (k).

MANDIBULAR LANDMARKS (Fig. 6-5B)

1. In the mandibular impression, again we find that the frenum attach-

ments form notches (a), and the residual ridge forms the alveolar groove.

2. The mucous membrane reflections in the vestibule are more active than are the maxillary ones. Small lines may appear in the reflected impression material.

3. The external oblique line appears as a slight groove.

4. The buccal shelf is a broad, flat area extending from the external oblique line to the beginning of the slope of the residual ridge (b).

5. The distobuccal area of the impression will appear grooved or reflected superiorly; this is the masseter groove, the results of the masseter muscle pushing against the buccinator muscle (c).

6. The retromolar pad will appear as a pear-shaped depression at the distal ends of the alveolar grooves (d). The retromolar papilla will appear as a small pear-shaped depression just anterior to the retromolar pad.

7. The sublingual fold appears similar to the mucous membrane reflections when the impression is turned medially and superiorly (e). The reflections are uniform and smooth.

8. The mylohyoid attachment area from the bicuspids posteriorly forms a groove; below this groove is usually an undercut (f).

9. The lingual tuberosity forms a light depression or fossa.

10. The retromylohyoid space appears as an eminence (g).

Impression Objectives

In an impression technique for complete dentures, the procedures must strive for five primary objectives.

PRESERVATION

Preservation of the remaining residual ridges is one objective. It is physiologically accepted that with the loss of the stimulation of the natural teeth the alveolar ridge will atrophy or resorb. This process varies in individuals. However, it appears that this process can be hastened or retarded by local factors. Although other factors such as occlusion, interocclusal distance, and centric relation in harmony with centric occlusion are of great importance, the prosthodontist should keep constantly in mind the effect the impression technique and the impression material may have on the denture base and the effect the denture base may have on the continued health of both the soft and hard tissues of the jaws. Pressure in the impression technique is reflected as pressure in the denture base and results in soft tissue damage and bone resorption.

SUPPORT

Maximum coverage provides the "snowshoe" effect, which distributes applied forces over as wide an area as possible. This helps in preservation, stability, and retention.

STABILITY

Close adaptation to the undistorted mucosa is most important. Stability, or the resistance to horizontal movement, decreases with the loss of vertical height of the ridges or with the increase in flabby, movable tissue.

ESTHETICS

Border thickness should be varied with the needs of each patient in accordance with the extent of residual ridge loss. The vestibular fornix should be filled, but not overfilled, to restore facial contour.

RETENTION

Retention is too often given more consideration than is necessary. It should be readily seen that if the other objectives are achieved, retention will be adequate. Atmospheric pressure, adhesion, cohesion, mechanical locks, muscle control, and patient tolerance affect retention.

ATMOSPHERIC PRESSURE. Atmospheric pressure depends on peripheral seal. To insure this seal, denture borders should extend into, but not to the extent to damage, movable tissue.

ADHESION.   Adhesion is the attraction of saliva to the denture.

COHESION. Cohesion is the attraction of molecules of saliva to each other.

MECHANICAL LOCKS. Mechanical locks of undercuts usually prove to be intolerable to the patient. The soft tissue is subject to damage during the insertion and removal of the denture.

MUSCLE CONTROL AND PATIENT TOLERANCE.   Muscle control and patient tolerance are often amazing influences. Dentures are often retained in the mouth and *appear* to be satisfactory, not because of the accuracy of conforming to the support but because of the adaptability of the muscles of the lips, tongue, and cheeks and patient tolerance.

Impression Materials

One or a combination of impression materials is not the panacea for making acceptable impressions in differing situations. The character and position of the tissues to be reproduced in the impression, the technique employed, and the purpose for which the impression is made dictate the choice of the material. A material should be selected because its properties are suitable to obtain specific results in specific situations and not because the prosthodontist considers that it works best in his hands. The validity of clinical results can be determined only by comparing the results of one operator with those of other operators. If the results from using similar materials under similar conditions are not consistent, the material or procedures should be more thoroughly evaluated.

The type of submucosa and the relation of the supporting bone to the denture bases determine how best to record the soft tissues and what properties the impression materials must possess to make them desirable for use.

The oral mucosa with a *tightly attached submucosa* covers the crest and slopes of the residual alveolar ridges and the anterior two thirds of the palate. When this type of mucosa is displaced in an impression and a denture is constructed on a cast made from this impression and the denture is seated, the tissue will attempt to return to its undisplaced position. This effort of the tissue creates objectionable forces that produce pressure to the supporting bone and dislodging pressure against the denture. It is not desirable to record this type of tissue in a displaced position; therefore, use an impression material that flows and allows the tissues to assume their undisplaced position before it sets. After setting, the material should remain dimensionally stable until the cast is made.

The oral mucosa that covers the soft palate and lines the vestibular fornix has a *loosely attached submucosa*. When this mucosa is displaced with selective pressure procedures, the pressure is not directed to the supporting bone. The displaced tissue does not exert any appreciable force in an attempt to return to its undisplaced form. This type of tissue can be used for denture border seal. The impression material of choice is one that will displace the tissue and hold it in the displaced position as it sets. The impression material should remain dimensionally stable after set until a cast is poured.

The oral mucosa with a *differentiated submucosa* is located in the posterior third of the hard palate and in the retromolar pads. It is not desirable to displace the palatal mucosa in an impression, as the pressure is directed at the bony support. A border seal can be developed in the anterior margin of the retromolar pad and the force can be directed in a horizontal direction, away from the supporting bone.

Impression materials that harden by chemical reaction are plaster of paris, zinc oxide-eugenol paste, irreversible hydrocolloid alginate, mercaptan rubber, and silicone rubber.

Other impression materials—modeling compound, reversible hydrocolloid, and waxes—are *thermoplastic*. They require heat for softening and harden or gel upon cooling.

GYPSUM PRODUCTS

Plaster of paris, a gypsum product, to which modifiers have been added to regulate the setting time and control the setting expansion is used in impression making. Some impression plasters are flavored or colored. Sometimes potato starch is added to make them more soluble. Plaster of paris is most frequently used in an individualized tray of modeling composition or acrylic resin as a refining "wash." However, if border refining is not required in the technique, it is used in a stock tray.

Some of the advantages in using plaster of paris are (1) minimal tissue distortion, (2) accurate record of tissue detail, (3) quick flow, (4) absorption of palatal secretions during set, (5) speedy handling, (6) easy manipulation.

One disadvantage of plaster of paris as an impression material is that the pores in the plaster must be sealed before stone is poured in the impression to form the cast. The sealing of these pores obliterates some of the detail and sometimes results in inaccuracies. A second disadvantage is the possibility of warpage in the palate position if the plaster is used in an impression tray that will not allow the plaster to expand in the flange areas during setting. A third is that plaster is brittle and subject to breakage; therefore, it is not suitable for reinserting to adjust or check for the accuracy of fit. Another disadvantage is that saliva washes the material and distorts the surface when a mandibular impression is made. Yet another is that although plaster of paris is easy to manipulate, it is untidy to handle. In addition, the resulting dehydration of the tissues allows the plaster to cling tightly to the tissues, and the impression may be inaccurate. Furthermore, the separation of stone cast from the impression is tedious and time-consuming. Finally, plaster of paris will not record undercuts without breaking upon removal from the mouth.

ZINC OXIDE EUGENOL PASTE

The basic composition of the zinc oxide-eugenol paste impression materials, regardless of the manufacturer, is zinc oxide and eugenol. Plasticizers, fillers, and other additives are incorporated to alter certain properties such as smoothness of mix, adhesiveness, hardness when set, and setting time. Zinc oxide-eugenol pastes have many advantageous properties. Fluidity aids accurate recording of tissue detail. Minimal tissue distortion results when the paste is allowed to flow with minimal pressure applied. Other advantages are ready flow, speed of handling, and ease in beading and boxing for pouring a cast and in separating from the cast. When an impression of the mandibular arch is made, this material is not washed out by saliva. The property of dimensional stability after setting is most desirable in any impression material, and the zinc oxide-eugenol pastes have no significant dimensional change subsequent to hardening. The impression can be preserved indefinitely without a change in shape from relaxation or other causes of warpage. Zinc oxide-eugenol paste is used as a refining material in combination with other materials; therefore the stability of the tray material must be considered. It is best to pour casts as soon as practical.

Some of the disadvantages are that the setting time is not easily controlled by inexperienced operators; temperature and humidity influence the setting time; the paste does not absorb the secretions in the palate, and therefore if the secretions are profuse, distortion results; it is untidy to handle, difficult to control at the borders, and may distort when removed from undercuts.

REVERSIBLE HYDROCOLLOID

The reversible hydrocolloid is an impression material made from agar-agar. Hydrocolloid *sols* possess the property of changing to *gels* under certain conditions. The application of heat to a reversible colloidal *gel* returns the *gel* to the *sol* condition. When the *sol* is cooled, it returns to the *gel*.

The reversible hydrocolloids accurately reproduce detail in hard objects. However, the accuracy in reproducing detail of hard objects is not necessarily valid when reproducing soft tissues. Any material that must be seated with positive pressure and held rigidly until the material hardens or gels is capable of displacing soft tissue. If the tissues are to be reproduced in their undistorted position, such distortion is not considered desirable. Another disadvantage of reversible hydrocolloid for complete denture impressions is that gels are invariably subject to changes in dimension by syneresis and imbibition;

therefore, the impression must be poured in stone immediately upon removal from the mouth. They are also easily distorted as a result of movement during the gelation period. A rapid cooling may cause a concentration of stress near the tray during gelation; the releasing of this stress after removal from the mouth results in distortion. Distortion may also result from varying thickness of material during gelation. In addition, the reversible hydrocolloid requires special water-cooled trays and equipment, and the tray must be held rigidly in place during gelation. The gel is not easy to manipulate, and beading and boxing are difficult. The primary advantage of reversible hydrocolloid is that it will reproduce accurately undercut areas.

IRREVERSIBLE HYDROCOLLOIDS

Irreversible hydrocolloids are those in which the sol is changed to the gel by chemical reaction. When this reaction is complete, the material cannot be changed again to a sol, hence the "irreversible" classification. This reaction does not appear to damage soft tissue, nor does the reaction cause discomfort to the patient. The soluble alginates dissolve in water and form viscous sols. The viscous sol is placed in either a perforated or a rim lock tray and placed over the tissues. The gelation takes place first where the material is in contact with tissue.

The advantages of these materials for preliminary impressions are simplicity of equipment needed, ease of manipulation, little discomfort to the patient, short chair time, and accurate reproduction of undercut areas.

The disadvantages are the same as those of reversible hydrocolloid. According to Skinner et al., "the irreversible hydrocolloids are not as accurate in recording detail of hard objects as the reversible or rubber impression materials."[27] In addition, the composition of the alginate radically affects its gel strength. The alginates deteriorate rapidly at elevated temperatures; material stored for a month at 65°C or over is unsuitable for dental use. The powder should be weighed, not measured. The alginates also affect the hardness of the surface of stone. One method advocated to overcome this is immersing the impression in a hardening solution for not more than 15 minutes. A 2 per cent solution of potassium sulfate is recommended if the manufacturer has not added a chemical for this purpose.

RUBBER IMPRESSION MATERIALS

Two types of rubber base—polysulfide and silicone—are employed as impression materials in dentistry. Polymers of either are mixed with suitable fillers to a paste consistency. In making an impression, this paste is cured to a semisolid rubber by combining it with a suitable catalyst. These materials, like the hydrocolloids, are used primarily when impressions of hard objects, such as teeth, are to be made. Some of the properties seem favorable for both preliminary and refined impressions for the edentulous situations. Rubber impression materials accurately reproduce hard objects, remain dimensionally stable for about an hour, do not affect the hardness of the surface of stone, and are easy and tidy to handle. The silicone base is pleasing in color and odor, and it records undercuts accurately.

Other properties are unfavorable. The tray must be held rigidly for accuracy for from 8 to 12 minutes for setting. Proper mixing is essential; if the mass is not homogenous, the impression will distort. The ratio of materials is also critical; if the ratio is not accurate, the mechanical properties may be changed.

The impression must be poured within one hour after removal from the mouth. The polysulfide base is untidy to handle, and the odor is objectionable. Complete adhesion to a prefabricated tray is essential.

MODELING COMPOUND

Modeling compound is a thermoplastic material that is made either as a tray or as an impression material. The cake form is used primarily as a tray material, whereas the stick form is used primarily as an impression material. The tray material requires a higher heat to soften, does not record detail accurately, and is rigid when it is hardened. The impression material is less viscous when softened, softens at lower temperatures, and records detail more accurately. The impression materials are used for hard impressions of individual teeth and for border refining. The trays that are made from the modeling compound are refined at the borders and further refined over the entire surface with other more fluid materials—plaster of paris, zinc oxide-eugenol paste, reversible hydrocolloid, and/or the injection type of rubber materials.

The thermal conductivity of modeling compound is very low. The outside softens first; the inside last. When the material is hardening, the tissue side is the last to be affected. Failure to attain a complete hardening of the compound prior to removing the impression may result in serious distortion. The lower the temperature of the compound at the time the impression is made the less the error from the linear thermal coefficient of expansion.

American Dental Association specifications for the compounds for impression making allow a flow of 6 per cent at mouth temperature. The compounds produced for tray material are allowed a flow of 2 per cent at mouth temperature.

Skinner and Philips state:

The flow of impression compound can be beneficial or it can be a source of error. After the compound has softened and during the period it is pressed against the tissues, a continuous flow is desired; the material should flow easily to conform to the tissues so that every detail and landmark is reproduced accurately. Once the compound has solidified, any deformation should be completely elastic, so that the impression can be withdrawn without distortion or flow. Actually, such a condition cannot be realized with this type of material.*

The modeling compounds are subject to distortion during and after removal from the mouth. Warpage results when the mass is not thoroughly set prior to removal from the mouth. Warpage also results when the individual stresses are released. To minimize the error produced by this lack of stability, the compound impressions should be poured within the hour. This lack of stability should be considered when modeling compound is used as the tray material. Modeling compounds should be softened with "dry" heat in an oven or similar container. When a flame is used, care should be exercised not to overheat, boil, or ignite the compound, as this results in a change in the properties owing to the loss of important constituents. When a large mass of compound is used for an impression, it is usually softened in a water bath. There are several disadvantages to this method: (1) prolonged heating makes the compound more brittle and grainy, and (2) manipulation of the compound in preparation to placing it in the tray may incorporate water with a resulting increase in flow.

*Skinner, E. W., and Philips, R. W.: *The Science of Dental Materials.* 5th ed. Philadelphia, W. B. Saunders Co., 1962, pp. 59–67.

Some of the advantages of modeling compound are (1) the surface can be corrected, (2) the impression can be reinserted in the mouth for evaluation of fit, (3) the surface does not have to be treated before pouring the stone cast, (4) the material can be beaded and boxed for cast pouring, and (5) the impression stick compounds are convenient to use and tidy; they can be controlled and will reproduce sufficiently accurately for border refining a tray.

IMPRESSION WAXES

The low fusing impression waxes are not sufficiently accurate for a final impression for complete dentures. As a corrective material for a small area and as a border refining material for a tray, they are extremely satisfactory.

Impression Techniques

Many techniques in impression making are used and discarded. Different concepts relative to the position of the supporting soft tissues when they are recorded in the impression, as well as the human desire to develop a procedure that is easier, faster, and cheaper, account for many of the techniques. The variety can *not* be attributed to changes in the biologicals, for the anatomic, psychologic, and physiologic entities remain fairly constant. When properly evaluated, the easy, fast, and cheap procedures rarely produce satisfactory results. It is not implied that one technique will produce satisfactory results, as there are many approaches to a desirable end product. Not all techniques are applicable in all situations. An impression technique that produces satisfactory results for a preliminary impression may not be acceptable for a final impression. An impression technique that requires border refining for the extension of the denture borders into the loosely attached mucosa for a border seal may not be acceptable if the borders are not extended.

The techniques developed in making preliminary impressions have not varied appreciably. However, the materials used have varied. Waxes and plaster are very infrequently used, modeling compound is used, the mercaptan and silicone rubber impression materials are suggested for use, but the irreversible hydrocolloids (alginates) are fast replacing the other materials. Modeling compound is a thermosetting material and is difficult to use. Once the compound is removed from the tempering bath, it begins setting, and its lack of flow does not always allow the tissues to be recorded in the rest position. If the rest position is desirable in the impression, modeling compound would not be the material of choice. The mercaptan silicone rubbers do not appear to have any advantages over the irreversible hydrocolloids, and they are more expensive. The irreversible hydrocolloids record the tissues without distortion, they are accurate, are not difficult to use, do not require elaborate equipment, and are not time consuming. These factors are the reasons for the acceptance of this material, and the reasons for presenting a technique for its use.

Preliminary Impressions

When a preliminary impression is made for the construction of a custom tray for final impressions, the objectives are to record all areas to be covered by the impression surface of the denture and the adjacent landmarks with an impression material that is accurate and incorporates the minimum of tissue displacement. The maxillary impression should include the *hamular notches, fovea palatina, entire buccal vestibule,* including the aforementioned retro-tubercle sulcus, frenum attachments, palate,* and *entire labial vestibule* (Fig. 6-6A). The mandibular impression should include the *retromolar pads,* the *buccal shelf areas,* the *external oblique ridges, frenum attachments, sublingual space, retromylohyoid space,* the *posterior mucous membrane floor of the mouth to include and be below the mylohyoid line* and the *entire labial and buccal vestibules* (Fig. 6-6B).

EQUIPMENT

No prosthodontist should try to perform a service or carry out a procedure without the proper equipment. Not only is it necessary to have all the essential equipment, but the equipment should be arranged so that it will be readily accessible.

The following materials and equipment should be available for preliminary impressions:
1. Perforated impression trays
2. Utility wax
3. X-ray time clock
4. Irreversible hydrocolloid, preferably packaged
5. Water at 70°F
6. Water measurer
7. Thermometer
8. Plaster bowl
9. Plaster spatula

This list may vary with the individual requirements from clinic to clinic or dentist to dentist.

SEATING THE PATIENT

The patient should be seated upright in a comfortable position with the *occiput* resting firmly in the head rest. Gravity influences the position of the tissues, and since dentures are, in most instances, constructed for patients who will use them while in an upright position, the tissues should be recorded in the impression at this position.

It is much easier to make impressions

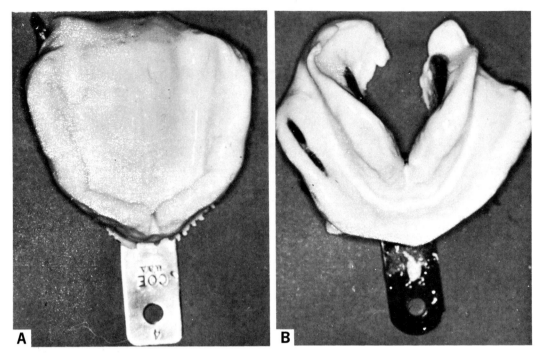

FIG. 6-6. *Preliminary impressions.* **A.** *The maxillary arch.* **B.** *The mandibular arch.*

if the patient is seated in this position and relaxed. The dentist should instruct the patient in the procedures, prior to impression making, and assure him of the ease of the procedures so that the patient will work with and not against him.

IMPRESSION FOR THE
MANDIBULAR ARCH

1. Select a slightly oversized per-forated impression tray. The mandibular tray should be refined at its posterior borders with utility wax to carry the impression material to place (Fig. 6-7).

2. Mix the irreversible hydrocolloid impression material according to the manufacturer's specifications. In this step of the procedure time, temperature of water, and quantity of material are critical. A time clock should be used.

3. Just before inserting impression material, instruct the patient to irrigate his mouth with astringent mouthwash to reduce viscosity of saliva.

4. Load the tray from the side slightly over level full.

5. Using mouth mirror, place a small amount of impression material in the right and left retromylohyoid spaces.

6. Seat the tray in the mouth. In-struct the patient to raise his tongue and let it fall slightly forward. Vibrate the tray to place until the material flows out into the labial and buccal reflection areas.

7. Hold the tray in place for three minutes. Remove from the mouth, rinse under gentle stream of tap water, dry, and pour immediately with dental plaster or stone.

IMPRESSION FOR THE
MAXILLARY ARCH

1. Select proper sized tray and, using utility wax, extend across the posterior

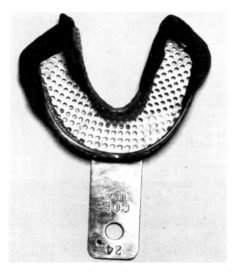

FIG. 6-7. *A perforated impression tray for the mandibular arch. Wax has been applied to the posterior borders to hold the cheek laterally and allow the impression material to flow into the masseter groove area, to avoid hurting the patient if excessive pressure is applied, and to direct the impression material into the retromylohyoid space.*

5. Place the tray in the mouth so that the impression material in the tray attaches itself to the impression material in the mouth.

6. Vibrate the tray and seat until the impression material flows out into the buccal and labial reflection areas and over the posterior palatal seal area. As the tray is being seated, instruct the patient to keep his eyes open, relax, take short breaths through the nose, and flex the head forward.

7. Hold the impression material in place for three minutes, remove from the mouth, rinse with tap water, dry, and pour immediately with dental plaster or stone.

border and the distal termination of the buccal flange area (Fig. 6-8). If necessary, the labial flange may be altered with utility wax. When the patient has a very high vault, utility wax may be added to this area in the tray (Fig. 6-9). These alterations are accomplished to carry the impression material more accurately to place and insure the same bulk throughout the palate.

2. Immediately prior to mixing the impression material, wipe the posterior palatal seal area of the hard palate and the soft palate with gauze to remove excessive saliva.

3. Mix impression material as above. Load the tray from the side.

4. Using the mirror or index finger as a carrier, place the remaining material in the *vault of the palate* and the *buccal vestibule.*

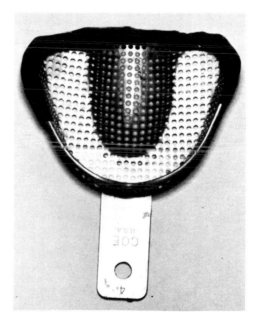

FIG. 6-8. *Perforated impression tray for the maxillary arch. The wax is applied to hold the cheek laterally and allow the impression material to flow into the distobuccal vestibular space and to retain the impression material in the tray and hold it in intimate contact with the soft palate.*

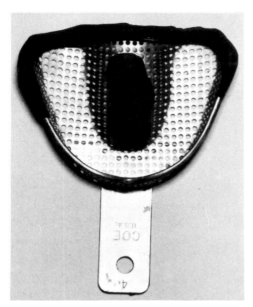

FIG. 6-9. *An impression tray for a patient with a high vault. Notice that utility wax has been added to this area in the tray. An equal thickness of impression material results in a more accurate impression.*

CASTS FOR ACRYLIC RESIN IMPRESSION TRAYS

To make an outline one must know how to interpret the anatomic landmarks on the cast. The outline for the mandibular individualized tray is somewhat more difficult than the outline for the maxillary tray.

MAXILLARY CAST (Fig. 6-10)

1. With an indelible pencil, draw a line transversely across the posterior border connecting the two hamular notches, Points A, in such a manner that the connecting line passes just posterior to the fovea palatinus, Point B. (Note: This is not a straight line, but one that follows the hard palate.)

2. Draw a line outlining the muco-buccal fold at the point where the buccal reflection leaves the lateral wall of the alveolar ridge. Carry the outline well above the frenum attachments, Points C.

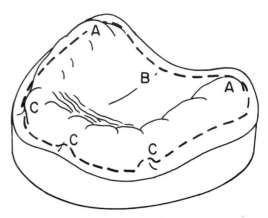

FIG. 6-10. *Maxillary cast outlined for impression tray: hamular notches (**A**); fovea palatinus (**B**); frenum attachments (**C**).*

3. All trays are subject to refinement in the mouth when tissue is displaced by the borders. Displacement should be checked in the patient's mouth prior to making the border refining impression.

MANDIBULAR CAST (Fig. 6-11)

1. With an indelible pencil, draw a line distal to the retromolar pad, Points A. Continue this line buccally in an

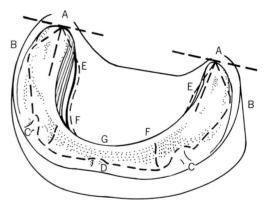

FIG. 6-11. *Mandibular cast outlined for impression tray: line distal to retromolar pad (**A**); external oblique ridge (**B**); buccal frenum (**C**); labial frenum attachment (**D**); lingual tuberosity (**E**); mylohyoid ridge (**F**); lingual frenum attachment (**G**).*

inferior and anterior direction following the masseter groove to the beginning of the external oblique ridge, Points B.

2. Progressing anteriorly, follow the oblique ridge to the buccal frenum attachment.

3. Carry outline well above the frenum attachment and end at the buccal frenum, Points C.

4. Connect Point C with Point C on the opposite side, following the mucolabial reflection and allowing space for the labial frenum attachment, Point D.

5. On the lingual border area drop a line inferiorly from Point A to the lingual tuberosity, Point E.

6. From Points E extend line anteriorly and inferiorly to the mylohyoid ridge but 2 or 3 mm short of the mucous membrane floor of the mouth reflection to a point opposite the cuspid eminence, Points F.

7. Connect Point F with Point F on the opposite side, following the sublingual mucous membrane reflection and allowing space for the lingual frenum attachment, Point G.

CASTS AND IMPRESSION TRAYS OF ACTIVATED ACRYLIC RESIN

1. Eliminate undercuts with a *thin* coat of wax (Fig. 6-12A).

2. Paint cast with tinfoil substitute (Alginate Compound) and allow to dry. Apply another coat of Alginate Compound and start "the sprinkle-on acrylic" technique.

3. Place acrylic resin powder (polymer) in a container with a perforated top (like a salt shaker). Place the monomer in a Dappen dish.

4. Shake the polymer on the border area. With a glass medicine dropper, add monomer to the saturation point. Continue to build this over the entire denture bearing area to a thickness that will yield a rigid tray—a minimum of 2.5 mm.

5. Just before the final polymerization, remove the tray, reseat on the cast, and allow complete polymerization.

6. Reduce the borders to coincide with the outline on the cast (Fig. 6-12C).

7. Roughen the ridge areas on top of the tray and apply sticky wax to this

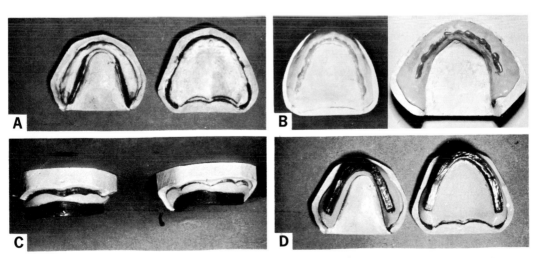

FIG. 6-12. *Procedures for the construction of individualized impression trays.* **A.** *Place wax in undercut areas prior to painting the cast with alginate compound.* **B.** *Apply sticky wax to the roughened areas.* **C.** *Reduce the borders and apply compound rims.* **D.** *Contour the rims in the approximate position that will be occupied by the teeth.*

area (Fig. 6-12B). The compound rims must be rigidly attached to the impression tray.

8. Using softened impression compound, mold a rim over the roughened ridge areas. (Flame the sticky wax and the compound prior to placing the compound on the tray.) This rim will occupy the space on the tray where normally we would place the artificial teeth and should be 9 mm high and 7 mm wide in the molar area. In the anterior section the rim should be 11 mm in length and 4 mm in thickness. On the maxillary tray this rim acts as a handle and also as a seat for the fingers when making the refined impression. The mandibular rim is used for these reasons, also. It strengthens the tray and acts as a guide for the patient in his tongue movements during border refinements (Fig. 6-12D).

CHECKING IMPRESSION TRAYS
THE MAXILLARY TRAY

1. With tray in place have the patient open his mouth wide. If this action causes displacement, the tray is overextended in the hamular notch area.

2. While the jaws are separated, have the patient protrude and move the mandible to right and left lateral positions; if this movement unseats the tray, the thickness distal to the alveolar tubercle area is being contacted by the anterior border of the ramus of the mandible.

3. By inspecting the buccal flanges one can note if the tray is 2 to 3 mm shy of the tissue reflection.

4. Gently move the cheek anteroposteriorly to observe clearance for the buccal frenum attachments.

5. Extend the lip directly forward and observe clearance of labial frenum attachment and the labial flanges. The labial flanges should be 2 to 3 mm shy of mucous membrane reflection.

THE MANDIBULAR TRAY

1. With tray in place have the patient separate jaws widely. As the patient attempts to close, exert slight pressure downwards on the tray and note masseter groove area. Reduce tray to allow space 2 or 3 mm shy of buccinator muscle action.

2. Check buccal flanges to see if they are 2 or 3 mm medial to the external oblique line. If the finger is moved gently from the inferior border upward and the external border of the tray is contacted enough to displace it, this is usually an indication of overextension.

3. Have the patient place tongue in right buccal vestibule. Dislodgement of the tray will indicate overextension of lingual flange on the left side in the posterior one third. Repeat on other side.

4. Have patient place tongue well back in the palate and check for overextension of anterior two thirds of lingual flange.

5. Have patient separate jaws and place tip of tongue on margin of upper lip. Check tray at lingual frenum attachment.

6. With patient's lower lip relaxed, grasp lip with forefinger and thumb and extend directly forward. This checks the labial frenum attachment and labial flanges.

7. Gently move cheek anteroposteriorly to observe clearance for buccal frenum attachment.

Final Impressions

The basic differences in techniques for final impressions can be resolved as those which record the soft tissues in a functional position and those which record the soft tissues in the undisplaced or rest position.

FUNCTIONAL POSITION

Closed mouth techniques record the tissues in their functional position. The patient applies pressure by closing against occlusion rims or teeth that are attached to the impression trays. In this closed jaw relation, the patient exerts pressure and executes muscle actions such as swallowing, grinning, or pursing the lips while the impression material flows. One of the first materials used in this technique was impression compound. Waxes that flowed at mouth temperature were used at a later date. Recently the use of "soft liners" has been advocated. The principles are the same; only the materials are different.

Soft tissues that are displaced and recorded in this displaced position will attempt to return to their undisplaced position when the forces are released. The dentures will be unseated from their bases by this tissue action. When tissues are held in a displaced position, the pressure limits the normal blood flow. When hard tissues are deprived of their normal blood supply, the result is resorption.

REST POSITION

Open mouth techniques are those that record the tissues in their undisplaced position. The techniques for the open mouth have varied more than those for the closed mouth.

EXTENSION. The *extension* of the denture flanges into the undercuts in the distolingual third of the mandibular arch and high into the distobuccal vestibule in the maxillary arch has been advocated, but excessive extensions into the loosely attached mucosa are not tolerated. The use of undercut areas for retention has disadvantages. The insertion and removal procedures damage

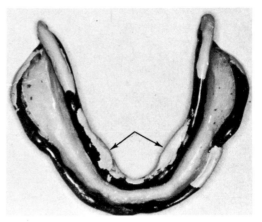

FIG. 6-13. *The borders are refined with anteroposterior extensions in the anterior lingual sulcus prior to making the final impression. Walter Hall termed this extension "butterfly wings." Arrows point to the extensions.*

the mucosa, resulting in tissue atrophy. The excessive retention also allows the patient to function in masticatory acts such as biting apples and corn on the cob or chewing sticky foods. These acts are potentially damaging to the supporting tissues. Anteroposterior extensions in the anterior lingual sulcus in selected situations have been used successfully (Fig. 6-13).

PASSIVE TECHNIQUE. The *passive technique* derives its name from the passive position of the oral mucous membranes when the jaws are at rest. This technique is also referred to as a non-pressure or mucostatic technique. The impression is made in an oversized or spaced tray with no border seal or border refining. The completed denture borders are usually reduced to the stress-bearing mucosa. This deprives the denture of maximum coverage within tissue tolerance. The procedure results in close adaptation of the denture base to the undistorted mucosa for stability but does not incorporate the retentive features of a border seal.

CONTROLLED SUBATMOSPHERIC PRESSURE. *Controlled subatmospheric pressure* is a technique using individualized impression trays to which are attached small rubber hoses. Through these hoses a vacuum is created in the tissue side of the tray. The borders are refined, using an impression material such as Adaptol.* A refining of this impression is accomplished by using other free-flowing plastic materials. This technique is in the investigational stage and requires further evaluation.

SELECTIVE PRESSURE. The *placement pressure technique* or *selective pressure technique* is a combination of extension for maximum coverage within tissue tolerance with light pressure or intimate contact with the movable, loosely attached tissues in the vestibules. The impression is refined with a minimum of pressure.

IMPRESSION COMPOUND TRAY AND ZINC OXIDE-EUGENOL PASTE

The principle of selective pressure is utilized when an impression compound is used to make an impression tray. A preliminary impression is made in a stock edentulous tray (Fig. 6-14A). The borders are refined and a space is created over the denture-bearing areas by scraping away some of the hardened compound (Fig. 6-14B,C,D). Escape holes are placed in the vault of the palate, and a refined impression of zinc oxide-eugenol impression paste is made (Fig. 6-14E,F).

This technique is used frequently for the maxillary arch and less frequently for the mandibular arch. It is considered particularly desirable when the patient is not available for numerous appoint-

*Manufactured by Jelenko and Co., 170 Pleasantville Road, New Rochelle, N. Y. 10801

ments. The properties of impression compound for a preliminary impression tray have been discussed earlier in this chapter. The impression should be poured in stone immediately after the zinc oxide-eugenol paste impression material is set.

The technique that is described in detail in this chapter combines the principles of extension for maximum coverage within tissue tolerance. Allowing freedom but not exaggerated movements, the borders of the impression are extended to make intimate contact with the loosely attached mucosa in the vestibular fornix and soft palate to furnish a border seal, and the remaining soft tissue support is recorded as nearly as possible in its rest or undisplaced position. When registering border movements and securing an accurate registration of the peripheral denture border areas, one must take care not to exceed the movements falling within the envelope of normal function. Exceeding the movements will produce an *underextended* denture, which is as undesirable as an *overextended* one.

Individualized impression trays fabricated on casts made in an impression that recorded the soft tissues of the crest, slopes of the ridges, and palate in their undistorted positions are used. When borders of the individualized trays are shortened, a border extension and refining with a low fusing impression material are allowed. After the borders have been refined, the trays are altered to allow space and escapes for a free flowing zinc oxide-eugenol impression paste to record the supporting tissues in their undistorted positions. This technique allows for minor corrections with waxes that flow at mouth temperature. It is designed not only to produce an acceptable negative likeness of the residual ridges, but also to require a minimum number of hours in the chair.

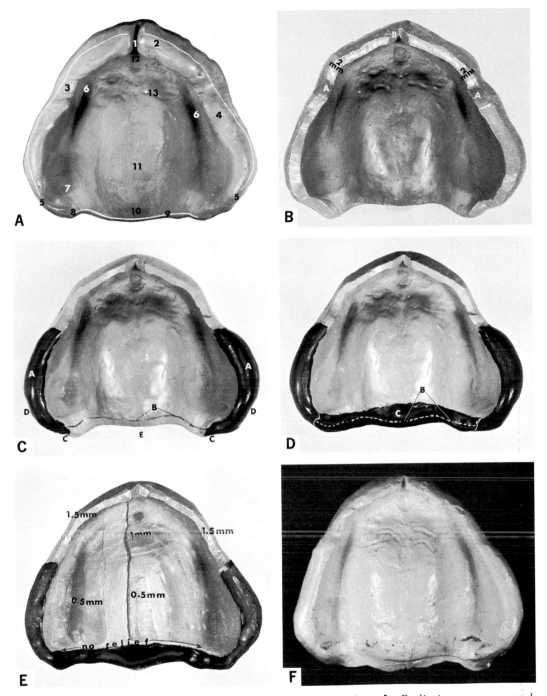

FIG. 6-14. *A technique for making a maxillary impression.* **A.** *Preliminary compound impression: labial frenum* (**1**), *labial vestibule* (**2**), *buccal frenum* (**3**), *buccal vestibule* (**4**), *distobuccal space* (**5**), *crest of the residual alveolar ridge* (**6**), *alveolar tubercle* (**7**), *hamular notch* (**8**), *posterior palatal seal area* (**9**), *fovea palatinus* (**10**), *midpalatal suture* (**11**), *incisal papilla* (**12**), *and rugae area* (**13**). **B.** *The preliminary impression is removed from the tray, and the borders are reduced.* **C.** *The distobuccal flange and hamular notch areas are border refined.* **D.** *The posterior palatal seal area is developed as a border, not as the posterior palatal seal.* **E.** *Space is provided to allow the tissues to return to rest position. An escape is provided to prevent trapping air.* **F.** *The refined impression of zinc oxide-eugenol paste. (Courtesy of A. L. Martone, Medical Towers, Norfolk, Virginia.)*

EQUIPMENT

When final impressions are made, the following equipment should be readily accessible.

1. Water bath with wax pot attached
2. Alcohol torch
3. Bunsen burner
4. Indelible pencil
5. Glass slab
6. Impression trays—individualized
7. Modeling compound knife
8. Modeling compound—green stick and grey stick
9. Mouth mirror, 10 Stellite spatula
10. Ice water
11. Zinc oxide-eugenol impression paste with mixing paper and spatula
12. Physiologic type impression wax
13. Modeling compound knife, preferably the type having a replaceable Bard Parker blade—very sharp
14. Petrolatum

REFINING

The refinement of the final impression is divided into two steps—border refining of the mandibular and maxillary impression trays and refining of the tissue-bearing area.

BORDER OF THE MANDIBULAR
IMPRESSION TRAY

1. The buccal shelf area should be developed bilaterally. This bilateral procedure will insure the proper seating of the tray as the rest of the borders are refined. Using low fusing impression compound, apply bulk enough to retain molding consistency from the distal of the buccal frenum attachment to the distal of the retromolar papilla both right and left sides. Soften the impression compound with flame from alcohol torch, temper in water, 115°F to 128°F, seat to place, and have patient separate jaws, then close, while the operator applies pressure in a downward direction. This action forces the masseter

muscle into action, and the masseter in turn forces the buccinator in the direction of the retromolar papilla to create the masseter groove (Fig. 6-15A 1).

2. The distolingual and post mylohyoid areas should be developed bilaterally. Place bulk of impression compound on the lingual flange opposite the buccal and extend it distally to join the distal to the retromolar papilla. Soften, temper, and seat. Have patient place the tongue in the distal part of the palate in right and left buccal vestibules. Remove the tray, chill it, and trim the excess. Repeat this procedure if anatomic landmarks do not appear definite enough for accurate trimming (Fig. 6-15A 2).

3. The sublingual flange area is developed in its entirety. Place a sufficient bulk of impression compound on the remainder of the underdeveloped lingual flange. Have the patient place his tongue in the anterior part of palate and then gently wipe his upper lip with tip of his tongue. Remove the tray, chill it, and trim the excess (Fig. 6-15A 3).

4. The labial flange is developed unilaterally. If it is done bilaterally, lip interference distorts the impression material. During these procedures if the impression compound flows into the tray on the slope or crest of the residual ridge, it should be removed before proceeding (Fig. 6-15A 4-5).

BORDER OF THE
MAXILLARY IMPRESSION TRAY

1. Add impression compound to the buccal flange, beginning distal to the buccal frenum attachment area, extending distally to and including the hamular notch and across the posterior palatal seal area. Soften with Hanau torch flame, temper, and set to place. Have patient open his mouth wide as in yawning, then protrude, and move mandible to the right and left. This combined action develops the distal extent

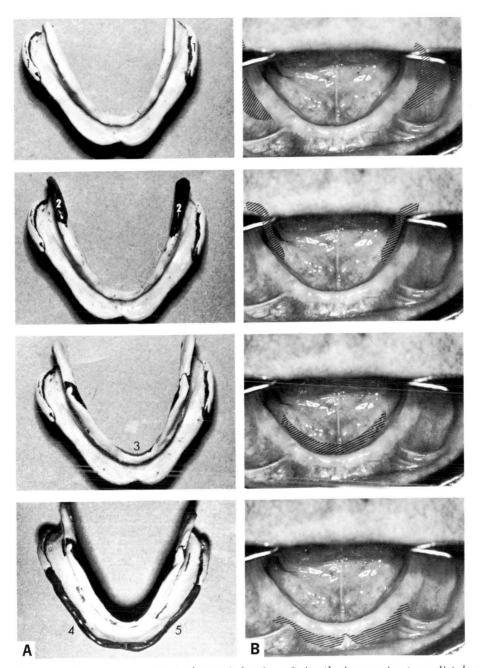

Fig. 6-15. *Mandibular arch.* **A.** *Clinical steps in border refining the impression tray: distobuccal flange (**1**) and buccal shelf area (**2**); distolingual flange and retromylohyoid space (**3**); anterior lingual sulcus (**4**); remainder of buccal flange and labial flange, left side (**5**); remainder of buccal and labial flanges; right side.* **B.** *Photographs of patient's mandibular arch with areas shaded.*

of the denture in the hamular notch and also develops the space between the anterior border of the ramus and the tubercles. The impression compound across the posterior palatal seal area maintains contact with the tissues in this area. It is not the seal.

The border refining should be done bilaterally to insure proper seating of the tray while the remainder of the posterior borders are refined (Fig. 6-16A 1). A systematic procedure saves time.

2. Add bulk of impression compound at the buccal frenum attachment (unilaterally). Flame, temper, and seat to place. Gently massage the upper lip in a superior-inferior direction. Remove the tray and chill it (Fig. 6-16A 2).

3. Repeat for opposite side (Fig. 6-16A 3).

4. Soften impression compound in the buccal frenum area (unilaterally).

5. Add compound in the labial flange area to join the refined buccal border and seat. Have the patient suck gently on your finger. Repeat for opposite side (Fig. 6-16A 4–5).

6. Soften impression compound in the labial frenum area, seat, grasp upper lip, and extend directly forward.

TISSUE-BEARING AREA. Many different materials are used to refine the tissue-bearing areas. Of these the zinc oxide-eugenol paste has many advantages.

The tissue-bearing areas of the individualized impression trays are made 2 to 3 mm thick for a purpose. When a plastic impression material, like zinc oxide-eugenol paste, is placed in the impression tray and then seated in the mouth, the movable tissue is displaced. If the tray is perforated or a space is created in the tray as the impression material flows, the tissues will rebound to their undistorted position.

1. After the borders have been refined, the tissues are examined and palpated with a ball burnisher, and the tray is relieved with an acrylic bur to a depth approximating the displaceability of the tissue (Fig. 6-17). In extreme cases of pendulous and displaceable tissue in the mandibular arch, it is advisable to perforate the tray in that area with a #8 round bur. In the maxillary arch, in addition to creating the space, three holes about the size of a #8 round bur are placed in the tray in the anterior section of the rugae area and two holes in the posterior area (Fig. 6-17B). These holes assure no trapping of air in the vault.

2. Apply petrolatum to the patient's face, as the impression material is sticky and will be hard to remove.

3. Mix the impression material according to manufacturer's instructions. Load the trays, including the borders, to a uniform thickness.

4. Place the loaded trays in the patient's mouth; seat them with positive pressure until the impression material is seen to flow from the borders. After the loaded tray for the mandibular denture has been seated, the patient is instructed to place the tip of his tongue on the tip of the upper lip and to breathe through his nose. *All* pressure is released, and the index and middle fingers are rested one on each side on the superior surface of the compound occlusion rim in the bicuspid area.

In seating the loaded maxillary tray, the posterior palatal seal area and the holes in the rugae area should be observed. When the impression material flows over and through these areas, all pressure should be released and the index and middle fingers rested lightly, one on each side, on the occlusion rims about the bicuspid area. The patient is instructed to flex his head forward and breathe through his nose.

In seating both the loaded maxillary and mandibular trays, it is usually better to seat the anterior section first. If a pa-

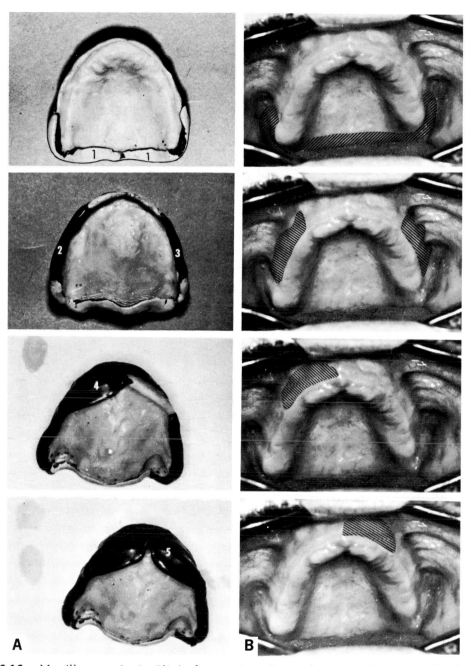

FIG. 6-16. *Maxillary arch.* **A.** *Clinical steps in refining the impression tray: distobuccal flange, hamular notch, and posterior palatal seal area* (**1**); *buccal flange, left* (**2**), *right* (**3**); *labial flange, left* (**4**), *right* (**5**). **B.** *Photographs of patient's maxillary arch with areas 1, 2, 3, 4, and 5 shaded.*

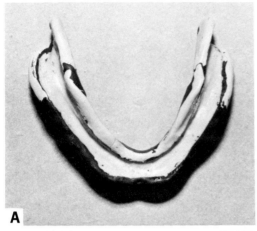

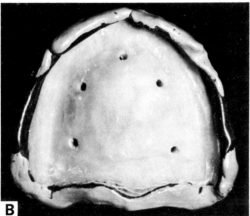

FIG. 6-17. *Creating space in the impression trays to allow the tissues to assume an undistorted position.* **A.** *The mandibular tray has been relieved over the crest and slopes of the ridge.* **B.** *The maxillary tray has also been relieved and has been perforated to allow air to escape.*

tient evidences moderate mucous secretions in the posterior palatal seal area of the palate, the area should be wiped dry with gauze just before inserting the loaded tray. In cases of excessive mucous secretion, plaster gum or plaster impression material is advisable.

5. When the zinc oxide-eugenol impression paste is thoroughly set, the refined impression is removed from the mouth, washed with tap water, dried with a gentle application of air, and

inspected. If desired, the impression can be reseated and checked for retention and stability.

6. The impressions should be beaded, boxed, and poured as soon as practical. Baseplate wax, one sheet cut in half lengthwise, is used to form the container for the Hydrocal from which the stone casts are formed. The maxillary impression is seated, tray side down, in a soft mixture of half pumice and half dental plaster in water. When the mixture is set, the shoulders are contoured approxi-

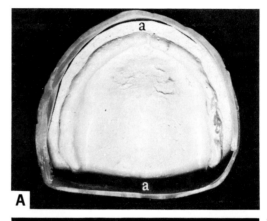

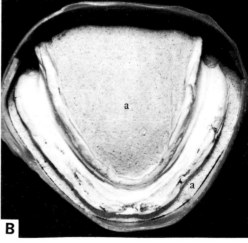

FIG. 6-18. *Refined impression trays prepared for pouring Hydrocal to form the stone casts.* **A.** *Maxillary impression.* **B.** *Mandibular impression. The shoulders (**a**) in both impressions have been contoured.*

mately 3 mm below the borders and 4 mm in width (Fig. 6-18A). The mandibular tray also is seated tray side down in the pumice and dental plaster mixture, and the shoulders are contoured in the same manner, except that there is a solid mass of the hard mixture between the lingual flanges (Fig. 6-18B).

Descriptions of specific techniques may present tedious reading for the student. However, it is essential to know how a procedure is accomplished, what materials are used, and above all *why* the procedures were followed and *why* the materials were selected. It is not implied that the impression materials used in the techniques in this chapter are the only materials that can be used successfully. A knowledge of the basic principles of making complete denture impressions will enable the operator to evaluate techniques and materials and to select those best adapted to each patient.

REFERENCES

1. Asgarzadeh, K., and Peyton, F. A.: Physical properties of corrective impression pastes. J. Prosth. Dent., 4:555, 1954.
2. Blanchard, E. H.: Eyes in your fingers. J. Prosth. Dent., 4:739, 1954.
3. Bohannon, H. M.: A critical analysis of the mucostatic principles. J. Prosth. Dent., 4:232, 1954.
4. Booth, J. M.: Reversible hydrocolloid and plastics in complete denture construction. J. Prosth. Dent., 6:24, 1956.
5. Boucher, C. O.: A critical analysis of mid-century impression technique for full dentures. J. Prosth. Dent., 1:472, 1951.
6. ———: Fundamental approach to the problems of impressions for complete dentures. D. Pract., 8:162, 1958.
7. Buckley, G. A.: Diagnostic factors in the choice of impression material and methods. J. Prosth. Dent., 5:145, 1955.
7a. Carlile, E. F.: Functional adaptation of lower denture bases. J. Prosth. Dent., 1:662, 1951.
7b. Collett, H. A.: Final impressions for complete dentures. J. Prosth. Dent., 23:250, 1970.
8. Clark, R. J., and Philips, R. W.: Flow studies of certain dental impression materials. J. Prosth. Dent., 7:259, 1957.
9. Collett, H. A.: Peripheral control with alginate full denture impressions. J. Prosth. Dent., 4:739, 1954.
10. ———: Complete denture impressions. J. Prosth. Dent., 15:603, 1965.
11. Denen, H. E.: Impressions for full dentures. J. Prosth. Dent., 3:737, 1952.
12. DeVan, M. M.: Basic principles of impression making. J. Prosth. Dent., 2:26, 1952.
13. Dresen, O. M.: The rubber base impression material. J. Prosth. Dent., 8:14, 1958.
13a. Ellinger, C. W.: Minimizing problems in making a complete lower impression. J. Prosth. Dent., 30:553, 1973.
13b. Fisher, R. D.: Fundamental rules for making full denture impressions. J. Prosth. Dent., 1:135, 1951.
13c. Frank, R. P.: Analysis of pressures produced during maxillary edentulous impression procedures. J. Prosth. Dent., 22:400, 1968.
13d. Frankewicz, C. A., and Boles, G. G.: An impression procedure. J. Prosth. Dent., 1:648, 1951.
13e. Freeman, S. P.: Impressions for complete dentures. J.A.D.A., 80:1173, 1970.
14. Friedman, S.: Edentulous impression procedures for maximum retention and stability. J. Prosth. Dent., 7:14, 1957.
14a. Heartwell, C. M., Jr., et al.: Comparison of impressions made in perforated and nonperforated rimlock trays. J. Prosth. Dent., 27:494, 1972.
14b. Herfort, T. W., Gerberich, W. W., Macosko, C. W., and Goodkind, R. J.: Viscosity of elastomeric impression materials. J. Prosthet. Dent., 38:396, 1977.
15. Jamieson, Charles: A complete denture impression technique. J. Prosth. Dent., 4:17, 1954.
15a. Joglekar, A. P., and Sinkford, J. C.: Impression procedures for problem mandibular complete dentures. J.A.D.A., 77:1303, 1968.
15b. Kabcenell, J. L.: More retentive complete dentures. J.A.D.A., 80:116, 1970.
15c. Kaiser, D. A., and Nicholis, J. I.: A study

of distortion and surface hardness of improved artificial stone casts. J. Prosth. Dent., *36*:373, 1976.

16. Klein, I. E.: Complete denture impression technique. J. Prosth. Dent., *5*:739, 1955.

16a. Levin, B., Gamer, S., and Francis, E. D.: Patient preference for a mandibular complete denture with a broad or minimal base: A preliminary report. J. Prosth. Dent., *23*:525, 1970.

16b. Logan, T. E.: Principles involved in impression making. J. Prosth. Dent., *29*:594, 1973.

16c. Luthra, S. P.: Measurement of the area of the maxillary basal seat for dentures. J. Prosth. Dent., *30*:25, 1973.

17. McCracken, W. L.: Impression materials in prosthetic dentistry. Dent. Clin. N. Amer., November, 1958, p. 671.

17a. Marmour, D., and Hebertson, J. E.: The use of swallowing in making complete lower denture impressions. J. Prosth. Dent., *19*:208, 1968.

17b. Milligen, J. D. V.: Movement of mandibular sulci during normal tongue and mouth movements. J. Prosth. Dent., *27*:4, 1972.

18. Millsap, C. H.: The posterior palatal seal area for complete dentures. Dent. Clin. N. Amer., November, 1964, p. 663.

19. Moses, C. H.: Physical considerations in impression making. J. Prosth. Dent., *3*:449, 1953.

20. Myers, C. E., and Peyton, F. A.: Clinical and physical studies of the silicone rubber base impression materials. J. Prosth. Dent., *9*:315, 1959.

21. —— and Stockman, D. C.: Factors that affect the accuracy and dimensional stability of the mercaptan rubber-base impression materials. J. Prosth. Dent., *10*:525, 1960.

22. Nealor, Frank H.: The effect of temperature on the flow of alginates. J. Prosth. Dent., *3*:814, 1953.

23. Page, H. L.: *Mucostatics—A Principle Not A Technique.* Harry L. Page, Chicago, 1946.

24. Pleasure, M. A.: Impression procedures for stability of complete dentures. Dent. Clin. N. Amer., November, 1964, p. 653.

25. Porter, C. G.: Mucostatics—panacea or propaganda. J. Prosth. Dent., *3*:464, 1953.

25a. Reisbick, M. H., and Matyas, J.: The accuracy of highly filled elastomeric impression materials. J. Prosth. Dent., *33*:67, 1975.

26. Roberts, A. L.: Principles of full denture impression making and their application in practice. J. Prosth. Dent., *1*:213, 1951.

26a. Rudd, K. D., and Morrow, R. M.: Premedication: An aid in obtaining accurate complete denture impressions. J. Prosth. Dent., *18*:86, 1967.

26b. —— and Morrow, R. M.: A simplified method for mixing dental stone. J. Prosth. Dent., *32*:675, 1974.

26c. Simmonds, C. R., and Jones, P. M.: A variation in complete mandibular impression form related to an anomaly of the mylohyoid muscle. J. Prosth. Dent., *34*:384, 1975.

27. Skinner, E. W., Cooper, E. N., and Ziehm, H. W.: Some physical properties of zinc oxide-eugenol impression pastes. J.A.D.A., *41*:449, 1950.

27a. —— and Chung, P.: The effect of surface contact in the retention of a denture. J. Prosth. Dent., *1*:229, 1951.

27b. Springmann, W., and Vieira, D. F.: Changes in physical properties of joined gypsum fragments. J. Prosth. Dent., *37*:50, 1977.

27c. Starcke, E. N., Jr., et al.: Physical properties of tissue conditioning materials used in functional impressions. J. Prosth. Dent., *27*:111, 1972.

27d. Stockhouse, J. A.: A comparison of elastic impression materials. J. Prosth. Dent., *34*:305, 1975.

28. Sussman, B. A.: Upper and lower impression technique as developed at Mt. Sinai hospital dental department. J.A.D.A., *31*:1346, 1944.

29. Swenson, M. G.: Anatomy in relation to edentulous impressions for full dentures. J.A.D.A., *20*:1078, 1933.

30. Tylman, S. D.: Hydrocolloid impression materials. Dent. Clin. N. Amer., November, 1958, p. 713.

31. Vieira, D. F.: Factors affecting the setting of zinc oxide-eugenol impression pastes. J. Prosth. Dent., *9*:7, 1959.

31a. Walsh, J. F., and Walsh, T.: Muscle-formed complete mandibular dentures. J. Prosth. Dent., *35*:254, 1976.

31b. Walter, J. D.: Composite impression procedures. J. Prosth. Dent., *30*:385, 1973.

32. Woelfel, J. B.: Contour variations in impressions of one edentulous patient. J. Prosth. Dent., *12*:229, 1962.

33. Young, J. M.: Surface characteristics of dental stone: Impression orientation. J. Prosth. Dent., *33*:336, 1975.

Mandibular Movements, Maxillomandibular Relations, and Concepts of Occlusion

7

Maxillomandibular * relations and occlusion create more controversy than any other dental subjects. Since these subjects are considered the meeting ground for all the disciplines in dentistry, dissension is to be expected. Several factors contribute to this situation: (1) differences in the interpretation of definitions, (2) usage of terminology that is not universally understood, (3) differences in the interpretation of clinical results, (4) enthusiasm created in sincere efforts to produce mechanical instruments that will record and reproduce exact movements of living tissue, and (5) differences in the evaluation of jaw relations and occlusion of natural teeth and relating and applying these findings to the completely edentulous patient.

The last factor *must* be understood and considered, for the difference between the influence of natural teeth and that of dentures on maxillomandibular relations, mandibular movements, jaw relation records, and occlusion is important. Complete denture bases rest on tissue that is movable and displaceable in varying degrees and in different

areas. The natural teeth are supported by bone and are movable only to the extent of the periodontal attachments under favorable forces. Unfavorable forces can move natural teeth beyond the normal limits of the periodontal attachments. The natural teeth can act singly or as a unit, whereas the teeth in a denture must act as a unit. A premature contact existing between natural teeth affects the involved teeth and adjacent support, whereas premature contact between artificial teeth affects the entire base in its relation to the supporting tissue. As a result of their relatively fixed positions in the bone, natural teeth have a greater influence in mandibular movements than do artificial teeth on their movable bases.

This chapter will review briefly mandibular movements and maxillomandibular relations, define and discuss terminology used in occlusion, and analyze the concepts of occlusion. One must understand these factors before recording maxillomandibular relations, transferring casts to articulators, or developing an occlusal scheme that will be acceptable as a substitute for the missing natural teeth.

*Jaw relations (used synonymously).

Mandibular Movements

The condyles articulate with the temporal bones and are located in the elliptical concave depressions called the *glenoid fossae* in which they travel forward, from side to side, and in some instances slightly backward. Between the dome-shaped concavities in the temporal bones and the condyles are interposed the interarticular fibrocartilages, the menisci, which are attached at their margins to the articular capsules. The menisci divide the joints into upper and lower compartments. Normally, the movement in the upper compartment is chiefly a gliding anteroposterior motion in which the condyles and the cartilage move as a unit; the movement in the lower compartment is hingelike. Because of its peculiar form and the manner of its attachments, the mandible is *capable of,* and *subject to, a great variety of movements.* So free and varied are these that, unless carefully considered, they may appear to lack coordination. Four movements of prime importance to complete denture service are (1) the *hingelike* movement used in opening and closing the mouth for the introduction of food and, to a limited degree, for the crushing of certain types of brittle food, (2) a protrusive movement used in the grasping and incision of food, (3) *right* or *left lateral* movements for use in the reduction of fibrous as well as other types of food, and (4) *Bennett* movement—the bodily side shift of the mandible which, when it occurs, may be recorded in the region of the rotating condyle on the working side.

The importance of Bennett movement cannot be overly emphasized in reproducing the cusps of the teeth. Its direction and timing influence the freedom of movement to and from the centric and eccentric jaw positions through the corresponding sulci of their antagonists. Precise fashioning or carving of fossae and sulci allows eccentric movements that do not introduce lateral stress. Balanced gliding occlusion will be difficult to achieve if the direction and timing of Bennett movement is not accurately recorded and transferred to an articulator capable of reproducing the movement.

Functional mandibular movements include all natural or characteristic movements occurring during mastication, swallowing, speech, and yawning. Although not all of the factors involved in the release of nervous tension are understood, movements that occur in the clenching, tapping, or grinding of the teeth are *parafunctional* movements and are not natural, or characteristic.

Investigators have learned that the teeth of some individuals rarely contact during mastication and that those of others make frequent contacts. The size, type, and consistency of the bolus of food and the vigor with which a person masticates influence these contacts. Teeth make many contacts in the absence of food during speech and swallowing. Since eating requires about one hour a day for most individuals, it can be assumed that the contacting of the teeth in nonmasticatory mandibular movements, whether considered to be functional or parafunctional, is of more concern to the dentist than those contacts made during mastication.

Not all dentists are in a position to investigate the entities involved in mandibular movements; however, terminology and definitions should be understood. This understanding permits the dentist to interpret investigations and findings and use the results to advantage.

Mandibular movements are related to three planes of the skull—horizontal, frontal, and sagittal—and are usually described as three-dimensional. *Dimension* is defined as "magnitude measured in a particular direction, or along a diameter or principal axis."* The rotational centers for mandibular movements are the transverse, sagittal, and vertical axes (Fig. 7-1). A trained individual can open and close about the transverse axis in a hinge action; lateral movement takes place about a vertical axis; and opening other than hinge action includes movement about the sagittal axis. Unguided mandibular movements are a combination of rotations and glidings, and the rotational centers move and change. These movements include bruxism and bruxomania.[56]

Only if instruments that duplicate pantographic tracings are used can a fourth dimension—time—be incorporated in the study of mandibular movements. Gnathological findings have demon-

Random House Dictionary of the English Language.

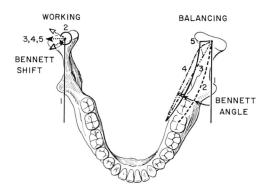

FIG. 7-2. *Bennett movement is recorded on the rotating side; the Bennett angle is measured on the gliding side.*

strated the time at which the Bennett movement occurs in the opening and closing movements (Fig. 7-2).

The knowledge of the elements of mandibular movements is the key to the choice and use of articulators in developing occlusion. The transverse axis can be transferred to an articulator that is capable of receiving a kinematic type of face-bow. The centers of lateral motion can be transferred to an articulator that can be adjusted for intercondylar distance (Fig. 7-3).

BORDER POSITIONS

A mandibular element to be understood before recording maxillomandibular relationships and making tooth arrangements for complete denture service is border position. *Border* refers to the boundary of a surface and may imply the limiting line. *Border positions* of the mandible can be defined as the extreme positions of the mandible in any direction in which it moves. The border positions are limited by nerves, bones, muscles, teeth when present, and ligaments. The limiting is not a simple mechanical stoppage but a physiologic control through the neuromuscular system. The recording of border positions in the absence of some of these factors

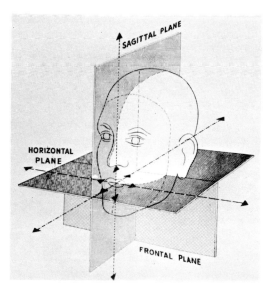

FIG. 7-1. *The three planes of the skull. (From Posselt, U.: Physiology of Occlusion and Rehabilitation. Oxford, Blackwell Scientific Publications, 1966.)*

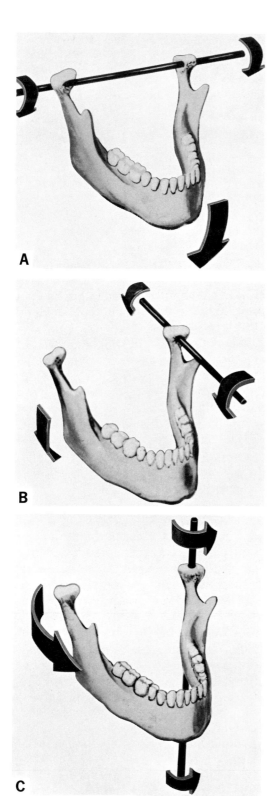

A

B

C

does not indicate that the factor was not an aid in limiting the position when it was present.

The envelope* of motion of the mandible in the border positions has been recorded in three planes—horizontal, frontal, and sagittal (Fig. 7-4). The envelope of motion during masticatory functions has been recorded and found to be within the envelope of border movements (Fig. 7-5). It has been demonstrated that the envelope of mandibular movements during the process of chewing is variable, since the movements are influenced by the size and resistance of the bolus, number and size of the teeth, excess or lack of saliva, the musculature, and the vigor of the stroke. Although the envelope takes similar form, the occlusal form of the tooth influences the character of the chewing cycle (Fig. 7-6).

The *functional range* refers to the full extent over which something is effective. This range of movement of the mandible may or may not include border positions; however, border positions are invaluable when making jaw relation records, as they are the only consistently repeatable positions. The *terminal hinge axis* represents a border position that can be repeated and recorded (Fig. 7-7).

CONDYLE PATH

The condyle path is a controlling factor in mandibular movement and is peculiar to each individual patient. It is the path traveled by the condyles in the temporomandibular joints during the

---

*In geometry, "the envelope is the locus of the ultimate intersections of a series of curves or surfaces."

FIG. 7-3. A. *Transverse axis.* **B.** *Sagittal axis.* **C.** *Vertical axis.* (*Courtesy of the J. M. Ney Co., Hartford, Connecticut.*)

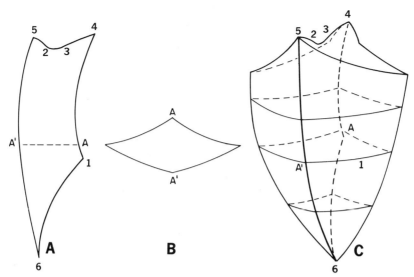

FIG. 7-4. *Schematic drawings of motion in the sagittal plane. In the three figures note the horizontal cross section at a given degree of maxillomandibular separation (A and A′). Horizontal cross sections at varying degrees of maxillomandibular separation differ in size but not in form.* **A.** *Average movements in the sagittal plane (left profile): 4 to 1, the terminal hinge movement, a border movement; 1 to 6, opening exceeding hinge movement, another border movement; 6, maximal opening; 4, the retruded contact position (centric occlusion) or maximum intercuspation with the mandible in terminal hinge position; 4 to 3, tooth contact from centric occlusion in straight protrusion following the cingulae of the maxillary anterior teeth; 3 to 2, edge to edge contact; 2 to 5, protrusion of mandibular anterior teeth beyond the maxillary anterior teeth; 4 to 5, guided by tooth contact (intraborder); 5, contact between the teeth in the maximal protruded relation; 5 to 6, mandibular movement from the maximal protruded contact to maximal opening. The anterior border opening is not a hinge movement.*

*   **B.** *A horizontal movement area at a definite level of maxillomandibular separation.*

*   **C.** *A composite of average movement area in the sagittal plane with horizontal movement areas at three levels of maxillomandibular separation. (After Posselt, U.: Physiology of Occlusion and Rehabilitation. Oxford, Blackwell Scientific Publications, 1966.)*

various mandibular movements. In completely edentulous patients condyle paths are determined by (1) the bony fossae, (2) the tone of the muscles responsible for mandibular movements and their nerve controls, (3) the limitations imposed by the attached ligaments, and (4) the shape and movements of the menisci. The path cannot be altered by the prosthodontist.

The condyle path does not follow a straight line but follows the contour of the tissue-lined bony surroundings.

It is not recorded when a protrusive or lateral protrusive record is made at a static point in the path. The path therefore is not recorded with an articulator in which the condylar elements travel in a straight slot or on a flat surface. Such articulators travel in a straight line (Fig. 7-8). Articulators that have individually ground condyle paths refined to pantographic tracings recorded in three planes can travel in the path recorded in the tracings (Fig. 7-9).

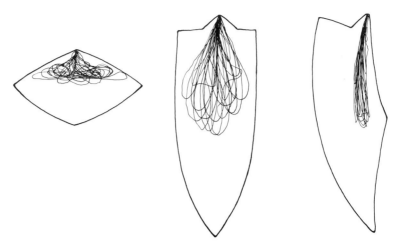

FIG. 7-5. *Graphic drawing of movements of the mandible during masticatory function. They are within the space envelope. Masticatory movements vary as a result of consistency, bulk, and type of food. (Courtesy of J. Marvin Reynolds, Dept. of Occlusion, Medical College of Georgia, School of Dentistry.)*

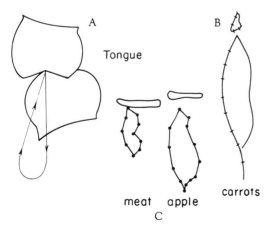

FIG. 7-6. *Graphic representation of electro-myographic study of mandibular movements.* **A.** *The "tear drop" movement. (From Nagle and Sears, Denture Prosthetics, Complete dentures. 2nd ed. St. Louis, The C. V. Mosby Company, 1962, p. 21.* **B.** *The chewing stroke with carrots, not exactly a tear drop. (From Hickey, J. C., Stacey, B. W., and Rinear, L. L.: Mandibular movements in three dimensions. J. Prosth. Dent., 13:89, 1963.)* **C.** *The mandibular movements are different, yet similar. (From Jankelson, B., Hoffman, G., and Hendron, J.: The physiology of the stomatognathic system. J.A.D.A., 46:381, 1953.)*

The question of the immutability of the condyle path cannot be considered of any clinical significance during the construction of a denture. In the absence of pathosis, a change would not be expected to be rapid or dramatic. It is

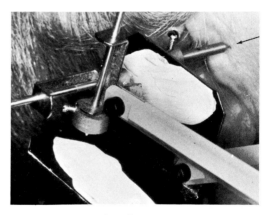

FIG. 7-7. *Recording hinge movement. Arrow designates the point on the skin where hinge movement was recorded and repeated. Trained individuals can execute pure hinge movement at different degrees of protrusion. Pure hinge movement with both condyles in terminal hinge position is the only hinge movement that is definitive.*

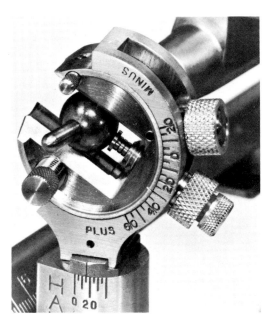

FIG. 7-8. *The Hanau articulator travels in a straight path. (Courtesy of the Hanau Engineering Company.)*

significant that the condyles can be rotated in their path. Although this action may be advantageous in many instances, it can result in inaccuracies in maxillomandibular relation records. One sees this clinically when using interocclusal recording materials of unequal resistance bilaterally in making jaw relation records. It is possible to make an accurate anteroposterior record and not have equal vertical pressure bilaterally. The result in occlusion of artificial teeth when arranged to this record will be premature tooth contact on the side of the more resistant material. This phenomenon can also be a result of the unequal displacement of the supporting soft tissues on the two sides.

Maxillomandibular Relations

CENTRIC RELATION

Centric relation is "the most retruded physiologic relation of the mandible to the maxillae to and from which the individual can make lateral movements. It . . . can exist at various degrees of jaw separation. It occurs around the terminal hinge axis."*

An analysis of this definition reveals that centric relation is an anteroposterior bone-to-bone relation, that of the maxillae and mandible. It is an unstrained position in which an individual can assume the most posterior relation voluntarily and by reflex action without stretching the muscles to their utmost to reach the position. Neither force nor

*Glossary of Prosthodontic Terms.

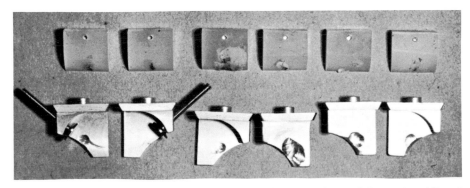

FIG. 7-9. *The Stewart instrument has individually ground condyle paths. (Courtesy of C. H. Stewart, D.D.S.)*

pressure has been applied to alter the shape or the position of the muscles or stretch them to their utmost. McCollum defines this position as "the most retruded position of the idle condyles in the glenoid fossae."[53] Idle means inactive. An object that is inactive is passive. Passive objects are not considered to be resisting forces that would stretch or force them beyond the normal, customary, or legitimate limits. It is possible to apply unequal vertical force bilaterally with a recording medium and cause a change in the form or size of tissues and produce strain. Although lateral movements can be made from the position of centric relation, it is impossible to make pure lateral movement if the jaws are separated to the maximum open position. There is controversy regarding a more retruded position, as many investigators think that the mandible can be forced into a more retruded position than that from which lateral movement is possible. Other investigators do not consider a more retruded position possible. It is questionable if a record could be made and repeated at a more retruded position. The usable valid record of centric relation in complete denture construction is *repeatable*.

The mandible has *a most* retruded relation to the maxillae at varying degrees of jaw separation. Records that will coincide with centric relation can be made at these varying vertical positions. These records are obtainable without teeth being present, with occlusion rims, or with teeth. Stuart and Stallard define centric relation of the mandible as "the rearmost, midmost, untranslated hinged position. It is a *strained* relation as are all border relations. It is the only maxillomandibular relation that can be statically repeated."[92]

According to Posselt[64] the border movements of the mandible are reproducible, and all other movements take place within the framework of the borders. When the mandible is held in the most retruded position by the patient or the operator, a hinge movement can be recorded in the sagittal plane at the incisor point. The movement is referred to as *terminal hinge movement*. The relation of the mandible is referred to as *centric relation*, hinge position, or retruded position. It is a *bone-to-bone* relation.

Posselt also demonstrated a disparity between the contacting tooth surfaces when the mandible was in a terminal hinge position and when the teeth were in maximum intercuspal relation. To provide maximum intercuspation the mandible must be moved in a combination of forward and lateral direction. This slide was demonstrated in adults with good dentition, in successfully treated orthodontic patients,[23] and in children.[44]

If these findings are accepted by the dental profession to be normal, the term *centric,* if used to define the retruded relation of the mandible and the maxillae, should be restricted when used with occlusion to maximum intercuspation when the mandible is in terminal hinge position. The use of *centric* to define a tooth-to-tooth relation and also a bone-to-bone relation creates confusion.

Regardless of whether the maxillomandibular relation is strained or unstrained, whether lateral movements can be made from this relation, or whether it is the most retruded position to which the mandible can be forced, these observations about centric relation are significant in complete denture construction:

1. It is a definite learned position.
2. The patient can voluntarily and reflexly return to this position.

3. It can be recorded and repeated.

4. In mounting the cast on an articulator, the anteroposterior relation of the maxillary and mandibular casts becomes a definite entity.

5. This position can be verified, as other records can be made in the mouth, and the articulator will accept the records.

6. Centric relation is a reference point in recording maxillomandibular relations and a starting point for developing occlusion. It is a *point of return.*

ECCENTRIC RELATIONS

Any relation of the mandible to the maxillae other than centric relation is an *eccentric relation.* The eccentric relations that are recorded and used in complete denture construction are protrusive and right and left lateral.

Protrusive relation is the relation of the mandible to the maxillae when the mandible is thrust forward. If the motion in every part of the mandible as it is thrust forward has simultaneously the same velocity and direction, the motion could be correctly termed *translatory.* The movement in the joint is downward and forward. The condyles and menisci are guided downward by the articular eminences of the glenoid fossae. The angle of glide varies from patient to patient and from side to side in the same patient. The muscles responsible for a straight protrusive movement are the external pterygoid muscles acting simultaneously. Protrusive relation is a bone-to-bone relation, which can be recorded.

Right and *left lateral maxillomandibular relations* are the relations of the mandible to the maxillae when the mandible is moved either to the right or to the left side. The movement of the mandible is the result of the contraction of one external pterygoid muscle. When the external pterygoid of one side contracts, the corresponding side of the mandible is pulled forward while the other side remains comparatively fixed. The side that is pulled forward is termed the "nonworking or balancing side," whereas the side that remains comparatively fixed is termed the "working or rotating side." The movements that take place in the nonworking side are downward and forward. The downward and forward movement may be accompanied by a movement in a medial direction. The movement is both gliding and rotary. The movements that take place when the mandible is moved to the working side are those of rotation. The rotation may also be accompanied by a side shift, Bennett movement with a forward, backward, upward, or downward component. Lateral maxillomandibular relations can be recorded.

The question of necessity for eccentric records is one of controversy, since the problem of accuracy exists in the recording methods and the capabilities of the articulator to receive and reproduce the record. These factors contribute to inaccuracy: (1) unstability of records, (2) resiliency and displaceability of denture-bearing tissues, (3) materials used in record making, (4) equipment used in record making, (5) lack of muscle coordination by the patient, and (6) the use of articulators that do not accurately adjust to all lateral interocclusal check records.

The controversy about the merits of eccentric records will exist as long as there are differences in the concepts of occlusion and posterior tooth form required for complete dentures. Dentists who prefer a cusp form posterior tooth and *balanced occlusion* in *eccentric* jaw positions or *organic* occlusion will require eccentric maxillomandibular relation records. Dentists who prefer a noncusp form posterior tooth and *balanced occlusion* in *centric* jaw position will not require eccentric maxillomandibular relation records.

There are no scientific data to support advantages of one concept over the other. We do not know how much accuracy is required in many of the procedures in complete denture construction to assure success. Each situation must be analyzed, and the method of choice is the method that is the most accurate.

PHYSIOLOGIC REST POSITION

The position assumed by the mandible when the head is in an upright position, the muscles are in equilibrium in tonic contraction, and the condyles are in a neutral, unstrained position, is the physiologic rest position of the mandible (Fig. 7-10). There is considerable controversy about the anteroposterior position of the condyles in relation to the glenoid fossae and the anteroposterior relation of the maxillae and mandible at rest position. In some individuals the condyles are in their most posterior unstrained position and the maxillae and mandible are in their most retruded relation. If this is correct, the closure from rest position to centric occlusion would be hingelike. It has also been shown that closure from rest position to occlusal contact is not usually a hinge closure. It is possible that closure varies with individuals; therefore, neither premise must be accepted as applicable in all situations. Sicher states that "the rest position is constant in each individual due to the individually fixed and only slightly variable tonus of the masticatory muscles, which, in their 'relaxation,' allow the mandible to drop slightly. The rest position is therefore not dependent on the presence of teeth or on their shape or position but on the musculature and on muscle balance

only."[86] In spite of all the changes of the residual alveolar ridges because of atrophy, accident, etc., the rest position of the mandible remains fairly stable throughout the life of an individual, unless it is changed by severe chronic illness.

The studies of Thompson, Niswonger, Gillis, Shanahan, Boos, Shpuntoff, Neuakari, Silverman, and many others furnish valuable information regarding physiologic rest position, and their findings should be reviewed when considering this subject.

The significance of physiologic rest position to the dentist is that (1) it is a bone-to-bone relation in a vertical direction, (2) in the absence of pathosis the relation is fairly constant throughout life, (3) the position can be recorded and measured within acceptable limits, and (4) it is used in determining the vertical dimension of occlusion.

VERTICAL DIMENSION

The vertical dimension refers to the length of the face. It is maintained either by the occlusion of the teeth or the balanced tonic contraction of the opening and closing muscles of mandibular movements. These two measurable lengths of the face are important guides in making maxillomandibular relation records and are referred to as (1) the vertical dimension of physiologic rest position (Fig. 7-10) and (2) the vertical dimension of occlusion (Fig. 7-11).

The *vertical dimension of physiologic rest position* is the vertical separation of the jaws when the opening and closing muscles of the mandible are at rest in tonic contraction. It is measured on the face, but its value in maxillomandibular relation records is that these measurements are used to determine the vertical distance between the occluding surfaces of teeth on occlusion rims and/or the crests of the residual ridges.

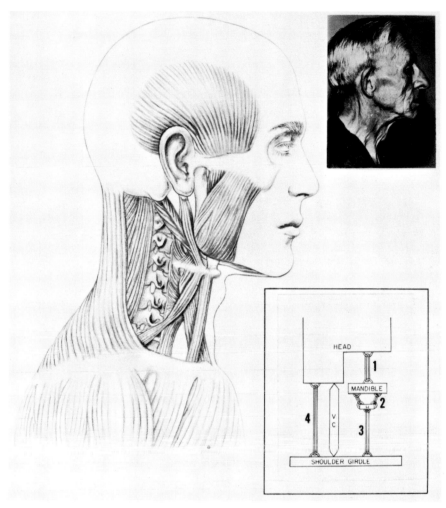

FIG. 7-10.   *The vertical dimension of physiologic rest position is recorded when the elevator and depressor muscles attached to the mandible are in tonic equilibrium. (From Martone, A. L.: Anatomy of facial expression and its prosthodontic significance. J. Prosth. Dent., 12:1036, 1962.)*

The *vertical dimension of occlusion* is the vertical separation of the jaws when the teeth are in occlusion. It is generally conceded that the teeth should not be in contact when the jaws are at the vertical dimension of rest position. The distance between the teeth is the interocclusal distance frequently referred to as the "freeway space." This distance is not the same for all individuals and therefore must be established for each patient. A variation of 3 millimeters between the vertical dimension of physiologic rest position and the vertical dimension of occlusion is not applicable to all patients and should not be relied upon in the construction of dentures.

Failure to provide *adequate* interocclusal distance produces *excessive* interarch distance when the teeth are in occlusion. This position does not allow the muscles that elevate the mandible

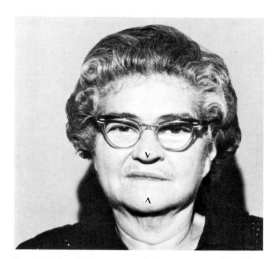

FIG. 7-11. *The vertical dimension of occlusion is measured with the teeth in maximum intercuspation. Points of reference can be placed on the nose and the chin or on the forehead and the chin.*

flabby instead of firm and full. The etiology of angular cheilitis is sometimes attributed to overclosure of occlusion or excessive interocclusal distance (Fig. 7-12). It should not be in the planned treatment to create an error; however, if an error in the establishment of the interocclusal distance is made, a slight excess appears to be more acceptable than an inadequacy. Deliberately to allow excessive interocclusal distance to favor a resorbed ridge or damaged supporting tissues in one arch is not advisable. To establish the occlusal plane at a different vertical position than existed with the natural teeth may result in more damage than protection.

The terms *open bite* or *closed bite* have no scientific or grammatical place in this phase of dental terminology as the

to complete their contraction. The muscles will continue to exert force to overcome this obstacle, and as a result the supporting tissues will be resorbed until the proper distance is returned. Fortunately, the premature contacting of the teeth also results in a clicking noise, and this unpleasant sound is one of the guides in determining the proper interocclusal distance. Inadequate distance results in facial distortion because the individual has difficulty in closing the lips. In addition, swallowing is difficult.

Excessive interocclusal distance results in a *reduced* interarch distance when the teeth are in occlusion. This overclosure in occlusion is potentially damaging to the temporomandibular joint. The normal tongue space is limited. Facial distortion appears more noticeable with overclosure than with the slightly opened closure, as the chin appears to be closer to the nose, the commissure of the lips turns down, and the lips lose their fullness. The muscles of facial expression lose their tonicity, and the face appears

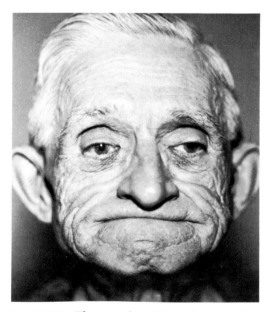

FIG. 7-12. *The muscles of facial expression are distorted when there is excessive interocclusal distance. (From Martone, A. L., and Edwards, L. F.: The face. In The Phenomenon of Function in Complete Denture Prosthodontics. Reprinted from J. Prosth. Dent., St. Louis, The C. V. Mosby Company, 1961, 1962, 1963.)*

word *bite* is defined as "to seize, grip or cut with as with the teeth."

OCCLUSION

Occlusion is an anatomic and physiologic complex present when the opposing teeth are in contact. It consists of the positional relations, the stresses directed to the supporting structures, their resistance to stresses, the form and the arrangement of the teeth, the influencing factors of the components of the temporomandibular joints, and the neuromuscular mechanism responsible for mandibular movements.

The *Glossary of Prosthodontic Terms* defines occlusion as "the relationship between the occlusal surfaces of the maxillary and mandibular teeth when they are in contact." This is a static position, and the jaws can be in either centric or eccentric relation. The static contacting of teeth should be differentiated from *gliding occlusion.*

Gliding occlusion is the contacting of teeth in motion. Dynamic as opposed to static, it is related to energy or physical force in motion. Gliding occlusion occurs when the occlusal surfaces of the teeth make contact when the mandible is moving to and from eccentric and centric jaw relations.

Centric occlusion (Fig. 7-13) is the relation of opposing occlusal surfaces that provides the maximum planned contact and/or intercuspation. In complete dentures it is desirable that the occluding surfaces of the teeth be in the maximum planned contact and/or intercuspation when the jaws are in *centric* relation. Centric occlusion with teeth present is a *tooth*-to-*tooth* relation, whereas centric relation, a static position, is a bone-to-bone relation.

Eccentric occlusion is the contacting of teeth or occluding surfaces when the jaws are in any other relation than centric relation. The contacting of teeth

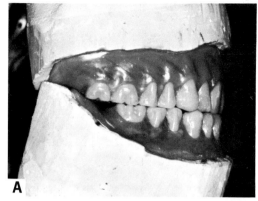

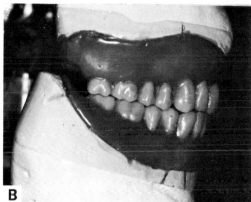

FIG. 7-13. *Centric occlusion does not depend upon the posterior tooth form.* **A.** *Noncusp form posterior teeth in maximum contact.* **B.** *Cusp form posterior teeth in maximum contact. The casts were mounted with a maxillomandibular relation record taken with the jaws in terminal hinge position.*

in eccentric occlusion can occur with the jaws in a static relation or with the jaws in motion.

Balanced occlusion (Fig. 7-14) is the simultaneous contacting of the maxillary and mandibular teeth on the right and left and in the anterior and posterior occlusal areas when the jaws are in either centric or eccentric relation. Teeth can be arranged in these static positions and observed on positional, semiadjustable, and adjustable articula-

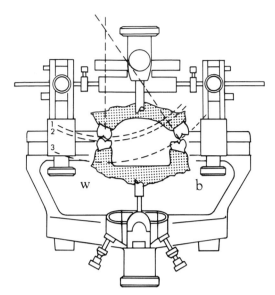

FIG. 7-14. *Schematic interpretation of balanced occlusion: 1 and 2, contacts on the working side* (**w**); *3, contact on the balancing side* (**b**).

tors; and assuming that the maxillomandibular relation records are accurate, the contacts will be repeated in the mouth.

Balanced gliding occlusion is the even contacting of teeth as the mandible moves to and from eccentric and centric maxillomandibular relations. The teeth can be arranged in these dynamic positions and observed on positional and adjustable articulators, but the contacting in the mouth will not be the same. Instruments that accept pantographic tracings and whose condylar paths have been contoured in harmony with the tracings would be expected to duplicate many of these contacts.

Concepts of Occlusion

Occlusion must satisfy physiologic requirements and be acceptable to the patient. When one considers the concepts of occlusion, he must review certain factors before deciding which will govern a satisfactory arrangement of teeth for complete dentures.

Natural teeth are surrounded by bone. Except for movement within the limits of their periodontal attachments, they can be considered as fixed. Stability and retention of the dentition does not depend upon the contact of a tooth in one part of the arch to balance tooth contact in another part of the arch.

Artificial teeth are attached to a movable base resting on soft tissues that can be displaced. The displacement of tissue varies in the same individual. Stability and retention of dentures are partially dependent upon the contact of a tooth in one part of the arch to balance tooth contact in another part of the arch.

When natural teeth are present, bone receives stimulation, tensile in nature, through the pull of the periodontal attachments. Tensile stimulation contributes to normal bone physiology. Dentures do not replace this stimulation.

When the teeth are supported by a denture base resting on and exerting forces to the bone, which is covered with vascular tissue, resorption results.

There is no scientific proof that any one concept of occlusion will satisfy all of the requirements of a complete denture in all patients.

There is likewise no scientific proof that one tooth form is more efficient than other tooth forms.

It has not been scientifically proved that one material for artificial teeth has any significant advantages over other materials or that one tooth form is more esthetically acceptable than other tooth forms.

It is almost impossible to conduct a scientific investigation that will give definite predictable results of the reactions of the basal seat to dentures. Clinical observation and evaluation are not always reliable. Competent prosthodontists differ in their evaluations.

Occlusion is often confused with articulation. Occlusion is bringing the mandibular teeth up into contact with the maxillary teeth. This is a static* position when the jaws are centrically or eccentrically related. Hanau used the term *articulation* to define the contacting of teeth as the mandible moved to and from centric relation and eccentric relation. This is dynamic.† In time, the term *gliding occlusion* will be used to describe this phenomenon, but until that time the learner will be confused when he reads that balanced occlusion on an adjustable articulator can be repeated in the mouth. On the contrary, he finds that *balanced articulation* on the same articulator is not necessarily balanced articulation in the mouth. Hanau recognized this and contended that the resiliency of the supporting tissues and the resiliency of the tissues in the temporomandibular joints compensated for some of the discrepancy. Hanau also recognized that this compensation does not always occur and suggested that the final adjustment of the occlusion must be accomplished in the mouth.

Until scientific proof of these factors is available, clinical results must be evaluated in an objective manner and claims for any specific occlusal arrangement must be restrained. Developing the occlusion is an important phase in denture construction, but the other procedures are also important. Overenthusiasm in one phase of the procedures can lead to neglect and less precision in another phase. The most important procedure in complete denture service is the procedure that one is doing at the time.

The concepts of occlusion for complete dentures fall into two broad disciplines: (1) balanced occlusion and (2) nonbalanced occlusion.

BALANCED OCCLUSION

Balanced occlusion is generally associated with cusp form posterior teeth and nonbalanced occlusion with noncusp form posterior teeth. Organic occlusion, which is used by students in gnathology, employs cusp form posterior teeth that are not arranged in protrusive and bilateral balance.

Balanced occlusion involves a definite arrangement of the teeth to provide simultaneous contact of all posterior teeth in harmony with mandibular movements.

Balanced gliding occlusion involves the arrangement of the teeth to provide even tooth contacts between posterior and anterior teeth as the mandible moves to and from centric and eccentric positions. The purpose of this arrangement of the teeth is to provide stabilizing forces to the denture bases on their basal seat when the teeth make contact and the jaws are in centric or eccentric relation. It is to maintain these stabilizing forces as the mandible moves the teeth to and from centric occlusion and eccentric occlusion.

To accept the concept of balanced occlusion is to accept the concept that the mandible makes eccentric movements during function and, more *precisely,* that the teeth make contact when the mandible is in eccentric relation to the maxillae. From cinefluorographic studies Jankelson and his associates concluded that "centric occlusion is the only tooth contact of significance that occurs during stomatognathic function."[45] Hickey, et al. stated, "The teeth were a guiding factor in only a few instances

---

*Static: not moving or progressing; at rest; inactive; stationary

†Dynamic: relating to energy or physical force in motion; opposed to static.

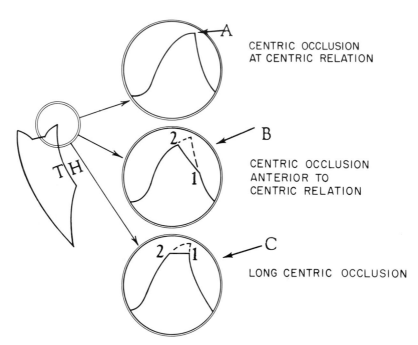

FIG. 7-15. *A schematic interpretation of mandibular movements from terminal hinge position on the sagittal plane related to concepts of occlusion. The terminal hinge position* (**TH**) *at varying vertical dimensions of opening.* **A.** *The most retruded position of the mandible with the posterior teeth in maximum intercuspation at a given vertical dimension.* **B.** *Centric occlusion anterior to centric relation: the first position of tooth contact (1); maximum intercuspation of the posterior teeth (2). This is often referred to as acquired centric occlusion with natural teeth, but the use of the term* centric *is confusing.* **C.** *Long centric occlusion: position of first tooth contact (1). The fossae of the teeth are altered to allow freedom of movement between points 1 and 2 in an anteroposterior direction. To complete the concept of long centric occlusion, the fossae of the posterior teeth are altered mediolaterally and the cingulae of the anterior teeth are altered in harmony with the freedom of movement.*

as the jaws opened from centric occlusion during mastication."[38] Adams and Zander, using radio transmitters, established that actual tooth contact takes place both in centric, lateral, and protrusive occlusion.[1] The type of food, size of the particle, and chewing cycle influenced the duration of and the increase or decrease in tooth contacts. Not only are the contacts of teeth during mastication important, but the contacts of teeth during the abnormal mandibular movements such as bruxism (centric and eccentric), clenching, and tapping, direct forces to the support that must be considered in any concept of occlusion.

Posselt, Glickman, Arstad, Yurkstas, and others have demonstrated that maximal intercuspal relation of the teeth is anterior to terminal hinge position in approximately 90 per cent of the analyzed individuals with full complements of natural teeth. Although these demonstrations were made with natural teeth, the findings cannot be overlooked when the occlusal concepts of artificial teeth are considered (Fig. 7-15).

When artificial cusp form teeth are arranged for complete dentures, it is possible that the occlusal surface of the teeth should be altered to allow freedom of tooth movement in harmony with the rotation when it takes place in the fossae. The freedom of tooth contact is accomplished by altering the fossae of the teeth both anteroposteriorly and mediolaterally. When a noncusp form posterior tooth is used, this freedom exists. In both situations the anterior teeth are arranged or altered to allow this freedom of movement. The anterior teeth are not arranged in contact when the jaws are in centric relation.

This concept of the occlusion is similar to the alterations of natural teeth to develop freedom in centric or the long centric relation and includes the concept of balanced occlusion.

This concept is not interpreted to imply that centric relation (bone to bone) is an area. It means that centric occlusion (tooth to tooth) for some individuals may be an area.

In the application of the terminology, the failure to distinguish between *balanced centric* and *eccentric occlusion, balanced occlusion,* and *gliding balanced occlusion* contributes to a misunderstanding for the learner.

NONBALANCED OCCLUSION

When the requirements for *balanced centric* and *eccentric occlusion* and *balanced gliding occlusion* are accepted as requisites for *balanced occlusion,* it follows that all other occlusal arrangements are *nonbalanced* occlusion. The arrangement of teeth according to the spherical theory, organic occlusion, occlusal balancing ramps for protrusive balance, transographics, and on a plane may be classified as nonbalanced occlusion.

Nonbalanced occlusion is an arrangement of teeth with form or purpose. Stansbery, an advocate of balanced occlusion, used the term to mean balance in the entire functional range of mandibular movement.[90] Kurth refers to balanced occlusion, meaning balance when the mandible is in centric relation

to the maxillae.[49] He disregards incisal and condylar guidance, eccentric balance, and sets noncusp form teeth with a reverse compensating curve. DeVan's concept of neutrocentric occlusion embodies the centralization of occlusal forces which act on the basal seat when the mandible is in centric relation to the maxillae.[22]

In *organic* or organized occlusion, the aim is to relate the occlusal elements of teeth so that the teeth will be in harmony with the muscles and joints in function. The muscles and joints should determine the mandibular position of occlusion without tooth guidance. The mandibular position of occlusion is terminal hinge position. In function the teeth should always be passive to the paths of mandibular movement, never dictate them.

Organic occlusion has three phases of mutually interdependent protection: (1) The posterior teeth should protect the anterior teeth in the centric occlusal position. (2) The maxillary incisors should have vertical overlap sufficient to provide separation of the posterior teeth when the incisors are in end-to-end contact. (3) In lateral mandibular positions outside the masticatory cyclic movements, the cuspids should prevent contact of all other teeth.

In transographics, eccentric balancing contacts are not considered, since balancing contacts are believed to be outside of the functional range. According to Schweitzer, "This theory agreed in principle with the tenets of gnathology, but differed in its concept of the problem."[78]

To accept the concept of nonbalanced occlusion includes acceptance of the following: (1) The character of the supporting foundation makes it almost impossible to harmonize tooth arrangement with mandibular movements in the eccentric relations to the maxillae and maintain this harmony. (2) The contacting of teeth during masticatory and nonmasticatory mandibular movements takes place when the mandible is in centric relation to the maxillae. (3) The artificial teeth should not contact when the mandible is in eccentric relations to the maxillae; for, when the jaws are eccentrically related and the teeth contact, horizontal and torquing forces are directed to the support. These forces are unstabilizing and potentially destructive to the supporting tissue. (4) When the jaws are in centric relation and the contact of the teeth produces no discomfort to the supporting tissues or the joints, the patient is encouraged to make similar maxillomandibular relations repeatedly.

Schematic drawings 7-16 through 7-25* represent factors of occlusion and

*Prepared in collaboration with J. Marvin

the relations of mandibular movements, condylar guidances, and incisal guidance. The labels represent the following:

W—working side
T—balancing (idling for natural teeth)
R—rotating condyle (side toward which a lateral jaw movement is made)
O—orbiting condyle (opposite condyle)
W′—path taken by a maxillary lingual cusp over the occlusal surface of a mandibular tooth on the working side during a lateral jaw movement
B—path taken by a maxillary lingual cusp over the occlusal surface of a mandibular tooth on the balancing side during a lateral jaw movement
h—horizontal
v—vertical

Reynolds, D.D.S., Department of Occlusion, Medical College of Georgia, School of Dentistry.

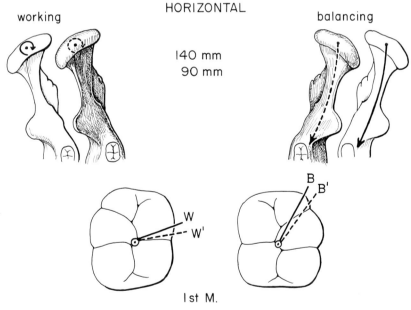

FIG. 7-16. *Effect of intercondylar distance on cusp paths. The greater the intercondylar dimension, the more distal are the working and balancing cusp paths on the mandibular teeth and the more mesial they are on the maxillary teeth. The lesser the intercondylar dimension, the more mesial are the working and balancing cusp paths on the mandibular teeth and the more distal they are on the maxillary teeth.*

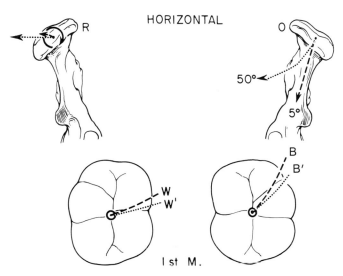

FIG. 7-17. *Effect of Bennett movement on cusp paths. The more the side shift (Bennett movement), the more mesial are the working and balancing cusp paths on the mandibular teeth and the more distal they are on the maxillary teeth. The less the side shift, the more distal are the working and balancing cusp paths on the mandibular teeth and the more mesial they are on the maxillary teeth.*

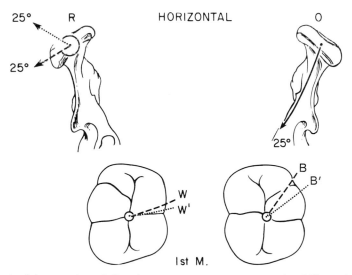

FIG. 7-18. *Effect of forward and distal components on cusp paths. When the side shift has a forward component, the more distal are the working and balancing cusp paths on the mandibular teeth and the more mesial they are on the maxillary teeth. When the side shift has a distal component, the more mesial are the working and balancing cusp paths on the mandibular teeth and the more distal they are on the maxillary teeth.*

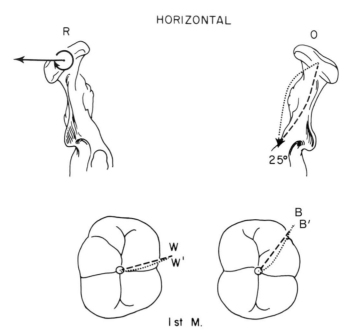

FIG. 7-19. *Effect of speed on cusp paths. The more rapid the side shift initially, the more mesial is the cusp path on mandibular teeth and the more distal it is on maxillary teeth.*

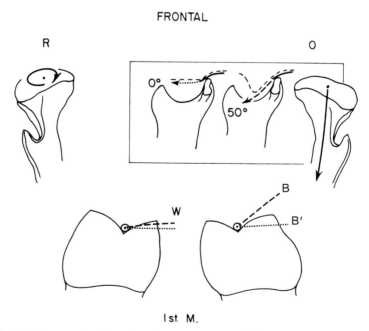

FIG. 7-20. *Effect of the angle of eminentia on cusps and fossae. The lesser the angle of the eminentia, the shorter the cusps and shallower the fossae must be. The greater the angle of the eminentia, the longer the cusps and deeper the fossae may be.*

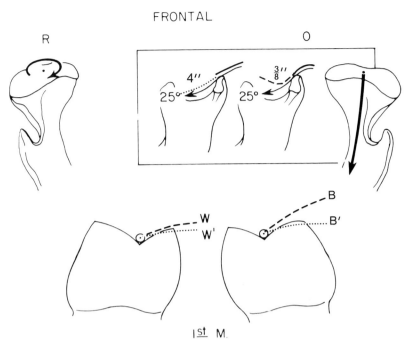

FIG. 7-21. *Effect of curve on the eminentia on cusps and fossae. The less curved the eminentia, the shorter the cusps and shallower the fossae must be. The more curved the eminentia the longer the cusps and deeper the fossae may be.*

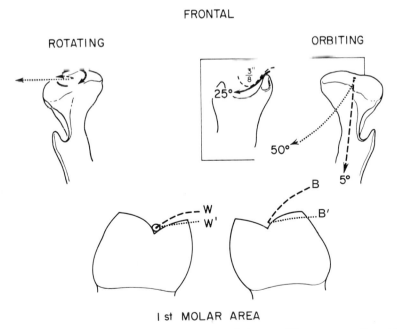

FIG. 7-22. *Effect of frontal side shift on cusps and fossae. The greater the side shift, the shorter the cusps and shallower the fossae must be. The lesser the side shift, the longer the cusps and deeper the fossae may be.*

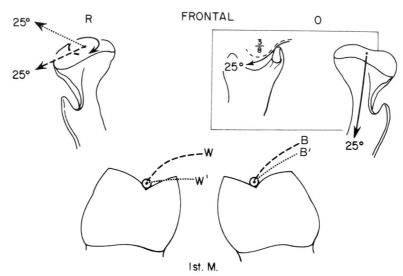

FIG. 7-23. *Effect of upward and downward component on cusps and fossae. When the side shift has an upward component, the shorter the cusps and shallower the fossae must be. When the side shift has a downward component, the longer the cusps and deeper the fossae may be.*

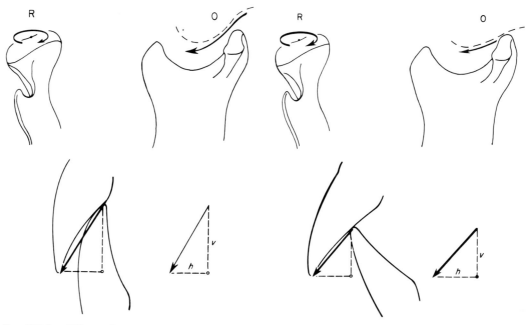

FIG. 7-24. *Effect of increase in the angle of eminentia on lingual concavity. The greater the angle of the eminentia, the lesser the lingual concavity of the upper anterior teeth may be. Expressed another way, the greater the vertical overlap, the lesser the horizontal overlap of the anterior teeth may be. This results in a steep incisal guide angle.*

FIG. 7-25. *Effect of decrease in the angle of eminentia on concavity. The lesser the angle of the eminentia, the greater the concavity of the upper anterior teeth must be, or the lesser the vertical overlap and greater the horizontal overlap of the anterior teeth must be. This results in a less steep incisal guide angle.*

REFERENCES

1. Adams, S. H., and Zander, H. A.: Functional tooth contacts in lateral and in centric occlusion. J.A.D.A., *69*:465, 1964.

2. Artman, H. R.: The role of occlusion in preservation and prevention in complete denture prosthodontics. J. Prosth. Dent., *25*:12, 1971.

3. Arstad, T.: The influence of the lips on mandibular rest position in edentulous patients. J. Prosth. Dent., *15*:27, 1965.

4. Atwood, D. A.: A review of fundamentals in rest position and vertical dimension. Int. Dent. J., *9*:1, 1959.

4a. Azarbal, M.: Comparison of myo-monitor centric position to centric relation and centric occlusion. J. Prosth. Dent., *38*:331, 1977.

5. Bear, P. N.: An analysis of physiologic rest position, centric relation, centric occlusion. J. Periodont., *27*:181, 1956.

6. Beck, H. O., and Morrison, E. W.: A method for reproduction of movements of the mandible. J. Prosth. Dent., *12*:873, 1962.

7. Bell, D. H., Jr.: Sagittal balance of the mandible. J.A.D.A., *64*:486, 1962.

8. Boos, R. H.: Intermaxillary relation established by biting power. J.A.D.A., *27*:1192, 1940.

9. ———: Occlusion from rest position. J. Prosth. Dent., *2*:575, 1952.

10. ———: Vertical, centric and functional dimensions recorded by gnathodynamics. J.A.D.A., *59*:682, 1959.

11. Boswell, J. V.: Practical occlusion in relation to complete dentures. J. Prosth. Dent., *1*:307, 1951.

12. Boucher, C. O.: Maxillomandibular relations. Dent. Pract., *13*:427, 1963.

13. Boucher, L. J.: Limiting factors in posterior movements of mandibular condyles. J. Prosth. Dent., *11*:23, 1961.

14. ———: Anatomy of the temporomandibular joint as it pertains to centric relation. J. Prosth. Dent., *12*:464, 1962.

15. ———, and Jacoby, J.: Posterior border movements of the human mandible. J. Prosth. Dent., *11*:836, 1961.

16. Brotman, N. D.: Contemporary concepts of articulation. J. Prosth. Dent., *10*:221, 1960.

16a. Calagna, L. J., Silverman, S. I., and Garfinkel, L.: Influence of neuromuscular conditioning on centric relation registrations. J. Prosth. Dent., *30*:598, 1973.

17. Clayton, J. A., Katowicz, W. E., and Myers, G. E.: Graphic recordings of mandibular movements: Research criteria. J. Prosth. Dent., *25*:287, 1971.

18. Christensen, F. T.: The compensating curve for complete dentures. J. Prosth. Dent., *10*:637, 1960.

19. Cohen, S.: A cephalometric study of rest position in edentulous persons: Influence of variations in head position. J. Prosth. Dent., *7*:467, 1957.

20. D'Amico, A.: Origin and development of the balanced occlusion theory. J. South. Cal. State Dent. Ass., *28*:10, 1960.

21. DePietro, A. J.: Concepts of occlusion—A system based on rotational centers of the mandible. Dent. Clin. N. Amer., November, 1963, p. 607.

22. DeVan, M. M.: Synopsis. Stability in full denture construction. Penn. Dent. J., *22*:8, 1955.

22a. Dyer, E. H.: Importance of stable maxillomandibular relation. J. Prosth Dent., *30*:241, 1973.

23. Eggleston, W. B., and Echelberry, J. W.: An electromyographic and functional evaluation of treated orthodontic cases. M.S. Thesis, University of Michigan, 1961.

24. Fedi, P. F., Jr.: Cardinal differences in occlusion of natural teeth and that of artificial teeth. J.A.D.A., *64*:482, 1962.

25. Friedman, S.: An effective pattern of occlusion in complete artificial dentures. J. Prosth. Dent., *1*:402, 1951.

26. ———: A comparative analysis of conflicting factors in the selection of the occlusal pattern for edentulous patients. J. Prosth. Dent., *14*:30, 1964.

27. Garnick, J., and Ranfjord, S.: Rest position, an electromyographic and clinical investigation. J. Prosth. Dent., *12*:895, 1962.

28. Gibbs, C. H., et al.: Functional movements of the mandible. J. Prosth. Dent., *26*:604, 1971.

28a. ———, Suit, S. R., and Benz, S. T.: Masticatory movements of the jaw measured at angles of approach to the occlusal plane. J. Prosth. Dent., *30:*283, 1973.

29. Gillings, B. R. D.: Photoelectric mandibilography: A technique for studying jaw movements. J. Prosth. Dent., *17:*109, 1967.

30. Gillis, R. R.: Setting up the full denture: Producing a balanced articulation. J.A.D.A., *17:*228, 1930.

31. Glickman, I., Pameijer, H. N., and Roeber, F. W.: Intraoral occlusal telemetry, Part I. A multifrequency transmitter for registering tooth contacts in occlusion. J. Prosth. Dent., *19:*60, 1968.

32. Granger, E. R.: Centric relation. J. Prosth. Dent., *2:*160, 1952.

33. Hall, W. A., Jr.: Important factors in adequate denture occlusion. J. Prosth. Dent., *8:*764, 1958.

34. Hanau, R. L.: Occlusal changes in centric relation. J.A.D.A., *16:*1903, 1929.

35. Hardy, I. R., and Passanorti, G.: A method of arranging artificial teeth for Class II jaw relations. J. Prosth. Dent., *13:*606, 1963.

36. Harris, E.: Occlusion. J. Prosth. Dent., *1:*301, 1951. Hodge, L. C., and Mehan, P. E.: A study of mandibular movement from centric occlusion to maximum intercuspation. J. Prosth. Dent., *18:*19, 1967.

37. Hickey, J. C.: Centric relation—A must for complete dentures. Dent. Clin. N. Amer., November, 1964, p. 587.

38. ——— et al.: Mandibular movements in three dimensions. J. Prosth. Dent., *13:*72, 1963.

39. ———, Stacey, R. W., and Rinear, L. L.: Electromyographic studies of mandibular muscles in basic jaw movements. J. Prosth. Dent., *7:*565, 1957.

40. ———, ———, and ———: Electromyographic analysis of jaw movements. J. Prosth. Dent., *10:*688, 1960.

41. ———, Williams, B. H., and Woelfel, J. B.: Stability of mandibular rest position. J. Prosth. Dent., *11:*566, 1961.

42. Hildebrand, G. V.: Studies in the masticatory movements of the human lower jaw. Scand. Arch. Physiol., *61:*190, 1931.

43. Hughes, G. A., and Reglies, C. P.: What is centric relation? J. Prosth. Dent., *11:*16, 1961.

44. Ingernall, B.: Retruded contact position of the mandible. A comparison between children and adults. Odont. Rev., *15:*130, 1964.

45. Jankelson, B., Hoffman, G., and Hendron, J.: The physiology of the stomatognathic system. J.A.D.A., *46:*386, 1953. Kouats, J. J.: Overclosure of the jaws; a clinical syndrome. J. Prosth. Dent., *18:*311, 1967.

46. Jarabak, J. R.: An electromyographic analysis of muscle behavior in mandibular movements from rest positions. J. Prosth. Dent., *7:*682, 1957.

47. Jerge, C. R.: The neurologic mechanism underlying cyclic jaw movements. J. Prosth. Dent., *14:*667, 1964.

47a. Kantor, M. E., Silverman, S. I., and Garfinkel, L.: Centric relation recording techniques: A comparative investigation. J. Prosth. Dent., *30:*604, 1973.

47b. Kelly, E.: Centric relation, centric occlusion, and posterior tooth forms and arrangement. J. Prosth. Dent., *37:*5, 1977.

48. Kingery, R. H.: The maxillo-mandibular relationship of centric relation. J. Prosth. Dent., *9:*922, 1959.

49. Kurth, L. E.: Balanced occlusion. J. Prosth. Dent., *4:*150, 1954.

50. Landa, J. S.: A study of the temporomandibular joint viewed from the standpoint of occlusion. J. Prosth. Dent., *1:*601, 1951.

51. LaVere, A. M.: Lateral interocclusal positional records. J. Prosth. Dent., *19:*350, 1968.

51a. Levy, P. H.: A form and function concept of occlusion and maxillomandibular relationship. J. Prosth. Dent., *33:*149, 1975.

52. Lucia, V. O.: Centric relation—theory and practice. J. Prosth. Dent., *10:*849, 1960.

52a. Lundeen, H. C.: Centric relation records: Effect of muscle action. J. Prosth. Dent., *31:*244, 1974.

53. McCollum, B. B.: Mandibular hinge axis and a method of locating it. J. Prosth. Dent., *10:*431, 1960.

54. Mann, A. W., and Pankey, L. D.: Concepts of occlusion—the P-M philosophy

of occlusal rehabilitation. Dent. Clin. N. Amer., November, 1963, p. 621.

55. Messerman, T.: A means of studying mandibular movements. J. Prosth. Dent., *17*:36, 1967.

56. Miller, S. C.: *Oral Diagnosis and Treatment Planning.* Philadelphia, Blakiston Co., Inc., 1936.

57. Millstein, P. L., Kronman, J. H., and Clark, R. E.: Determination of the accuracy of wax interocclusal registrations. J. Prosth. Dent., *25*:189, 1971.

58. Moyers, R. E.: Some physiologic considerations of centric and other jaw relations. J. Prosth. Dent., *6*:183, 1956.

58a. Nairn, R. I.: Sources of confusion in study of occlusion. J. Prosth. Dent., *30*:488, 1973.

58b. ———: Maxillomandibular relations and aspects of occlusion. J. Prosth. Dent., *31*:361, 1974.

58c. Neiburger, E. J.: Flat-plane occlusion in development of man. J. Prosth. Dent., *38*:459, 1977.

59. Neuakari, K.: An analysis of mandibular movement from rest to occlusal position. Acta Odont. Scand., *14*, Suppl. 19, 1956.

60. Niswonger, M. E.: The rest position of the mandible and centric relation. J.A.D.A., *28*:430, 1941.

60a. Noble, W. H.: Anteroposterior position of myo-monitor centric. J. Prosth. Dent., *33*:398, 1975.

60b. Owens, S. E., Lehr, R. P., and Biggs, N. L.: The functional significance of centric relation as demonstrated by electromyography of the lateral pterygoid muscles. J. Prosth. Dent., *33*:5, 1975.

61. Page, H.: A critical appraisal of centric relation. Dent. Dig., *59*:342, 1953.

61a. Parker, M. L., Hemphill, C. D., and Regli, C. P.: Anteroposterior position of mandible as related to centric relation registrations. J. Prosth. Dent., *31*:262, 1974.

62. Payne, H. S.: A study of posterior occlusion in duplicate dentures. J. Prosth. Dent., *1*:322, 1951.

63. ———: Diagnostic factors which influence the choice of posterior occlusion. Dent. Clin. N. Amer., March, 1957, p. 203.

64. Posselt, U.: Studies in the mobility of the human mandible. Acta Odont. Scand., *10*: Suppl. 10, 1952.

65. ———: Movement areas of the mandible. J. Prosth. Dent., *7*:375, 1957.

66. ———: An analyzer for mandibular positions. J. Prosth. Dent., *7*:368, 1957.

67. Pound, E., and Murrell, G. A.: An introduction to denture simplification. J. Prosth. Dent., *26*:570, 1971.

68. Preiskel, H. W.: Some observations on the postural position of the mandible. J. Prosth. Dent., *15*:625, 1965.

69. ———: Considerations of the check record in complete denture construction. J. Prosth. Dent., *18*:98, 1967.

70. ———: Lateral translatory movements of the mandible: Critical review of investigations. J. Prosth. Dent., *28*:46, 1972.

71. Rader, A.: Centric relation is obsolete. J. Prosth. Dent., *5*:333, 1955.

72. Ransfjord, S. P.: Bruxism: A clinical and electromyographic study. J.A.D.A., *62*:21, 1961.

72a. Remien, J. C., and Ash, M. M.: Myo-Monitor Centric: An evaluation. J. Prosth. Dent., *31*:137, 1974.

73. Ricketts, R. M.: Occlusion, the medium of dentistry. J. Prosth. Dent., *21*:39, 1969.

74. Saizar, P.: Centric relation and condylar movement, anatomic mechanism. J. Prosth. Dent., *26*:581, 1971.

75. Sauser, C. W.: Posterior occlusion in complete denture construction. J. Prosth. Dent., *7*:456, 1957.

76. Schuyler, C. H.: Problems associated with opening bite which would contraindicate it as common practice. J.A.D.A., *26*:734, 1939.

77. ———: Factors of occlusion applicable to restorative dentistry. J. Prosth. Dent., *3*:772, 1953.

78. Schweitzer, J. M.: Concepts of occlusion. Dent. Clin. N. Amer., November, 1963, p. 649.

79. Shanahan, T. E. J.: Physiologic vertical dimension and centric relation. J. Prosth. Dent., *6*:741, 1956.

79a. Sharry, J. J.: An essential question of occlusion. J. Prosth. Dent., *30*:509, 1973.

80. Sheppard, I. M.: Movements of mandible. J. Prosth. Dent., *14*:898, 1964.

81. ——— and Sheppard, S. M.: Denture occlusion. J. Prosth. Dent., 26:468, 1971.
82. Sheppard, S. M., and Sheppard, I. M.: Incidence of lateral excursions during function with complete dentures. J. Prosth. Dent., 26:258, 1971.
83. Sherman, H.: Phonetic capability as a function of vertical dimension in complete denture wearers: A preliminary report. J. Prosth. Dent., 23:621, 1970.
84. Shpuntoff, H., and Shpuntoff, W.: A study of physiologic rest position and centric position by electromyography. J. Prosth. Dent., 6:621, 1956.
85. Sicher, H.: Positions and movements of the mandible. J.A.D.A., 48:620, 1954.
86. Sicher, H.: *Oral Anatomy*, 3rd ed. St. Louis, The C. V. Mosby Co., 1960.
87. Silverman, M. M.: Vertical dimension must not be increased. J. Prosth. Dent., 2:188, 1952.
88. Smith, D. E.: The reliability of preextraction records for complete dentures. J. Prosth. Dent., 25:592, 1971.
88a. Smith, H. F.: A comparison of empirical centric relation records with location of terminal hinge axis and apex of Gothic arch tracing. J. Prosth. Dent., 33:511, 1975.
89. Standard, S. G., and Lepley, J. B.: The free-way space and its relation to the temporomandibular articulation. J. Prosth. Dent., 5:20, 1955.
90. Stansbery, C. J.: Balanced occlusion in relation to lost vertical dimension. J.A.D.A., 24:288, 1932.
91. Storey, A. T.: Physiology of a changing vertical dimension. J. Prosth. Dent., 12:912, 1962.
91a. Stuart, C. E.: The contributions of gnathology to prosthodontics. J. Prosth. Dent., 30:607, 1973.
92. ——— and Stallard, H.: *A Syllabus on Oral Rehabilitation and Occlusion*, vol. I. San Francisco, University of California San Francisco Medical Center, 1959.
93. Swerdlow, H.: Vertical dimension literature review. J. Prosth. Dent., 15:241, 1965.
94. Thompson, J. R.: Concepts regarding function of the stomatognathic system. J.A.D.A., 48:626, 1954.
95. ———: Rest position of the mandible and its significance to dental science. J.A.D.A., 33:15, 1946.
96. Trapozzano, V. R.: Current concepts of occlusion. J. Prosth. Dent., 5:764, 1955.
97. ———: Occlusion in relation to prosthodontics. Dent. Clin. N. Amer. March, 1957, p. 313.
98. ———: Test of balanced and nonbalanced occlusions. J. Prosth. Dent., 10:476, 1960.
99. ———: Laws of articulation. J. Prosth. Dent., 13:34, 1963; Boucher, C. O.: Discussion of "laws of articulation." J. Prosth. Dent., 13:45, 1963.
100. Turrell, A. J. W.: Clinical assessment of vertical dimension. J. Prosth. Dent., 28:238, 1972.
101. Urictorin, L., Hedegard, B., and Lundberg, M.: Cineradiographic studies of bolus position during chewing. J. Prosth. Dent., 26:236, 1971.
102. Vierheller, P. G.: A functional method for establishing vertical and tentative centric maxillomandibular relations. J. Prosth. Dent., 19:587, 1968.
103. Weinberg, L. A.: Rationale and technique for occlusal equilibration. J. Prosth. Dent., 14:74, 1964.
103a. ———: Temporomandibular joint function and its effect on concepts of occlusion. J. Prosth. Dent., 35:553, 1976.
103b. ———: Temporomandibular joint function and its effect on centric relation. J. Prosth. Dent., 30:673, 1973.
104. Yurkstas, A. A.: The masticating act. J. Prosth. Dent., 15:248, 1965; Shanahan, T. E. J.: Discussion of "the masticating act." J. Prosth. Dent., 15:261, 1965.
105. Zeibert, G. J., and Knap, F. J.: Effect of jaw guidance on retruded stroke as recorded in the sagittal plane. J. Prosth. Dent., 29:594, 1973.

Gnathology

8

This chapter is a brief outline of the concepts and philosophies of dentists who subscribe to the research findings and disciplines of gnathology. The terminology is that used by students of gnathology and was proposed by Stallard, an orthodontist with a Doctor of Languages. Unfortunately, the adoption of new terms may delay acceptance of the principles presented. All dentists are not students of language, and terminology that does not appear in the majority of current dental literature may be confusing.

The meaning of terminology is always a problem in accurately communicating concepts in a discipline, and as Kurth remarked, "It is to be regretted that a new terminology (to me, at least) was used to denote movement, as 'detrusion' for downward; 'surtrusion' for upward; 'medistrusion' for downward, forward and medially; and 'laterotrusion' for backward, upward and laterally. These terms can be confusing until their definitions are known."[2]

Gnathology deals with the whole apparatus of mastication. According to Stallard, "it was proposed as a science that would concentrate on the gnathic system—gnathology—to emphasize how important the knowledge of gnathodynamics is in caring for teeth."[4] When gnathology was proposed, it was primarily concerned with the recusping of the natural teeth. In recent years a technique for complete dentures has incorporated the recusping of artificial posterior teeth with gold and contouring the cingulae of anterior teeth to conform to the concept of organic occlusion.

Historically, the science and use of gnathology came about slowly. When studies in gnathology were instituted, it was accepted that balanced occlusion was the answer to occlusal problems. This concept was applied to both natural and artificial dentition. It was assumed that the only way to balance teeth was to have teeth with cusps.

Gysi suggested the research tool that McCollum used in 1920 to locate the opening and closing axis position and to transfer a patient's maxillomandibular relations to an articulator. For his research McCollum fastened the Snow face-bow rigidly to the lower teeth and located the axis position. When he had done this, he discovered other facts.

1. When the patient closed on a hard object on the anterior or posterior teeth, the point of the stylus did not change position. He concluded that an articulator of metal could be made to simulate mandibular joint movements.

2. Translation on the horizontal axis made constant paths.

3. The axis remained constant to the mandibular teeth when the jaws were in protrusion during the opening and closing of the jaws if the openings were not excessive.

4. The coincidence of repeated terminal hinge positions was so regular that it indicated that the terminal hinge axis position is constant.

When McCollum concluded his investigation with the face-bow, he and Wadsworth developed an articulator that could be narrowed and widened (adjustable intercondylar width). McCollum and Warner made a sturdier instrument that could be set by lateral interocclusal records. However, the instrument would not reproduce mandibular movements and probably did not accept pantograms recorded in three planes. In the 1920's McCollum learned how to test the accuracy of an articulator, and in 1927 he undertook to test for balanced occlusion. It took another three years and the making of many instruments to obtain one that could be used as an aid in balancing occlusion. It took about twenty years for Stuart to conclude that balanced occlusion is not suitable for natural teeth and probably not suitable for dentures.

Stuart designed his first articulator in 1928–29 but decided not to promote it out of deference to McCollum. After Stallard had made a three-plane plastic articulator device to study laterotrusion (Bennett movement) and record roentgenographically the shift on the three planes of the skull, Stuart saw the possibilities of making an articulator that could be adapted to reproduce the jaw writings (pantograms).

The jaw writings are recorded by a *pantograph*, a mechanical device for reproducing a map and drawing on the same or a different scale. It consists of a framework of jointed rods roughly in the form of a parallelogram. A pantogram is the tracing that the device writes or draws. The graphic tracings recorded in three planes are all the writings necessary to reproduce mandibular movements in order to develop a satisfactory occlusion. The gnathologist uses these graphic tracings to adjust the articulator, which is designed to receive and reproduce the mandibular movements.

The purpose of the mandibular recorder (pantograph) is to locate the centers of mandibular movement and at the same time record the paths of motion that these centers take in relation to a given plane in the face. The axis-orbital plane is the one most often used. This is valuable information, regardless of the type of occlusion to be developed.

In 1947 the concept of organic occlusion was introduced by Stuart and Stallard to replace the concept of balanced occlusion. Organic occlusion is the concept that any jaw movements away from centric occlusion will result in disocclusion (separation) of all posterior teeth on both sides of the arch. This is made possible by contouring the cingula of the anterior teeth. These gnathologists found that balanced occlusion was disagreeable to the patient with sound periodontium and decided the findings should warn against applying it to teeth that have weak periodontium.

However better organic occlusion may be, it will not solve all of the problems in constructing complete dentures. The hope of this type of occlusion is to contour the teeth so that patients can eat well without being conscious of having teeth. However, the direction of the ridges and grooves, the dimensions of the cusps, the organizations of the disocclusions, and the cusp to fossae occlusal contacts are not dictated by an articulator or by "chew-in" techniques (page 274). The articulator must be adjusted to the pantograms. Furthermore, the operator must have knowledge of mandibular movements and know how to interpret the pantograms before he can place the grooves and ridges and contour the teeth.

Stallard reported that Swab and Harrington independently found that patients given organic occlusion to replace balanced occlusion in their dentures voluntarily commented about absence of weariness in the pterygoid and masseter muscles. These patients also felt that they had much less tooth substance in their mouths.[5]

The evaluation of the concepts of occlusion based solely on the opinions of patients may lead to methods of treatment that destroy, rather than preserve, the supporting structures. Until dentures using organic occlusion are constructed in sufficient quantity and are tested with different age groups and with varying systemic conditions, this concept of occlusion cannot be accepted. The physiologic acceptance by the supporting tissues must be compared with results under similar conditions and situations from dentures constructed in other concepts. The use of organic occlusion developed on an articulator that receives pantograms in three planes is worthy of support and further investigation.

Stallard summarized the possibilities for gnathology in caring for natural teeth and gave the following advice to gnathologists:

1. Become proficient by learning the movements of the condyles and the effects of these movements upon cusp heights, cusp sizes, and cusp paths;
2. Master the technique by gathering the necessary data to put into an articulator which will reproduce the necessary jaw relations;

3. Acquire an understanding of the anatomy and physiology of the mandibular joints;
4. Comprehend how the neuromuscular system assists us to fix teeth for the best arch automation;
5. Give greater attention to the nature, structure, and health of the periodontium.[5]

This advice for gnathologists may be extended to complete denture construction; however, instead of giving attention to the periodontium, the prosthodontist should give great attention to the reactions of the supporting tissue (physiologic tolerance) and very little attention to the patient's expressions (patient tolerance).

Figures 8-1 through 8-6 illustrate procedures required to write pantograms and interpret the writings and the purpose for which the writings are made.

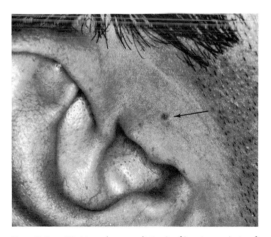

FIG. 8-1. *Tattoo (arrow) to indicate point of terminal hinge axis. (The point has been accentuated for photographic purposes.)*

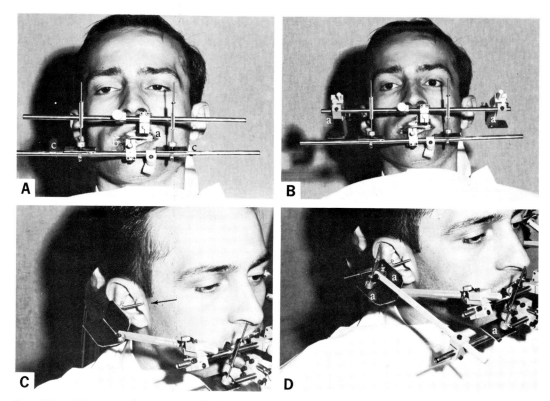

FIG. 8-2. *The recorder is assembled.* **A.** *The clutches are rigidly attached to the teeth (a). The recorder bars are rigidly attached to the stems of the metal clutches (b). The anterior recording plates and styli are secured in place (c).* **B.** *The vertical and horizontal recording plates, at condyle level, are secured in place (a).* **C.** *The recorder is oriented to the terminal hinge axes. Note arrow.* **D.** *All styli are adjusted (a).*

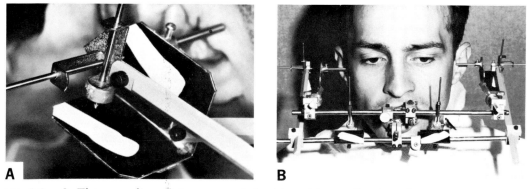

FIG. 8-3. **A.** *The recording plates are coated with a thin application of a pressure sensitive material.* **B.** *The styli remain retracted as the patient is rehearsed in the procedure.*

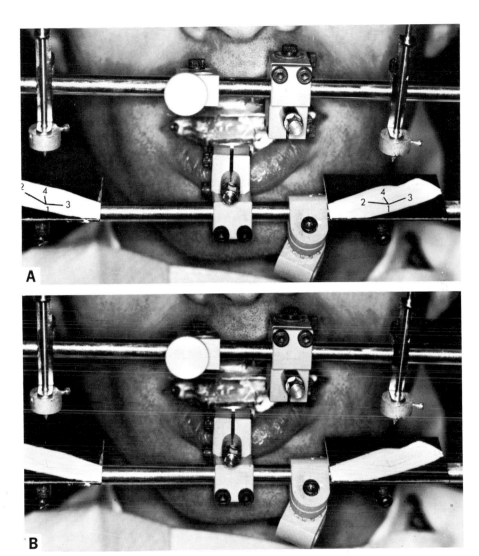

FIG. 8-4. *Pantograms.* **A.** *The graphic tracings on the anterior horizontal plates are accentuated for analysis and interpretation. The tracings are projections from the centers of lateral rotation: Point 1, centric relation (terminal hinge position), is a border position. Point 2, the left lateral mandibular border movement. Point 3, the right lateral mandibular border movement. Point 4, the straight protrusive mandibular movement.*

Lines 1–2 are the effects of the condyle disc movements during a guided left lateral mandibular movement. The left condyle is rotating, and the right condyle is gliding.

Lines 1–3 are the effects of the condyle disc movements during a guided right lateral mandibular movement. The right condyle is rotating, and the left condyle is gliding.

Lines 1–4 are the effects of a straight, unguided protrusive movement. Both condyles are gliding in a uniform motion in a straight line (translating).

Movements between 1 and 2 and 1 and 3 are guided border movements. The operator is manually guiding the mandible. Movement between 1 and 4 is made by the patient and is not guided by the operator.

B. *The styli meet a minimum of resistance as they move across the tracing plate. Therefore, the tracings are delicate fine lines.*

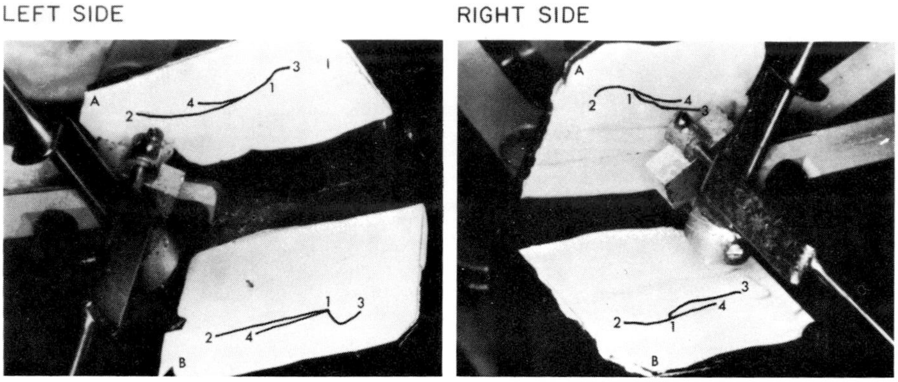

LEFT SIDE   RIGHT SIDE

FIG. 8-5. *Graphic tracings of the left and right sides at condyle level: vertical recording plates* (**A**); *horizontal recording plates* (**B**). *The tracings are accentuated for photographic purposes. The centric relation (terminal hinge position) is at 1. The tracings are oriented to the transverse hinge axis of the mandible (Point 1 on vertical plates* (**A**)).

Analysis of Tracings on the Left Side:

Line 1–2 on the vertical plate (**A**) denotes the projected movement of the transverse hinge axis as the gliding condyle moves forward, downward, and medially in a protrusive right lateral movement.

Line 1–2 on the horizontal plate (**B**) denotes the projected movement of the vertical axis of the gliding condyle as it moves forward, downward, and medially in a protrusive right lateral movement.

Line 1–3 on the vertical plate (**A**) denotes the projected movement of the transverse hinge axis of the rotating condyle during a protrusive left lateral movement.

Line 1–3 on the horizontal plate (**B**) denotes the projected movement of the vertical axis of the rotating condyle during a left lateral movement.

Lines 1–4 on the vertical (**A**) and horizontal (**B**) plates are the effect of the projected condylar movements during a straight protrusive movement.

Lines 1–2 and 1–3 are guided movements—guided by the operator. Line 1–4 is a learned movement made by the patient with the central bearing pin in contact with a heavy plate in the maxillary arch.

Analysis of Tracings on the Right Side:

Lines 1–2 and 1–3 are tracings made during a protrusive right and left lateral movement.

Lines 1–3 on the right side are the same projected movements as lines 1–2 on the left side.

Lines 1–4 on the vertical (**A**) and the horizontal (**B**) plates are the same as line 1–4 on the left side.

Compare line 1–2 on the right horizontal (**B**) plate with line 1–3 on the left horizontal (**B**) plate. There is very little Bennett movement (side shift) of the mandible during the protrusive right lateral movement, line 1–2. There is extensive Bennett movement during the protrusive left lateral movement, line 1–3.

Then compare lines 1–2 and 1–4 on the left vertical plate (**A**). The protrusive right lateral movement, line 1–2, and the straight protrusive movement, line 1–4, initially have the same character. Compare the character of these lines with lines 1–3 and 1–4 on the right vertical plate (**A**). The condyle paths appear different as the mandible is moved in left lateral protrusion and straight protrusion.

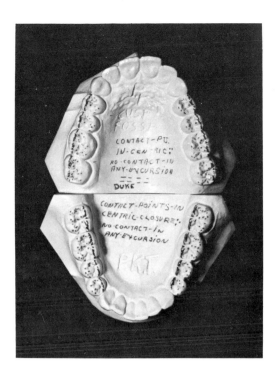

FIG. 8-6. *Casts of teeth contoured in the concept of organic or organized occlusion. The dots on the occlusal surfaces of the posterior teeth denote the contact points when the mandible is in terminal hinge position and is elevated to tooth contact.*

The occluding surfaces of the opposing cusps are contoured to permit glide paths for the opposing paths that will be concentric to the movements of the rotational centers.

The occlusion of the posterior teeth is developed when the mandible is in terminal hinge position. The occlusal contacts are made between convex surfaces around the cusp tips and ridges that rim opposing fossae. The posterior teeth do not contact in any eccentric mandibular movement. For the preparation of such casts students of gnathology recommend an instrument that will reproduce the writings obtained with a pantograph. (Courtesy of Peter K. Thomas, Beverly Hills, California.)

REFERENCES

1. Contino, R. M., and Stallard, H.: Instruments essential for obtaining data needed in making functional diagnosis of the human mouth. J. Prosth. Dent., 7:66, 1957.
2. Kurth, L. E.: Discussion of condylar determinants of occlusal patterns, Part I. Statistical report on condylar path variations, Part II. J. Prosth. Dent., 15:847, 1965.
2a. Lundeen, H. C., Shryock, E. F., and Gibbs, C. H.: An evaluation of mandibular border movements. J. Prosth. Dent., 40:442, 1978.
3. Shaw, D. M.: Form and function in teeth and a rational unifying principle applied to interpretation. In Stuart, C. E., and Stallard, H. A.: A Syllabus on Rehabilitation and Occlusion, Vol. I. San Francisco, University of California San Francisco Medical Center, 1959.
4. Stallard, H.: Forty years of gnathology. Read before the First International Congress of Gnathology, Mexico City, April 16, 1964.
5. ———: The future of gnathology. Read before the First International Congress of Gnathology, Mexico City, April 19, 1964.
6. Stuart, C. E.: The growth of gnathology. Read before the First International Congress of Gnathology, Mexico City, April 19, 1964.
7. ———: Why should dental restorations have cusps? In A Syllabus on Oral Rehabilitation and Occlusion, Vol. 1, San Francisco, University of California San Francisco Medical Center, 1959.
8. Stuart, C. E., and Stallard, H.: Principles involved in restoring occlusion to natural teeth. In A Syllabus on Oral Rehabilitation and Occlusion, Vol. 1. San Francisco, University of California San Francisco Medical Center, 1959.
9. ———: What kind of occlusion shall we give to toothborne restorations? Read before the Mid-Atlantic Conference in Dentistry, Buck Hill Falls, Penn., April, 1959.

Record Bases
and Occlusion Rims

9

When all or part of the natural teeth are present, they are used in the recording of the maxillomandibular relations. The teeth are fixed in bone and, for recording purposes, are considered *immovable*. They are used to retain the recording medium or device and to act as guides. In the completely edentulous situation, other means must be provided to retain the recording medium or device and to keep it in its proper position in relation to the support. The majority of the procedures in recording maxillomandibular relations use record bases to which occlusion rims, other recording mediums, or devices are attached. The record bases rest on the soft tissue covering of the residual ridges and extend into the adjacent mucosa. The supporting tissues are displaceable; therefore, for recording purposes the record bases are considered *movable*.

Record Bases

A record base or baseplate is a temporary form representing the base of a denture. It is used in recording maxillomandibular relations and in the arrangement of teeth. After the teeth are arranged, they are returned to the mouth on the same record bases that were used to record the maxillomandibular relations. At this time, centric relation and centric occlusion are verified, eccentric maxillomandibular relations are recorded, and the arrangement of anterior teeth is evaluated for esthetic acceptance.

The temporary form representing the denture base must have rigidity, accuracy, and stability. The borders should be developed in the same manner as the borders of the finished denture. All surfaces that contact the lips, cheeks, and tongue should be smooth, rounded, and polished. The crest and labial and/or buccal slopes should be thin to provide space for tooth arrangement.

The accuracy of maxillomandibular relation records is affected by the rigidity, stability, and the movability of the record bases. The smoothness of the polished surfaces contributes to the comfort of the patient. The more comfortable and compatible the record bases are to the tissues, the more normal are the jaw movements.

MATERIALS AND METHODS

It is generally agreed that maxillomandibular relations are difficult to record accurately on poorly fitting bases fabricated from bulky material and from material that is subject to distortion and dimensional change. Record bases or baseplates are made of several different materials, including shellac and acrylic resin.

SHELLAC. The shellac record base forms are manufactured in the shapes of the maxillary and mandibular arches. The forms are softened with an open flame and molded to the cast with an instrument or the fingers. While the material is in a softened state, the excess is removed with scissors. After hardening, the borders are smoothed but as a rule will not take a polish.

Although shellac record bases are easily and quickly adapted, they are not considered satisfactory. They warp, do not fit accurately, distort easily, lack rigidity, become brittle and break, and will not permit polishing of the borders.

REINFORCED SHELLAC. The manufactured form of shellac is softened as above with an open flame. A flattened wire is contoured and adapted across the posterior palatal seal area of the maxillary record base and incorporated in the base. In the mandibular arch the flattened wire is contoured and adapted to the lingual flange and incorporated in the base. Tinfoil is burnished over the surface of the cast. A thin layer of zinc oxide-eugenol impression paste is spread over the tissue side of the base and is seated on the tinfoiled cast in the manner of making an impression. After the paste has been allowed to set, the excess flash is removed and the borders are smoothed.

Although this procedure results in a base that is more rigid and stable than shellac is, the record base is still subject to distortion and breakage. It is bulky, the odor and taste of the paste are objectionable to some patients, and it is unsuitable for the arranging of teeth, par-ticularly in situations of limited interarch space.

PROCESSED ACRYLIC RESIN. A wax pattern is applied to the unaltered final cast in a manner similar to that used when waxing the cast for the finished denture. The vestibules are filled, and the palate and lingual flanges are contoured and waxed to the contour and thickness desired for the completed denture. The crest area and the labial and/or buccal slopes are either thinly waxed or reduced after polymerization. The thickness in these areas influences the arrang-

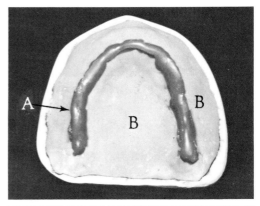

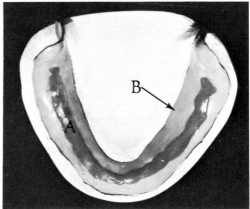

FIG. 9-1. *Baseplates made of processed acrylic resin: top, maxillary; bottom, mandibular. A sticky wax is applied to the unpolished ridge crest areas (A). The surfaces that will contact the tongue and cheeks are polished (B).*

ing of teeth and will be governed by the available interarch space. The cast and pattern are flasked, the wax is eliminated, acrylic resin is packed and heat processed. The processed base is removed from the cast, smoothed, and polished at the borders. The slopes and crest are allowed to remain unpolished, as occlusion rims will be attached in these areas (Fig. 9-1).

Although record bases fabricated in this manner require considerable time and are more expensive than some others, they are considered to be excellent. They are rigid, accurate, stable, not subject to distortion, not easily broken, and suitable for the arrangement of teeth. After the maxillomandibular relations have been verified and the teeth have been finally arranged and waxed, the teeth are processed to the base. Any processing error in this part of the denture base does not affect the accuracy of occlusion.

CHEMICALLY ACTIVATED OR SELF-CURING ACRYLIC RESIN. Self-curing acrylic resin is an acrylic resin to which an activator and catalyst have been added. The result is an acrylic resin requiring no externally applied heat for polymerization. Three methods are commonly used in fabricating a record base from this material.

1. Noncompression Dough Method

Any undercuts present in the final cast are altered by flowing wax from above the greatest convexity down and into the undercut (Fig. 9-2). This method, which does not completely eliminate the undercut but allows the removal of the base without damaging the cast, will result in a more accurate fit. Tinfoil or tinfoil substitute is applied to the cast to act as a separating medium. The self-curing resin is mixed according to the manufacturer's directions. When it

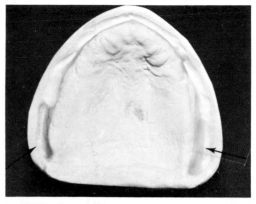
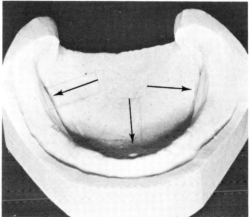

FIG. 9-2. *Final casts: top, maxillary; bottom, mandibular. The arrows point to undercut areas. It is possible to damage the casts if the undercuts are not properly altered. It is not necessary to eliminate the undercuts completely if the wax is flowed from above the greatest convexity.*

reaches a doughlike stage, it is pressed into molds shaped like the maxillary and mandibular arches. The molds, which are provided by the manufacturer, assure the correct shape and an even thickness of material (Fig. 9-3). The resin is removed from the mold with a stainless steel instrument, such as a cement spatula, and molded to the cast with the instrument or the fingers. The acrylic resin is allowed to polymerize to the consistency that will allow it to be raised but not removed from the cast. It is reseated immediately and allowed to

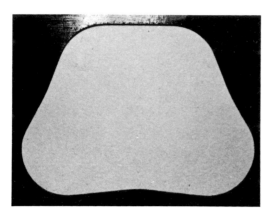

FIG. 9-3. *The use of a mold aids in the conservation of material.*

polymerize completely. Polymerization may be hastened by placing the cast in a pressure cooker in hot water for twenty minutes under twenty-four pounds of pressure.

2. Compression Molded Dough Method

The procedure for fabricating compression molded autopolymerizing record bases is essentially the same procedure used for processed acrylic resin for dentures. The resin is packed when in a doughlike consistency; the flasks are closed and allowed to remain under pressure of the clamps or press as the resin self-cures.

A compression molded self-curing record base of acrylic resin is processed to become a part of the denture. The advantage advanced for this procedure is that it requires less time and therefore is less expensive than the processed denture base acrylic resin. The processed denture base acrylic resin is still the material of choice.

3. Sprinkle On Method

The final cast is prepared in the manner used in the noncompression dough method. The monomer and polymer are applied alternately. It is most desirable to keep excess polymer when applying the monomer and the polymer, as excessive monomer is conducive to dimensional changes. To provide additional rigidity a slight excess in thickness can be tolerated on the lingual flange of the mandibular and in the palate of the maxillary base. Before complete polymerization, the record base should be unseated from the cast but not removed and then reseated immediately. To hasten polymerization and eliminate excess monomer, place the cast and base in a pressure cooker in hot water for twenty minutes under twenty-four pounds of pressure.

A record base made by the shake on method is preferred to the dough methods. The bases are rigid, stable, not easily broken or warped, fit accurately except at the undercut areas, can be contoured and polished for compatibility with the surrounding oral environment, and are relatively inexpensive. They require more time to fabricate than the dough method.

Occlusion Rims

Occlusion rims are occluding surfaces constructed on record bases or permanent denture bases to be used in recording jaw relations and for arranging teeth. Baseplate wax and modeling compound are the materials commonly used for occlusion rims. Combinations and alterations of these materials are often used to meet the requirements of a special procedure. Wax is used more frequently, since it is easier to manage in the registrations and in the arranging of the teeth.

The positions of the lips and cheeks are important in the recording of maxillomandibular relations. The proper contouring of the occlusion rims for lip and cheek support allows the muscles of facial expression to act in a normal manner. Facial contours act as guides in some of the techniques of recording jaw relations. The borders of the record bases and the polished surfaces of the occlusion rims should be smooth and rounded, since smooth, rounded surfaces are conducive to patient comfort and relaxation. An uncomfortable, tense patient is not in a favorable state to undergo the procedures involved in recording jaw relations; therefore, errors can occur in records taken under these conditions.

The basic fabrication of occlusion rims is a laboratory procedure. The final altering and contouring is usually accomplished at the dental chair prior to and during the recording of maxillomandibular relations. The contouring, as well as the materials used, varies with the method of record making. The functional methods of recording jaw relations usually require occlusion rims of compound to which recording devices can be attached; pantographic tracings require clutches that can be rigidly attached to the record bases; static methods usually require occlusion rims of wax.

MAXILLARY OCCLUSION RIM

In contouring the maxillary occlusion rim the anteroposterior dimension of the labial vestibule can be visually determined if the relaxed lip is gently moved in an anteroposterior direction. The anterior extension of the occlusion rim should go no further than the anterior border of the labial flange of the record base. Viewed in profile, the contour from the labial vestibule to the relaxed lip line should be in harmony with the profile of the face. The contour from cuspid eminence to cuspid eminence follows the contour of the arch if there has not been excessive loss of bone. Proper contouring between these points assures support to the lips. When the natural teeth were present, the labial surfaces of the maxillary

cuspids supported the upper lip at the corners of the mouth; the labial surfaces of the maxillary central incisors supported the upper lip in the midsection; and when the teeth were together in occlusion, the labial incisal third of the six maxillary anterior teeth supported the superior border of the lower lip.

The best anatomic guides to aid in determining the proper contouring of the anterior section of both occlusion rims are the nasolabial sulcus, the mentolabial sulcus, the philtrum, and the commissure of the lips. When support is absent, the nasolabial and mentolabial sulci become more deep, the philtrum is flattened, and the commissures droop. When oversup-

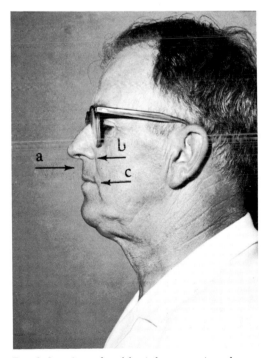

Fig. 9-4. *A study of facial expression shows the effects of the position of teeth. The occlusion rims should be contoured to support the lips and cheeks. The philtrum (a), nasolabial sulcus (b), and commissure of the lips (c), are excellent guides in determining proper contour.*

ported, the nasolabial and mentolabial sulci are distorted and shallow, the philtrum is partially, if not totally, obliterated, and the commissures are distorted laterally (Fig. 9-4).

The contouring of the buccal surface of the posterior section of the maxillary occlusion rim begins just distal to the cuspid. The buccal surface of wax is slanted slightly toward the palate to create an acceptable space between the cheeks and the rim (Fig. 9-5). This space, the buccal corridor, is created between the buccal surface of the posterior teeth and the corner of the lips when the patient smiles.

The vertical length of the maxillary occlusion rim in the anterior region extends approximately 2 millimeters below the relaxed lip (Fig. 9-6). When most individuals with natural teeth say "five fifty-five," the incisal edges of the maxillary central incisors contact the vermillion border of the lower lip at the junction of the moist and dry mucosa. The occlusion rim is reduced in length until the inferior border makes similar contact with the lower lip.

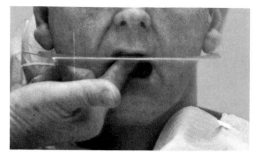

FIG. 9-6. *Maxillary occlusion rim. The occlusion rim has been reduced to the low lip line, and the Fox plane guide is used to determine the vertical contour in the posterior region.*

Another method used to establish the vertical length is to record a horizontal line which extends between the commissures of the lips coinciding with the position of the inferior border of the upper lip during serious speaking or relaxation. This is termed the *low lip line*. The lip positions are essentially the same, but the method of determining it is different. Some patients can be encouraged to speak seriously; others can

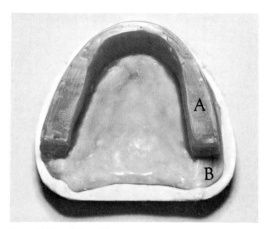

FIG. 9-5. *Maxillary occlusion rim. Space exists between the buccal surfaces of the posterior teeth and the cheeks. Contour the occlusion rim at (A) to allow space. Allow space (B) over the alveolar tubercles. This space is not occupied by a tooth.*

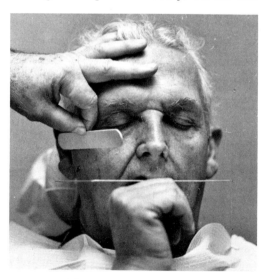

FIG. 9-7. *The occlusion rims are contoured so that the occluding surfaces of the maxillary rim are parallel with Camper's line. A tongue blade is placed on Camper's line and compared with the Fox plane guide.*

be encouraged to relax. A patient will not relax easily if he is conscious of being observed. There are some patients for whom these procedures must be carefully analyzed, as the action of the muscles of the cheeks and lip is influenced by malrelated jaws and/or malpositioned teeth.

The length of the occlusion rim is reduced to coincide with the recorded line. The *posterior* vertical length and occlusal plane are made to coincide with a line from the inferior border of the ala of the nose to the superior border of the tragus of the ear, Camper's line (Fig. 9-7). The vertical length at the first molar is established at one fourth of an inch below the orifice of Stensen's duct. The posterior distal extension of the maxillary rim should terminate slightly anterior to the alveolar tubercle.

MANDIBULAR OCCLUSION RIM

From the right mandibular cuspid to the left mandibular cuspid the mandibular occlusion rim should occupy the space over the crest of the residual ridge. The labial fullness should not extend over one half the width of the labial vestibule. The labiolingual thickness should be approximately 4 millimeters (Fig. 9-8).

Buccolingually in the posterior regions the rims should be placed over the crest of the residual ridge. In a buccal direction the rim should extend one eighth of an inch, in a lingual direction the rim should extend to but not exceed the medial extension of the border of the lingual flange of the record base (Fig. 9-8).

The anterior height should be approximately 10 millimeters; the posterior height should not exceed half the height of the retromolar pad. The distal extension should terminate 2 or 3 millimeters anterior to the retromolar papilla (Fig. 9-8).

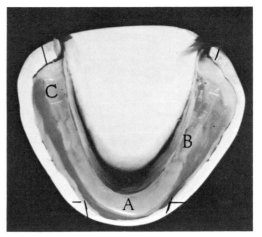

FIG. 9-8. *The mandibular occlusion rim. The labiolingual thickness (A) is excessive. The buccolingual position (B) is over the crest of the residual ridge. The distal extension (C) is shy of the retromolar papilla.*

The dimensions used in contouring the occlusion rims are subject to alterations to meet the requirements of the individual patient and the different methods for recording jaw relations.

USEFUL GUIDE LINES

Guide lines placed on the maxillary wax occlusion rims are useful for orientation purposes when recording maxillomandibular relations and later for arranging the teeth.

THE MIDLINE.   Several methods are used to determine the midline:

1. Bisect the philtrum of the lip with a flexible ruler and record a line on the labial surface of the rim to coincide with the margin of the ruler.

2. Extend a string from the center of the forehead downward, bisecting the face, and record a line on the labial surface of the rim to coincide with the string (Fig. 9-9).

3. Extend a line onto the rim inferiorly from the labial frenum (Fig. 9-9B).

4. Extend a line from the midpalatal

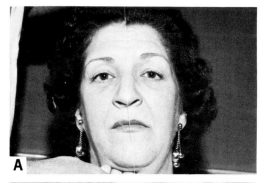

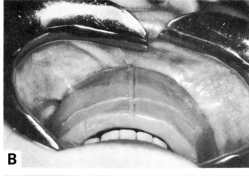

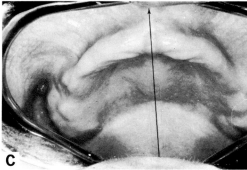

FIG. 9-9. *The midline.* **A.** *Using a string to locate the midline.* **B.** *The remnant of the labial frenum is used as a guide.* **C.** *Bisecting the palate and the incisal papilla is usually quite accurate.*

suture bisecting the incisal papilla onto the occlusal rim. (Fig. 9-9C).

THE LOW LIP LINE. The speaking line, relaxed lip line, or low lip line is used to determine the vertical incisal length (Fig. 9-10A). The method for determining it was described on page 262.

THE GUM LINE, HIGH LIP LINE, SMILING LINE. The smiling line, high lip line, or gum line is almost a straight line with a slight upward component and is used as a guide in the arrangement of teeth (Fig. 9-10B). The extent to which the teeth and gums are revealed superiorly and laterally will depend on the type of smile of the individual. The personalities of individuals influence the smiling line. Some individuals have a broad smile, others not so broad, and still others a rare smile.

It is not always easy to elicit a natural smile. A forced smile reveals the extent of lip separation. Some patients smile normally at request, others elevate and spread the lips as in smiling when they say "cheese," and others require ingenuity on the part of the den-

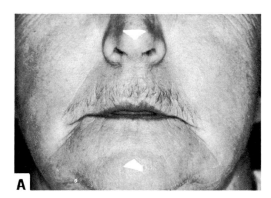

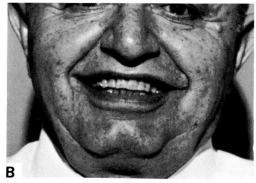

FIG. 9-10. **A.** *The low lip line. The maxillary occlusion rim is visible below the relaxed lip.* **B.** *The smiling or high lip line.*

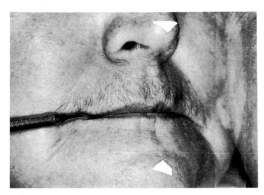

FIG. 9-11. *Recording the approximate position of the cuspid. Note the marker at the commissure of the lips.*

tist to elicit a smile. To ask a patient to repeat a thought-provoking, tongue-twisting sentence with record bases and occlusion rims in the mouth often invites a smile.

THE CUSPID LINE. The *cuspid line* is also used as a guide in arrangement and selection of teeth. With the occlusion rims seated in the mouth and in occlusion a pointed instrument, such as a straight pin, is passed medially on a line parallel to the pupils of the eyes at the corners of the mouth. Vertical lines recorded at this point will be approximately the distal extension of the cuspids (Fig. 9-11).

REFERENCES

1. Bailey, L. R.: Permanent-type bases for transferring records to an articulator. Dent. Clin. N. Amer., November, 1964, p. 623.
2. Block, L. S.: Preparing and conditioning the patient for intermaxillary relations. J. Prosth. Dent., 2:599, 1952.
3. Elder, S. T.: Stabilized baseplates. J. Prosth. Dent., 5:162, 1955.
4. Harris, L.: Facial templates and stabilized baseplates with the new chemical set resins. J. Prosth. Dent., 1:150, 1951.
5. ————: An advanced use of impression trays. J. Prosth. Dent., 3:150, 1953.
6. House, M. M.: The correction of malocclusion in artificial dentures. J.A.D.A., 7:339, 1920.
7. ————: Art of fundamentals in denture prosthesis. J.A.D.A., 24:407, 1937.
8. Keyworth, R. C.: Monson technic for full denture construction. J.A.D.A., 16:130, 1929.
9. Kingery, R. H.: A review of some of the problems associated with centric relation. J. Prosth. Dent., 2:307, 1952.
10. Kyes, F. M.: Pitfalls in a full denture. J.A.D.A., 43:651, 1951.
10a. La Vere, A. M., and Freda, A. L.: Accurate-fitting record bases. J. Prosth. Dent., 32:335, 1974.
11. McCracken, W.: Auxiliary uses of cold curing acrylic resins in prosthetic dentistry. J.A.D.A., 47:298, 1953.
12. Ringsdorf, W. M.: Ideal baseplates. J.A.D.A., 50:66, 1955.
13. Schoen, P. E., and Stewart, J. L.: The effect of temporary bases on the accuracy of centric jaw-relation records. J. Prosth. Dent., 18:211, 1967.
14. Silverman, S. I.: The management of the trial denture base. Dent. Clin. N. Amer., March, 1957, p. 231.
15. Trapozzano, V. R.: A comparison of the equalization of pressure by means of the central bearing point and wax check bites. J.A.D.A., 38:586, 1949.
16. ————: Occlusal records. J. Prosth. Dent., 5:325, 1955.
17. Wright, W. H.: Impression taking and materials. J.A.D.A., 20:1611, 1933.

Hinge Axis and Facebow

10

Hinge Axis

The *hinge axis* is an imaginary line around which the condyles can rotate without translation. The *opening axis* is an imaginary line around which the condyles may rotate during the opening and closing movements of the mandible. The significance of these definitions is that they say there is an imaginary axis around which all opening and closing movements of the mandible can or may occur. The condyles are not restricted to any one position in the fossae when this action occurs.

Terminal hinge position is the most retruded hinge position. Movement from this position, a conditioned response, is always less than median full-mouth opening. The terminal hinge position is significant because it is a learnable, repeatable, and recordable position that coincides with the position of centric relation. The limits of hinge movement in this position have been determined to be about 12 to 15 degrees from maximum intercuspation or about 19 to 20 millimeters at the incisal edges. The condyles are in a *definite* position in the fossae during terminal hinge movements.

REVIEW OF THE LITERATURE

The hingelike action in the lower compartment of the temporomandibular joint was described in the earliest editions of *Gray's Anatomy.* Snow recognized the importance of the hinge axis in mandibular movements and developed a face-bow to be used to transfer the position of the axis to the articulator. In 1921 McCollum, Stuart, and others reported discovery of the first positive method of locating the axis. Since 1921, investigators have differed in their findings; therefore, their conclusions about the location of the hinge axis have varied.

Sloane stated:

"The mandibular axis is not a theoretical assumption, but a definitely demonstrable biomechanical fact. It is the axis upon which the mandible rotates in an opening and closing function when comfortably, not forcibly retruded."[18]

Sicher said:

"The hinge position, or terminal hinge position, is that position of the mandible from which or in which pure hinge movement of a variably wide range is possible."[17]

According to Brekke, in reference to a single intercondylar transverse axis of rotation,

"Unfortunately, this optimum condition does not prevail in the mandibular apparatus, which is asymmetric in shape and size, and has its condyloid process joined at the symphysis, with no connection directly at the condyles. The assumption of a single intercondylar transverse axis is, therefore, open to serious question."[4]

Trapozzano and Lazzari concluded:

These findings indicate that, since multiple condylar hinge axis points were located, the high degree of infallibility attributed to hinge axis points may be seriously questioned.[21]

After further investigation, Trapozzano and Lazzari reached these conclusions:

1. The presence of multiple hinge axes has been established.
2. The technique for locating terminal hinge axes requires two operators.
3. Relaxation of the patient during the making of terminal hinge axes recordings is essential.
4. Because of the presence of multiple hinge axes points, increasing or decreasing the vertical dimension on the articulator is contraindicated unless a new interocclusal record is made on the patient at the desired occlusal vertical dimension.
5. The concept that only one terminal hinge axis exists is fallacious.[23]

Lucia concluded:*

"The centers in the terminal hinge position provide a definite starting position relation of the mandible to the maxillae (or their duplicates on an articulator).—How the teeth are arranged when the mandible and maxillae are so related will depend on one's beliefs about centric occlusion and centric relation—whether these two factors should be in harmony or whether centric occlusion should occur slightly in front of centric relation. By having the centric relation of the mandible to the maxillae properly related on the articulator, the dentist can develop the centric occlusion accurately according to his own specifications."[13]

Controversy has arisen as to the presence of a single axis, the methods used

*Lucia, V. O.: *Modern Gnathological Concepts.*

to locate the axis, the method and validity of recording the positions on the skin for future reference, and the relation of the terminal hinge position to the position of centric relation. These differences exist in concepts and interpretations of findings. Each dentist must evaluate his own findings and the findings of others and decide for himself which are valid and which are applicable to the present situation.

The differences in findings and interpretations are understandable. Mechanical equipment must be used to record movements involving living tissues; the vision and the judgment of different individuals introduce variables; and different concepts have a way of influencing human evaluations. There seems to be general agreement that when the mandible is in its most posterior unstrained position from which lateral movements can take place, a trained individual can voluntarily open and close the mandible in a hinge movement. Sicher came to this conclusion:

"An edentulous patient is an individual whose mandibular musculature has lost its precise guiding signals, especially in the closing movements of the jaws. It is this loss of periodontal proprioceptors that causes the wavering uncertain pattern of the 'bite' of the edentulous patient. . . . The patient is taught to move his mandible into the most posterior position that his own muscles can achieve, then suddenly a new and precise pattern of proprioceptive stimuli is established, because now some parts of the capsule of the temporomandibular joints are in an extreme, though unstrained, and therefore, unique tension."[17]

This biologic phenomenon is reenacted when a record of centric relations is made; therefore, it can be assumed that the anteroposterior relation of the mandible to the maxillae at the terminal hinge position is the same as centric relation. It is a repeatable border position; therefore, it is a *point of return.*

HINGE AXIS LOCATION TECHNIQUE

The technique for locating the terminal hinge axis position is essentially the same for the dentulous and the edentulous patient, but the methods of attaching the clutch to the mandible are quite different. The clutch is a mechanical device made to be rigidly attached to the mandibular teeth or the mandibular residual ridge to which a hinge axis bow is attached.

The construction of the clutch for the dentulous patient is illustrated in Figure 10-1.

1. Make an accurate impression of the

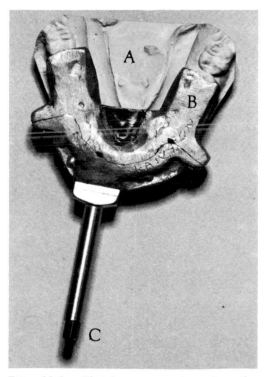

FIG. 10-1. *Clutch construction for the dentulous patient: accurate cast* (**A**); *two-piece clutch* (**B**); *the stem* (**C**).

mandibular arch and pour a stone cast (A).

2. Construct a two-piece custom-built metal clutch to fit the mandibular cast, or use a stock clutch fitted to the cast (B).

3. Parallel to the sagittal plane, attach a stud or stem to the center of the labial surface of the clutch (C). The hinge-bow will later be attached to this stud.

4. Attach the clutch firmly to the teeth with a zinc oxide-eugenol impression paste (Fig. 10-2).

The clutch for the edentulous patient is shown in Figure 10-3.

1. Make an accurate impression of the mandibular basal seat and pour an accurate stone cast (A).

2. On the cast make an accurate record base of self-curing or processed acrylic resin (B).

3. Attach compound occlusion rims firmly to the record base and secure a specially designed bite fork to the rims, with the stem extending forward parallel to the sagittal plane (C).

4. Attach this assembly to the mandible with chin clamps or chin straps (Fig. 10-4).

Movements between the teeth and the clutch or between the alveolar mucosa and the clutch may produce inaccurate styli rotations. Attach the hinge-bow to the stem and adjust the styli to the locations of the condyles. The condyles are located by placing marks 13 millimeters from the external auditory meatus on a line from the outer canthus of the eye to the superior border of the tragus of the ear. Place the patient in a semisupine position with the headrest tilted slightly backward. Assist or guide the patient in making hinge openings and closings. When the rotational centers have been located and verified, secure the styli. Place the patient in an upright position with the head unsupported. Move the styli to the side of the face and record

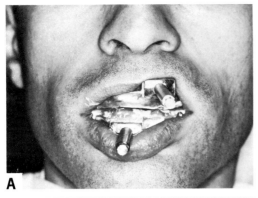

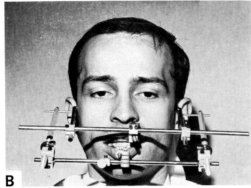

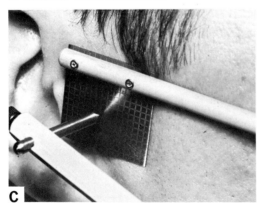

FIG. 10-2. *Positioning the hinge axis locator on a dentulous patient.* **A.** *Clutch attached with impression paste.* **B.** *Hinge axis bow attached to stem of clutch.* **C.** *Stylus and grid in place.*

the points with a dye. These points should be tattooed (Fig. 8-1).

TERMINAL HINGE AXIS

The procedures in registering the terminal hinge axis are not complicated,

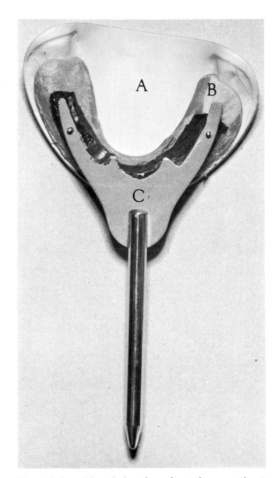

FIG. 10-3. *Clutch for the edentulous patient: the edentulous cast* **(A)**; *accurate record base* **(B)**; *specially designed bite fork* **(C)**.

but in many edentulous situations they are difficult to perform accurately. Investigators, particularly those in gnathological study groups, are exploring ways and means of accomplishing this procedure accurately for the edentulous patient. These studies should be followed and evaluated. Pre-extraction locations of the terminal hinge axis offer a more accurate point of reference than the arbitrary locations; unfortunately, they are not always available.

ARBITRARY HINGE AXIS

The relation of the maxillary cast to the axis of rotation of the articulator

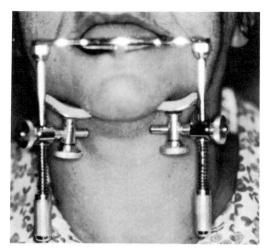

FIG. 10-4. *A chin clamp is used to stabilize the clutch for an edentulous patient. (Courtesy of Almore Mfg. Co., Portland, Oregon.)*

must be the same relation that exists between the maxillae and the terminal hinge axis in the skull. This is necessary in order to develop on the articulator certain occlusal schemes that will need minimum adjustment in the mouth. The errors produced by not using a hinge axis can be demonstrated and are considered negligible. Any error that can be eliminated in denture construction will make physiologic acceptance of the dentures easier. It is estimated that the use of condyle points as arbitrary centers of rotation will place them within 6 mm of the true center of the opening axis. When the method of locating the individual hinge axis is analyzed and considered in relation to the displaceable tissue and movable record bases in the edentulous patient, the arbitrary location may be more acceptable. Future developments in these procedures should be closely observed and evaluated.

Face-bow

The *face-bow* is a caliper-like device used to record the relationship of the maxillae to the temporomandibular joints (Fig. 10-5). The purpose of this instrument is to orient the maxillary cast to the articulator in the same relationship to the opening and closing axis of the articulator as exists between the maxillae and the opening and closing axis in the temporomandibular joints. When the cast is oriented to the articulator, the face-bow retains the cast in its correct relation until it is attached to the upper member with plaster.

REVIEW OF FACE-BOWS

In 1880 Hayes used a tonglike device which he called "Caliper." This instrument was not used as the face-bow is used today, but it did relate the median incisal point to its distance from the condyles.

About the turn of the century Gysi developed an instrument similar to a face-bow primarily to record the paths of the condyles. However, it was also used to transfer the maxillary cast to the articulator. About the same time Snow introduced the Snow face-bow. The majority of the face-bows used today are modifications of the Snow (Fig. 10-5).

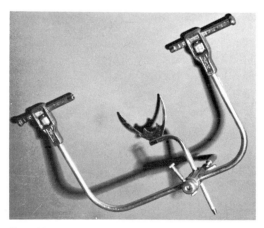

FIG. 10-5. *Hanau face-bow and bite fork. (Courtesy of the Hanau Engineering Company, Buffalo, New York.)*

The Snow type of bow utilizes arbitrarily located marks on the skin at the condyle points as the hinge axis positions. For this reason this type of face-bow is called an arbitrary bow. The condylar rods are adjusted to these points. There are no adjustments to compensate for asymmetric hinge points either vertically or horizontally. Therefore, if the terminal hinge rotational centers are to be located, a face-bow capable of being adjusted to any asymmetric location must be used.

Another type of arbitrary face-bow is similar to the Hayes' Caliper. The depressions anterior and medial to the tragus of the ears are used as the hinge axis points. Specially contoured inserts on the condylar ends of the bow are placed in the external auditory meatus. The bow arms are secured anteriorly either by clamps or springs. The inserts are held in position until the bow is secured to the stem of the bite fork (Fig. 10-6).

A *hinge axis* (kinematic) face-bow is a hinge-bow used to record the center

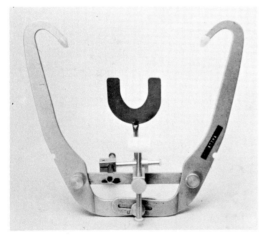

FIG. 10-6. *Caliper type of face-bow. The bite fork has wide, flat prongs. The plastic attachment is used for the third point of reference. (Courtesy of the Whip Mix Corporation, Avery-Louisville, Kentucky.)*

of rotation at the hinge axis points and transfer the cast to the articulator in accurate relation to these points (Fig. 10-7). The *hinge axis* bow can also be used to transfer the maxillary cast to arbitrarily located hinge axis points.

DISCUSSION OF FACE-BOW USE

The face-bow is considered a waste of time by some dentists and essential by others. This is understandable, for some articulators are not designed for use with the face-bow, a face-bow is not needed for some concepts of occlusion for complete dentures, and some dentists question the validity of articulators that require the use of a face-bow. However, some articulators are designed to receive a face-bow transfer and some concepts of occlusion for complete dentures require the rotational centers of mandibular movements to be transferred to the rotational centers of the articulator as accurately as possible. Those who use these articulators and believe in the face-bow also believe that failure to use the face-bow will result in errors of occlusion to a greater extent, depending upon the variations in position in mounting the cast.

Articulators developed in accord with Monson's spherical theory were not designed for use with the face-bow. Positional articulators and many hinge articulators have no accommodations for attaching a face-bow. The Class I and Class II, Type 3, articulators are designed to receive a face-bow, and it will be needed if these instruments are to be used to the full extent of their capabilities.

Some dentists contend the face-bow is not necessary under the following conditions:

1. When monoplane teeth are arranged on a plane in occlusal balance and the mandible is in the most retruded rela-

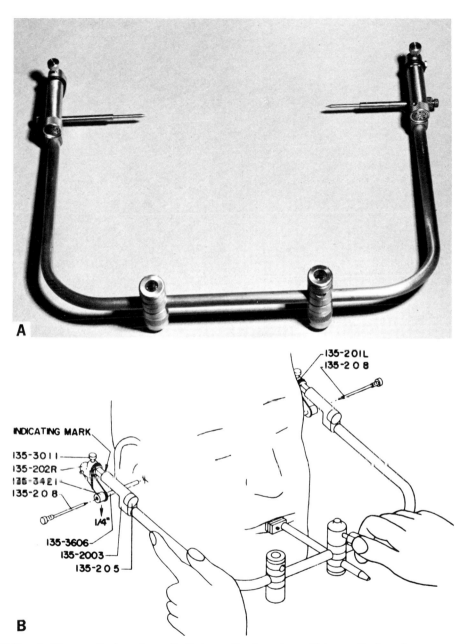

FIG. 10-7. **A.** *Kinematic face-bow.* **B.** *Schematic drawing of kinematic face-bow assembled.* *(Courtesy of the Hanau Engineering Company, Buffalo, New York.)*

tion to the maxillae at an acceptable vertical dimension of jaw separation.

2. No alterations of the occluding surfaces of the teeth that would neces-

sitate changes in the vertical dimension of the occlusion originally recorded.

3. No interocclusal check records that would be at a different vertical

dimension from that in the original interocclusal record.

4. When articulators that are not designed to accept a face-bow transfer are used in the denture procedures.

When these conditions are analyzed, several factors should be considered.

1. It is questionable if one occlusal form of posterior tooth is indicated for all edentulous patients.

2. Electromyographic, laminographic, cinefluoroscopic, and mechanical methods of studying the contacts of the occluding surfaces of the teeth and muscle function indicate that teeth do make contact when the jaws are eccentrically related.

3. Changes do occur in the vertical dimension of occlusion as a result of waxing, flasking, processing, and mounting procedures. Resorption of the bone and changes in the soft tissues that form the basal seat for the dentures alter the vertical dimension of occlusion.

4. Dentists use interocclusal check records to verify articulator mountings.

5. The occluding surfaces of the teeth are altered to correct for changes in the vertical dimension of occlusion.

6. There is no scientific proof that the errors when the face-bow is not used are within the acceptable physiologic range in all individuals.

7. When an articulator with rotational centers that can be adjusted to conform to the rotational centers of mandibular movements is used, the face-bow is an accurate method of relating the casts to these centers.

Blind orientation of the maxillary cast on an articulator may result in an error so slight that a face-bow appears to be unnecessary. However, since the procedure is not complicated nor time-consuming, the chances of incorporating an error should not be taken. If the convenience of mounting the cast were the only reason for the use of the face-

bow, it is questionable if it should be used. The mounting jig is more convenient for cast mounting. However, if the maxillary cast is mounted on the articulator in terminal hinge position (Fig. 10-8), the opening and closing path of movement recorded on the mid-sagittal plane can be duplicated.

The elimination of errors that can be produced by failure to use the face-bow where indicated justifies the time required and the procedures involved in the face-bow transfer. Disharmony in centric occlusion can result from these errors in mounting the casts on the articulator: (1) anterior or posterior and/or superior or inferior to the axis when the vertical dimension recorded is not maintained, (2) below and posterior to the rotational center so that the distal cusp inclines of the mandibular teeth make premature contact with the mesial cusp inclines of the maxillary teeth, or (3) above and anterior to the rotational center so that the mesial cusp inclines of the mandibular teeth make premature contact with the distal cusp inclines of the maxillary teeth.

When the disharmonies in occlusion

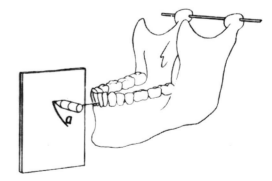

FIG. 10-8. *Maxillary cast mounted in terminal hinge position. The path of movement is recorded on the median plane (***a***) during the terminal hinge movement. (From Posselt, U.: Physiology of Occlusion and Rehabilitation. 2nd. ed. Oxford, Blackwell Scientific Publications, 1966.)*

resulting from failure to use the face-bow are analyzed, it can be concluded that the face-bow should be used when (1) cusp form teeth are used; (2) balanced occlusion in the eccentric positions is desired; (3) a definite cusp fossa or cusp tip to cusp incline relation is desired; (4) interocclusal check records are used for verification of jaw positions; or (5) the occlusal vertical dimension is subject to change, and the alterations of tooth occlusal surfaces are necessary to accommodate the change.

FACE-BOW TRANSFER PROCEDURE

When a face-bow is used, the procedure can be accomplished at the same sitting at which jaw relations are recorded. Although this procedure is performed at the same sitting, it is *not* to be confused with maxillomandibular jaw relation records. Although the purpose of using the face-bow would be nullified, it is possible to make the transfer in the absence of a mandible. The lower jaw is a reference for maxillo-mandibular records but not for a face-bow transfer of the maxillary cast to the articulator. In this procedure the points of reference for the rotational centers are arbitrarily located.

PRELIMINARY STEPS

1. Seat the patient in a comfortable position in the dental chair with the backrest extending to slightly below the scapula. The patient's head should be in an upright position with the headrest supporting the occiput (a, Fig. 10-9A).

2. Locate the axis points by measuring 12 millimeters anterior to the middle of the tragus of the ear on a line drawn from the outer canthus of the eye to the middle of the tragus of the ear. Record

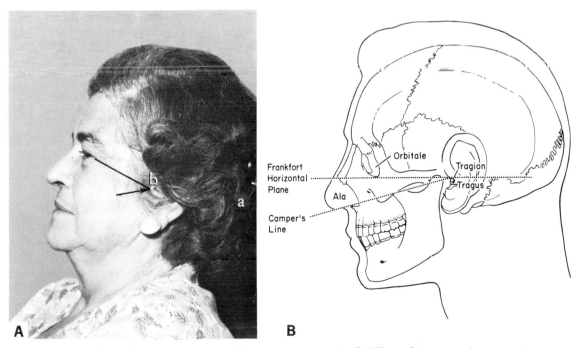

A   B

FIG. 10-9.   **A.** *The arbitrary location of the transverse axis.* **B.** *The arbitrary axis was not established by an arbitrary point on the skin but by anatomic landmarks to establish average points.*

points on the skin or on adhesive tape placed in the area (b, Fig. 10-9A).

3. Contour the maxillary occlusion rim; establish the occlusal plane; place the guide lines for the arranging of teeth on the labial section and a mounting index on the occlusal surface in the regions of the first molars. Make the index by placing transversely a step that is approximately 2 millimeters deep anteriorly, tapering distally to nothing (Fig. 10-10).

4. Apply a thin layer of petrolatum to the occlusion rims to facilitate separating from the wax on the bite fork.

5. Reduce the mandibular occlusion rim to allow adequate interocclusal distance for the fork and attached wax.

6. Adjust the condyle rods to the face for centering the bow by placing the ends over the condyle points so that the ends lightly touch the skin or tape. Secure either the right or left condyle rod; lock and remove the bow from the face.

FACE-BOW RECORD

1. Soften a sheet of low fusing baseplate wax and roll together in the shape of a horseshoe.

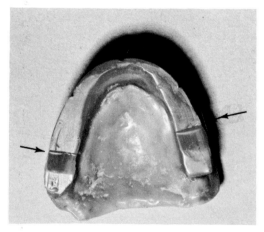

FIG. 10-10. *A contoured maxillary occlusion rim. The arrows designate the indices, which aid in repositioning the occlusion rims in a record.*

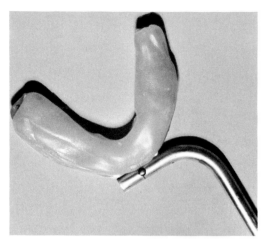

FIG. 10-11. *Wax adapted to the bite fork. When the procedures are followed systematically, the wax will remain soft, and an accurate record will be made.*

2. While the wax is soft, imbed the prongs of the bite fork in it. Fold the wax over at the margins to secure it to the fork. The thickness of the wax should be approximately 6 mm (Fig. 10-11).

3. Place the prongs of the bite fork with the attached soft wax between the occluding surfaces of the occlusion rims. Adjust the midline of the fork to coincide with the midline on the occlusion rim. Extend the stem of the fork forward and parallel to the sagittal plane.

4. Instruct the patient to close the jaws until both occlusion rims are imbedded in the soft wax to a depth that insures a stable seat. The relation of the mandible to the maxillae is of no importance except to place favorable pressure to stabilize the maxillary record base.

5. Slide the stem of the fork through the opening in the clamp of the bow and adjust the condyle rods to the arbitrary axis points (Fig. 10-12A).

6. Adjust the width of the condyle rods equidistant bilaterally and secure the clamp of the bow to the stem of the bite fork. Asymmetrical setting of the

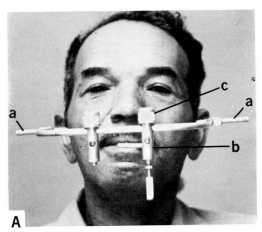

A

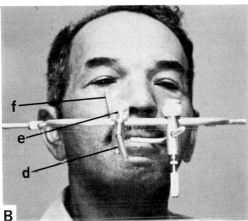

B

FIG. 10-12. *Face-bow record.* **A.** *Securing bite fork to face-bow. The condyle rods (***a***) are adjusted to the arbitrary axis points and the bite fork stem (***b***) is securely clamped, using the adjustment on the bow (***c***).* **B.** *Using the infraorbital notch as the anterior point of reference. The pointer (***d***) is secured by the face-bow clamp (***e***) after the pointer has been placed on the infraorbital notch (***f***).*

condyle rods within the accommodating range of the articulator width will not result in error if the bow is arranged symmetrically on the articulator.

7. Slide the condyle rods from the skin. Extend the condyle rods back to the axis points to check against displacement that may have occurred when the clamp was secured.

8. When the infraorbital notch is used as the anterior point of reference, the pointer should be placed in the clamp provided for it on the bow. Palpate the infraorbital notch and mark it with a skin marker. Place the point of the pointer over the mark and secure the clamp to the pointer (Fig. 10-12B). Remove the assembly from the face and allow the wax to set hard before removing the bite fork and face-bow record from the occlusion rims.

The method of attaching wax to the bite fork and having the patient close into the softened wax is advocated for several reasons: (1) the patient is in a comfortable position with the jaws closed and the arms at rest; (2) the maxillary record base is accurately seated and not subject to tipping; (3) the patient's hand is not required to hold the record base in place; therefore, the hand is not in the way of adjusting the bow assembly; (4) the assembly is held rigidly and is stable.

When it is desirable, mount the maxillary cast at this time.

FACE-BOW MOUNTING   (Fig. 10-13)

1. Set the sliding condylar rods (A) symmetrically on both sides until the bow gently springs over the articulator condyle shaft, provided the rods are adjusted symmetrically on the face. If the rods were not symmetrically adjusted on the face, shift the rods equidistantly in opposite directions until the bow gently springs over the ends of the articulator shaft.

2. Raise or lower the face-bow (B) to adjust for the vertical position until the low lip line, which was recorded on the labial surface of the occlusion rim, is on a level with the groove marked around the incisal pin (C). If an infraorbital pointer is used, adjust the pointer to touch the pointer plate attached to the maxillary bow of the articulator.

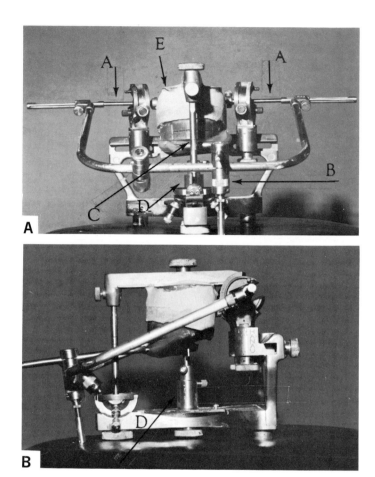

FIG. 10-13.   *A face-bow mounting.* **A.** *Frontal view of an articulator to which a maxillary cast is attached. The condylar rods (**A**) are extended to accept the arms of the face-bow. The vertical height of the occlusion rim is adjusted (**B**) so that the line on the incisal pin (**C**) is even with the low lip line of the occlusion rim. The face-bow fork is supported by the metal support (**D**), and the plaster (**E**) is used to attach the cast to the mounting ring.* **B.** *Lateral view. Notice the metal support (**D**) to avoid depressing the face-bow fork and wax record.*

3. Support the face-bow securely in position with the face-bow support (D).

4. Soak the maxillary cast in water for at least five minutes to insure adhesion of the plaster to the stone.

5. Secure the incisal guide pin with its top flush with the top of the maxillary bow of the articulator. Open the maxillary bow of the articulator and apply a creamy mix of dental plaster to the top of the articulator until the incisal guide pin is stopped on the guide table and the

mounting plate on the maxillary bow is imbedded in the plaster.

6. Carefully remove the excess plaster. Allow the plaster to harden before removing the face-bow assembly. The maxillary cast is related to the opening axis in the articulator in the same anteroposterior and horizontal position as the maxillae in the skull are related to the arbitrarily located opening axis in the temporomandibular joints (E).

When the record bases, occlusion

rims, and interocclusal relations are satisfactory for further records, proceed with making the tentative centric relation record with the jaws at the vertical dimension of occlusion. Chapter 11 discusses procedures for recording centric relation and centric occlusion.

REFERENCES

1. Aull, A. E.: A study of the transverse axis. J. Prosth. Dent., *13*:469, 1963.
2. Borgh, O., and Posselt, U.: Hinge axis registration on the articulator. J. Prosth. Dent., *8*:35, 1958.
3. Brandrup-Morgsen, T.: The face bow, its significance and application. J. Prosth. Dent., *3*:618, 1953.
4. Brekke, C. A.: Jaw function. Part II, hinge axis, hinge axes. J. Prosth. Dent., *9*:936, 1959.
5. Brotman, D. N.: Hinge axis, Part I. The transverse hinge axis. J. Prosth. Dent., *10*:436, 1960.
6. ———: Hinge axis, Part II. Geometric significance of the transverse axis. J. Prosth. Dent., *10*:631, 1960.
7. ———: Hinge axis, Part III. Vertical and sagittal rotational centers. J. Prosth. Dent., *10*:873, 1960.
8. Christiansen, R. L.: Rationale of the face-bow in maxillary cast mounting. J. Prosth. Dent., *9*:388, 1959.
9. Craddock, F. W., and Symmons, H. F.: Evaluation of the face bow. J. Prosth. Dent., *2*:633, 1952.
9a. Graser, G. N.: An evaluation of terminal hinge position and neuromuscular position in edentulous patients. Part I. Maxillomandibular recordings. J. Prosth. Dent., *36*:491, 1976.
9b. ———: An evaluation of terminal hinge position and neuromuscular position in edentulous patients. Part II. Duplicate mandibular dentures. J. Prosth. Dent., *37*:12, 1977.
10. Lauritzen, A. G., and Bodner, C. H.: Variations in location of arbitrary and true hinge axis points. J. Prosth. Dent., *11*:224, 1961.
11. Lauritzen, A. G., and Wolford, L. W.: Hinge axis location on an experimental basis. J. Prosth. Dent., *11*:1059, 1961.
12. Lazzari, J. B.: Application of the Hanau model "C" facebow. J. Prosth. Dent., *5*:626, 1955.
13. Lucia, V. O.: Centric relation—theory and practice. J. Prosth. Dent., *10*:855, 1960.
14. McCollum, B. B.: The mandibular hinge axis and a method of locating it. J. Prosth. Dent., *10*:428, 1960.
14a. McNamara, D. C., and Henry, P. J.: Terminal hinge contact in dentitions. J. Prosth. Dent., *32*:405, 1974.
15. Posselt, U.: Terminal hinge movement of the mandible. J. Prosth. Dent., *7*:787, 1957.
15a. Renner, R. P., and Lau, V. M. S.: Hinge-axis location and facebow transfer for edentulous patients. J. Prosth. Dent., *35*:352, 1976.
15. Posselt, U.: Terminal hinge movement of the mandible. J. Prosth. Dent., *7*:787, 1957.
16. Sheppard, I. M.: The effect of hinge axis clutches on condyle position. J. Prosth. Dent., *8*:260, 1958.
17. Sicher, H.: The biologic significance of hinge axis determination. J. Prosth. Dent., *6*:616, 1956.
18. Sloane, R. B.: Recording and transferring the mandibular axis. J. Prosth. Dent., *2*:172, 1952.
19. Stansbery, C. J.: The futility of the face-bow. J.A.D.A., *15*:1467, 1928.
20. Teteruck, W. R., and Lundeen, H. C.: The accuracy of an ear face bow. J. Prosth. Dent., *16*:1035, 1966.
20a. Thorp, E. R., Smith, D. E., and Nicholls, J. I.: Evaluation of the use of a facebow in complete denture occlusion. J. Prosth. Dent., *39*:5, 1978.
21. Trapozzano, V. R., and Lazzari, J. B.: A study of hinge axis determination. J. Prosth. Dent., *11*:858, 1961.
22. ———: The physiology of the terminal rotational position of the condyles in the temporomandibular joints. J. Prosth. Dent., *17*:122, 1967.
23. ———: Terminal rotational position of condyles. J. Prosth. Dent., *17*:132, 1967.
24. Villa, A. H.: Circular rotations in mandibular movements. J. Prosth. Dent., *11*:1053, 1961.
25. Weinberg, L. A.: The transverse hinge axis: real or imaginery. J. Prosth. Dent., *9*:775, 1959.
26. ———: An evaluation of the face bow mounting. J. Prosth. Dent., *11*:32, 1961.

Recording Maxillomandibular Relations

11

Maxillomandibular relation records made during the *diagnostic evaluation* in complete denture procedures show the vertical and horizontal relationships of the jaws. A face-bow is used to mount the maxillary cast on the maxillary bow of the articulator. The mandibular cast is then related to the maxillary cast with a centric relation record and is attached to the mandibular bow of the articulator. The centric relation record is made with the jaws in a vertical relation that provides adequate interocclusal distance between physiologic rest position and the position of occlusion.

In the *construction procedures* for complete dentures additional eccentric maxillomandibular relation records are made to dictate setting of the articulator controls for the arrangement of the artificial teeth in an acceptable occlusal scheme. Definite repeatable points of reference are necessary to orient the cast on an articulator to duplicate or similate the relations of the mandible as related to the maxillae. The records made of these relations must be capable of capturing these points of reference in a material that will retain the reference points until the casts are attached to the articulator. In healthy individuals the points of reference are subject to slight variations; however, these points are considered constant enough to be used for the construction of dentures.

Dentures are not permanent; therefore, as the need for alterations or for new dentures occurs, the points of reference must be re-evaluated. Repeatable points of reference make it possible to obtain check records to verify the initial or subsequent records. Records are of no value unless the articulator is capable of accurately accepting the records.

Vertical Relations

The physiologic rest position of the mandible as related to the maxillae and the relations of the mandible to the maxillae when the teeth are in occlusion are the two dimensions of jaw separation of primary concern in complete denture construction.

REST POSITION

The vertical dimension of jaw separation at rest occurs when the maxillofacial musculature is in a state of tonic equilibrium. It is a more involved phenomenon than the definition of rest position indicates. Not only the opening and closing muscles of the mandible are involved, but also the muscles responsible for the actions in masticating, speaking, swallowing, and breathing. These physiologic functions aid in determining the vertical dimension of rest and occlusion.

The vertical dimension of rest is a measurable distance, a repeatable reference within an acceptable range, and a useful reference when establishing the vertical dimension of occlusion. At present no scientific mechanical methods of proven validity are available for extensive use in recording rest position. Electromyography may lead to a practical usable method. When used as a reference point in recording the vertical dimension of occlusion, rest position must first be established. Some techniques do not use rest position in establishing the vertical dimension of occlusion.

For those who do use the rest position as a reference there are several pertinent factors to be considered.

1. The position of the mandible is influenced by gravity; therefore, mandibular positions are postural. The patient sitting upright or standing with the head erect looks straight ahead when jaw relation records are made, rest position is determined, or the occlusion is adjusted intraorally.

2. Rest position is a relaxed position of the mandible. When a patient is tense, under strain, nervous, tired, or irritable, the value of the measurements is questionable. The procedure is advisably postponed and repeated when conditions are more favorable. When the dentist is under strain, nervous, tired, or irritable, this condition can influence the patient's reaction.

3. It is difficult to determine maxillomandibular relations on patients who suffer from neuromuscular disturbances. With these patients the dentist must be very considerate and patient. He must

also be willing to devote considerable time to the procedure.

4. Rest position is a position in space, not to be maintained for definite periods of time. The duration is usually short; therefore, the dentist should be prepared to make measurements without delay when the position is assumed.

5. No one method for determining rest position can be accepted as being valid for all patients; therefore, it is advisable to use several methods and compare the results.

6. Space between the teeth is essential when the mandible is at rest. If no space is present between teeth in dentures, discomfort, pain, and generalized hyperemia result until resorption of the bone establishes the necessary interocclusal distance. Failure to establish rest position as a reference point may result in a lessened or excessive interocclusal distance; both are potentially damaging either to the support or to the temporomandibular joint.

RECORDING REST POSITION

Facial measurements after swallowing and relaxing, tactile sense, measurements of anatomic landmarks, speech, and facial expression are methods of recording the vertical dimension of rest position.

FACIAL MEASUREMENTS. Instruct the patient to stand comfortably upright with the eyes looking straight ahead at some object which is on the same level. Insert the maxillary record base with the attached contoured occlusion rim. With either an indelible marker or a triangle of adhesive tape, place a point of reference on the end of the patient's nose and another on the point of his chin (Fig. 11-1). Instruct the patient to wipe his lips with his tongue, to swallow, and to drop his shoulders. When the mandible drops to rest position, measure between the

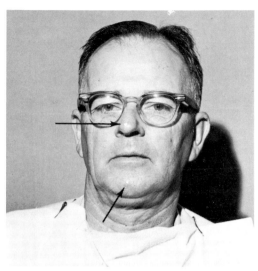

FIG. 11-1. *A patient in a comfortable upright position. Gravity influences the position of the mandible. Arrows designate tape used as points of reference.*

points of reference. A millimeter ruler is convenient and will not alarm the patient as it is seen being positioned against the face (Fig. 11-2). Repeat this procedure until the measurements are consistent. Such measurements are helpful but cannot be considered as absolute. This method is also used with the patient seated comfortably in the dental chair with the head upright and the feet flat on the base of the foot rest.

TACTILE SENSE. Instruct the patient to stand erect and open the jaws wide

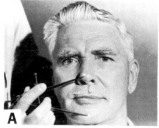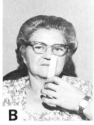

FIG. 11-2. *Measuring between the points of reference.* **A.** *Dividers can be used.* **B.** *A ruler is preferred.*

until strain is felt in the muscles. When this opening becomes uncomfortable, ask him to close slowly until the jaws reach a comfortable, relaxed position. Measure the distance between the points of reference and compare with the measurements made after swallowing.

PHONETICS. Speech is used in several different ways as an aid in establishing rest position. Two of these methods are as follows:

1. Have the patient repeat the name *Emma* until he is aware of the contacting of the lips as the first syllable *em* is pronounced. When the patient has rehearsed this procedure, ask that he stop all jaw movement when the lips touch. At this time measure between the two points of reference.

2. Engage the patient in a conversation that will divert his attention from conscious participation in the procedure. A pause in speech, followed by relaxation as indicated by a drop of the mandible, is indication for another measurement.

FACIAL EXPRESSION. The experienced dentist learns the advantage of recognizing the relaxed facial expression when a patient's jaws are at rest (Fig. 11-3). In normally related jaws the lips will be even anteroposteriorly and in slight contact. The lips of the patient with a protruded mandible will not be evenly related anteroposteriorly; the lower lip will be anterior to the upper lip and not in contact. The lips of the patient with a retruded mandible will not be even; the lower lip will be distal to the upper and not in contact. The skin around the eyes and over the chin will be relaxed. Relaxation around the nares reflects unobstructed breathing. These evidences of rest position of the maxillomandibular musculature are the indications for recording a measurement of the vertical dimension of rest.

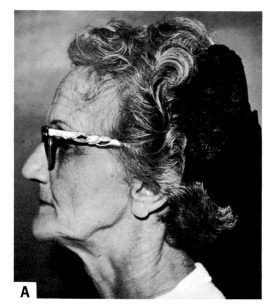

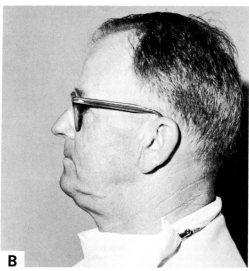

FIG. 11-3. *Profile photographs.* **A.** *A patient who was not conscious of being observed.* **B.** *A patient who had difficulty relaxing.*

ANATOMIC LANDMARKS. Measurement of anatomic landmarks of the face is another method of recording the vertical dimension of the rest position. The Willis guide is designed to measure the distance from the pupils of the eye to the rima oris and the distance from the anterior nasal spine to the lower border of the mandible. When these measurements are equal, the jaws are considered at rest. The asymmetry of faces makes the value of average measurements using anatomic landmarks questionable.

OCCLUSION POSITION

The vertical dimension of jaw separations when the teeth or occlusion rims are in contact is not like the vertical dimension of jaw separation when the jaws are at rest. When the mandible is at rest, it is hanging in space and is not in a completely static position; but when the mandible is braced against the maxillae with the teeth as intermediaries, the position is static and can be maintained for an indefinite time. When the vertical dimension of occlusion is established for use in the construction of dentures, the jaws are in centric relation. When natural teeth are in maximum occlusion, the jaws are not necessarily in centric relation. For this reason, all pre-extraction records must be carefully evaluated. The horizontal relations of the jaws influence facial measurements.

RECORDING OCCLUSION

Pre-extraction records, measurements with former dentures, and wax occlusion rims are used to determine the vertical dimension of occlusion. Neuromuscular perception and power point are methods suggested for edentulous patients with no pre-extraction records or dentures.

PRE-EXTRACTION RECORDS

Profile Photographs. Profile photographs (Fig. 11-3) are made and enlarged to life size. Measurements of anatomic landmarks on the photograph are compared with measurements using the same anatomic landmarks on the face. These measurements can be compared when the records are made and again when the artificial teeth are tried in. The photographs should be made with the teeth in maximum occlusion, as this position can be maintained accurately for photographic procedures.

Profile Silhouettes. An accurate reproduction of the profile in silhouette can be cut out in cardboard or contoured in wire. The silhouette can be repositioned to the face after the vertical dimension has been established at the initial recording and/or when the artificial teeth are tried in.

Radiography. The two types of radiographs advocated are the cephalometric profile and the condyles in the fossae. The inaccuracies that exist in either the technique or the method of comparing measurements make these methods unreliable.

Articulated Cast. After accurate casts of the maxillary and mandibular arches have been made, the maxillary cast is related in its correct anatomic position in an articulator with a face-bow transfer. An occlusal record with the

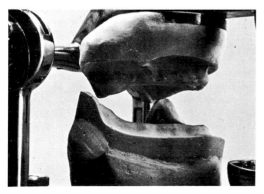

FIG. 11-4. *Accurately articulated casts have many uses in complete denture procedures. The distance between the residual ridges of the articulated edentulous casts can be compared with that of casts mounted prior to the extraction of the teeth.*

jaws in centric relation is used to mount the mandibular cast (Fig. 11-4). After the teeth have been removed and edentulous casts have been mounted on the articulator, the interarch measurements are compared. This method is valuable with patients whose ridges are not sacrificed during the removal of the teeth or resorbed during a long waiting period for denture construction.

Facial Measurements. The patient is instructed to close his jaws into maximum occlusion after two tattoo points have been placed—one on the upper half of the face and the other on the lower half. The distance is measured, and these measurements are compared with measurements made between these points when the artificial teeth are tried in.

Closest-speaking Space. Silverman suggested this method and described it as follows:

The closest-speaking space which measures the vertical dimension in this phonetic method must not be confused with the freeway space of the physiologic method reported by Niswonger (1934) and Thompson (1946). The closest-speaking space is not the free-way space. These two measurements, by two different methods based on different principles, should not be confused. The free-way space establishes vertical dimension when the muscles involved are at complete rest, or in physiologic tonus and the mandible is in its rest position. The closest-speaking space measures vertical dimension when the mandible and muscles involved are in physiologic function of speech. In one method everything involved is still (static) and in the other method everything is moving (dynamic or functional).[29]

The "F" or "V" and "S" Speaking Anterior Tooth Relation. Incisive guidance is established by arranging the anterior teeth in the occlusion rims before recording the vertical dimension of oc-

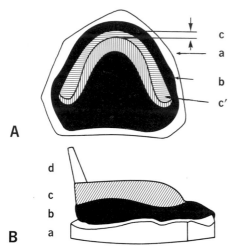

FIG. 11-5 *Casts (a) with record bases (b) and occlusion rims (c) for "f" or "v" and "s" speaking anterior tooth relation. A. Maxillary cast. The width of the hard wax rim is approximately the width of the anterior (c) and posterior (c') teeth. B. Mandibular cast. Note the inclination of the "speaking wax" (d). (Redrawn from Pound and Murrell: An introduction to denture simplification. J. Prosth. Dent., 26:570, 1971.)*

clusion in a technique developed by Pound and Murrell. The position of the artificial maxillary anterior teeth is determined by the position of the maxillae when the patient says words beginning with "f" or "v"; the mandibular anterior teeth by the position of the mandible when the patient says words beginning with "s" as follows:

1. Make stable record bases over accepted stone casts of the maxillary and mandibular arches.

2. Using hard baseplate wax, contour the maxillary occlusion rim (Fig. 11-5A). Keep the labiopalatal and buccopalatal width the same as that of the anterior and posterior teeth.

3. After applying hard baseplate wax to a height of 2 or 3 mm over the superior surface of the mandibular record base, place a section of beeswax about ¾ inch high in the estimated location of the four

anterior teeth (Fig. 11-5B). The section of beeswax is referred to as "speaking wax."

4. Place the maxillary record base with the attached occlusion rim in the patient's mouth. Adjust the occlusion rim to provide lip support. When the "f" and "v" sounds are articulated, the incisal edges of the maxillary anterior teeth create a seal on the moist area of the vermilion border of the lower lip.

5. Have the patient repeat the word "first" or "Victor" and contour the wax to create the seal. The seal can be checked by having the patient repeat or read the numbers "five" and "fifty-five."

6. Record the midline on the wax rim and arrange the two artificial central incisors, one on each side of the midline, with the incisal edges at right angles to the long axis of the face at the determined incisal length for lip seal (Fig. 11-6). The incisal edges form a seal by contacting the lower lip.

7. Remove the record base from the mouth and arrange the artificial lateral incisors and cuspids. A template may be used at the workbench as an aid to arrangement.

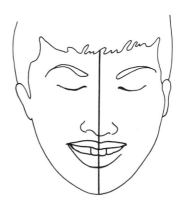

FIG. 11-6. *Vertical line designating the midline that serves as a guide for placement of the two central incisors. (Redrawn from Pound and Murrell: An introduction to denture simplification. J. Prosth. Dent., 26:570, 1971.)*

8. Place the incisal edges of the artificial lateral incisors and cuspids at the same level as the central incisors. Keep the labial surfaces in harmony with the contoured occlusion rim. This may or may not follow the form of the arch to give lip support.

9. Return the maxillary record base to the mouth and make any changes necessary for natural appearance. The incisal edges should follow the curvature of the lower lip.

10. Seat the mandibular record base with the attached "speaking wax." Have the patient repeat the numbers 6 and 65 and adjust to the "s" position. When the "s" sounds are articulated, the mandible moves forward. The incisal edges of the anterior teeth do not make contact (Fig. 11-7). Merely having the patient pronounce words beginning with "f" or "s" will bring forth conscious speech patterns that are not adequate for determining the position. Unconscious, more natural speech patterns with the words recurring fairly quickly can be produced by asking the patient to read a newspaper article or a poem.

CLASS	"S" Position	Retrusion	Closure
I			
II			
III		none	

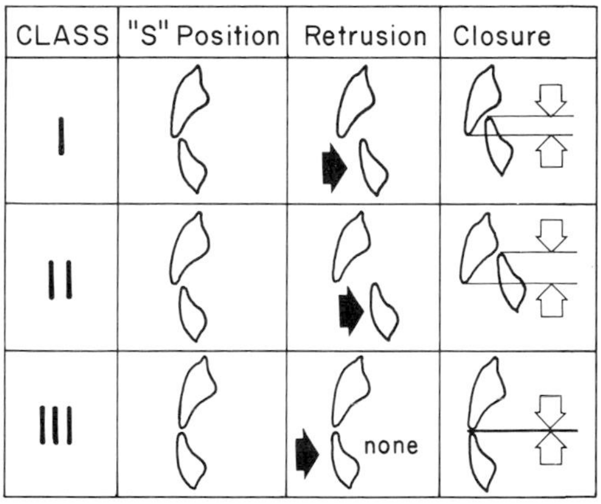

FIG. 11-8. *Relation of the anterior teeth at the "s" position for three classified jaw relations, for retrusion, and for closure. (Redrawn after Pound and Murrell: An introduction to denture simplification. J. Prosth. Dent., 26:570, 1971.)*

11. Record the center line on the wax rim to coincide with the midline of the maxillary central incisors.

12. After removing the mandibular record base from the patient's mouth, remove the "speaking wax" from one side of the center line. Replace the wax with the central and lateral incisors, with the necks of the artificial teeth inclined toward the crest of the residual ridge. Then remove the remaining wax and arrange the other artificial central and lateral incisors.

13. Return the mandibular base to the mouth and refine the four artificial teeth to the "s" position (Fig. 11-8). This position represents the protrusive phase of incisal guidance.

14. Adjust the hard wax rim on the maxillary record base to parallel Camper's line (Fig. 9-7). Place notches in it to aid in repositioning the vertical dimension and central occlusal records (Fig. 11-9).

15. Place soft recording wax* on the

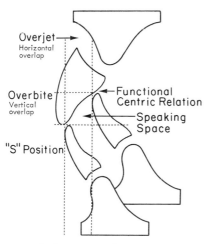

FIG. 11-7. *"S" position for anterior mandibular teeth. (Redrawn from Pound and Murrell: An introduction to denture simplification. J. Prosth. Dent., 26:570, 1971.)*

Overjet
Horizontal overlap

Overbite
Vertical overlap

Functional
Centric Relation

Speaking
Space

"S" Position

*Synthetic Occlusal Plane Wax, Harry J. Bosworth, Chicago, Illinois.

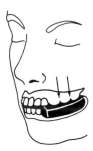

FIG. 11-9. *Notches (arrows) placed in the maxillary hard wax rim as an aid in repositioning. (Redrawn from Pound and Murrell: An introduction to denture simplification. J. Prosth. Dent., 26:570, 1971.)*

posterior superior surface of the mandibular base to a height that exceeds the anticipated vertical dimension of occlusion (Fig. 11-10). Seal it to the hard wax.

16. Place the maxillary record base with the attached teeth on the wax rim in the mouth and assure that it is stable and is retained.

17. Seat the mandibular record base in the patient's mouth. Ask the patient to retrude his mandible from the "s" position to a comfortable retruded relation and then to close vertically until a firm posterior contact is encountered (Fig. 11-11).

18. Remove the record from the patient's mouth and check for alignment and sufficiency. Correct any discrepancies and remove excess wax.

19. Reinsert the record base and re-

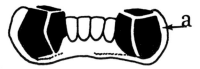

FIG. 11-10. *Synthetic occlusal wax (a) placed on posterior section of the mandibular record base. Note that it is higher than the central and lateral incisors. (Redrawn from Pound and Murrell: An introduction to denture simplification. J. Prosth. Dent., 26: 570, 1971.)*

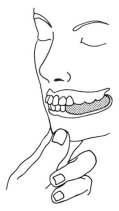

FIG. 11-11. *Mandible in a repeatable retruded relation to the maxillae with closure at an acceptable vertical dimension of occlusion. (Redrawn from Pound and Murrell: An introduction to denture simplification. J. Prosth. Dent., 26:570, 1971.)*

peat step 4 until the incisal edges of the mandibular anterior teeth contact firmly against the maxillary teeth or the palate. The latter can occur in some Class II related jaws in which the mandible has a retruded relation to the maxillae. Firm contact at this point does not mean that the teeth will be in contact when arranged in centric occlusion.

According to Pound and Murrell, their technique will be acceptable for 80 per cent of edentulous patients provided with dentures. A record made following this technique, however, may incorporate undue pressure. If the patient is instructed to open and then make light contact without pressure, the anterior teeth may not contact as they did. To assure that the record does not incorporate excess pressure, the patient must be instructed to return to the retruded position, again close into the record with pressure, and then to open and close lightly. Because less wax is compressed on each closure, repeating this procedure will develop an acceptable record of the jaws in terminal relation at the correct vertical dimension of occlusion with minimal pressure, except in some of the extreme Class II relations. In most situations this posterior contact represents the posterior contact of incisal guidance. It also determines the patient's original class of occlusion.

An alternate technique, not suggested by Pound and Murrell, is to use Tenax wax made passive by applying dry heat, plaster, softened impression compound, or zinc oxide-eugenol paste as the recording material. The patient is instructed to retrude from the "s" position to the terminal relation and close until the anterior teeth make contact. This procedure has been used with acceptable results when the correct remount procedures are instituted for selective grinding (page 385).

FORMER DENTURES. Methods for the natural teeth present and in occlusion can also be used when the patient has dentures. The most common method is a comparison of measurements made with the former dentures with measurements made during the record-making procedure. It is advisable to use other methods and establish the vertical dimension of occlusion in the occlusion rims and then compare the measurements between reference points with the former dentures in occlusion.

There are several reasons for not accepting the measurements made with former dentures without thoroughly checking. Loss of the ridges under the dentures results in an increase in interocclusal distance. Patients can shift the mandible, or the denture can be shifted on its support to accommodate for errors in occlusion. Inaccurate adaption of the denture base to the support results in displacement of the denture.

EDENTULOUS PATIENTS. Often edentulous patients have no pre-extraction records or former dentures available. For these patients the following methods can determine the vertical dimension of occlusion.

Neuromuscular Perception (as suggested by Lytle[19]). A central bearing device attached to accurately adapted record bases permits the patient to experience through neuromuscular perception the different vertical relations.

Step 1—Accurately mount the casts (Fig. 11-4).

Step 2—Mount central bearing plates directly on the accurately adapted record bases, adapting the plates to the patient's interarch distance. (Fig. 11-12A, B,C,D).

Step 3—Adjust the bearing pin (Fig. 11-12E) until the mouth is opened beyond the physiologic rest position (Fig. 11-12F). Lower the pin a half turn at a time, having the patient make two sharp contacts each time, until the patient signifies he has closed too far. Turn the pin back a half turn and record the number of turns on the pin.

Step 4—Repeat the procedure, starting from an overclosed position (Fig. 11-12H). Open the pin a half turn and have the patient make two sharp contacts of the pin against the metal plate after each adjustment. When the patient signifies he has reached excessive opening, turn the pin back a half turn.

Step 5—When the records in steps 3 and 4 do not correspond, the patient may choose one of them. Then he may choose between this adjustment and one halfway between steps 3 and 4. Recheck the record by repeating steps 3, 4, and 5.

Step 6—Relate the mandible to the maxillae in the most retruded relation (centric relation). Instruct the patient to close until the central bearing pin is in contact with the metal plate and to retain the contact (Fig. 11-12G). Inject soft fast-setting plaster (Fig. 11-12I) to secure the relation. This record is considered

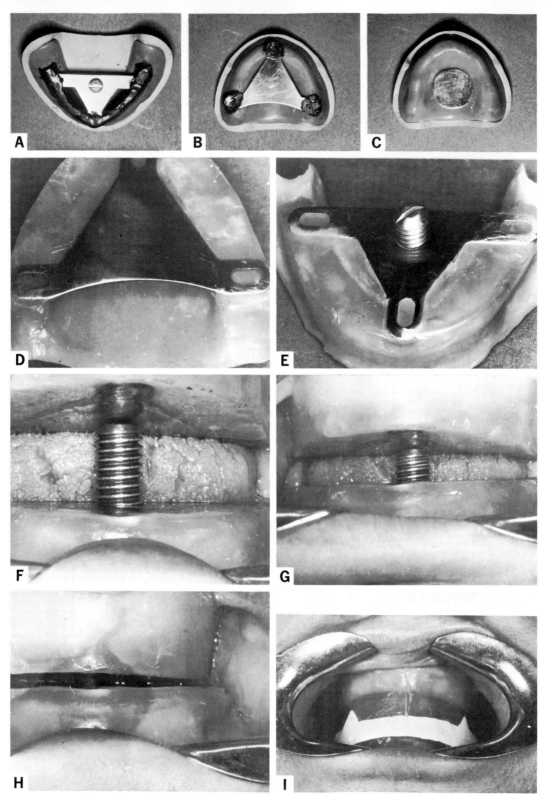

FIG. 11-12. *Procedures for neuromuscular perception of vertical dimension of occlusion.* **A.** *and* **B.** *Central bearing plate mounted directly on base with compound for patients with average interarch distance.* **C.** *Flat plate mounted in palate for patient with little interarch space.* **D** *and* **E.** *Plate mounted in occlusion rims for patients with adequate or excessive interarch space.* **F.** *Adjustment with mouth opened beyond physiologic rest position.* **G.** *Adjustment with mouth in correct closure.* **H.** *Adjustment with mouth in over closed position.* **I.** *Central bearing device made secure with fast-setting plaster.* (*After Lytle, R. B.: Vertical relation of occlusion by the patient's neuromuscular perception. J. Prosth. Dent.,* 14:12, 1964.)

tentative, as are most centric relation records that are made in the absence of teeth.

Step 7—Transfer the record to an articulator and arrange the artificial teeth. At the try-in appointment re-evaluate the procedure and evaluate the position and arrangement to meet the physiologic requirements in speech and swallowing and esthetics.

Power Point (as suggested by Boos[3]). Attach the Bimeter to an accurately adapted mandibular record base. Attach a metal plate in the vault of an accurately adapted maxillary record base to provide a central bearing point. Adjust the vertical distance by turning the cap (Fig. 11-13). The gauge indicates the pounds of pressure generated during closure at different degrees of jaw separation. When the maximum power point is determined, lock the set nut. Make plaster registrations and transfer the cast to an articulator.

WAX OCCLUSION RIMS. It is possible to obtain *tentative* records with wax occlusion rims attached to accurately adapted record bases. The final evalua-

tion is determined after the casts have been mounted on the articulator with a *tentative* centric relation record that was made at the *tentative* vertical dimension of occlusion. The artificial teeth are then arranged for both the functional and the esthetic requirements, and the wax is contoured to simulate the finished denture base.

The following technique uses wax occlusion rims as the medium and employs physiologic phenomena in making the records. This technique is used for establishing both the tentative vertical dimension of occlusion and the tentative centric relation of the jaws. It may also be used for accurately mounting casts for diagnostic evaluation. After the casts have been mounted on the articulator, a tracing device can be attached to the occlusion rims for use in graphic tracings. The final evaluation uses facial expression and esthetics as a guide after the teeth have been arranged for the trial denture.

1. Establish the vertical dimension of rest and record the distance between the points of reference placed on the nose and chin (page 262).

2. The maxillary occlusion rim contoured to the tentative occlusal plane for the face-bow transfer (Chapter 10) is not altered unless absolutely necessary. At times the interarch space is so limited that the maxillary rims must be altered. When they must be, reduce the rim distal to the cuspid and retain the guides for positioning the anterior teeth. Make the interocclusal distance approximately 4 or 5 millimeters less than the interocclusal distance at rest position. When accurate recording of measurements is difficult, use facial expression.

3. Thinly coat the maxillary occlusion rim with petrolatum. Seat the maxillary record base with the attached rim securely in place. If it is determined that the record base does not have

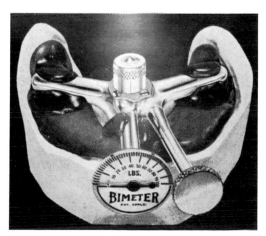

FIG. 11-13. *The Bimeter. (From Swenson's Complete Dentures, C. Boucher, ed. St. Louis, The C. V. Mosby Company, 1937.)*

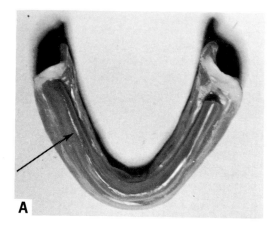

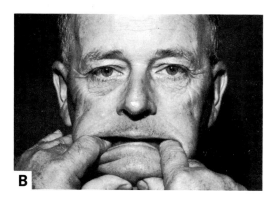

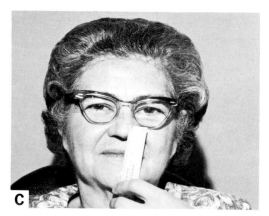

FIG. 11-14. *Making tentative records with wax occlusion rims.* **A.** *Arrow indicates the roll of softened (passive) wax attached to the mandibular rim.* **B.** *Index fingers placed on buccal flanges to stabilize the dentures. They also serve as reminders that there are two temporomandibular joints.* **C.** *Measuring the vertical dimension of occlusion in millimeters.*

adequate retention, apply a very *thin* dusting of denture adhesive powder to the tissue side of the base. Excessive denture adhesive is *not* necessary. Too much will cause an error in the vertical relation record.

4. Make a roll of Tenax wax about one third the diameter of a lead pencil and attach it to the occlusal surface of the mandibular occlusion rim (Fig. 11-14A). Soften the roll of wax in a water bath at 130°F and contour it in a triangular shape with the base on the occlusion rim. Resoften the Tenax wax in the water bath or with a controlled alcohol torch flame. Seat the mandibular record base in the mouth and place the tips of the index fingers bilaterally on the buccal flanges in the area of the second bicuspids to assure that the record base is stable when the jaw is moved (Fig. 11-14B). Request the patient to retrude the mandible and close on the back teeth but to stop closing the jaw when he feels that the closure is sufficient (tactile sense). The experienced dentist can feel with his fingers and see with his eyes when the contraction of the elevator muscles begins to diminish. This should coincide with the patient's perception of adequate closure.

Allow the wax to harden before removing the tentative record from the mouth. Reinsert the record and have the patient close to maximum occlusion. Measure the distance between the points of reference and compare with the measurements made with the mandible at rest (Fig. 11-14C). If the measurement is less than the measurement at rest and the Tenax wax was not penetrated through to make occlusion rim contact, the record is acceptable. This is a *tentative* record of centric relation obtained with the jaws separated at the *tentative* vertical dimension of occlusion. This record can be verified with methods that involve the patient's tactile sense, phonetics, swallowing, and esthetics. However, these check methods are more valid after teeth have been arranged on the record bases and the wax has been contoured.

PREPARING FOR EVALUATION

1. Relate the mandibular cast to the face-bow mounted maxillary cast with this record and attach the mandibular cast to the articulator with plaster.

2. Orient the plane of occlusion and arrange the anterior and posterior artificial teeth (page 349) to meet the functional and esthetic requirements in centric occlusion.

3. Contour the wax in the form of the finished denture. Have the patient return for the try-in. This is necessary to evaluate the record of the vertical dimension of occlusion with the mandible in centric relation and to make other records of centric and eccentric relations of the jaws. The arrangement of teeth for esthetics is also evaluated at this sitting.

EVALUATING VERTICAL DIMENSION

The following are methods used to evaluate the *vertical dimension of occlusion.*

PATIENT'S TACTILE SENSE. Place the trial dentures in the patient's mouth and determine that they are stable. Instruct the patient to open and close until the teeth contact. Ask the patient if the teeth appear to touch too soon, if the jaws seem to close too far before they touch, or if the teeth feel just right. This method is not very effective with senile patients or with those who have impaired neuromuscular coordinations.

SWALLOWING FOLLOWED BY RELAXING. With the dentures in place instruct the patient to wipe the lips with the tip of the tongue, swallow, and let the shoulders drop in a relaxed position. Watch the reference points and ask the patient to close the teeth together. If the teeth are together it can indicate that no interocclusal distance exists. However, some patients may force their teeth together, thinking that is what is expected.

Another method that can be used with either occlusion rims or teeth is based on the theory that the teeth make contact at or near centric occlusion. Two small cones of a soft wax are placed, one in each central sulcus of the mandibular first molars. Encourage the patient to swallow several times. If the vertical dimension of occlusion is correct, the wax will be penetrated and reduced to tooth contact.

PHONETICS. The use of speech in evaluating the vertical dimension of occlusion for patients receiving their first dentures is of dubious value. The awkwardness of those patients often defeats the purpose. However, in patients for whom subsequent dentures are constructed, phonetics is a useful aid. In using phonetics, the enunciation of words is not of primary interest.

The position of the tongue and the relation of the teeth are important. Have the patient repeat "three thirty-three"; there should be enough space for the tip of the tongue to protrude between the anterior teeth. Have the patient repeat "fifty-five". The incisal edges of the maxillary central incisors should contact the vermilion border of the lower lip at the junction of the moist and dry mucosa. When the patient repeats the words *Emma* and *Mississippi,* the teeth should not contact.

Centric Relation Record

The most difficult record to make and the most important maxillomandibular relation in complete denture construction is the centric relation of the mandible to the maxillae. If an accurate record of this relation is not used to relate the casts on the articulator, it is impossible to harmonize the positions of the teeth with mandibular movements. In the absence of pathology, the relationship is stable and reproducible. A record that cannot be repeated is not acceptable. A maxillomandibular relation record that must be repeated appears to be more difficult to make than one that does not have to be repeated.

Relaxation of muscles attached to the mandible is essential in the procedure. Psychic or emotional tensions, pain or discomfort in any part of the stomatognathic system, and built-in muscle memory contribute to the problem of record making. The normal physiologic response to characteristic stimuli is different from the response to abnormal stimuli. The physiology of the neuromuscular system must be considered in making a centric relation record. It is not sufficient to assume that because a ligament is inelastic movements are limited only by mechanical means. Centric relation in the normal individual is considered to be a ligamentous position, but this does not rule out the functions of the other entities in the joint. All of these factors have contributed to the development of various techniques and the use of different materials to achieve an accurate record that can be repeated.

The three primary requirements for making a centric relation record are (1) to record the correct horizontal relation of the mandible to the maxillae, (2) to exert equalized vertical pressure, and (3) to retain the record in an undistorted condition until the casts have been accurately mounted on the articulator or until a previous record can be verified. Retruding the mandible establishes the horizontal position

anteroposteriorly and mediolaterally. The recording medium should be of uniform consistency. In the act of the vertical closure of the jaws, if a recording medium resists the forces exerted by the muscles to an unequal extent on the right or left, tissues can be displaced, the condyle can be rotated in its path, or both can occur, and the result will be an inaccurate record. Recording mediums or instruments must retain the record in an undistorted condition, for it is possible to have made an accurate record and then to destroy its accuracy. This is particularly significant if the mandible moves when one uses a central bearing device or waxes, because wax distorts before it breaks.

Methods used to make the centric relation record are the functional, the graphic, and the tactile or interocclusal check.

FUNCTIONAL (Chew-in)

The Patterson technique and the Needles-House technique are examples of the functional, or chew-in, method. Both are based on the same principle. The patient produces a pattern of mandibular movements by moving the mandible to protrusion, retrusion, and right and left lateral.

The Needles-House method uses compound occlusion rims with four metal styli placed in the maxillary rim (Fig. 11-15). When the mandible moves with the styli contacting the mandibular rim, the styli cut four diamond-shaped tracings. The tracings incorporate the movements in three planes, and the records are placed on a suitable articulator to receive and duplicate the record. The record can also be used as a centric relation record on other types of articulators.

The Patterson method uses wax occlusion rims. A trench is made in the mandibular rim and a mixture of half

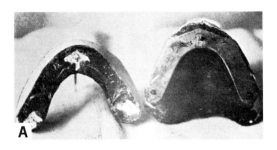

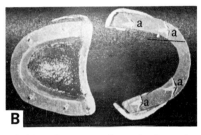

FIG. 11-15. *Compound occlusion rims for central relation records by Needles-House method.* **A.** *The use of three styli as suggested by Needles. (From Nichols, I.: Prosthetic Dentistry, St. Louis, The C. V. Mosby Company, 1930, p. 167.)* **B.** *The House modification with four styli to make the needle point tracings (a). (From Anthony, L. P.: American Textbook of Prosthetic Dentistry, 7th ed. Philadelphia, Lea & Febiger, 1942.)*

plaster and half carborundum paste is placed in the trench. The mandibular movements generate compensating curves in the plaster and carborundum (Fig. 11-16). When the plaster and carborundum are reduced to the predeter-

mined vertical dimension of occlusion, the patient is instructed to retrude the mandible and the occlusion rims are joined together with metal staples.

Both of these methods require a tentative interocclusal wax record of centric relation at the tentative vertical dimension of occlusion to prepare the recording devices. Both methods adjust the recording mediums at a height of vertical jaw separation which is in excess to the predetermined dimension of occlusion. The correct vertical dimension of occlusion is established as the patient closes the mandible.

The functional methods of recording centric relation require very stable record bases. Forces which can dislodge the record bases occur in any method that requires the mandible to move into eccentric jaw positions with the recording medium in contact. The record will not be accurate unless the bases are stable. The displaceable basal seat tissues, the resistance of the recording mediums, and the lack of control of equalized pressure in the eccentric relations contribute to inaccuracy in these methods. Patients not only must have good neuromuscular coordination to participate in the functional methods of recording centric relations but also must be capable of following instructions if accurate records are to be obtained.

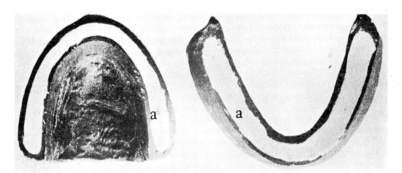

FIG. 11-16. *The Patterson occlusion rims: pumice and plaster (a). (From Anthony, L. P.: American Textbook of Prosthetic Dentistry. 7th ed. Philadelphia, Lea & Febiger, 1942.)*

GRAPHIC METHODS

The graphic methods record a tracing of mandibular movements in one plane, an arrow point tracing. It indicates the horizontal relation of the mandible to the maxillae. The apex of a properly made tracing presumably indicates the most retruded relation of the mandible to the maxillae from which lateral movements can take place (Fig. 11-17). Do not confuse this with other graphic tracings that are made in additional planes. Pantographic tracings, for example, are made in three planes.

Graphic methods are either intraoral or extraoral, depending upon the placement of the recording device. The intraoral tracings cannot be observed during the tracing; therefore, the method loses some of the value of a visible method. Since the intraoral tracings are small, it is difficult to find the true apex. The tracer must be definitely seated in a hole at the point of the apex to assure accuracy when injecting plaster between the occlusion rims. If the patient moves the mandible before the occlusion rims are secured, the records shift on their basal seat; this destroys the accuracy of the record. The extraoral tracings are larger than the intraoral because they are made further from the centers of rotation, and the apex is more discernible (Fig. 11-17). The extraoral tracings are visible while the tracing is being made. Therefore, the patient can be directed and guided more intelligently during the mandibular movements. The stylus can be observed in the apex of the tracing during the process of injecting plaster between the occlusion rims, and no hole is required.

When any graphic tracing is made, these factors are important: (1) Displacement of the record bases may result from pressure if the central bearing point is off center when the mandible moves into eccentric relations to the maxillae. (2) If a central bearing device is not used, the occlusion rims offer more resistance to horizontal movements. (3) It is difficult to locate the center of the true arches to centralize the forces with a central bearing device when the jaws are in favorable relation and far more difficult if the jaws are in excessive protrusive or retrusive relation. (4) It is difficult to stabilize a record base against horizontal forces on tissues that are pendulous or otherwise easily displaceable. (5) It is difficult to stabilize a record base against horizontal forces on residual ridges that have no vertical height. (6) It is difficult to stabilize a record base or bearing device with patients who have large awkward tongues. (7) Recording devices are not usually considered compatible with normal physiologic stimulation in mandibular movements. (8) The tracing is not acceptable unless a pointed apex is developed; a blunted apex usually indicates an acquired functional relation-

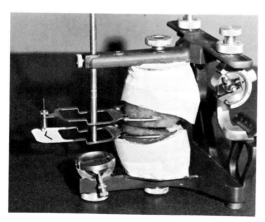

Fig. 11-17. *An extraoral tracing recorded in the horizontal plane near the incisal point. The tracing has been accentuated for photographic purposes. The stylus was attached to the maxillary arch.*

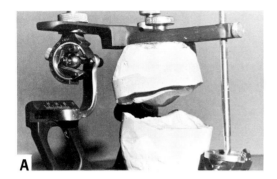

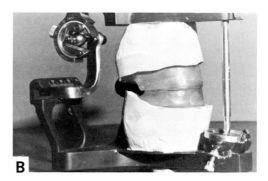

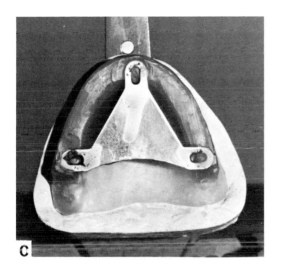

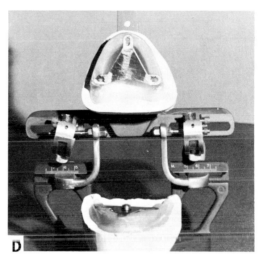

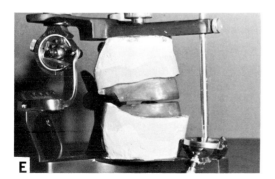

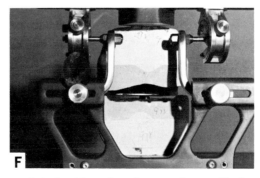

FIG. 11-18. *Extraoral tracing.* **A.** *Maxillary cast related with a face-bow and mandibular cast mounted with a centric relation record.* **B.** *Wax occlusion rims mounted in the casts and attached to the articulator with plaster. Note they are in contact at the vertical dimension of occlusion.* **C, D, E,** *and* **F.** *Central bearing device.*

ship, and a sharp apex usually indicates the position of centric relation. (9) Double tracings usually indicate lack of co-ordinated movements or recordings at a different vertical dimension of jaw separation. In either event, additional tracings are necessary. (10) A graphic tracing to determine centric relation is made at the predetermined vertical dimension of occlusion. This harmonizes centric relation with centric occlusion and the anteroposterior bone-to-bone relation with the tooth-to-tooth contact. (11) Graphic methods can record eccentric relations of the mandible to the maxillae. (12) Graphic methods are the most accurate visual means of making a centric relation record with mechanical instruments; however, all graphic tracings are not necessarily accurate.

TECHNIQUE FOR GRAPHIC METHOD. The technique for an *extraoral arrow point tracing* using a Hight tracing device follows.

1. Make accurate, stable maxillary and mandibular record bases (Chapter 9).

2. Attach occlusion rims of hard baseplate wax (Chapter 9).

3. Contour the wax occlusion rims (Chapter 9).

4. Establish the vertical dimension of jaw separation with the mandible at physiologic rest (pages 261–264).

5. Reduce the mandibular occlusion rim to provide excessive interocclusal distance (Chapter 9).

6. Make a face-bow transfer and mount the maxillary cast (Chapter 10 and Fig. 11-18A).

7. With soft wax make a tentative centric relation record at a predetermined vertical dimension of occlusion.

8. Adjust the articulator with the condylar elements secured against the centric stops.

9. Relate the maxillary occlusion rims in the soft wax record and attach the mandibular cast to the articulator with plaster (Fig. 11-18B).

10. Mount a central bearing device. Exercise care to center the central bearing point in relation to the plate, both anteroposteriorly and laterally (Fig. 11-18C,D,E,F).

11. Mount the tracing device. Be sure to attach the devices securely to the occlusion rims. The stylus is attached to the maxillary rim and the recording plate to the mandibular rim. This arrangement develops an arrow point tracing with the apex anteriorly. The reverse develops an arrow point tracing with the apex posteriorly (Fig. 11-19).

12. Seat the patient, with head upright, in a comfortable position in the dental chair.

13. Seat the record bases with the attached recording devices. Inspect the record bases and recording devices for stability. Make sure that there is no interference between the occlusion rims when the mandible is moved in any direction. Lower the stylus to the recording plate and determine that the

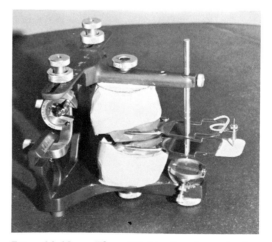

FIG. 11-19.   *The Hight tracing device mounted. The device is extraoral with the stylus attached to the maxillary bow* (**a**).

stylus maintains contact with the recording plate during mandibular movements (Fig. 11-20).

14. Retract the stylus and conduct training exercises with the patient. Place the tips of the index fingers under the mandible in the bicuspid areas. Place the tip of the thumb under the mandible near the chin. Calmly and quietly instruct the patient to move the jaw forward, backward, and to the right

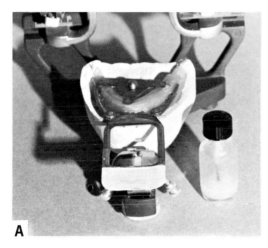

A

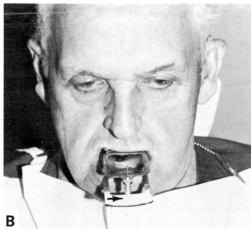

B

FIG. 11-20. *Making an extraoral tracing.* **A.** *Recording plate coated with a solution made by dissolving precipitated chalk in denatured alcohol.* **B.** *Stylus contacting recording plate (arrow). Note the patient is seated in a comfortable upright position.*

and left while gently applying guiding pressure with the thumb. It is possible to dislodge the mandibular record base by improperly placing the thumbs or by exerting excessive pressure. The Ney Excursion Guide is an aid in training the patient (Fig. 11-21).

15. When the patient is proficient in executing the mandibular movements, prepare the tracing plate to record the tracing. A thin coating of precipitated chalk in denatured alcohol applied evenly with a brush provides a medium that offers no resistance to the movement of the stylus and produces a clearly visible tracing.

16. Develop an acceptable tracing by dropping the stylus to the record plate (Fig. 11-22).

17. When a definite arrow point tracing with a sharp apex is made, have the patient retrude the mandible to centric relation. The point of the stylus should be at the point of the apex of the arrow point tracing. Inject quick setting dental plaster between the occlusion rims and allow the plaster to harden. (Fig. 11-23 A,B).

18. Remove the assembly and mount the mandibular cast with the new record (Fig. 11-23C).

This record is a *tentative* record and will be checked with an interocclusal check record when the teeth are arranged and the wax is contoured.

TACTILE OR INTEROCCLUSAL
CHECK RECORD METHOD

The tactile or interocclusal check record method is referred to as a physiologic method. The normal functioning of the patient's proprioception and tactile sense is essential in the making of an accurate record. The patient's proprioception is information provided about the movements and the positions of the body and its parts by receptors in the muscle spindles, tendon organs of Golgi,

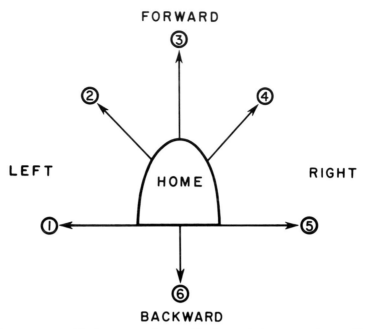

FIG. 11-21. *The Ney mandibular excursion guide for training procedures. Place the guide in a convenient position for the patient to see. Some patients respond more readily to the request to move the lower jaw to the right, left, forward, or backward than to position 1, 2, 3, 4, 5, or 6. Home is the most retruded comfortable position.*

pacinian corpuscles, and some free nerve endings. The kinesthetic sense or muscle sense helps to direct movements of parts of the body through space.

The visual acuity and the sense of touch of the dentist also enter into the making of a centric relation record using the physiologic method. This phase of the procedure is developed with experience and is exceedingly difficult to teach to another individual.

Factors that influence interocclusal check records are as follows:

1. The amount and equalization of pressure depends upon the uniform consistency of the recording material. The accuracy of the vertical component of the record is in direct proportion to the equalization of the pressure exerted on the displaceable supporting tissue and the joints.

2. The comfort of the patient depends on the stability and compatibility of the record bases and attached recording surfaces. Artificial teeth arranged in their correct anteroposterior, vertical, and mediolateral positions in relation to the lips, tongue, cheeks, and basal seat are more compatible to normal physiologic mandibular movements than occlusion rims.

3. An interocclusal check record with multiple points of reference made by styli or cusp tips is more satisfactory than one using occluding surfaces of wax or noncusp form teeth.

The interocclusal check record is particularly indicated in situations of abnormally related jaws, supporting tissues that are excessively displaceable, large awkward tongues, and uncontrollable or abnormal mandibular move-

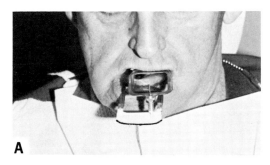

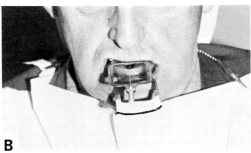

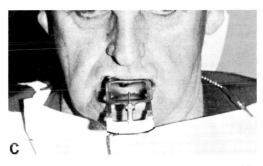

FIG. 11-22. *Extraoral tracing.* **A.** *Mandible moved to patient's right.* **B.** *Mandible moved to the left.* **C.** *Mandible moved to terminal hinge position.*

fusing, offer very little resistance to jaw closure when soft, and will harden quickly. Waxes are capable of making a record upon contact, and the jaws can be separated at once. This is advantageous when the muscular control of the mandible is poor. The compounds, plaster, and zinc oxide and eugenol paste must be maintained in contact until they are hard. If the mandible

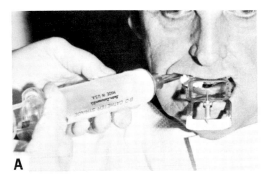

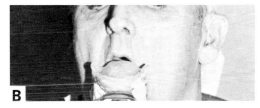

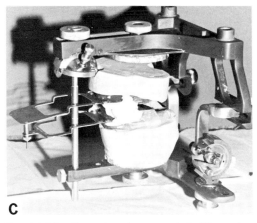

FIG. 11-23. *Securing the record.* **A.** *The point of the stylus at the apex of the tracing. Fast-setting plaster is being injected.* **B.** *Removal of the occlusion rims.* **C.** *The mandibular cast related to mount on the articulator.*

ments. The interocclusal record is also indicated to check the occlusion of the teeth in existing dentures. The dentures can be remounted to compare the occlusion to the jaw relationship. It is the most practical acceptable method to check teeth that have been arranged as trial dentures.

Some of the recording materials used in the interocclusal check record method are (1) waxes, (2) impression compounds, (3) dental plaster, and (4) zinc oxide and eugenol paste. The waxes are low

moves before the material sets, the record is not acceptable. The setting or hardening time can be controlled to some extent with plaster, less with zinc oxide and eugenol paste, and not at all with compounds.

Waxes are easily distorted, and, unless *extreme* care is exercised when the records are positioned, an error occurs. Compound, zinc oxide and eugenol paste, and plaster will break before they will distort. This is particularly true with plaster.

Plaster and zinc oxide and eugenol paste offer the same resistance to closure throughout the mass. Waxes and compound harden on the surface before they become hard throughout. The waxes require less time and equipment, and, if care is exercised in the procedure, acceptable records can be made. Plaster and zinc oxide and eugenol paste offer some advantage over waxes when noncusp form posterior teeth are used. Occlusal indicator wax in combination with red articulating paper (page 379) is an acceptable method for check records with teeth present.

TECHNIQUE FOR TACTILE OR INTEROC- CLUSAL CHECK RECORD METHOD. The technique for a tactile check record is divided into two steps: (1) tentative records using occlusion rims attached to accurate stable record bases; (2) interocclusal check records with the teeth arranged for try-in.

The procedure using *occlusion rims* was described in detail (pages 271–273) when the tentative record of the vertical dimension of occlusion was discussed. The technique includes these steps:

1. Seat the patient comfortably with the head upright.

2. Contour the maxillary occlusion rim, lip lines, distal cuspid points, and occlusal plane. Place the notch to aid in seating records.

3. Establish the vertical dimension of jaw separation with the mandible at rest and measure the distance.

4. Reduce the mandibular occlusion rim to allow excess interocclusal distance.

5. Make a face-bow transfer record (Chapter 10).

6. Using Tenax wax, make a tentative centric relation record by having the patient retrude and close the jaws until he feels the closure to be at the tentative vertical dimension of jaw separation.

7. Compare the measurements of the face at vertical dimension of occlusion with the vertical dimension of rest position. The measurement must be less for the vertical dimension of occlusion.

8. Adjust the condylar elements of the articulator and secure them against the centric stops.

9. Mount the maxillary cast, using the face-bow transfer record.

10. Secure the centric relation record to the maxillary occlusion rim and position the mandibular cast.

11. Attach the mandibular cast to the articulator with plaster.

Steps to be followed at the time of try-in of teeth are as follows:

1. Seat the patient comfortably with the head upright and supported by the headrest under the occiput.

2. Seat the maxillary record base. If the retention is not adequate, apply a fine dusting of denture adhesive to the wet tissue surface of the maxillary record base.

3. Seat the mandibular record base. *Do not* let the patient make tooth contact. If a premature tooth contact exists with the jaws in centric relation, the patient's proprioception may not direct the return to this identical position. Place two cotton rolls bilaterally between the maxillary and mandibular posterior teeth and have the patient close the teeth on the cotton and hold

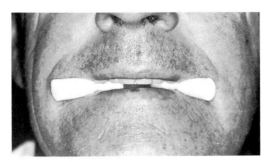

FIG. 11-24. *Maxillary denture seated with cotton rolls in place between the occlusal surfaces to prevent tooth contact.*

them together for several seconds (Fig. 11-24). *Do not* fatigue the patient in this position. This procedure allows the maxillary record base to seat properly to the supporting tissues.

4. Remove the mandibular record base and rehearse the patient in protruding and retruding the lower jaw.

5. Dry the mandibular posterior teeth.

6. Adapt two thicknesses of softened Tenax wax to the occlusal surfaces of the bicuspids and molars and extend over the buccal and lingual surfaces. Exercise care *not* to trap air under the wax. Resoften the wax with a controlled flame from an alcohol torch or in a water bath at 130°F.

7. Seat the mandibular record base. Place the tips of the index fingers on the buccal flanges of the record base in the area of the second bicuspids and rest the tips of the thumbs under the border of the mandible at the chin point (Fig. 11-25). The fingers help stabilize the record base, and the thumbs are used as guides. Calmly ask the patient

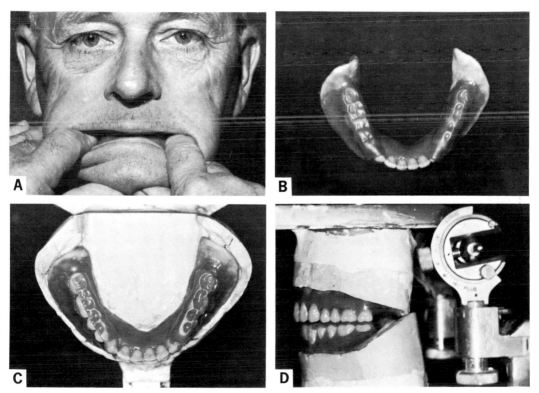

FIG. 11-25. A. *Recording centric relation.* **B.** *The wax record is not penetrated by tooth contact.* **C.** *The record is prepared for checking.* **D.** *The condylar element is against the centric relation stop.*

to move the lower jaw back and close on the back teeth. Ask him to stop closing when contact is made.

8. Allow the wax to harden. Remove and dry the occlusal surface of wax with a gentle stream of cool air.

9. Inspect the record to see that no cusp tip penetrated to make tooth-to-tooth contact. If the original record was accurate in the vertical direction, the cusp tips should penetrate the wax equally on both sides (Fig. 11-25B).

10. Remove the maxillary record base, dry the occlusal surfaces of the posterior teeth with air, and place it on the maxillary cast.

11. Release the horizontal condylar guide locks on the articulator.

12. Place the mandibular record base and attached record on the mandibular cast. The buccal third of the record is carefully removed to expose the cusp tips (Fig. 11-25C).

13. Carefully seat the maxillary teeth in the record.

14. Observe the condylar elements. If the record is the same as the original record, the condylar elements will rest against the centric stops in the same position as when the casts were originally mounted. (Fig. 11-25D).

15. If one or both condylar elements are not against the stops, then one or the other record is inaccurate.

Failure to make check records that repeat will necessitate a new mounting and further verification of the accuracy of the new mounting record with check records until three records agree.

Occlusal indicator wax is another method of checking the articulator mountings for accuracy. This method is particularly advantageous when arranging noncusp form posterior teeth. The technique for the use of occlusal indicator wax follows.

1. Place the trial dentures on the mounted cast.

2. Dry the occlusal surfaces of the posterior teeth with a stream of warm air.

3. Raise the incisal guide pin from the incisal guide table and secure it.

4. Place red articulating paper over the occlusal surfaces of all mandibular posterior teeth.

5. Secure the condylar elements in the centric relation position.

6. Tap the teeth together to record the tooth contacts. (Fig. 11-26A).

7. Place one thickness of occlusal indicator wax over the incisal edges and occlusal surfaces of the mandibular teeth.

8. Insert the trial dentures and instruct the patient to tap on the posterior teeth. In difficult situations it may be necessary to guide the patient.

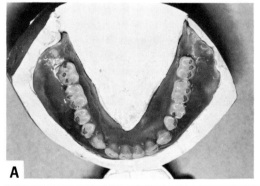

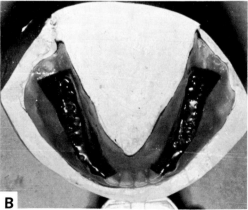

FIG. 11-26. **A.** *Contacts are visible on the teeth.* **B.** *The contacts are visible through the occlusal indication wax.*

9. Remove the mandibular trial denture and inspect the indicator wax. If the mounting is accurate, the wax will be penetrated to expose the red markings (Fig. 11-26B).

Eccentric Relation Records

An eccentric maxillomandibular relation is any relationship of the mandible to the maxillae other than centric position.

When an articulator that adjusts to protrusive and to right and left lateral movements is used, the purpose in making an eccentric relation record is to adjust the horizontal and lateral condylar inclinations so that the articulator jaw members perform eccentric movements equivalent, but not identical, to the relative movements of the mandible to the maxillae. These adjustments permit the condylar elements to travel to and from the centric and eccentric positions and make it possible to arrange the teeth for complete dentures in *balanced occlusion*.

One must remember these points:

1. The condyle path cannot be altered by the dentist and is not reproduced by a protrusive or lateral static record.

2. The condyles do not travel in a straight path in eccentric jaw movements but follow the contour of the bony fossae.

3. Articulators with condylar elements that travel in a straight slot, an "average" curved slot, or on a flat surface do not travel the same path as the condyle path.

4. Lateral maxillomandibular relation records furnish additional information by establishing other points of reference; however, the majority of articulators for the construction of dentures will not accurately receive lateral records nor do they provide the basis for their use.

5. The condylar elements of articulators with individually ground condyle paths refined to pantographic tracings in three planes can travel in the path traveled by the condyles as the tracing was made.

The eccentric positions to be recorded are protrusive and right and left lateral. Because the shapes of the mandibular fossae vary, they have been likened to the concave surface of a potato chip. In the sagittal plane, the shape is like an ogee curve.

Protrusive and lateral maxillomandibular relation records made by functional, graphic (one plane), and tactile methods are within the functional range and do not include the border limits. Most articulators do not adjust accurately to a protrusive record that is made to a protrusive position of less than 5 to 6 millimeters. An articulator on which the teeth are to be arranged in balanced occlusion must accurately receive an eccentric maxillomandibular relation record and adjust to the information the record contains. Otherwise, the record is useless.

Most adjustable articulators for complete denture procedures will receive a protrusive interocclusal relation record, and the horizontal condylar inclination will adjust so that the instrument jaw members perform protrusive movements equivalent, but not identical, to the relative movements of the mandible to the maxillae. The positional interocclusal records made in space rarely are repeated by the same patient. The variations in registrations will be a result of lack of stability of record bases in eccentric positions and differences in the resiliency of the supporting tissues and in the resistance offered by the recording medium. The horizontal condylar inclinations obtained with soft materials are usually steeper than those obtained with more resistant material. An individual's capability to move the mandible forward right or left to the same horizontal position, to close the jaws to the same vertical position, and to exert the same amount of pressure repeatedly is almost physically impossible.

The value in making several records and taking an average of these to adjust the articulator is questionable. When the asymmetry in records appears more than is expected, a variation of more than plus or minus five on the calibrations for horizontal adjustment necessitates another record. When repeated records show similar asymmetrical information, adjust the articulator to *one* of the records.

Technical procedures that use arrow point or Gothic arch tracings and a central bearing device cannot be accepted as being accurate if the central bearing devices are attached to record bases resting on displaceable tissue. The difficulty in locating a central bearing point and the shifting of the record bases was discussed on pages 276–277. Extraoral tracings with a central bearing device offer several advantages over other graphic methods if the bases to which the recording devices are attached are stable. The same vertical jaw separation and the same horizontal relationship is repeatable. The recording medium is injected with a syringe to eliminate any resistance factor of the medium that might influence the accuracy of the record.

The methods for eccentric maxillomandibular relation records may be classified in a manner similar to the methods for centric maxillomandibular relation records:

1. Functional or chew-in procedures are exemplified by Needles-House and Patterson techniques. A description of these methods appears on pages 274–275. After the record has been used to mount the mandibular cast in centric relationship to the maxillary cast, the articulator is adjusted to the eccentric records.

2. Graphic methods are exemplified by the extraoral arrow point or Gothic arch tracings made on one plane.

3. Tactile or direct check record methods are basically the same. The recording materials are different. Wax, compound, plaster, and zinc oxide and eugenol paste used on the wax occlusion rim before the teeth are arranged for try-in are considered tentative records. The preferred time to make eccentric maxillomandibular relation records is after all the teeth have been arranged for try-in. Arrange the anterior teeth for esthetics and the posterior teeth for centric occlusion. Seat the patient in a comfortable upright position and (a) verify the relationship of the maxillary and mandibular casts with a centric relation record (page 273); (b) check the plane of occlusion (page 264), (c) check the anteroposterior and mediolateral positions of the teeth for compatibility with the lips, tongue, and cheeks (page 311); (d) verify the vertical dimension of occlusion (page 261) and (e) determine the patient's acceptance of the esthetics of the teeth.

TECHNICAL PROCEDURES. The *graphic method* of making eccentric maxillomandibular relation records is performed at the same sitting and with the same equipment used to make the centric relation record.

After the mandibular cast has been mounted on the articulator in centric relation, reseat the recording devices in the patient's mouth. Proceed as follows:

1. Measure a distance of 5 or 6 mm from the apex of the arrow point tracing on the protrusive tracing and mark this point (Fig. 11-27A).

2. Instruct the patient to protrude

until the point of the stylus rests in the marked point.

3. Inject quick setting dental plaster between the occlusion rims, allow the plaster to harden, and remove the cast from the mouth (Fig. 11-27B).

4. Free the horizontal condylar adjustments on the articulator by releasing the locknuts.

5. Raise the incisal guide pin about one-half inch from the top of the guide table.

6. Carefully seat the record bases on the cast. Using the locknuts as handles, manipulate one side, then the other. An accurate seating of both record bases must be secured without forcing so that the protrusive record is not destroyed (Fig. 11-27C).

7. Secure the locknuts with positive finger pressure.

8. Record the right and left calibrations of the horizontal inclinations on the plaster mounting. This record is useful if the settings are accidentally moved.

The most common method to make a protrusive relation record is the *tactile* or *direct check record* using a soft wax.

1. Seat the patient in a comfortable upright position.

2. Having ascertained that the teeth are set in an acceptable arrangement, rehearse the patient in the procedure. Seat the dentures and support the mandibular base with the tips of the index fingers with the thumb tips under the mandible at the chin point in the same way as when making the centric relation record (Fig. 11-23A). Instruct the patient to protrude the lower jaw for approximately 5 or 6 mm. *Do not* use any recording medium at this time. Observe the midline between the maxillary central incisors to determine if it coincides mediolaterally with the midline of the mandibular central incisors. It is often necessary to guide the patient's mandi-

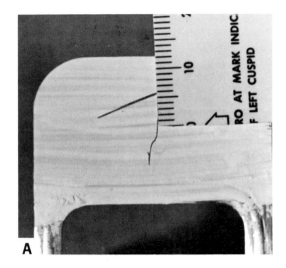

A

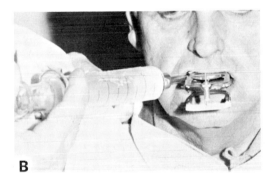

B

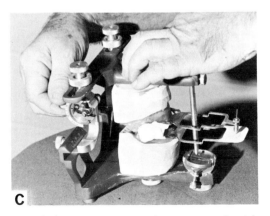

C

FIG. 11-27. *Protrusive relation record with extraoral graphic tracing.* **A.** *Measuring from apex of arrow point tracing on the protrusive tracing.* **B.** *Injecting fast-setting plaster.* **C.** *Adjusting the condylar elements.*

ble until a protrusive movement is learned. Gentle pressure is usually all that is needed to guide the mandible, and unnecessary manipulations should be avoided.

3. When the patient has learned the protrusive position, remove the mandibular trial denture.

4. Place four layers of soft wax over the mandibular teeth and seal the wax on the lingual and buccal surfaces of the posteriors and the lingual and labial surfaces of the anterior teeth.

5. Soften the wax with a controlled open flame or water at 135°F.

6. Reinsert the trial denture and instruct the patient to protrude the lower jaws and close until the upper teeth contact the wax. Allow the wax to harden before removing the trial denture and attached record (Fig. 11-28A).

7. Set the condylar post of the articulator at 0° on the lateral calibrations.

8. Inspect the wax record for evenness of contact. Records that lack contact in isolated areas or have uneven contacts are recontoured, and new records are made (Fig. 11-28B).

9. Release the horizontal condylar adjustments by freeing the locknuts. Raise the incisal guide pin one-half inch from the incisal guide table.

10. Place the maxillary and mandibular trial dentures in their respective mounting casts in the articulator.

11. Carefully relate the maxillary teeth to the wax protrusive records.

12. Examine the condylar elements to see that protrusion was 5 to 6 mm.

13. Using the horizontal condylar locknuts as handles, manipulate one side and then the other until all teeth

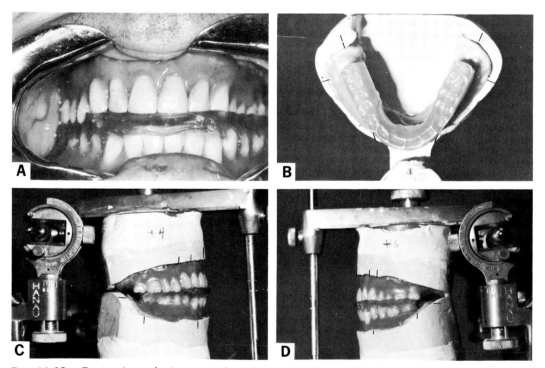

FIG. 11-28. *Protrusive relation record with wax.* **A.** *Interocclusal wax record inserted and mandible protruded about 5 to 6 mm.* **B.** *A wax record with even contacts.* **C** and **D.** *Horizontal inclinations recorded on the right and left plaster mountings.*

are accurately seated in the record. Do not use force.

14. Secure the horizontal condyle adjustment locknuts with finger pressure.

15. Record the horizontal right and left inclinations on the plaster mounting. This record is useful if the settings are accidentally moved (Fig. 11-28C,D).

Lateral Relation Records

When an articulator accurately receives and adjusts to a lateral maxillomandibular relation record, the additional points of reference are valuable. The more accurate the points of reference supplied in adjusting the articulator the more harmony will exist between mandibular movements and cusp inclines.

TECHNICAL PROCEDURES. Execute the *graphic methods* in the same manner as the protrusive relation record with the following exceptions: Two records are required—one of right lateral and one of left lateral. The articulator is adjusted as each record is made. When an interocclusal record of wax is made, additional layers of soft wax are placed on the balancing side to accommodate for the difference in the vertical jaw separation between the balancing and working sides.

Although the mechanics of making lateral jaw relation records appear simple, it is recognized that in complete denture construction the procedure is difficult and many inaccuracies occur. Hanau held the opinion that the setting of a lateral indication by an anatomic record offers no particular advantages and the required over-protrusion can be determined on the finished case in the mouth, by records, observation, and interpretations of symptoms on the ridges.* He recommended the following formula to arrive at an acceptable lateral indication:

$$L = \frac{H}{8} + 12.$$

L = lateral condyle indication in degrees; H = horizontal condyle indication in degrees as established by the protrusive relation record. The value of the formula has not been proved or disproved.

*Hanau, R. L.: *Full Denture Prosthesis—Intraoral Technique for Hanau Model H Articulator.* Rochester, N. Y., 1922.

REFERENCES
1. Armstrong, J. L.: A scientific method of establishing normal vertical dimension. J.A.D.A., *30*:1742, 1943.
1a. Atwood, A. A.: A critique of research of the posterior limit of the mandibular position. J. Prosth. Dent., *20*:21, 1968.
2. Berman, N. H.: Accurate interocclusal record. J. Prosth. Dent., *10*:620, 1960.
3. Boos, R. H.: Intermaxillary relations established by biting power. J.A.D.A., *27*:1192, 1940.
3a. _____: Condylar path by roentgenograph. J. Prosth. Dent., *1*:387, 1951.
4. Boucher, L. J.: Limiting factors in posterior movements of mandibular condyles. J. Prosth. Dent., *11*:23, 1961.
5. Cohn, L. A.: Two techniques for interocclusal records. J. Prosth. Dent., *13*:438, 1963.
6. Craddock, F. W.: The accuracy and practical value of records of condyle path inclination. J.A.D.A., *38*:697, 1949.
7. Downs, B.: The capture and use of centric relations. Dent. Clin. N. Amer., November, 1964, p. 611.
8. Durrer, G. T.: Use of the central bearing point for balancing full upper and lower dentures. Dent. Dig. *52*:19, 1946.
9. El-Aramany, M. A., George, A. W., and Scott, R. H.: Evaluating the needle point tracing as a method for determining centric relation. J. Prosth. Dent., *15*:1043, 1965.

9a. Feldman, S., Leupold, R., and Staling, L. M.: Rest vertical dimension determined by electromyography with biofeedback as compared to conventional methods. J. Prosth. Dent., 40:216, 1978.

10. Fountain, H. W.: Seating the condyles for centric relation records. J. Prosth. Dent., 11:1050, 1961.

10a. Frazier, Q. Z., et al: The relative repeatability of plaster interocclusal eccentric records for articulator adjustment in complete denture construction. J. Prosth. Dent., 26:448, 1971.

10b. Gattozzi, J. G., Nicol, B. R., Somes, G. W., and Ellinger, C. W.: Variations in mandibular rest positions with and without dentures in place. J. Prosth. Dent., 36:159, 1976.

11. Gillis, R. R.: Establishing vertical dimension in full denture construction. J.A.D.A., 28:433, 1941.

11a. Gonzalez, J. B., and Kingery, R. H.: Evaluation of planes of reference for orienting maxillary casts on articulators. J.A.D.A., 76:329, 1968.

11b. Grasso, J. E., and Sharry, J. J.: The duplicability of arrow-point tracings in dentulous subjects. J. Prosth. Dent., 20:106, 1968.

11c. Heartwell, C. M.: The effect of tissue resiliency on occlusion in complete denture prosthodontics. J. Prosth. Dent., 34:602, 1975.

12. Hickey, J. C.: Centric relation—a must for complete dentures. Dent. Clin. N. Amer., November, 1964, p. 587.

13. Hight, F. M., and Clapp, G. W.: Some essentials in full denture construction (adjusting the condyle paths of the articulator and checking the finished dentures). Dent. Dig., 37:810, 1931.

13a. Ismail, Y. H., and George, W. A.: The consistency of the swallowing technique in determining occlusal vertical relation in edentulous patients. J. Prosth. Dent., 19:230, 1968.

13b. ———, et al.: Cephalometric study of the changes occurring in the face height following prosthetic treatment. J. Prosth. Dent., 19:321, 1968.

13c. Javid, N. S.: A technique for determination of the occlusal plane. J. Prosth. Dent., 31:270, 1974.

13d. Joniot, B.: Physiologic mandibular resting posture. J. Prosth. Dent., 31:4, 1974.

14. Jordan, L. G.: Rest space, vertical dimension of intermaxillary space. *Prosthodontic Syllabus*. United States Army Institute of Dental Research, 1963.

15. Kapur, K. K., and Yurkstas, A. A.: An evaluation of centric relation records obtained by various techniques. J. Prosth. Dent., 7:770, 1957.

16. Kingery, R. H.: A review of some of the problems associated with centric relation. J. Prosth. Dent., 2:307, 1952.

17. Kurth, L. E.: Methods of obtaining vertical dimension and centric relation: a practical evaluation of various methods. J.A.D.A., 59:669, 1959.

18. ———: From mouth to articulator: static jaw relations. J.A.D.A., 64:517, 1962.

18a. Langer, A., and Michman, J.: Evaluation of lateral tracings of edentulous subjects. J. Prosth. Dent., 23:381, 1970.

18b. Long, J. H.: Location of the terminal hinge axis by intraoral means. J. Prosth. Dent., 23:11, 1970.

18c. Lundquist, D. O., and Luther, W. W.: Occlusal plane determination. J. Prosth. Dent., 23:489, 1970.

19. Lytle, R. B.: Vertical relation of occlusion by the patient's neuromuscular perception. J. Prosth. Dent., 14:12, 1964.

19a. McKewitt, F. H.: The measured vertical dimension and denture adhesive materials. J. Prosth. Dent., 1:393, 1951.

19b. Mehringer, E. J.: Physiologically generated occlusion. J. Prosth. Dent., 30:373, 1973.

20. Michman, J., and Lanzer, A.: Comparison of three methods of registering centric relation for edentulous patients. J. Prosth. Dent., 13:248, 1963.

20a. Mood, G. N.: Centric occlusion, centric relation, and the mandibular posture. J. Prosth. Dent., 20:292, 1968.

21. Niswonger, M. E.: The rest position of the mandible and the centric relation. J.A.D.A., 21:1572, 1934.

22. Olsen, E. S.: Vertical dimension of the face. Dent. Clin. N. Amer., November, 1964, p. 611.

23. Posselt, U., and Skytting, B.: Registration of the condyle path inclination:

variations using the Gysi technique. J. Prosth. Dent., *10*:243, 1960.

24. ———, and Franzen, G.: Registration of the condyle path inclination by intraoral wax records: variations in three instruments. J. Prosth. Dent., *10*:441, 1960.

25. ———, and Neustedt, P.: Registration of the condyle path by intraoral records: its practical value. J. Prosth. Dent., *11*:47, 1961.

25a. Pound, E.: Controlling anomalies of vertical dimension and speech. J. Prosth. Dent., *36*:124, 1976.

25b. Robinson, M H.: Centric position. J. Prosth. Dent., *1*:384, 1951.

26. Schuyler, C. H.: Intraoral method of establishing maxillomandibular relation. J.A.D.A., *19*:1012, 1932.

27. Shanahan, T. E. J.: Physiologic jaw relations and occlusion of complete dentures. J. Prosth. Dent., *5*:319, 1955.

28. ———, and Leff, A.: Interocclusal records. J. Prosth. Dent., *10*:842, 1960.

28a. Sheppard, I. M., and Sheppard, S. M.: Vertical dimension measurements. J. Prosth. Dent., *34*:269, 1975.

28b. ———: The relationship of vertical dimension to atypical swallowing with complete dentures. J. Prosth. Dent., *38*:249, 1977.

28c. Shirinian, G. H., and Strem, B. E.: Interocclusal distance: A comparison between American caucasians and negroes. J. Prosth. Dent., *37*:394, 1977.

29. Silverman, M. M.: Accurate measurements of vertical dimension by phonetics and the speaking centric space. Dent. Dig. *57*:261, 1951.

30. Simpson, H.: Registration of centric relations in complete denture prosthesis. J.A.D.A., *26*:1682, 1939.

31. Stuart, C. E.: Accuracy in measuring functional dimensions and relations in oral prosthesis. J. Prosth. Dent., *9*:220, 1959; Boucher, C. O.: Discussion of "Accuracy in measuring functional dimensions and relations in oral prosthesis." J. Prosth. Dent., *9*:237, 1959.

32. Trapozzano, V. R.: Comparison of the equalization of pressure by means of the central bearing point and wax checkbite. J.A.D.A., *38*:586, 1949.

33. ———: Occlusal records. J. Prosth. Dent., *5*:325, 1955.

33a. Wagner, A. G.: Comparison of four methods to determine rest position of the mandible. J. Prosth. Dent., *25*:506, 1971.

34. Walker, R. C.: A comparison of jaw relation recording methods. J. Prosth. Dent., *12*:685, 1962.

35. Ward, B. L., and Osterholtz, R. H.: Establishing the vertical relation of occlusion. J. Prosth. Dent., *13*:432, 1963.

35a. Wilkie, N. D., Hurst, T. L., and Mitchell, D. L.: Radiographic comparisons of condyle-fossa relationships during maxillomandibular registrations made by different methods. J. Prosth. Dent., *32*:529, 1974.

35b. Temm, R., and Berry, D. C.: Passive control in mandibular rest position. J. Prosth. Dent., *22*:30, 1969.

36. Yurkstas, A. A., and Kapur, K. K.: Factors influencing centric relation records in edentulous mouth. J. Prosth. Dent., *14*:1066, 1964.

Tooth Selection

12

The selection of teeth for complete dentures is best understood if the anterior teeth are considered separately from the posterior teeth. The anterior teeth are primarily selected to satisfy esthetic requirements, whereas the posterior teeth are primarily selected to satisfy masticatory functional requirements. Both the anterior and posterior teeth must function in harmony with and be anatomically and physiologically compatible with the surrounding oral environment. Technically, the anterior teeth are composed of the six maxillary and six mandibular teeth; however, there are occasions when the maxillary bicuspids, particularly the first, must be considered more for esthetics than for masticatory function. Also, there are instances in which the maxillary cuspids assume a functional role by addition of lingual centric stops. This occurs in some situations when the mandible is in a retruded relation to the maxillae.

The selection of teeth and their arrangement to meet esthetic requirements demand artistic skill in addition to scientific knowledge. There are no rules of thumb for this procedure; however, there are anatomic landmarks and manufactured aids that can be used as guides. Teeth meet esthetic requirements when they look natural, and the best method of developing the skill required to attain natural appearances is by observing natural teeth (Fig. 12-1). Projected slides and television demonstrations are excellent ways to carry on this study. In a study of this nature the size, shape, form, color, and arrangement of the teeth should be associated with the size, shape, and form of the face, the physical features, the age, and the sex of the individual.

The manufacturers of artificial teeth have conducted extensive research to develop tooth and denture base materials that will appear natural and be acceptable to the profession and the patient. It is fortunate that the manufacturers have been progressive in this area, since few practicing dentists have the time to conduct the research necessary for this progress. Only a few dentists manufacture individualized teeth. The manufacturers have also prepared many aids and guides that are useful in the selection of teeth for form, shape, size, and color. Mold guides, mold selectors, shade guides for characterized or personalized teeth, shade guides for teeth not characterized, instructions in arranging teeth for the different concepts of occlusion, and instructions for selecting and arranging teeth for esthetics are available to aid dentists in the selection of teeth for complete dentures (Fig. 12-2).

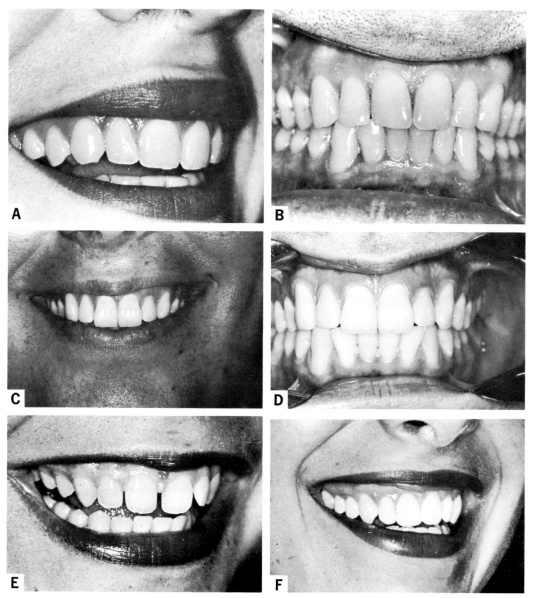

FIG. 12-1. *Studies of natural teeth.* **A.** *The maxillary lateral incisors of this female are in slight labial version to the maxillary central incisors. The incisal edges of the maxillary anterior teeth follow the curvature of the lower lip.*

B. *The prominence of the necks of the maxillary and mandibular cuspids produces the square arch form in this male. The maxillary central incisors are rotated slightly in a distal direction. The mandibular central and lateral incisors are not straight. Note the asymmetry of the midlines of the two dental arches.*

C. *The lips of this female have little curvature. The maxillary right lateral incisor is in labial version and the maxillary left lateral incisor is in palatal version. The medial surfaces of the maxillary central incisors are rotated in a palatal direction. The medial halves of the maxillary cuspids are in view. The incisal edges of the maxillary central incisors and the maxillary cuspids are on the occlusal plane, and the maxillary lateral incisors are above the occlusal plane.*

D. *Notice the square tooth form and square dental arches of this male. Two thirds of the labial surface of the maxillary cuspids is in view. The mandibular lateral incisors are not straight.*

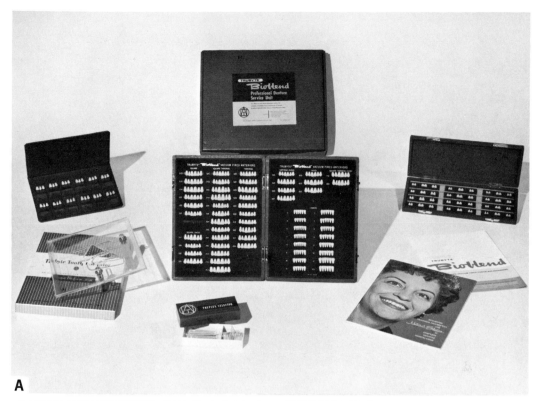

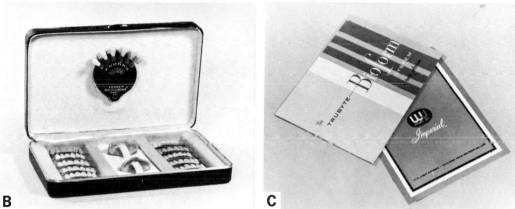

FIG. 12-2. *Aids for selecting teeth.* **A.** *Plastic tooth selector, tooth mold guides, shade guides for characterized and noncharacterized teeth, setup wax, and illustrated pamphlets on tooth arrangement. (Manufactured by the Dentists' Supply Company of New York.)* **B.** *A convenient tooth mold and shade guide kit. (Manufactured by Universal Dental Co.)* **C.** *Tooth mold guides in book form. (Courtesy of the Dentists' Supply Company of New York and H. D. Justi and Sons Inc.)*

FIG. 12-1. *Continued.*

E. *The diastema of the maxillary anterior teeth of this female looks natural and would be reproduced if and when dentures are necessary.*

F. *When this young female smiles, she exposes the maxillary teeth to include the medial half of the first molars. The curvature of the lips, the contour of the maxillary cuspids, the curved incisal angles of the central and lateral incisors, and the positions of the maxillary lateral incisors denote femininity.*

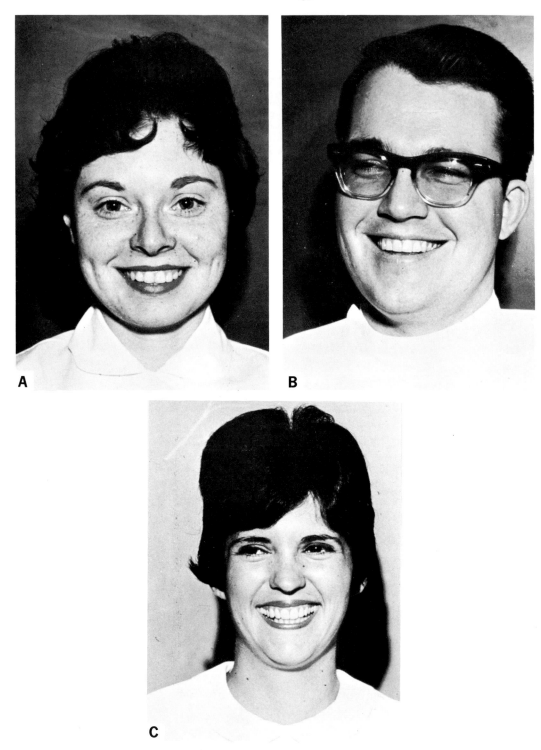

FIG. 12-3.   *Comparison of size of teeth of different persons.* **A.** *Female, height 4'8".* **B.** *Male, height 6'3".* **C.** *Female, height 5'4".*

Anterior Teeth

SIZE OF ANTERIOR TEETH

Seven anatomic entities are used as guides to selection of anterior teeth *for size.*

1. SIZE OF THE FACE. The average width of the maxillary central incisor is estimated to be one sixteenth of the width of the face measured between the zygoma. The size of the maxillary central incisors is important, for they are the most prominent teeth in the arches as an individual is viewed from a frontal position (Fig. 12-3). The maxillary lateral incisors vary more in size, form, and position than any other maxillary anterior tooth. This factor allows freedom in

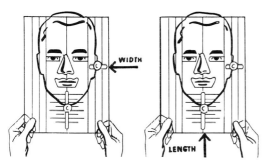

FIG. 12-4. *Using the Trubyte tooth indicator to determine the size of the upper central incisor. Place the indicator on the patient's face, allowing the nose to come through the center triangle. Center the pupils in the eye slots and hold the indicator with its center line coinciding with the median line. Slide the side indicator bar in until it touches the face; read the width of the upper central tooth in millimeters. Slide the bottom indicator bar up to position immediately underneath the chin with the lips at rest; read the indicated length of the upper central tooth in millimeters. When the lips are at rest, the reading of length will be approximately accurate, since the mouth would have to close 3/4" to lose 1 mm on the indicator, which is proportioned in a ratio of 16 to 1. (Courtesy of the Dentists' Supply Company of New York.)*

selecting the teeth from standard molds. The Trubyte Tooth Indicator* (Fig. 12-4) is useful in determining the size of the maxillary central incisors. The combined width of the six maxillary anteriors is slightly less than one third of the bizygomatic breadth of the face. The face-bow can be used as a caliper to record the bizygomatic breadth of the face.

2. SIZE OF THE MAXILLARY ARCH. The mold selector* can be used to make measurements of the maxillary cast. Accurately contoured occlusion rims are required. Make the measurements from the crest of the incisal papilla to the hamular notches and from one hamular notch to the opposite hamular notch. The combined length of the three legs of the triangle in millimeters is used on the selector. The circular slide rule indicates the tooth sizes, anterior and posterior, for both arches.

The Universal Dental Company provides a mold selector to be used in the selection of the anterior teeth manufactured by the company. The measurements are made from the midline on the maxillary occlusion rim to the distal of the cuspid eminence. An arrow or pointer designates on the selector which mold is indicated (Fig. 12-5).

It must be remembered that these are only guides in tooth selection and will not be usable in many situations, as spacing, rotating, and overlapping for esthetic purposes likewise influence the size of the anterior teeth. The excessive or unusual loss of bone may also influence the size, particularly the length. When discrepancies between face size and related arch size exist, the selection of anterior teeth should be governed more by face size than by

* Dentists' Supply Company of New York.

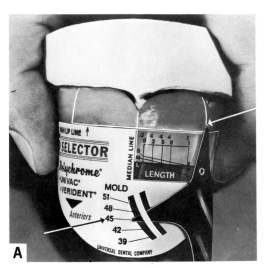
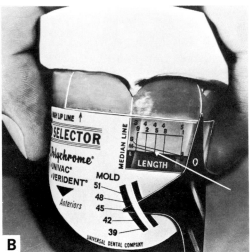
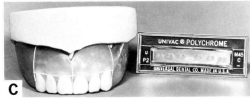

FIG. 12-5. *A mold selector.* **A.** *Superimpose the median line on the median line of the occlusion rim; bend the mold selector to conform with the contour of the occlusion rim. Move the scanner to the cuspid line (white arrow). The mold width of the anterior teeth is indicated on the lower scale (black and white arrow).*

B. *To determine the mold length—short (s), medium (m), or long (l)—of the anterior teeth, read through the transparent area marked "Length" to the point where the length line of the mold number intersects with the anterior occlusal plane (white arrow).*

C. *The teeth will occupy the space between the cuspid lines. For esthetic reasons it may be desirable to mix the molds. (Courtesy of Universal Dental Company.)*

arch size, since resorbed tissues can lead one astray.

3. INCISAL PAPILLA AND THE CUSPID EMINENCES OR THE BUCCAL FRENUM. If the cuspid eminences are discernible, a line can be placed on the cast at the distal termination of the eminence. If the cuspid eminences are not discernible, the attachments of the buccal frenum can be used. A line placed slightly anterior to the frenum attachment will be distal to the eminence. Measure the distance from the distal of one cuspid eminence to the distal of the other with a flexible ruler. The ruler should follow

the contour of the ridge, and as it reaches the midline, it should be placed on the anterior border of the incisal papilla because the maxillary central incisors are situated labially to the papilla. The combined width of the six maxillary anterior teeth is determined in millimeters (Fig. 12-6).

Another method to locate the distal of the cuspid eminences is to use the maxillary occlusion rim. After the occlusion rim has been properly contoured and the vertical length of the anterior section has been established, the rim is placed to position in the mouth. The patient is requested to relax

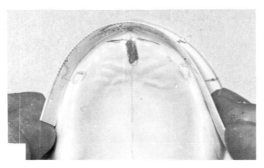

FIG. 12-6. *Flexible ruler properly positioned in the labial vestibule for maxillary cast measurements. It should not be placed on the lines designating the anterior border of the incisal papilla.*

with the lips touching. A pointed instrument used as a marker is passed to the occlusion rim at each corner of the lips, and a mark is recorded (Fig. 12-7). The marker is passed on a line parallel to the pupils of the eyes. The distance between the marks following the contour of the arch measured in millimeters is the combined width of the six maxillary anterior teeth.

4. MAXILLOMANDIBULAR RELATIONS. Any disproportion in size between the maxillary and the mandibular arches influences the length, the width, and the position of the teeth. The sizes and the

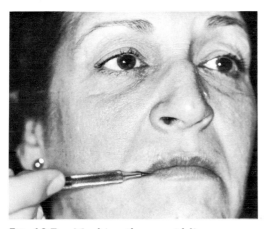

FIG. 12-7. *Marking the cuspid line.*

positions of the teeth will have to vary from the accepted normal if the teeth in one arch are to complement the teeth in the other arch. In instances of protruded mandibles the mandibular anterior teeth are frequently larger than normal. If the mandibles are retruded, the mandibular anterior teeth are frequently smaller. In protrusion, the face is usually longer, and longer faces frequently require longer teeth. Accurately articulated casts with the jaws in centric relation are necessary for the satisfactory determination of maxillomandibular relations, since patients can shift the mandible and compensate for some of the malrelations.

5. THE CONTOUR OF THE RESIDUAL RIDGES. The artificial teeth should be placed to follow the contour of the residual ridges that existed when the natural teeth were present. The loss of contour as a result of resorption, accident, or surgery makes this a difficult task. A knowledge of the direction of resorption of the two arches will allow a fairly accurate visualization of the original contour. Resorption of the maxillae in the anterior segment of the arch is in a vertical and palatal direction; posteriorly the resorption is in a vertical and medial direction.

The resorption of the mandible in the anterior segment of the arch is in a vertical and lingual direction; posteriorly the resorption is in a vertical and slightly lingual direction. However, as resorption occurs, because of the morphology, the maxillary arch appears smaller and the mandibular arch larger.

A square arch with the eminences present will be ovoid or tapering in their absence.

6. THE VERTICAL DISTANCE BETWEEN THE RIDGES. The length of the teeth is determined by the available space between the existing ridges. When the

space is available, it is more esthetically acceptable to use a tooth long enough to eliminate the display of the denture base. Teeth are more attractive in appearance than denture base materials, even those denture bases fabricated to simulate the oral mucosa. Denture bases that simulate the oral mucosa are referred to as characterized, personalized, or natural appearing. Teeth that are not in harmony in length and breadth are not natural appearing, but there will be times when the characterized denture bases will be more acceptable than disharmony in length and breadth (Fig. 12-8).

7. THE LIPS.   When the lips are relaxed and apart, the labial surfaces of the maxillary anterior teeth support the upper lip. Frequently the incisal edge extends inferior to or slightly below the lip margin. This extension will vary in relation to the fullness of the lip. When the teeth are in occlusion and the lips are together, the labial incisal third

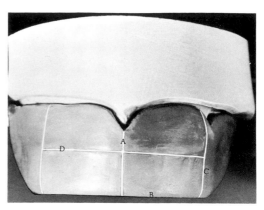

FIG. 12-9.   *Accurately contoured occlusion rims with recorded information derived from the anatomy of the mouth are invaluable aids in the arrangement of teeth; midline (A), low lip line (B), cuspid line (C), high lip line (D).*

of the maxillary anterior teeth supports the superior border of the lower lip. This support can be demonstrated by pressing against the lower lip when the teeth are in occlusion. In speech the incisal edges of the maxillary anterior teeth contact the lower lip at the junction of the moist and dry surfaces of the vermilion border. This is best demonstrated when the letter *F*, as in fifty-five, is pronounced. The properly contoured maxillary occlusion rim will include this position as the incisal edge position and will aid in determining the length of the teeth (Fig. 12-9).

FORM OF ANTERIOR TEETH
Three factors are used as guides in the selection of anterior teeth *for form.*

1. THE FORM AND CONTOUR OF THE FACE. The form of the face and the form of natural teeth are so varied that it would be impossible to develop a system of geometric figures that would be adequate for all individuals. In nature the most pleasing appearing sights or objects are those whose form is in harmony with the surrounding environment. A lack of

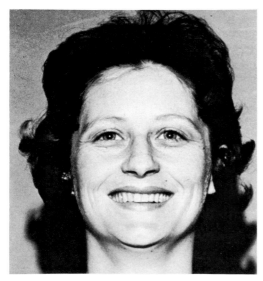

FIG. 12-8.   *This patient has a full smile. She exposes her teeth and is pleased with their appearance.*

harmony presents a contrast, and a marked contrast is not always pleasing. Artificial teeth will not present a pleasing appearance if they draw attention away from the surrounding environment. The form of a tooth should conform to the contour of the face as considered from the labial, mesial, distal, and incisal aspects. The general outline of the tooth should conform to the general outline of the face when viewed from the frontal aspect. A tooth viewed from the mesial or distal should conform to the contour of the profile.

The geometric figures—square, tapering, ovoid, and combinations thereof— serve as a starting point in selecting the tooth form as it is viewed from the

frontal aspect (Fig. 12-10). The indicator may be used in one of two ways to establish the facial outline.

a. Place the tooth indicator on the patient's face, allowing the nose to come through the center triangle. Center the pupils of the eye in the eye slots and hold the indicator with its center line coinciding with the median line of the face. The form of the face will be best observed by noting the particular characteristic of each form as it appears in comparison with the vertical lines of the indicator. In the square form the sides of the face will approximately follow the vertical lines of the indicator. In the square tapering form the upper third of the lower two thirds will taper

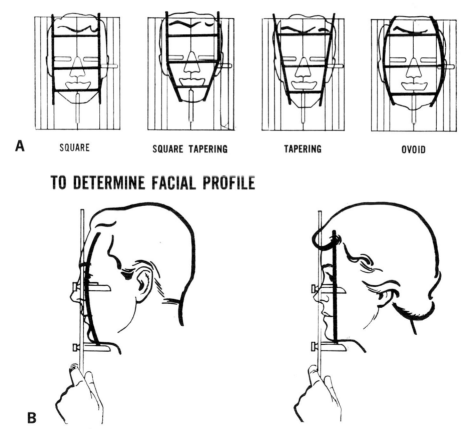

A SQUARE   SQUARE TAPERING   TAPERING   OVOID

TO DETERMINE FACIAL PROFILE

B

FIG. 12-10. *Determining the facial outline with the Trubyte tooth indicator.* **A.** *Frontal aspect.* **B.** *Facial profile. (Courtesy of the Dentists' Supply Company of New York.)*

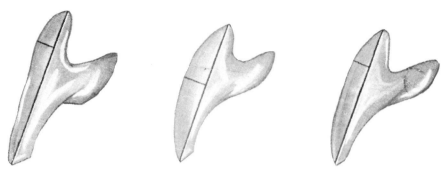

FIG. 12-11. *The labioincisal contour of the teeth usually conforms to the profile of the individual. (Courtesy of the Universal Dental Co., Philadelphia, Pa.)*

inward. In tapering faces, the side of the face from the forehead to the angle of the jaw will taper at an inward diagonal. Ovoid faces will be best determined by examination of the curved outline of the face against the straight vertical of the face against the straight vertical of the tooth indicator (Fig. 12-10A).

b. To determine the facial profile, observe the relative straightness or curvature of the profile. Check three points: the forehead, the base of the nose, and the point of the chin. If these three points are in line, the profile is straight. If the points of the forehead and of the chin are recessive, the profile is curved (Fig. 12-10B).

The dental assistant is very helpful in the evaluation of the general features and the face form of the patient. His impressions should be compared with those of the operator.

The terms flat, concave, and convex apply to the labial surfaces inciso-gingivally as viewed from the mesial or the distal (Fig. 12-11).

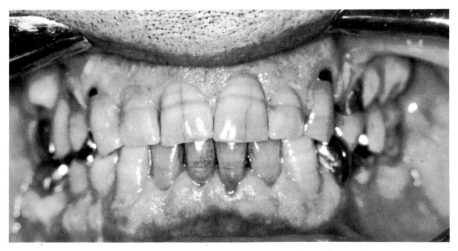

FIG. 12-12. *These natural teeth furnish excellent guides for selecting and arranging artificial teeth. Reproducing the wear at the incisal edges of the maxillary anterior teeth, the gingival recession at the neck of the maxillary lateral incisors and the mandibular left central incisor, the horizontal developmental lines, and the Class V restorations in the maxillary cuspids will make the artificial teeth appear natural.*

Form refers primarily to the outline of anything and *shape* is the quality of a thing that depends on the relative position of all points composing its outline. The facets, developmental grooves, grooves from wear or abrasion, cuppings and convexities are all points which compose the form of a tooth and are best copied from natural teeth. In the natural teeth these are not exaggerated but are subtle (Fig. 12-12).

2. SEX. Curved facial features are associated with femininity (Fig. 12-13A), and square features are associated with masculinity (Fig. 12-13B). Since there is harmony between tooth form and environment, it follows that the teeth of females are more ovoid or tapering than square. However, some males have female features and some females have male features, and the form of the teeth will vary as these features vary.

3. AGE. As the features change with the aging processes so does the form of the teeth. The lips lose their curves and cupid's bow, and the teeth wear at the incisal edges and interproximal sur-

faces. The labial surfaces seem flatter, and the outline form appears more square (Fig. 12-14). As the body of the female loses its curves, the teeth lose their curves. The teeth of the male become more square in form to complement added weight and squareness of body.

COLOR OR SHADE OF
ANTERIOR TEETH

Color is the sensation resulting from stimulation of the retina of the eye by light waves of certain lengths. Shade is the degree of darkness of a color with reference to its mixture with black. When a tooth is viewed for the purpose of determining its color, two principal colors—yellow and gray—are evident. The yellow is more prominent in the gingival third, and the gray is more prominent in the incisal third. The principal modifications are termed *hue*. The degree of intensity of the hue, as measured by its freedom from mixture with white, is saturation. Hue of the tooth is actually the quality that the dentist attempts to duplicate. One other slight modification appears in teeth with

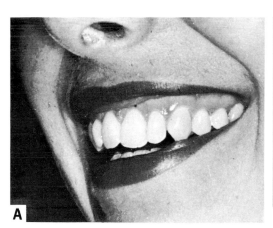 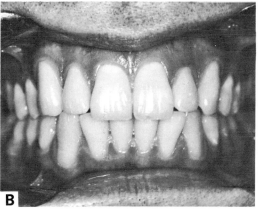

FIG. 12-13. **A.** *The curved teeth, the incisal edges of the maxillary anterior teeth following the curvature of the lower lip, and the curvature of the arch are in harmony with the curves of the female face.* **B.** *The square tooth and arch forms and the relation of the incisal edges of the maxillary anterior teeth to the incisal plane of occlusion are typical of the male.*

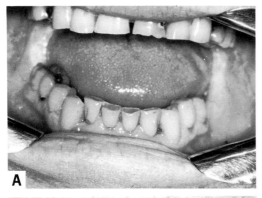

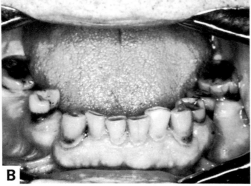

FIG. 12-14. *Teeth wear with use. To simulate or duplicate wear makes the artificial teeth appear more natural.* **A.** *Labial view of the maxillary and the mandibular teeth.* **B.** *Incisal and occlusal view of the mandibular teeth.*

thin incisal edges. The yellow disappears, and the edge appears blue-gray. This is the only place that blue appears in a tooth.

The position of the patient and the source of light are very important in color selection. The patient should be in an upright position. The dentist should be in a position so that the teeth are viewed in a plane perpendicular to the plane of his vision. The teeth should be viewed from different angles to make certain that the shadows do not influence the color. The patient's mouth should not be opened too wide but should remain a dark cavity as in

ordinary conditions. White light is considered suitable. White light may be secured from artificial sources if provided with the proper filters or from an overcast sky, preferably after ten o'clock in the morning and before two in the afternoon. Eyes fatigue to color perception very rapidly, and for this reason they should not be focused on a tooth more than a few seconds. If the proper shade (lightness or darkness) is hard to establish, the tooth and the shade guide should be viewed from a distance of six or eight feet. The dental assistant or the patient can hold the shade guide while the dentist views the tooth and the guide from the distant point.

The color of the teeth, like the form, must be in harmony with the surrounding environment if they are to appear pleasing. Harmony should exist between the color of the teeth and the color of the skin, hair, and eyes. The color of the skin or complexion of an individual is a more reliable guide than the hair. A female patient's cosmetics must be considered in the harmonizing with the complexion.

The changing color of the hair, particularly with the female, makes this guide unreliable; however, it should not be discarded as an aid. The support for dentures changes; therefore, dentures must be changed. Where it is ascertained that the hair color is natural, it should be used in the color scheme.

The color of the eyes is an excellent aid. Caucasians with blue, green, or light hazel eyes usually have light or blond hair and fair skin. Caucasians with black, dark brown, or dark hazel eyes usually have dark hair and a ruddy complexion.

The use of a single tooth from a shade guide is not very reliable when selecting the shade; however, if the teeth are allowed to remain in the guide holder held to one side of the nose of the patient, the tooth that is in harmony will be recognized.

To check the size, form, and shades, the anterior and posterior teeth of both arches should be arranged in their anatomic positions on accurately adapted record or trial bases (Fig. 12-15). The wax should be of an acceptable color to the oral mucosa and should be contoured to simulate the supporting soft tissues when natural teeth were present (Fig. 12-15D).

The vast number of combinations in face form and size, arch form and size, and the colors of hair, eyes, and complexion makes tooth selection anything but a menial task. These varying combinations are the reason set rules cannot be drawn for this procedure. Whenever possible, it is advisable to record the size, form, and color of the natural teeth before extracting them. It is unfortunate for the dentist that edentulous patients have such short memories of their natural teeth. The majority of edentulous patients remember only that their teeth were "small, white and were arranged in a straight row." The result of following that description is *small white pearls arranged like tombstones* (Fig. 12-16).

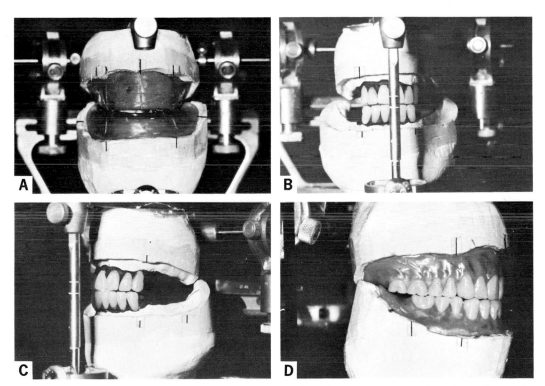

FIG. 12-15. *Steps in selecting teeth.* **A.** *Contoured occlusion rims are placed on the casts, and the guide lines are marked on the shoulders of the casts.* **B.** *Measurements are made (Fig. 12-5), and the teeth are arranged according to the guide lines that have been recorded on the cast.* **C.** *The anterior line on the mandibular cast designates the distal of the mandibular cuspid. The posterior line designates the ascending area of the mandible. The posterior teeth are selected to occupy this space.* **D.** *The teeth are arranged, and the wax is contoured for try-in. Note that the maxillary second molars were used. They help support the cheek and thereby prevent cheek biting.*

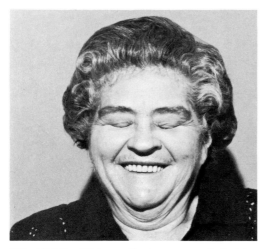

FIG. 12-16. *This patient requested "white pearls arranged like tombstones." Since she did not request that the teeth be positioned out of harmony with the functions of speech, swallowing, and masticating, her request was satisfied.*

COMPOSITION OF MATERIAL
OF ANTERIOR TEETH

Artificial teeth for complete dentures are made either of porcelain—a fused combination of various minerals, chiefly kaolin, feldspar, and quartz to which pigments are added—or of plastic—the processed acrylic resins.

The porcelain teeth are either air fired or vacuum fired. The vacuum fired are more dense than the air fired. Porcelain teeth are hard to abrade and will retain their finish. Acrylic resin teeth are not as hard as porcelain and can be abraded more readily. The porcelain teeth must be attached to the supporting base mechanically, usually by gold pins.[25] The acrylic resin teeth can be bonded to the denture base without mechanical means. This property allows extensive grinding in situations in which space is limited. The acrylic resin teeth can be contoured to become a part of the denture base, a particularly useful property in immediate complete denture restorations.

Although porcelain is easier to break, its hardness and resistance to abrasion from foods and brushing make it the material of choice for esthetic purposes when space is available.

Posterior Teeth

The selection of posterior teeth likewise involves shade, size, number, and form.

SHADE OF POSTERIOR TEETH

The shade of the posterior teeth should harmonize with the shade of the anterior teeth. As noted previously (page 293), the maxillary bicuspids are sometimes used more for esthetic than for functional purposes. Bulk influences the shade of teeth, and for this reason it is advisable to select a slightly lighter shade for the bicuspids if they are to be arranged for esthetics. They may be slightly lighter than the other posterior teeth but not lighter than the anterior teeth.

SIZE AND NUMBER OF
POSTERIOR TEETH

The size and the number of posterior teeth are closely related to usage. These characteristics are dictated by the anatomy of the surrounding oral environment and the physiologic acceptance by the supporting tissues. The posterior teeth must support the cheeks and tongue and function in harmony with the musculature in swallowing and speaking, as well as in mastication. It is considered desirable to have the buccolingual dimension of the artificial teeth less than that of the natural teeth to reduce the size of the food table. This reduction should not be accomplished at the expense of losing support for the cheeks. The buccolingual width should not be great enough to embarrass the tongue or encroach on a normal buccal corridor. The anteroposterior dimensions of the posterior teeth are determined by the edentulous area between the distal of the mandibular cuspids and the ascending area of the mandible (Fig. 12-15D). The ascending area of the mandible is usually situated slightly anterior to the retromolar pad. To place teeth on the ascending area of the mandible would be directing forces at an inclined plane. Forces directed to an inclined plane are more dislodging than forces directed at right angles to the support. This does not preclude the use of a tooth distal to this area for cheek support in the maxillary arch, neither does it require that the number of posterior teeth should equal those found with natural dentition.

FORM OF POSTERIOR TEETH

The occlusal surfaces are the primary concern in selecting the form of the posterior teeth. The proximal, lingual, and buccal surfaces should be contoured like the natural teeth so that they will feel natural, shed food, and be arranged in suitable contact.

The occlusal form will be decided by the type of occlusion to be developed. If the teeth are to be balanced in the centric and eccentric positions, a cusp form tooth is indicated. If the posterior teeth are to disocclude when an eccentric jaw movement occurs, either cusp or monoplane teeth can be used. If the posterior teeth are to be arranged on a plane and balanced in centric position only, monoplane teeth are used.

These advantages have been attributed to cusp posterior teeth.

1. They are considered more efficient in the cutting of food, thereby reducing the forces that are directed at the support during masticatory movements. Controversy exists over this claim.

2. They can be arranged in balanced occlusion in the eccentric jaw positions. If monoplane teeth are arranged for balance, they become a single long cusp.

3. When the cusps are making contact in the fossae at the correct vertical dimension of occlusion with the jaws in centric relation, the position is comfortable. This position is a definite point of return, as through proprioception the jaws will return to this position.

4. They look more like natural teeth and are therefore more acceptable esthetically.

5. The contours are more like natural teeth; therefore, they will be more compatible with the surrounding oral environment.

6. An attempted occlusion without cusps is disorganized because occlusion has depth; it is not a sudden closure of flat surfaces.

Some of the following advantages have been attributed to monoplane posterior teeth:

1. When the teeth are contacting in nonmasticatory mandibular movements, as in bruxism, the flat polished surfaces offer less resistance; therefore less force is directed to the support.

2. When the monoplane teeth are arranged to provide even contacting bilaterally with the vertical dimension of jaw separation in harmony with the jaws in centric relation, this position is comfortable. Through proprioceptive impulses the patient will return to this position reflexly.

3. In the absence of residual ridge or ridges there is no support present to resist dislodgement by horizontal or torquing forces. Monoplane teeth offer less resistance to these forces.

4. These teeth will allow a greater range of movement which is necessary in patients with malrelated jaws.

5. Where the neuromuscular controls are so uncoordinated that jaw relation records are not repeatable, the cusp form tooth cannot be balanced. Monoplane teeth are less damaging than cusp teeth not in balance.

Some of the same advantages and

disadvantages are listed for both cusp and monoplane teeth because there is no conclusive evidence from clinical or laboratory research that either tooth form is more efficient than the other. Patients have not experienced a deficiency in masticating with either form of tooth. Soreness and discomfort of the supporting tissues have not been appreciably different. The study of the bony support has not produced any difference either in quantity or quality. The many variables encountered in a study of the osseous structures have made it impossible to evaluate definitely the loss of, or the maintenance of, bone as related to the tooth form. Regardless of the posterior tooth form, the arrangement of the anterior teeth to present a natural appearance to satisfy the esthetic requirements is the same.

MATERIAL COMPOSITION OF POSTERIOR TEETH

Vacuum-fired porcelain teeth are more resistant to abrasion and therefore maintain their luster longer than acrylic resin teeth. Acrylic resin teeth can be altered and will bond with the denture base for retention in instances of limited interarch space.[25] When monoplane teeth are arranged on a plane, porcelain in one arch opposing acrylic resin in the other arch offers less resistance to horizontal or torquing forces, since unlike materials offer less resistance than like materials. Acrylic resin teeth are preferred when the teeth in the opposing arch have been restored with gold, as the porcelain has a higher coefficient of wear than gold.

REFERENCES

1. Bader, W. A.: Cutter bar technique. Dent. Dig., *63*:65, 1957.
1a. Beck, H. O.: Occlusion as related to complete removable prosthodontics. J. Prosth. Dent., *27*:246, 1972.
2. Boddicker, V. S.: Abrasion test for artificial teeth. J.A.D.A., *35*:793, 1947.
2a. Brewer, A. A.: Selection of denture teeth for esthetics and function. J. Prosth. Dent., *23*:368, 1970.
3. ———, Reibel, P. R., and Nassif, J. N.: Comparison of zero teeth and anatomic teeth on complete dentures. J. Prosth. Dent., *17*:28, 1967.
4. Brill, N., Schübeler, S., and Tryde, G.: Influence of occlusal patterns on the movements of the mandible. J. Prosth. Dent., *12*:255, 1962.
5. Carson, J. W.: Tooth form and face form, is it a "comedy of errors"? J. Prosth. Dent., *1*:96, 1951.
6. Clapp, G. W.: How the science of esthetic tooth-form selection was made easy. J. Prosth. Dent., *5*:596, 1955.
7. Clark, E. B.: An analysis of tooth color. J.A.D.A., *18*:2093, 1931.
8. ———: Tooth color selection. J.A.D.A., *20*:1065, 1933.
9. ———: Selection of tooth color for edentulous patient. J.A.D.A., *35*:787, 1947.
10. Coble, L. G.: A complete denture technique for selecting and setting up teeth. J. Prosth. Dent., *10*:455, 1960.
11. Frechette, A. R.: Masticatory forces associated with the use of various types of artificial teeth. J. Prosth. Dent., *5*:252, 1955.
11a. French, F. A.: The selection and arrangement of the anterior teeth in prosthetic dentistry. J. Prosth. Dent., *1*:586, 1951.
12. ———: The problem of building satisfactory dentures. J. Prosth. Dent., *4*:769, 1954.
13. Friedman, S.: A comparative analysis of conflicting factors in the selection of the occlusal patterns for edentulous patients. J. Prosth. Dent., *14*:30, 1964.
14. Hall, R. E.: The inverted cusp tooth. J.A.D.A., *18*:2366, 1931.
14a. Hardy, I. R.: The developments in the occlusal patterns of artificial teeth. J. Prosth. Dent., *1*:14, 1951.
14b. Harrison, A.: Clinical results of measurement of occlusal wear of complete dentures. J. Prosth. Dent., *35*:504, 1976.
14c. ——— and Huggett, R.: Measuring the rate of wear of artificial teeth in com-

plete dentures. J. Prosth. Dent., *33*:615, 1975.

15. Hodson, J. T.: Some physical properties of three dental porcelains. J. Prosth. Dent., *9*:325, 1959.

15a. Jones, P. M.: Monoplane occlusion for complete dentures. J.A.D.A., *85*:94, 1972.

16. Kapur, K. K., Soman, S. D., and Yurkstras, A. A.: Test foods for measuring masticatory performance of denture wearers. J. Prosth. Dent., *14*:483, 1964.

17. Kapur, K. K., and Soman, S. D.: The effect of denture factors on masticatory performance. IV. Influence of occlusal patterns. J. Prosth. Dent., *15*:662, 1965.

17a. Kelly, E. B.: Has the advent of plastics in dentistry proved of great scientific value? J. Prosth. Dent., *1*:169, 1951.

17b. Kelly, E. K.: Factors affecting the masticatory performance of complete denture wearers. J. Prosth. Dent., *33*:122, 1975.

18. Ketcham, H.: Color and the dental profession. J.A.D.A., *48*:396, 1954.

19. Klaffenback, A. O.: Vacuum fired porcelain. Iowa Dent. J., *41*:247, 1955.

19a. Koran, A.: Coefficient of friction of posterior tooth materials. J. Prosth. Dent., *27*:269, 1972.

19b. Lopuck, S., Smith, J., and Caputo, A.: Photoelastic comparison of posterior denture occlusions. J. Prosth. Dent., *40*:18, 1978.

19c. Machlick, J. A., Knap, F. J., and Ueiler, F. J.: Occlusal wear in prosthodontics. J.A.D.A., *82*:154, 1971.

20. Martins, E. A., Peyton, F. A., and Kingery, R. H.: Properties of custom-made plastic teeth formed by different techniques. J. Prosth. Dent., *12*:1059, 1962.

21. Moses, C. H.: Biomechanics and artificial posterior teeth. J. Prosth. Dent., *4*:782, 1954.

21a. ————: Tooth forms and masticatory mechanisms of natural and artificial teeth. J. Prosth. Dent., *19*:22, 1968.

22. Murphy, J. R.: Design for acrylic posterior teeth for full dentures. Brit. Dent. J., *84*:57, 1948.

23. Myerson, R. L.: Use of porcelain and plastic teeth in opposing complete dentures. J. Prosth. Dent. *7*:625, 1957.

23a. Nasr, M. F., et al.: The relative efficiency of different types of posterior teeth. J. Prosth. Dent., *18*:3, 1967.

24. Norman, R. L.: Frictional resistance and dental prosthetics. J. Prosth. Dent., *14*:45, 1964.

25. Paffenbarger, G. C., Sweeney, W. T., and Bower, R. L.: Bonding porcelain teeth to acrylic denture bases. J.A.D.A., *74*:1018, 1967.

26. Payne, S. H.: A study of posterior occlusion in duplicate dentures. J. Prosth. Dent., *1*:322, 1951.

27. ————: Selective occlusion. J. Prosth. Dent., *5*:301, 1955.

28. ————: Diagnostic factors which influence the choice of posterior occlusion. Dent. Clin. N. Amer., March, 1957, p. 203.

29. Pearson, W. D.: The extraoral tracing as an aid in tooth selection. J. Prosth. Dent., *10*:426, 1960.

30. Phillips, G. P.: Are anatomic teeth suited for full dentures? J.A.D.A., *22*:559, 1935.

31. Pleasure, M. A.: Anatomic versus nonanatomic teeth. J. Prosth. Dent., *3*:747, 1953.

32. Porter, C. G.: The cuspless centralized occlusal pattern. J. Prosth. Dent., *5*:313, 1955.

33. Pound, E.: Applying harmony in selecting and arranging teeth. Dent. Clin. N. Amer., March, 1962, p. 241.

34. Rapp, R.: The occlusion and occlusal patterns of artificial posterior teeth. J. Prosth. Dent., *4*:461, 1954.

34a. Roedema, W. H.: Relationship between the width of the occlusal table and pressures under dentures during function. J. Prosth. Dent., *36*:24, 1976.

34b. Saleski, C. G.: Color, light and shade matching. J. Prosth. Dent., *27*:263, 1972.

35. Schoonover, I. C., et al.: Bonding of plastic teeth to heat-cured denture base resins. J.A.D.A., *44*:295, 1952.

36. Schuyler, C. H.: Full denture service as influenced by tooth forms and materials. J. Prosth. Dent., *1*:33, 1951.

37. Sears, V. H.: What is the future status of nonanatomic posterior tooth forms in full denture prosthesis? J.A.D.A., *18*:662, 1931.

38. ————: Specifications for artificial posterior teeth. J. Prosth. Dent., *2*:353, 1952.

39. ————: Selection and management of

posterior teeth. J. Prosth. Dent., 7:723, 1957.

39a. Sexson, J. C., and Philips, R. W.: Studies on the effects of abrasives on acrylic resins. J. Prosth. Dent., 1:454, 1951.

40. Sobolik, C. F.: Observations on occlusal forms by an edentulous dentist. Dent. Items Interest, 60:672, 1938.

41. Somar, S., and Kapur, K.: Influence of the location of occlusal platform on the masticatory efficiency of dentures. I.A.D.R. Abst. 41st Meeting, Pittsburgh, 1963.

41a. Somter, J. B., and Bass, B. S.: Increasing the efficiency of resin posterior teeth. J. Prosth. Dent., 19:465, 1968.

42. Sosin, M. B.: Re-evaluation of posterior tooth forms for complete dentures. J. Prosth. Dent., 11:55, 1961.

43. Stuart, C. E.: Why dental restorations should have cusps. J. South. Cal. State Dent. Ass., 27:6, 1959.

44. Sweeney, W. T., Yost, E. L., and Fee, J. G.: Physical properties of plastic teeth. J.A.D.A., 56:833, 1958.

45. Thompson, M. J.: Masticatory efficiency as related to cusp form in denture prosthesis. J.A.D.A., 24:207, 1937.

46. Trapozzano, V. R.: Testing of occlusal patterns on the same denture base. J. Prosth. Dent., 9:53, 1959.

47. ———— and Lazzeri, J. B.: An experimental study of testing occlusal patterns on the same denture base. J. Prosth. Dent., 2:440, 1952.

48. Van Victor, A.: The mold guide cast—its significance in denture esthetics. J. Prosth. Dent., 13:406, 1963.

49. Villa, A. H.: Design of posterior teeth. J. Prosth. Dent., 9:814, 1959.

50. ————: Use of nonanatomic posterior teeth. J. Prosth. Dent., 12:63, 1962.

50a. Von Krammer, R.: Artificial occlusal surfaces. J. Prosth. Dent., 30:391, 1973.

50b. ————: Modified artificial occlusal surfaces. J. Prosth. Dent., 30:394, 1973.

51. Woelfel, J. B., Hickey, J. C., and Allison, M. L.: Effect of posterior tooth form on jaw and denture movement. J. Prosth. Dent., 12:922, 1962.

52. Wright, W. H.: Selection and arrangement of artificial teeth for complete prosthetic dentures. J.A.D.A., 23:2291, 1936.

53. Young, H. A.: Selecting the anterior tooth mold. J. Prosth. Dent., 4:748, 1954.

Tooth Arrangement

13

Patients can be quite demanding about the arrangement of their teeth. To meet the patient's demands at times would require placing teeth in positions unfavorable for physiologic compatibility. The dentist must decide the course of treatment and must have a thorough knowledge of all the factors involved.

Many factors enter into the arrangement of the artificial teeth in a denture. It is not simply a mechanical procedure of placing teeth to follow the form of the arch or to satisfy the laws of leverages; it requires dexterity and a knowledge of biology. The artificial teeth are attached to a movable base resting on movable and displaceable living tissue subject to damage. They act as a unit; therefore, they must be arranged to function as a unit. However, leverages, forces, vector of forces, discrepancies in residual ridges, maxillomandibular relationships, residual ridge relationships, functional and parafunctional mandibular movements, esthetic requirements, and preferences of patients vary. Exception to the rule is particularly applicable when considering the arrangement of teeth. A rule to satisfy one situation may have to be altered to satisfy another, but there are limits to alterations.

The arrangement of teeth must be physiologically and esthetically acceptable. Physiologically they must be in a position compatible with the lips, tongue, and cheeks whether the mandible is in a relaxed position or in motion. The teeth must function in harmony with the surrounding oral environment in masticating, swallowing, speaking, yawning, and all parafunctional mandibular movements.

The physiology of the supporting tissues must be considered. Although muscle tissue is very adaptable and bone is plastic, these properties should not encourage the indiscriminate placing of teeth in the hope that they will be tolerated. The residual ridge is bone covered by vascular tissue. Resorption results when much bone is subjected to pressure. Teeth must be arranged to act normally in their environment and to be acceptable to the patient. When the teeth are arranged to meet the physiologic requirements, their positions will contribute to preserving the supporting tissues, and they will appear natural in most situations.

Factors Governing the Positions of Teeth

The positions of the artificial teeth are influenced by (1) the functions of the surrounding structures, (2) the cellular structure of the basal seat tissues,

311

(3) the anatomic limits and (4) the mechanical aspects.

The four principal factors that govern the positions of the teeth for complete dentures are (1) the horizontal relations to the residual ridges, (2) the vertical positions of the occlusal surfaces and incisal edges between the residual ridges, (3) the esthetic requirements, and (4) the inclinations for occlusion. Esthetic requirements will be discussed in Chapter 14, and the inclinations for occlusion in Chapter 16.

HORIZONTAL POSITIONS

The horizontal positions of the teeth to the residual ridges involves placing the teeth anteroposteriorly and medio-laterally (1) to provide stability, (2) to direct the forces of occlusion to areas most favorable for support, (3) to support the lips and cheeks for esthetics, and (4) to be compatible with the functions of the surrounding structures.

Forces directed at right angles to the support are more stabilizing than forces directed at an inclined plane. An important point to remember is that when natural teeth are present the mandible moves in many directions. Masticatory movements are influenced by the resistance, size, and type of food, the vigor with which an individual chews, the quantity and consistency of the saliva, the quantity of water taken with the food, and habitual jaw motions.

In normal situations, with either the natural or artificial teeth, habit and comfort through proprioception and/or flexor reflexes guide the movements of the mandible. These movements result in tooth contacts at positions of greatest comfort. Protrusive and lateral movements involving tooth contacts result in forces directed toward inclined planes, and these forces are capable of dislodging the dentures. Unstable dentures are uncomfortable; un-

doubtedly many patients change their habitual jaw movements to a more vertical closure. This adjustment may not happen with patients who have a low reaction to pain. The dentist cannot always differentiate these patients. Therefore, all patients are instructed to crush their food by closing *up* and *down* and not from side to side and to cut food into small pieces with the knife and fork.

The character of the mucosa and sub-mucosa must be considered when the teeth are positioned. The forces of occlusion should not be directed to tissue incapable of withstanding the force. The differentiated submucosa in the distal two-thirds of the palate and in the retromolar pad is not capable of bearing stress. The loosely attached submucosa in the vestibular fornix provides a good denture seal area but should not be subjected to the stresses of occlusion.

The importance of positioning the artificial teeth for physiologic compatibility is illustrated by the acts of swallowing, speaking, masticating, or moistening the lips with the tongue. In the act of swallowing, the tip of the tongue is braced against the palatal surfaces of the maxillary anterior teeth and the anterior third of the palate. The teeth are clenched to prevent the food from escaping into the vestibular spaces. The rhythmic contractions of the tongue propel the trapped food up and backward. The orbicularis oris and attached muscles contract and force saliva and small particles of food from the vestibular spaces into the oral cavity and seal off the space distal to the last molar teeth. The artificial teeth must be placed in suitable horizontal positions to allow this muscle activity to occur naturally.

The positions of the teeth influence the phonetics as exemplified by the *f, ch,* and *sh* sounds. When the maxillary anterior teeth are placed too far posteriorly as related to the lower lip, the *f* sound may be muffled. It may be necessary to arrange the mandibular anterior teeth with more labial version to aid in the correct enunciations of the *ch* and *sh* sounds.

In mastication, the tip of the tongue reaches into the buccal and labial vestibules, gathers the food, and places it on the occlusal surfaces. When the teeth are placed too far in a lateral or anterior direction, the vestibular spaces are obstructed to the tongue. When the teeth are placed too far in a medial or posterior direction, the tongue will dislodge the mandibular denture in an attempt to reach over the teeth.

The tongue moistens the lips many times a day. The anteroposterior position of the teeth must be compatible with this action and all other actions to insure stability to the denture bases.

The positions of the *natural teeth* are not always compatible with the surrounding oral environment. It is difficult to determine which positions of natural teeth are acceptable. The positions of the clinical crowns of natural teeth may or may not have conformed to the pressures of the soft tissues to occupy a place in the dental arch compatible with function or esthetics. It is difficult to determine what effect the positions of the clinical crowns of the natural teeth contributed to their loss, if any. It may not be functionally or esthetically acceptable to place the artificial teeth in the exact positions formerly occupied by the clinical crowns of the natural teeth.

The crests of the *residual ridges* are aids in positioning the artificial teeth if the natural teeth were recently extracted and the cortical plates of bone remain intact. Unfortunately, the crests of the residual ridges do not remain in the same anteroposterior or mediolateral positions. Improper positioning of the teeth results from placing teeth over the crest of the residual ridge, particularly when the crest of the maxillary residual ridge is used. In 1967 Pietrokovski and Massler demonstrated that, viewed from the occlusal aspect, the crest of the residual alveolar ridge shifts lingually in the maxillae and in the mandible. Both arches are resorbed in a vertical and lingual direction. The anatomic topography of the bodies of the maxillae and the mandible is not the same. As absorption of the alveolar ridge progresses, the maxillary arch becomes narrower and the mandibular arch becomes broader (Fig. 13-1). The result of this difference is often improperly diagnosed as malrelation of the alveolar ridges, and the posterior teeth are arranged in reverse relationship in a mediolateral direction and the anterior teeth are arranged incisal edge to incisal edge.

Anatomic landmarks aid in relocating the original center of the mandibular alveolar ridge. For this reason, guide lines placed on the mandibular cast are reliable as guides for positioning the artificial

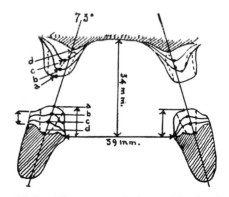

FIG. 13-1. *The crests of the residual ridges do not remain in their relative relations as resorption progresses. Lines a, b, c, and d designate horizontal and vertical positions of the crests at different time intervals during the resorption process. (After Gysi, in Nichols: Prosthetic Dentistry, St. Louis, The C. V. Mosby Company, 1930.)*

posterior teeth in horizontal relationship with the residual ridge. Guide lines are aids, however, and must not be considered ironclad rules. The anatomic landmarks are (1) the retromolar fossae, (2) the retromolar papilla, (3) the retromolar pad, and (4) the mandibular cuspid.

1. The *retromolar fossae* are triangles formed by the external oblique line and the mylohyoid line. The lines converge to form the apex at the base of the anterior border of the ascending ramus of the mandible. The third molar forms the base. The triangle is in a slightly posterior and lateral position to the molar teeth. The internal boundary, the *mylohyoid line,* is on a plane with the buccal surfaces of the mandibular posterior teeth. This point corresponds approximately with the middle of the retromolar pad in the medial lateral directions.

2. The *retromolar papilla* is a small pear-shaped area of gingival tissue that remains fused to the scar after the loss of the last molar tooth. This small, hard, pale pear-shaped tissue is situated at the base of the *retromolar pad,* approximately at the center of the alveolar residual ridge.

3. The *retromolar pad* is a triangular or pear-shaped soft pad of tissue located at the distal end of the mandibular ridge. It must be remembered that this pad of soft tissue contains glandular tissue, fibers from the buccinator muscle, and fibers from the superior pharyngeal constrictor muscle. The pterygomandibular raphe enters the pad at the superior medial corner, and the pad is displaceable. The retromolar pad is usually distorted in a medial or lateral direction in an impression. However, the vertical distance from the base of the pad to the superior border is a usable guide on the cast.

4. The *mandibular cuspid* is the turning point in the arch. The distal surface of the cuspid is usually rotated in a posterior direction in line with the center of the posterior alveolar ridge. The position of the distal surface of the cuspid is located by passing a marker, parallel to the pupils of the eyes, intraorally at the corners of the mouth. These two points, right and left, are recorded on the occlusion rims and then transferred to the mandibular cast. With these landmarks the crest of the alveolar posterior ridge is located and the guide lines (see Fig. 13-2), are placed on the cast.

LIMITS TO PLACING POSTERIOR TEETH. The mandibular arch determines the *posterior limit* for placing occluding posterior teeth. The mucosa considered capable of bearing stress terminates at the *retromolar papilla.* The stress-bearing mucosa in the mandibular arch is usually anterior to the stress-bearing mucosa of the maxillary arch. The distal of the most distal mandibular posterior tooth should not be placed in a more posterior direction to this area (Fig. 13-3). If the mandibular residual ridge has a steep ascent toward the anterior border of the ramus of the mandible, the distal of the most distal

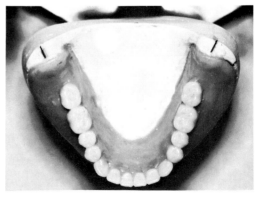

FIG. 13-2. *The guide lines on the margin of the cast designate the existing crests of the residual ridges.*

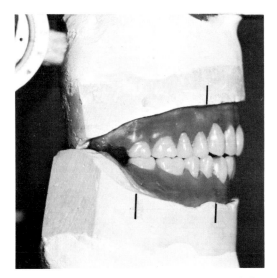

FIG. 13-3. *Guide lines on the margin of the mandibular cast aid in placing the last mandibular posterior tooth.*

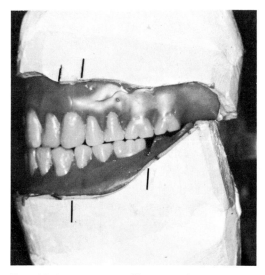

FIG. 13-4. *Last maxillary tooth in a more distal position than the last mandibular tooth. The distobuccal and lingual surfaces of the maxillary second molar may be reduced by grinding.*

mandibular posterior tooth is placed anteriorly to the ascent. When a tooth is placed over the ascending residual ridge, the forces are directed to an inclined plane. To support the cheek it is often desirable, in the *maxillary arch,* to place a posterior tooth in a more distal position than the last tooth in the mandibular arch (Fig. 13-4). When this is done, the tooth or teeth are not in an occluding relationship to the mandibular arch.

The medial extension of the mylohyoid ridge determines the medial limit in placing mandibular posterior teeth. If the teeth are placed more lingually than the extent of the ridge, elevating the tongue may dislodge the mandibular denture. A good guide to follow is that the lingual surfaces of the teeth are placed in a medial direction not to exceed the mylohyoid line. If one follows this rule, the posterior teeth will not be positioned in a medial direction more than the medial surface of the lingual flange of the denture base (Fig. 13-2). In situations of macroglossia this position

may have to be in a slightly lateral direction until the tongue alters to conform to the new confines (Fig. 13-5).

The actions of the tongue and the cheek and esthetics primarily determine the *lateral limits* of the mandibular posterior teeth. The size, shape, and relation of the maxillary arch to the mandibular arch influence the positions of the bicuspids. The maxillary bicuspids

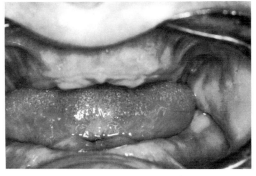

FIG. 13-5. *Compromises are often the rule. The size of this tongue must be considered.*

are considered in the arrangement of teeth for esthetics. The buccal surfaces are placed continuous with the arch of the anterior teeth. The mandibular bicuspids are placed in harmony with the arch of the mandibular anterior teeth. In normal ridge relations the lingual cusps of the maxillary posterior teeth occlude in the central fossae of the mandibular posterior teeth (Fig. 13-6). This tooth relationship places the buccal cusp of the maxillary posterior tooth lateral to (horizontal overlap) the buccal cusp of the mandibular posterior teeth. Posterior teeth arranged in this manner support the cheek and prevent cheek biting. When noncusp form posterior teeth are used in normal ridge relations, the horizontal overlap is greater.

When maxillomandibular or ridge relations are not normal, they dictate a different occlusal relation of the teeth; one must remember that the medial and lateral positions of the teeth must provide acceptable anatomic and physiologic limits. One must also consider mechanical factors. The teeth can be altered in form, shape, size, and to a limited position to accommodate for the malrelations of the jaws or residual ridges. When the maxillary arch is broader than the mandibular arch, the maxillary posterior teeth should not be moved medially over the palate to meet the mandibular posterior teeth and the mandibular posterior teeth should not be moved laterally into the vestibule to meet the maxillary posterior teeth. A limited alteration in the positions of the teeth in both arches may suffice, or altered position and larger teeth buccolingually may be required. When the maxillary arch is smaller than the mandibular arch, the buccolingual relations of the teeth are reversed from the relations when the arches are proportioned or when the maxillary arch is larger than the mandibular arch. Place the buccal cusps of the mandibular teeth lateral to the buccal cusps of the maxillary teeth.

The relations of the residual ridges may be classified in the same manner as the relations of the jaws. In a protruded residual ridge the maxillary and/or mandibular residual ridge is in a more anterior relation to the others. When both residual ridges are pro-

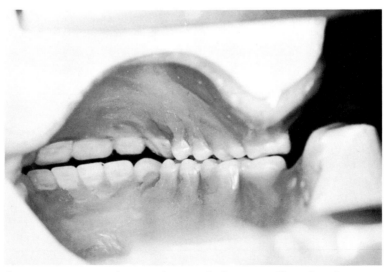

FIG. 13-6. *The arrangement of posterior teeth in normally related jaws. The lingual cusps of the maxillary teeth occlude in the central fossae of the mandibular teeth.*

truded, the arrangement of teeth is basically the same as for the normally related residual ridges. When the mandibular residual ridge is protruded, the disproportion may be so great that all the teeth are arranged in reverse positions in a mediolateral and anteroposterior direction when compared to those arranged for the normal relation. The disproportion may only require a reversed relation in the posterior arches and an incisal edge-to-edge relation in the anterior arch (Fig. 13-7).

If an underdeveloped mandible causes a retruded relation of the mandibular residual ridge to the maxillae, a disproportion exists in the posterior and the anterior arches. This presents a difficult situation, and when the jaws are in centric relation, the occlusion of two posterior teeth bilaterally is hard to achieve. It is fortunate that these patients have a wide range of mandibular movement and appear to function in an anterior direction to centric relation. However, it is an error to relate the cast on the articulator in a position other than centric relation or to place the teeth in unfavorable positions to compensate for the disproportion. The retruded mandible

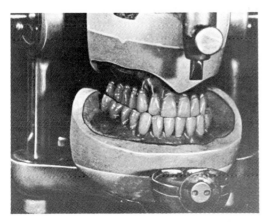

FIG. 13-7. *The reverse mediolateral relation of the posterior teeth is required. (From Swenson's Complete Dentures. 4th ed. St. Louis, The C. V. Mosby Company, 1937.)*

presents another problem, since the patient may demand teeth arranged as if the jaw were normally related. The patient must understand the problem, and the teeth must be arranged in their correct relation to the maxillary and mandibular residual ridges (Fig. 13-8).

LIMITS TO PLACING ANTERIOR TEETH. Placing anterior teeth in harmony with functional activity involves placing the teeth in an anteroposterior and mediolateral position in harmony with the action of the lips and the tongue. The artificial anterior teeth should not be used to incise food, and patients should be instructed to do their incising with a knife and a fork. It is desirable to establish horizontal overlap sufficient to prevent the anterior teeth from contacting when the posterior teeth are in centric occlusion (Fig. 13-9).

The artificial teeth are balanced in the protrusive jaw positions to stabilize the denture during the contacting of the anterior teeth in nonmasticatory movements. Forces exerted to the anterior teeth when the jaws are eccentrically related are inclined to dislodge the denture bases, thereby damaging the supporting tissues.

The mediolateral and anteroposterior positions of the anterior teeth influence sounds in speech. To make the *f* sound as in *fifty-five*, the incisal edges of the maxillary central incisors should barely contact the vermilion border of the lower lip at the junction of the moist and dry mucosa. The positions of the mandibular anterior teeth affect the *s* sound. When the mandibular incisors are set in a lingual direction, the *s* becomes softened away from the whistle sound. When a patient says the *th* sound, the tip of his tongue should make contact with the palatal surface of the maxillary anterior teeth. When the teeth are placed too far in a posterior direction, the contact is too great and

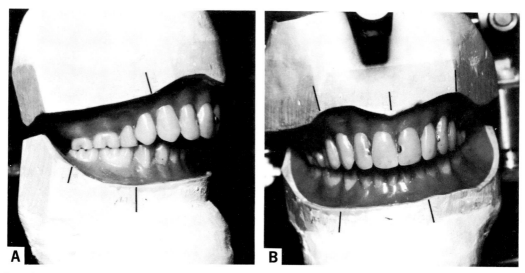

FIG. 13-8. *The mandible in a retruded relation to the maxillae presents a problem in esthetics.* **A.** *A right lateral view of the arrangement of the teeth. Note the extent of horizontal overlap of the anterior teeth.* **B.** *Frontal view of the arrangement of the teeth.*

the *th* sound is muffled. When the teeth are placed too far in an anterior direction, the *th* sound is distorted, since it is difficult for the tip of the tongue to make the proper contact with the teeth.

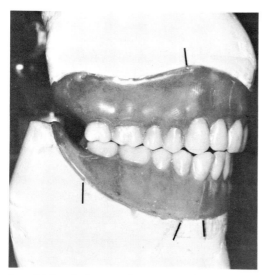

FIG. 13-9. *It is not always possible esthetically to arrange the anterior teeth with vertical and horizontal overlaps sufficient for balanced occlusion.*

When the anterior teeth are placed in favorable positions to support the lips, the normal muscle tonus is maintained. Placing the teeth too far in a posterior direction allows the muscle to go unsupported and the lips to sag. Placing the teeth too far in an anterior direction stretches the muscles and results in a smaller looking mouth.

When the maxillary natural teeth are present, the incisal papilla is located on the palatal side and between the necks of the central incisors. The artificial maxillary central incisors should be placed anterior to the incisal papilla regardless of the relation of the papilla to the existing residual ridge (Fig. 13-10). Most artificial maxillary central incisors are slightly larger anteroposteriorly at the neck of the tooth; therefore, the palatal surface may be placed slightly farther back than were the natural teeth. The labial surfaces of the maxillary anterior teeth infrequently extend in an anterior direction to a greater distance than the outer surface of the labial flange of the denture (Fig. 13-11).

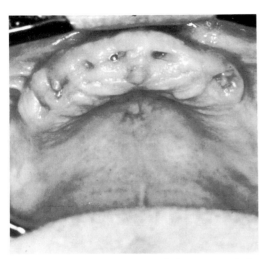

FIG. 13-10. *The relation of the roots of the maxillary central incisors to the incisal papilla is discernible.*

The anteroposterior space in the labial vestibules will vary with the quantitative loss of bone. The labial flange of the denture should fill the space and be contoured in harmony with the labial surface of the residual ridge. The incisogingival contour of the

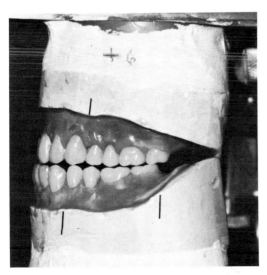

FIG. 13-11. *The labial surface of these maxillary anterior teeth is consistent with the labial flange of the denture and the profile of the patient. (The teeth are being evaluated for balance of protrusion.)*

maxillary anterior teeth and the vertical contour of the labial surface of the residual ridge are usually in harmony with the profile of the individual. The artificial teeth should be placed similarly (Fig. 13-12).

When natural teeth are present, the inclinations of the anterior teeth, as related to the crest of the alveolar ridge, are downward and forward. Usually this relationship is accentuated as resorption takes place. *One of the greatest errors in positioning artificial teeth* is the use of the crest of the maxillary anterior residual ridge to place the teeth. The upper lip is supported in the area of the philtrum by the labial surfaces of the maxillary anterior teeth and at the corners of the mouth by the cuspids. In normally related jaws when the teeth are in occlusion, the superior border of the lower lip is supported by the labial incisal third of the maxillary anterior teeth. When the maxillary anterior teeth are placed too far in a posterior direction, the lips are unsupported and lose tissue tone. When the teeth are placed too far in an anterior direction, the upper lip is stretched. The stretched lip is particularly noticed at the philtrum and the commissures. When the tissue tone is lost or the lip is stretched, the facial expressions of an individual are altered.

Definite anatomic landmarks to be used as guides in arranging the anterior teeth are (1) the incisal papilla, (2) the midsagittal suture, and (3) the cuspid lines. By locating these landmarks and recording their positions on the cast, one establishes points of reference indispensable to the correct arranging of the teeth.

Place maxillary cast guide lines as follows:

1. The *incisal papilla.* Place a ruler parallel to the anterior border of the incisal papilla and make a line on either

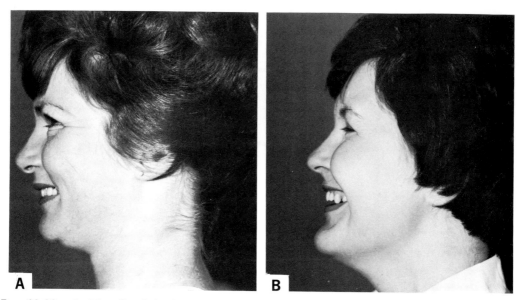

FIG. 13-12. **A.** *The flat labial surfaces of the central incisors are in harmony with the patient's profile.* **B.** *The convex labial surfaces of the central incisors are not in harmony with the patient's profile; however, they are pleasing in appearance.*

side of the margin of the cast parallel to this border (Fig. 13-13).

2. The *midsaggital suture*, the *incisal papilla*, and the *labial frenum*. These are guides to the *median line*. Draw a line anteroposteriorly bisecting these points and extend this line to the margin of the cast (Fig. 13-13). Compare this line with the median line which was made on the maxillary occlusion rim (page 244).

3. The *cuspid lines*. The six maxillary anterior teeth occupy the space between the distal of the right cuspid eminence and the distal of the left cuspid eminence. When the cuspid eminences are visible on the cast, a line coinciding with the posterior margin of the eminence coincides with the posterior surface of the cuspid. Record this line on the margin of the cast (Fig. 13-13). When the eminences are not visible, use the points that were recorded at the corners of the mouth on the mandibular occlusion rim as a reference (page 245).

The directions of resorption of the mandibular residual ridge cause the crest to become more anterior. This change in position is not very noticeable until the residual alveolar ridge is greatly resorbed. The positions of the clinical crowns of the natural mandib-

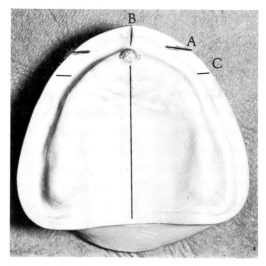

FIG. 13-13. *Maxillary cast guide lines.* **A.** *The anterior margin of the incisal papilla.* **B.** *The midline.* **C.** *The cuspid line.*

ular anterior teeth are more in line in a vertical direction with the alveolar process of the mandibular arch than the maxillary anterior teeth are related in a vertical direction with the alveolar process of the maxillae. These two factors explain why the crest of the mandibular anterior ridge is favorable as a guide for positioning the mandibular anterior teeth. The anteroposterior relations of the maxillary and mandibular ridges influence the amount of horizontal overlap between the maxillary and mandibular anterior teeth. The necks of the maxillary anterior teeth are placed anterior to the incisal papilla, and the necks of the mandibular anterior teeth are placed to direct a vertical force toward the crest of the anterior residual ridge. The labial and/or lingual version of the crowns is governed by the differing situations. Normally related and protruded ridge relations require different anteroposterior inclinations of the teeth. The underdeveloped mandible in a retruded relation to the maxillae and extremely protruded situations are examples of the extreme positions encountered.

The horizontal positions of the posterior and anterior teeth in dentulous situations usually follow the form and shape of the arch. Ideally, the shape of the arch has not been altered or destroyed by atrophy, resorption, accident, or surgical procedures.

Arch shapes may be classified as (1) square, (2) tapering, or (3) ovoid. Ordinarily, an unaltered arch supported natural teeth whose roots followed its shape. However, this position of the roots does not necessarily assure that the clinical crowns follow the same arch shape. Nor does it necessarily follow that the shape of the teeth conform to the shape of the arch. In the absence of other more definite information the arch shape is used as a guide for the initial arrangement of the teeth.

The size and shape of the head are reliable factors in determining arch shape. Long, narrow heads are associated with long, narrow palates, tapered arches, and a tapered anterior tooth arrangement. Round heads are associated with square arches and a broad, flat arrangement of the anterior teeth. The labial surfaces of the central incisors are in full view and the cuspids are prominent.

The arrangement of the anterior teeth for the tapered arch places the central incisors farther forward than the cuspids (Fig. 13-14A). The arrangement of the anterior teeth for the square arch places the central incisors more nearly horizontal with the cuspids (Fig. 13-14B). The arrangement of the anterior teeth for the ovoid arch places the six anterior teeth in a gentle curve (Fig. 13-14C).

VERTICAL POSITIONS

The arrangement of artificial teeth in the correct vertical positions involves

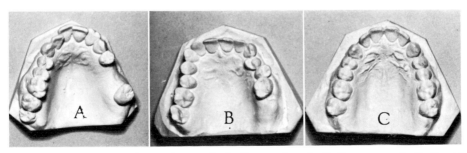

FIG. 13-14. *Arrangement of anterior teeth.* **A.** *Tapered arch.* **B.** *Square arch.* **C.** *Ovoid arch.*

placing the anterior and posterior teeth in an acceptable position between the two residual ridges in a vertical direction. As in correct horizontal positioning, correct vertical positioning of the teeth should provide (1) denture stability, (2) favorable forces, (3) support for the lips and cheeks, and (4) compatibility.

To place the occlusal surfaces of the posterior teeth and the incisal edges of the anterior teeth at the same vertical positions occupied by the natural teeth would be ideal if the natural teeth erupted and established physiologically satisfactory occlusal and incisal relations and if the relations were maintained until the teeth were removed. Natural teeth lose contact and migrate; they assume abnormal relations and positions when subjected to forces beyond the physiologic limits. Natural teeth extrude when the antagonists are removed, and at times the teeth and bone extrude as a unit. They can also be intruded. To place the artificial teeth in the exact positions occupied by the natural teeth may not be tolerated in functions involving mandibular movements even though the teeth appear natural. One must remember that artificial teeth are on a movable base and the natural teeth were fixed in bone. A compromise between appearance and function may have to be reached for a favorable prognosis.

When the mandibular teeth extend too high, the tongue cannot reach the labial or buccal vestibules to retrieve the food. When the mandibular teeth are too low, the tongue will not be supported at the lateral margins and will therefore enlarge in a lateral direction. The tongue apparently accommodates more readily for anteroposterior changes in position than for vertical changes in position.

The length and horizontal position of the central incisors should be such

that when an individual says "five" or "valve" the teeth should come into slight end-to-end contact with the center of the lower lip. This slight contact is rarely seen when maxillary anterior

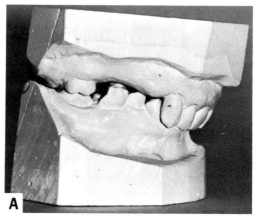

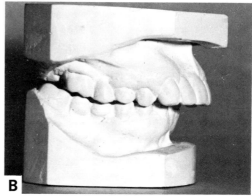

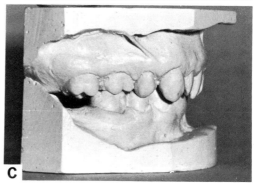

FIG. 13-15. *Arrangement of central incisors.* **A.** *Steep vertical overlap.* **B.** *The teeth of a thumb sucker.* **C.** *The maxillary anterior teeth tucked in a palatal direction.*

teeth erupt to a steep vertical overlap position, when the maxillary anterior teeth have migrated or been forced anteriorly, or when the clinical crowns are in palatal version (Fig. 13-15).

When the teeth are placed in a vertical position to favor a weak arch, any mechanical advantage gained may be overcome because the position is incompatible with the activities of the lips, cheeks, and tongue. When the teeth are improperly placed in a vertical direction, they may not look right to the patient (see Chapter 14.)

The anteroposterior occlusal plane is established when the mandibular posterior teeth are placed at their correct vertical length and the maxillary anterior teeth are placed at their correct vertical length on a plane (Fig. 13-16). The deviations of the individual teeth are discussed in Chapter 16.

VERTICAL POSITIONS OF MANDIBULAR POSTERIOR TEETH. Two anatomic guides to establish the vertical position of the occlusal surfaces of the posterior teeth are (1) the orifice of the duct of the parotid gland (Stensen's duct) and (2) the retromolar pad.

1. The occlusal surface of the maxillary first molar is measured approximately one-fourth inch below the orifice of the duct from the parotid gland (Stensen's duct). This measurement is based on averages, which are not always reliable (Fig. 13-17). Record the measurement on the lateral surface of the maxillary occlusion rim and reduce the length of the rim to the recorded point.

2. The occlusal surface of the last mandibular natural molars is on a plane approximately at the bottom of the upper third of the *retromolar pad*. This vertical position is usually compatible with the activities of the tongue and the cheeks. After the casts are properly attached to the articulator with a face-bow

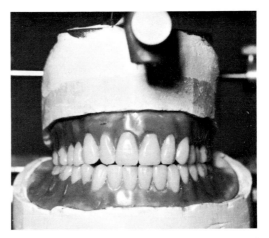

FIG. 13-16. *The anteroposterior occlusal plane is established by anatomic landmarks: the relaxed lip in the anterior and the retromolar pad in the posterior.*

transfer and a centric relation record has been made at the desired vertical dimension of occlusion, place a mark on the cast at the top of the retromolar pads. Extend a line from these points to the lateral borders of the casts to use as a guide (Fig. 13-18). The occlusal groove, on the inner surface of the cheek, is located opposite the occlusal plane of the natural mandibular posterior teeth. When this groove is present, it is a reliable guide to the position occupied by the

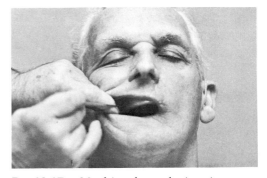

FIG. 13-17. *Marking the occlusion rim opposite the opening to Stensen's duct—an aid, not an ironclad rule.*

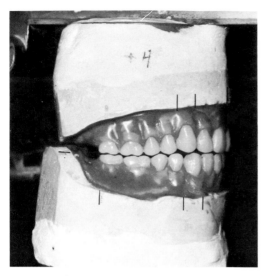

Fig. 13-18. *Anatomic landmarks to be used as guides in arranging artificial teeth are marked on the casts. The anterior line on the maxillary cast is an extension of the horizontal line that is placed at the anterior border of the incisal papilla. The posterior line on the maxillary cast is an extension from a point at the distal of the maxillary right cuspid eminence.*

The anterior line on the mandibular cast is an extension of the horizontal line that bisects the anterior residual ridge. The line corresponding with the distal surface of the mandibular cuspid is an extension of the mark that was placed on the mandibular occlusion rim to denote the distal surfaces of the mandibular cuspid. The line corresponding with the distal of the mandibular second molar denotes the area where the residual ridge begins to ascend toward the retromolar pad. The posterior line on the mandibular cast bisects the retromolar pad in a mediolateral direction.

occlusal surfaces of the natural mandibular posterior teeth and can be used as a guide to positioning the posterior artificial teeth in a vertical direction.

VERTICAL POSITIONS OF MAXILLARY ANTERIOR TEETH. Esthetics and phonetics are used to establish the vertical

position of the incisal edges of the maxillary anterior teeth. The patient is instructed to say "fifty-five," and the teeth are adjusted until the incisal edges of the maxillary central incisors contact the vermilion border of the lower lip at the junction of the moist and dry mucosa (Fig. 13-19). If this position is also esthetic, the vertical position of the anterior end of the occlusal plane is established.

The following are aids to establishing the vertical positions of the artificial teeth by using occlusion rims:

1. Attach hard wax occlusion rims to accurate, stable record bases.

2. Properly contour the occlusion rims in an anteroposterior and mediolateral direction.

3. Instruct the patient to say "fifty-five" and establish the vertical length of the occlusion rims in the anterior section of the maxillary arch.

4. Reduce the posterior occlusal surfaces until the surface is parallel to a line drawn from the ala of the nose to the tragus of the ear (Fig. 13-20.)

5. Make a face-bow transfer and a centric relation record and attach the casts to the articulator.

6. Record the top of the retromolar pad on the cast.

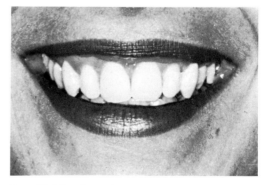

Fig. 13-19. *Junction of the moist and the dry mucosa. When in doubt, have the patient remove lip rouge. The junction will be more discernible.*

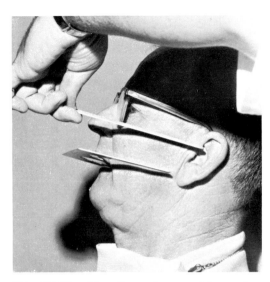

FIG. 13-20. *The Fox plane guide and a tongue blade are used to parallel the maxillary occlusion rim with Camper's line.*

7. Alter the occlusion rims so the posterior vertical positions of the mandibular rim are on a plane at the same level as the top of the retromolar pads and the anterior vertical position is in contact with the maxillary occlusion rims.

Remember that the use of the alatragus line is an expediency and is not a reliable indication for the occlusal surfaces of the teeth. The plane established in this manner is not used unless it coincides with the other guiding factors. Establish the plane, using the retromolar pad for the posterior and the incisal edge or low lip line for the anterior points of reference.

REFERENCES

1. Alsson, A., and Posselt, U.: Relationship of various skull reference lines. J. Prosth. Dent., *11:*1045, 1961.

1a. Beresin, V. E., and Schiesser, F. J.: Neutral zone in complete dentures. J. Prosth. Dent., *36:*356, 1976.

2. Bizzozero, G. A.: Importance of the over-jet in full denture construction. Dent. Dig., *51:*613, 1945.

3. Brotman, D. N.: Contemporary concepts of articulation. J. Prosth. Dent., *10:*221, 1960.

3a. Brudvik, J. S., and Wormley, J. H.: A method of developing monoplane occlusion. J. Prosth. Dent., *19:*573, 1968.

4. Coble, L. G.: A complete denture technique for selecting and setting up teeth. J. Prosth. Dent., *10:*455, 1960.

4a. Ellinger, C. W.: Radiographic study of the oral structures and their relation to anterior tooth position. J. Prosth. Dent., *19:*36, 1968.

5. Fedi, P. F., Jr.: Cardinal differences in occlusion of natural teeth and that of artificial teeth. J.A.D.A., *64:*482, 1962.

6. Frechette, A. R.: Comparison of balanced and nonbalanced occlusion of artificial dentures based upon distribution of masticatory force. J. Prosth. Dent., *5:*801, 1955.

6a. Friedman, S.: Principles of setups in complete dentures. J. Prosth. Dent., *22:*11, 1969.

6b. Goodland, R. J.: A practical approach to balancing complete denture occlusion. J. Prosth. Dent., *26:*85, 1971.

7. Hall, W. A., Jr.: Important factors in adequate denture occlusion. J. Prosth. Dent., *8:*764, 1958.

8. Hanau, R. L.: Articulation defined, analyzed, and formulated. J.A.D.A., *13:*1694, 1926.

9. Hardy, I. R.: Developing a correct occlusal pattern for a maxillary denture. Dent. Dig., *56:*526, 1950.

10. Hickey, J. C., et al.: A method of studying the influence of occlusal schemes on muscular activity. J. Prosth. Dent., *9:*498, 1959.

11. Hooper, B. L.: Functional factors in the selection and arrangement of artificial teeth. J.A.D.A., *21:*603, 1934.

12. Hughes, G. A.: Facial types and tooth arrangement. J. Prosth. Dent., *1:*82, 1951.

13. Landa, J. S.: Arrangement and placement of the anterior teeth from a mechanical standpoint. Amer. Prosthetics, *1:*7, 1946.

14. ———: Biologic significance of balanced

occlusion and balanced articulation in complete denture service. J.A.D.A., *65:* 489, 1962.

15. Maritato, F. R., and Douglas, J. R.: A positive guide to anterior tooth placement. J. Prosth. Dent., *14:*848, 1964.

16. Miller, R. H., Jr.: A posterior tooth combination. J. Prosth. Dent., *10:*260, 1960.

17. Moses, C. H.: Studies in articulation. J. Prosth. Dent., *2:*326, 1952.

18. ———: Human tooth form and arrangement from the anthropologic approach. J. Prosth. Dent., *9:*197, 1959.

19. Mumford, J. M., and Storer, R.: Modification of the occlusal table in restorative dentistry. J. Prosth. Dent., *12:*330, 1962.

19a. Nassif, N. J.: The relationship between the mandibular anterior teeth and the lower lip. J. Prosth. Dent., *24:*483, 1970.

20. Naylor, J. G.: Complete denture procedures in class II relations. J. Prosth. Dent., *8:*241, 1958.

21. Needles, J. W.: The problem of articulation. J.A.D.A., *11:*1220, 1924.

22. Nepola, S. R.: Balancing ramps in prosthetic occlusion. J. Prosth. Dent., *8:*776, 1958.

22a. Palmer, J. M.: Analysis of speech in prosthodontic practice. J. Prosth. Dent., *31:*605, 1974.

22b. Payne, A. G. L.: Factors influencing the position of artificial anterior teeth. J. Prosth. Dent., *26:*26, 1971.

23. Payne, S. H.: Posterior occlusion. J.A.D.A. *57:*174, 1958.

23a. Pietrokovski, J., and Massler, M.: Alveolar ridge resorption following tooth extraction. J. Prosth. Dent., *17:*21, 1967.

24. Pleasure, M. A.: Prosthetic occlusion— a problem in mechanics. J.A.D.A., (and Dental Cosmos), *24:*1303, 1937.

25. ———, and Friedman, S. W.: Practical full denture occlusion. J.A.D.A. (and Dental Cosmos), *25:*1606, 1938.

26. Pound, E.: Applying harmony in selecting and arranging teeth. Dent. Clin. N. Amer., March, 1962, p. 241.

27. Sauser, C. W.: Posterior occlusion in complete denture construction. J. Prosth. Dent., *7:*456, 1957.

28. Schiffman, P.: Relation of the maxillary canines to the incisive papilla. J. Prosth. Dent. *14:*469, 1964.

29. Schlosser, R. O.: The relation of physics and physiology to balanced occlusion. J.A.D.A., *15:*1108, 1928.

30. ———: Treatment of malocclusion and the loss of retention in full denture prosthesis. J.A.D.A., *20:*803, 1933.

31. Schuyler, C. H.: Discussion of "human tooth form and arrangement from the anthropologic approach." J. Prosth. Dent., *9:*213, 1959.

32. ———: Full denture service as influenced by tooth forms and materials. J. Prosth. Dent., *1:*33, 1951.

33. Schwartz, J. R.: Occlusion—what it means to the prosthodontist. New York J. Dent., *16:*142, 1946.

34. Shanahan, T. E. J.: Physiologic jaw relations and occlusion of complete dentures. J. Prosth. Dent., *5:*319, 1955.

35. Shaw, D. M.: Form and function in teeth and a rational unifying principle applied to interpretation. Int. J. Orthodont., *10:* Jan–Dec., 1924.

36. Stuart, C. E., and Stallard, H.: What kind of occlusion shall we give to toothborne restorations? Presented before the Mid-Atlantic Conference in Dentistry, Buck Hill Falls, Penn., April, 1959.

37. Swaggart, L. W.: Occlusal harmony in complete denture construction. J. Prosth. Dent., *7:*434, 1957.

38. Trapozzano, V. R.: Occlusion in relation to prosthodontics. Dent. Clin. N. Amer., March, 1957, p. 313.

39. Wright, W. H.: Anatomic influences on the establishment of balanced jaw relations and balanced occlusion. J.A.D.A., *15:*1102, 1928.

40. ———: Selection and arrangement of artificial teeth for complete prosthetic dentures. J.A.D.A., *23:*2291, 1936.

The Arrangement of Teeth for Esthetics

14

The arrangement of artificial teeth to make them appear natural requires study and training to differentiate between that which is natural and in good taste and that which is unnatural and in poor taste. Very few bodies are symmetrical. Faces are usually asymmetrical in size and shape; the shoulders are rarely the same shape or height; and it is unusual to see natural teeth that are symmetrical in size, form, or arrangement.

Arrangement to meet esthetic requirements is usually associated with the composition, size, shape, and color of the six anterior teeth. However, the horizontal and vertical positions of the posterior teeth are intimately involved in facial expression. In many situations the maxillary first and second bicuspids are as important to appearance as the central and lateral incisors as one sees when many people smile or laugh (Fig. 14-1). To arrange artificial teeth that will encourage the acts of smiling and laughing is a science and an art. These acts are encouraged when all of the artificial teeth are arranged in harmony with the surrounding features of an individual.

The general features and asymmetries should be observed and recorded during the first appointment with the patient.

The record should be enlarged as the patient is observed under different situations. Some of the factors influencing the size and form of the anterior teeth are (1) the size of the face, (2) the amount of available interarch space, (3) the measured distance between the distal of the right and left maxillary cuspids, using the arch and incisal papilla as measuring guides, (4) the length of the lips, and (5) the size and relation of the arches. The hue and the brilliance of teeth are influenced by (1) age, (2) habits, (3) complexion, and (4) color of the eyes. These factors were discussed in Chapter

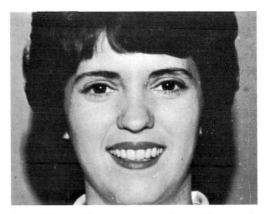

FIG. 14-1. *The number of visible teeth varies between individuals. Females usually expose more maxillary teeth than do males.*

12 and are summarized here as a reminder that the esthetic requirements involve size, form, and color, as well as arrangement.

The arrangement is influenced by (1) age, (2) sex, (3) personality, (4) cosmetic factor, and (5) artistic reflection.

Age

In each individual, *age* changes take place throughout the entire body, and the teeth are no exception. To arrange teeth in disharmony with these changes is in bad taste, and the resulting appearance will be unnatural.

As muscle tonus decreases, the positions of the teeth for support to the lips and cheeks are more critical. The lips and cheeks are supported by teeth, not by denture borders. The denture borders are contoured to fill the vestibules, and the teeth are arranged to support the lips and the cheeks (Fig. 14-2). If the

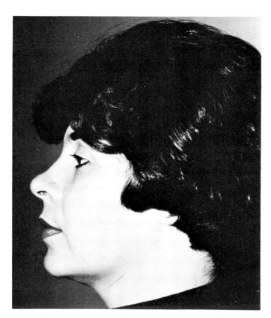

FIG. 14-2. *Denture borders and tooth positions must be compatible with the surrounding oral environment to provide support for this patient's lips and cheeks.*

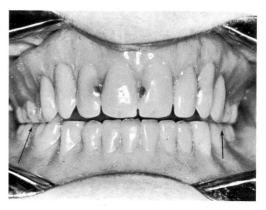

FIG. 14-3. *Horizontal overlap (arrows) for noncusp form posterior teeth.*

cheeks sag, the horizontal overlap of the posterior teeth is increased to prevent cheek biting (Fig. 14-3).

The interincisal distance increases with age; therefore, the mandibular teeth become more visible. That mandibular anterior teeth are more visible than maxillary anterior teeth does not necessarily indicate that the teeth have been positioned incorrectly in a vertical direction. Increased visibility can result from loss of muscle tonus, which can allow the lower lip to sag and the upper lip to drop.

Teeth abrade with age. The central and lateral incisors abrade in a straight line (Fig. 14-4A). The cuspids abrade in a curve (14-4B). The abrasion of the incisal edges of the anterior teeth flattens the arch. This is in harmony with the flattening of the lips as the Cupid's bow of the upper lip disappears, and the fullness of the lower lip diminishes with the aging processes (Fig. 14-4C).

The wearing away of the natural teeth at the contact points creates spaces between the teeth. The migration of teeth also creates spaces. To simulate the wear by positioning the artificial teeth creates a natural appearance. However, to position the artificial teeth in abnormal posi-

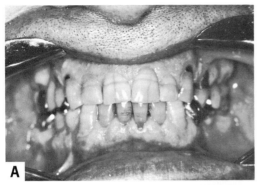

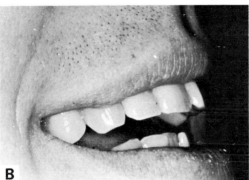

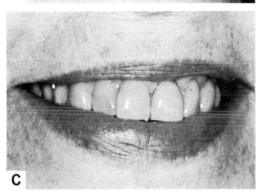

FIG. 14-4. *Abrasion of teeth.* **A.** *The central and lateral incisors are abraded in a straight line.* **B.** *The cuspid is abraded in a crescent.* **C.** *The flat lip and the abrasion of the central and lateral incisors are in harmony.*

they were visible when he was young may result in an improper vertical position of the occlusal plane (Fig. 14-6).

Gingival tissues recede with age. This recession can be reproduced by selecting a long tooth, contouring the wax, and positioning the tooth properly (Fig. 14-7).

The natural teeth of older persons have areas that support restorations. The restorations can be duplicated and

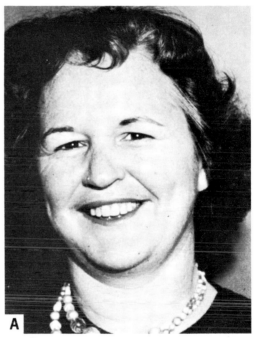

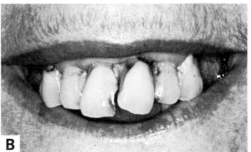

FIG. 14-5. *The original contour of the natural teeth was approximated. The positions of the teeth were not duplicated. Compare the contour and arrangement of the artificial teeth,* **A,** *with that of the natural teeth they replaced.* **B.**

tions that result from migration of the natural teeth may not be acceptable in function or in appearance (Fig. 14-5).

The smiling line is sharp in young people and less sharp in older people. To attempt to make the teeth of the older patient visible to the same extent

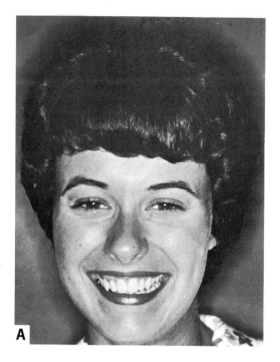

the teeth can be placed in a position to accentuate or lessen the effect.

Sex

The sex of an individual influences the arrangement of the artificial teeth. The contours of the bodies of males and females are different, and the individual contours and the arrangement of the teeth are different. Square features are associated with males and curved features are associated with the female (Fig. 14-8). The features vary; therefore, females may have some male features and males may have some female features. These variations are noted and considered when the teeth are arranged. The positions of the incisal edges, the prominence of the gingival portions of the necks of the teeth, and the positions of the body of the teeth reflect femininity and/or masculinity.

A study of the positions of natural teeth reveals the following.

1. Roundness of the arch form denotes femininity, and squareness denotes masculinity.

2. The incisal edges of the maxillary

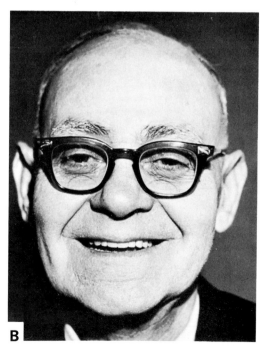

FIG. 14-6. A. *A natural smile.* **B.** *A forced smile. The lack of muscle tonus is evident.*

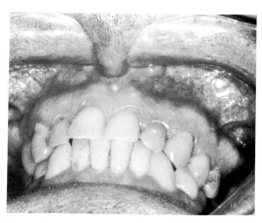

FIG. 14-7. *Natural contours of the gingiva were reproduced in the maxillary denture base.*

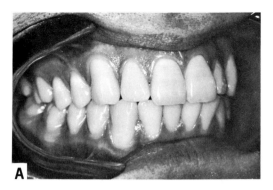

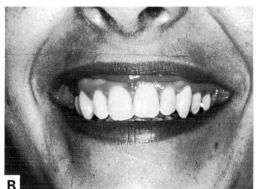

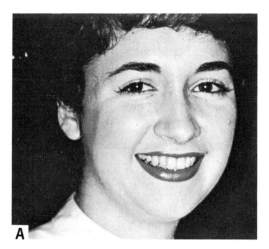

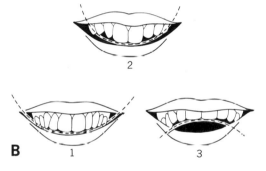

FIG. 14-8. **A.** *Square features of the male. Note the positions of the central and lateral incisors, the prominence of the cuspids, and the square arch.* **B.** *Curved features of the female. The curves of the angles of the teeth, the relations of the lateral and central incisors, and the rotations of the cuspids in a distal direction form a curved arch.*

anterior teeth of females follow the curve of the lower lip (Fig. 14-9).

3. The incisal edges of the maxillary teeth of males are related to the lower lip in the following manner: the central incisors are on a horizontal plane parallel with the lip, the lateral incisors are above the plane, and the cuspids are on the plane (Fig. 14-9C).

4. Viewed from in front, the distal surfaces of the central incisors of females are usually rotated in a posterior direction (Fig. 14-10A). The labial surfaces of the central incisors of males are not usually rotated (Fig. 14-10B).

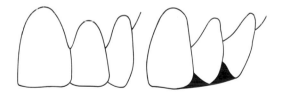

FIG. 14-9. *Incisal edges of maxillary anterior teeth.* **A.** *The incisal edges of the anterior natural teeth and the tips of the buccal cusp of the bicuspid in this female follow the curve of the lower lip.* **B.** *Acceptable curvature of lip (1 and 2) as guide for arranging artificial teeth for esthetics and function; unacceptable reverse curve (3).* **C.** *Comparison of the male (left) with the female (right) incisal edges.*

5. In the arrangement for females the mesial surface of the lateral incisor is often seen in an anterior relation to the distolabial surface of the central incisor. The distal surface of the lateral incisor is rotated in a posterior direction. The smile is softened as a result of this arrangement (Fig. 14-11A). For the male, the mesial surface of the lateral incisor is often hidden behind the distal surface of the central incisor. The distal surface of the lateral incisor is rotated very slightly in a posterior direction (Fig. 14-11B). The cuspid is made more prominent as a result of this arrangement.

6. The distal surfaces of the cuspids for females are rotated in a posterior direction; therefore, the mesial third of the labial surface is exposed when viewed

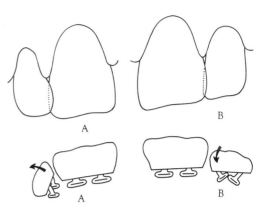

FIG. 14-11. *A diagrammatic arrangement of the maxillary central and lateral incisors for the female,* **A,** *and the male,* **B.**

from the front (Fig. 14-10A). The cuspids for males are rotated less in a posterior direction. As a result, the mesial two thirds of the labial surface is exposed when viewed from the front (Fig. 14-10B). In a lateral view the cuspids for both sexes are vertical to the occlusal plane; any deviation from this is in a posterior direction at the neck of the tooth (Fig. 14-12A). When viewed from the inferior direction, the necks of the cuspids are in a slightly more labial position than the incisal edges (Fig. 14-12B). The maxillary first bicuspids are contoured and positioned to conform with the cuspids (Fig. 14-12C). Frequently the main concern in arranging the first bicuspid in a maxillary denture for a female patient is esthetics rather than function because a woman usually exposes more maxillary teeth than a man when speaking, smiling, or laughing.

Personality

The *personality* of people is expressed in their habitual patterns and qualities of behavior. Their personalities can be influenced by the appearance of their teeth. The shy person may be shy because he is ashamed of the appearance

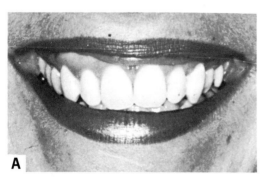

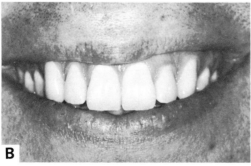

FIG. 14-10. *Compare the central incisors, the curvature of the lower lip, and the relation of the incisal edges and tips of the buccal cusps of the bicuspids with the lips of the female in* **A** *with those of the male in* **B.**

appearing artificial teeth. It is the obligation of the dentist to arrange the artificial teeth in a manner to encourage the development of an attractive personality (Fig. 14-13).

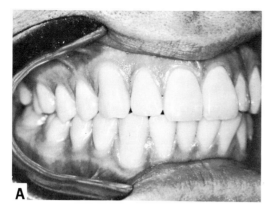

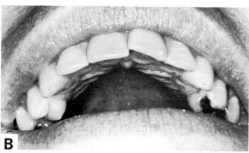

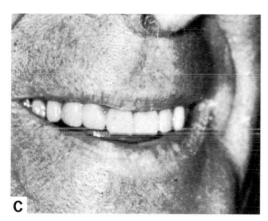

FIG. 14-12. **A.** *Lateral view showing the long axis of the cuspid slightly to the distal of its neck.* **B.** *Inferior view showing the neck of the cuspid more labial than its incisal edge.* **C.** *Maxillary first bicuspid arranged principally for esthetics.*

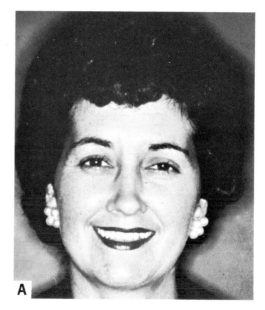

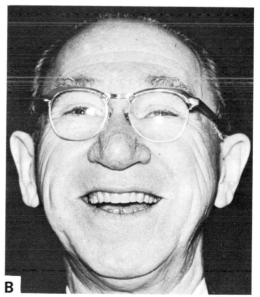

of his teeth. Self-consciousness is possible with either natural or artificial teeth. An unselfconscious person may have had natural teeth pleasant in appearance or dentures with natural

FIG. 14-13. *The personality of the patient and the esthetic arrangement of the teeth are in harmony for the attractive female in* **A** *and the happy male in* **B.**

Cosmetic Factor

The *cosmetic factor* involves personal grooming. When a person dresses neatly and keeps generally well-groomed, the dentist should arrange the artificial teeth in positions that will complement these efforts. However, it is ill-advised to select delicately curved teeth of matching hues and arrange them in a pleasing contour for the woman who uses no cosmetics and does not manicure her nails or keep her hair well-groomed. It is likewise inadvisable to strive for refinement in the arrangement of artificial teeth for the man with bushy, unkempt eyebrows and hair and with dirty or unpressed clothing. The teeth would not harmonize with their setting and would therefore appear more artificial. On the other hand, it would be a mistake for the dentist to confuse the patient who does not use cosmetics because of unsightly teeth with the habitually sloppy person. Attempts to beautify or improve the face with cosmetics may make poorly arranged teeth more noticeable. The dentist should not strive for too exact a reproduction of the arrangement of the natural teeth when he makes dentures for such a patient. Modifications of the natural arrangement may help to improve the patient's appearance.

Artistic Reflection

Artistic reflection is the arrangement of the teeth to reflect the dentist's concept of what he thinks appears natural for the patient. The artistic ability of the dentist is often taxed to achieve a composition of teeth that harmonizes with the surrounding features and is acceptable to the patient. It is not advisable to force a composition of teeth on a patient just because it meets your artistic taste. The dentist is in a position to advise and should be willing to discuss with the patient the advantages of placing teeth in particular positions. After the physiologic requirements have been satisfied, the patient's desires can be considered (Fig. 14-14). If the pa-

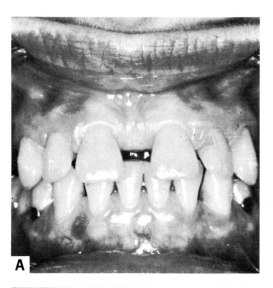

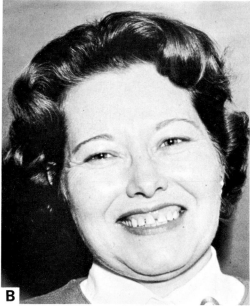

FIG. 14-14. A. *The diastema had been accepted for years as part of this patient.* **B.** *The diastema was reproduced in the teeth of the denture at the request of the patient.*

tient's wishes are not compatible with the physiologic requirements, the dentist must decide the course of the treatment.

Many positions in which the maxillary artificial anterior teeth may be placed will be harmonious with the other facial features.

1. Vary the slant of the long axis (Fig. 14-15).

2. Place the teeth so that the tips of the lateral incisors show when the patient speaks seriously; the amount depends on the age and sex, less for old than for young people and more for women than for men.

3. Create asymmetry in the divergencies of the proximal surfaces of the teeth from the contact points (Fig. 14-15).

4. Use an eccentric midline (Fig. 14-15).

5. Place one central and lateral incisor parallel to the midline and rotate the other central and lateral incisors slightly in a posterior direction (Fig. 14-15).

6. Place one maxillary central incisor slightly in an anterior direction to the other central incisor (Fig. 14-15).

7. Place the neck of one maxillary central incisor in a posterior direction and the neck of the other central incisor in an anterior direction (Fig. 14-15).

8. Create asymmetry for the maxillary right and left cuspids. Rotate one in a more posterior direction than the other (Fig. 14-16). Place the neck of one in a more labial direction than the other (Fig. 14-16).

9. Create a good smiling line by the

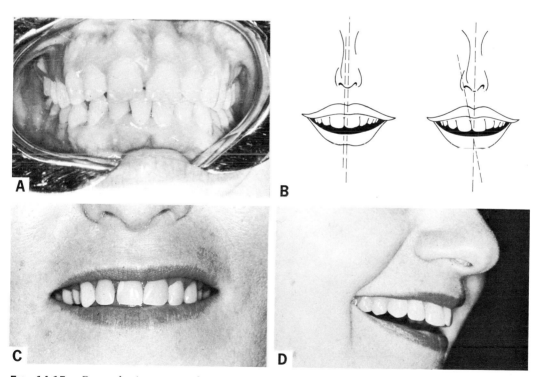

FIG. 14-15. *Reproducing natural arrangement of maxillary anterior teeth.* **A.** *Photograph of natural teeth. Note the asymmetry in the central incisors.* **B.** *Diagram illustrating asymmetry as related to the midline of the face.* **C** *and* **D.** *Front and side views of artificial teeth arranged to create asymmetry.*

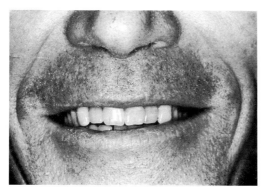

FIG. 14-16. *The maxillary cuspids are rotated to create asymmetry. Notice the space between the cheeks and the buccal surfaces of the posterior teeth. The posterior teeth are placed in harmony with the actions of the tongue and the cheeks.*

proper placing of the maxillary posterior teeth mediolaterally in relation to the cheek. When the teeth are placed too far laterally, the buccal corridor is eliminated, resulting in a harsh, ugly, and toothy appearance.

The similarity in shape and size of the mandibular anterior teeth presents a

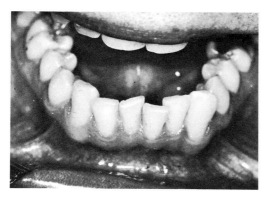

FIG. 14-17. *The mandibular anterior teeth are frequently overlooked in arrangements for esthetics. The incisal edges of the artificial teeth can be altered by grinding to appear like the incisal edges of these natural teeth. The artificial teeth can be rotated and overlapped in a manner similar to the natural teeth. Observe the asymmetry of the cuspids.*

problem in positioning for esthetics. The esthetic acceptance can be enhanced by (1) grinding the incisal edges (Fig. 14-17), (2) rotating and overlapping the teeth to give an irregular appearance (Fig. 14-17), (3) creating asymmetry in the divergencies of the proximal surfaces of the teeth from the contact points (Fig. 14-17), (4) creating a slight diastema between the lateral incisor and the cuspid on the one side (Fig. 14-18), (5) varying the direction of the long axis (Fig. 14-18).

The esthetic arrangement of teeth is a procedure so vital to a favorable prognosis that it must not be delegated to auxiliary personnel who have not studied the patient. Opinions of others, particularly of the patient's family or of people considered close associates, are valuable aids to composition of the teeth for esthetics. Facial features, mannerisms, facial expressions, and tooth positions are inherited. The position of a daughter's or a son's natural teeth can be an excellent guide when positioning the teeth for the parents. The dentist is the only one who has had an opportunity and the experience to evaluate all of these factors and can therefore meet the esthetic requirements of the patient.

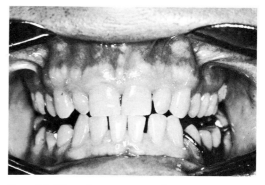

FIG. 14-18. *Asymmetry, diastema, and a variation in direction of the long axis are frequently seen in the arrangement of the natural teeth.*

REFERENCES

1. Beder, O. E.: The dental aspect of esthetics. J. Prosth. Dent., 9:722, 1959.
2. Beyron, H. L.: Occlusal changes in adult dentition. J.A.D.A., 48:674, 1954.
3. Bizzozero, G. A.: Importance of the overjet in full denture construction. Dent. Dig., 51:613, 1945.
4. Blanchard, C. H.: Transferring facial surfaces from the impression of the denture. J. Prosth. Dent., 4:621, 1954.
5. Clapp, G. W.: How the science of esthetic tooth-form was made easy. J. Prosth. Dent., 5:596, 1955.
6. Clark, W. D.: Aesthetics in full denture construction. J. Canad. Dent. Ass., 8:61, 1942.
7. De Van, M. M.: The appearance phase of denture construction. Dent. Clin. N. Amer., March, 1957, p. 285.
8. Dirksen, L. C.: Natural esthetic buccal and labial anatomic form for complete dentures. J. Prosth. Dent., 5:368, 1955.
9. Fisher, R. D.: Esthetics in denture construction. Dent. Clin. N. Amer., March, 1957, p. 245.
10. French, F. A.: Selection and arrangement of the anterior teeth in prosthetic dentistry. J. Prosth. Dent., 1:587, 1951.
11. Frush, J. P., and Fisher, R. D.: Introduction to dentogenic restorations. J. Prosth. Dent., 5:586, 1955.
12. ———: How dentogenic restorations interpret the sex factor. J. Prosth. Dent., 6:160, 1956.
13. ———: Age factor in dentogenics. J. Prosth. Dent., 7:5, 1957.
14. ———: The dyesthetic interpretation of the dentogenic concept. J. Prosth. Dent., 8:558, 1958.
15. ———: Dentogenics: its practical application. J. Prosth. Dent., 9:914, 1959.
16. Harper, R. N.: Incisive papilla—basis of a technic to reproduce the positions of key teeth in prosthodontics. J. Dent. Res., 27:661, 1948.
17. Hughes, G. A.: Facial types and tooth arrangement. J. Prosth. Dent., 1:82, 1951.
18. Kemnitzer, D. F.: Esthetics and the denture base. J. Prosth. Dent., 6:603, 1956.
19. Krajicek, D. D.: Natural appearance for the individual denture patient. J. Prosth. Dent., 10:205, 1960.
20. ———: Achieving realism with complete dentures, J. Prosth. Dent., 13:229, 1963.
20a. ———: Dental arts in prosthodontics. J. Prosth. Dent., 21:122, 1969.
20b. Lombardi, R. E.: A method for the classification of errors in dental esthetics. J. Prosth. Dent., 32:501, 1974.
20c. ———: Factors mediating against excellence in dental esthetics. J. Prosth. Dent., 38:243, 1977.
21. McGee, G. F.: Tooth placement and base contour in denture construction. J. Prosth. Dent., 10:651, 1960.
22. Martone, A. L.: Effects of complete dentures on facial esthetics. J. Prosth. Dent., 14:231, 1964.
22a. Mathews, T. G.: The anatomy of a smile. J. Prosth. Dent., 39:128, 1978.
22b. Murrell, G. A.: Occlusal considerations in esthetic tooth positioning. J. Prosth. Dent., 23:499, 1970.
23. Pound, E.: Esthetics and phonetics in full denture construction. J. Calif. Dent. Assoc., 26.179, 1950.
23a. ———: Esthetic Dentures and their phonetic values. J. Prosth. Dent., 1:98, 1951.
24. ———: Lost—fine arts in the fallacy of the ridges. J. Prosth. Dent., 4:6, 1954.
25. ———: Recapturing esthetic tooth position in the edentulous patient. J.A.D.A., 55:181, 1957.
25a. ———: Utilizing speech to simplify a personalized denture service. J. Prosth. Dent., 24:586, 1971.
25b. Smith, B. J.: The value of the nose width as an esthetic guide in prosthodontics. J. Prosth. Dent., 34:562, 1975.
25c. Tautin, F. S.: Denture esthetics is more than tooth selection. J. Prosth. Dent., 40:127, 1978.
26. Vig, R. G.: The denture look. J. Prosth. Dent., 11:9, 1961.

Arranging the Artificial Teeth for the Trial Denture

15

The technical procedures for arranging teeth are not considered in detail in this chapter. These procedures are explained in laboratory manuals. However, there are details that must be considered before the try-in appointment.

Teeth are tried in before processing them in acrylic resin (1) to verify the maxillomandibular records that were made without teeth (tentative records), (2) to test for the acceptance of the established vertical dimension of occlusion, (3) to determine if the positions of the teeth and the contours of the denture base are compatible with the surrounding oral environment, (4) to evaluate the arrangement for esthetic requirements, and (5) to make additional interocclusal maxillomandibular records if needed for further adjustment of the articulator.

The arrangement of the teeth for the try-in conforms to basic positions, with the understanding that these positions may be altered to meet the anatomic and physiologic variations that are encountered with different persons. The anterior teeth are arranged in basic positions, principally for esthetics (see Chapter 14). The posterior teeth are arranged in maximum planned inter-cuspation (cusp form) or occlusal contact (noncusp form) on a plane, but they are not inclined to meet any concept of balanced occlusion in eccentric mandibular positions until all the reasons for trying in the teeth have been satisfied.

Another detail must be clearly understood. The use of auxiliary personnel makes it possible to meet the dental needs of more people. However, when auxiliary persons are improperly used, dental needs are met only in a quantitative manner. When auxiliary personnel are properly used, dental needs can be met in both a quantitative and a qualitative manner.

A technician may arrange artificial teeth, but it is the responsibility of the dentist to verify the positions of the teeth. Personnel with little or no education in the biological sciences do not know and should not be expected to know the many intricate physiologic factors that are involved in the construction of dentures. The dentist must evaluate these factors before and during the try-in appointment. Such factors can be understood best through illustrations.

Figure 15-1 illustrates the mounted

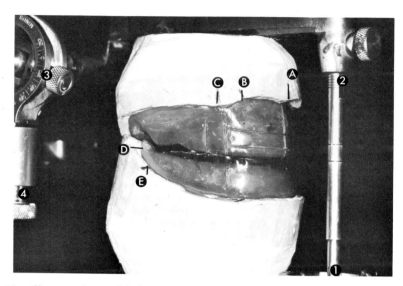

FIG. 15-1. *Maxillary and mandibular casts mounted on the articulator. The incisal guide pin is resting in the center of the incisal guide table (1). The calibrations on the incisal guide pin are recorded (2). The horizontal condylar lock is secured with the condylar element against the stop (3). The lateral condylar lock is secured (4). Guide lines are placed on the margins of the cast in positions that are visible when the record bases are seated: midline (A), point corresponding with the distal surface of the mandibular cuspid (B), point corresponding with the distal margin of the maxillary cuspid eminence (C), point designating half the height of the retromolar pad (D), and point designating the beginning of the ascent of the mandibular arch to the ramus (E).*

casts. The following procedures have been carried out:

1. The maxillary cast has been transferred to the articulator with a face-bow.

2. The mandibular cast has been mounted, using an interocclusal wax record. The record was a tentative record of the vertical dimensions of occlusion with the jaws in centric relation (terminal hinge position).

3. The low lip line has been adjusted to coincide with the low mark on the incisal guide pin.

4. The occlusal plane has been established between the low lip line in the anterior region and a point half the height of the retromolar pad in the posterior region.

Guide lines are then established to determine the positions of the artificial teeth (Fig. 15-2).

MAXILLARY CAST (Fig. 15-2A)

1. A line is drawn parallel to the frontal plane that touches the anterior margin of the incisal papilla.

2. The midline follows the midpalatal suture and bisects the incisal papilla. This line is perpendicular to line 1. When the cuspid eminences are present, the most distal extent is recorded with a line on the cast.

MANDIBULAR CAST (Fig. 15-2B)

1. A line is drawn parallel to the frontal plane, bisecting the residual ridge. The direction of the resorption of the residual ridge must be considered when this line is placed.

2. A point designates the distal of the mandibular cuspids. This point was recorded on the mandibular occlusion rim (Fig. 9-11).

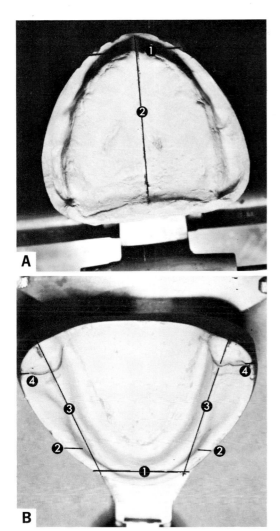

FIG. 15-2. *Guide lines aid in determining tooth position.* **A.** *Maxillary cast. The line designating the anterior margin of the incisal papilla (1) is the most valuable aid for positioning the maxillary anterior central incisors. The line designating the midline (2) is the division between the right and left quadrants of teeth.* **B.** *Mandibular cast. The line (1) bisecting the crest of the residual ridge aids in positioning the mandibular central incisors. The curve of the arch is followed for positioning the lateral incisors and the cuspids. The cuspid points (2) are the approximate points that designate the distal surfaces of the mandibular cuspids. The line following the crest of the residual ridge (3) from the cuspid point of the*

3. A line follows the crest of the residual ridge from the cuspid point to a point that bisects the retromolar pad at 4. This designates the guide for the buccolingual position of the mandibular posterior teeth.

4. A line that bisects the retromolar pad designates the posterior vertical occlusal plane.

The arrangement of the six maxillary anterior teeth is the third step (Fig. 15-3). The contoured occlusion rims, the incisal papilla, and the cuspid points are the guides (Fig. 15-3A). The labial surfaces of the central incisors should not be in a more anterior direction than the labial surface of the denture border that occupies the labial vestibule (Fig. 15-3B). When viewed from either the distal or the mesial, the long axis of the labial surfaces of the maxillary central incisors should harmonize with the profile of the patient (Fig. 15-3C). The left central incisor is placed in a slight anterior relation to the right central incisor (Fig. 15-3D).

In the arrangement of the mandibular anterior teeth an attempt is made to direct the *vertical* force toward the crest of the residual ridge (Fig. 15-4). This does not place the collar of the artificial teeth over the crest of the residual ridge.

Horizontal overlap is another consideration. It is determined by the anteroposterior and mediolateral relationship of the mandible to the maxillae (Fig. 15-5).

The mandibular posterior teeth are arranged before the maxillary posterior

---

retromolar pad is an aid in positioning the posterior teeth in an acceptable relation with the tongue and the cheeks. The line (4) that bisects the vertical height of the retromolar pad aids in establishing the vertical position of the occlusal surfaces of the posterior teeth.

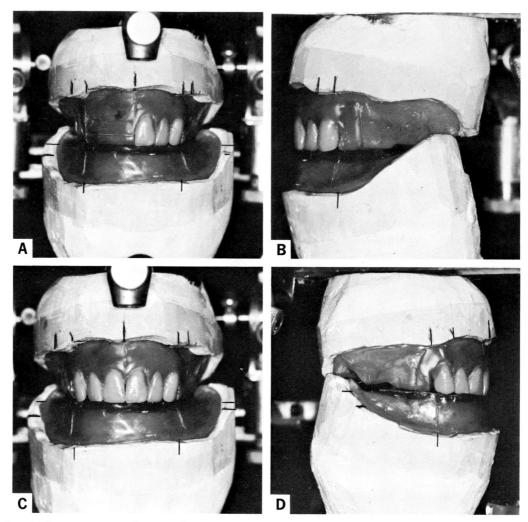

FIG. 15-3. *Arranging the maxillary anterior teeth.* **A.** *The central incisor, the lateral incisor, and the cuspid are arranged on one side before the contour of the occlusion rim on the other side is removed. This frontal view reveals the relation of the medial surface of the central incisor with the midline.* **B.** *This lateral view of the left maxillary anterior teeth shows the relation of the distal surface of the cuspid with the guide line that designates the distal margin of the maxillary cuspid eminence.* **C.** *The frontal view of all the maxillary anterior teeth reflects the symmetry of arrangement. This symmetry is retained at the try-in appointment.* **D.** *This lateral view points out the slight inclination of the neck of the cuspid in a distal direction.*

teeth for the following reasons (Fig. 15-6):

1. There are more anatomic landmarks to locate the guide lines in the mandibular arch.

2. The lingual surfaces of the mandibular posterior teeth are not placed more in a medial direction than is the medial surface of the lingual flange of the denture base.

3. The mandibular cuspids are the turning points in the arch.

4. The retromolar pad is used to determine the vertical height of the

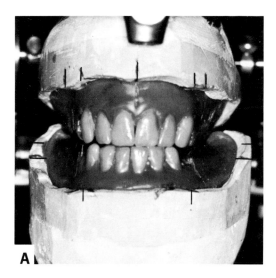

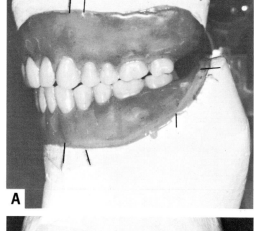

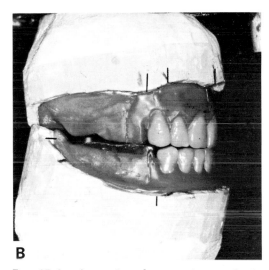

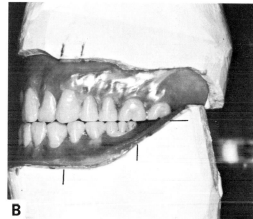

FIG. 15-4. *Arranging the anterior teeth.* **A.** *Frontal view depicting the relation of the mandibular to the maxillary anterior teeth. Note the asymmetry at the midline and the distal rotation of the cuspids toward the crest of the posterior residual ridge.* **B.** *Lateral view of the relation of the maxillary and mandibular cuspids. Note the guide lines for placing the distal slope of the incisal edge of the mandibular cuspid in the correct relation with the mesial slope of the incisal edge of the maxillary cuspid.*

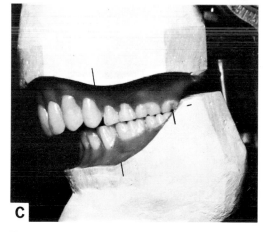

FIG. 15-5. *Variations in horizontal overlap.* **A.** *Normal maxillomandibular relations.* **B.** *Mandible in a protruded relation to the maxillae.* **C.** *Mandible in a retruded relation to the maxillae.*

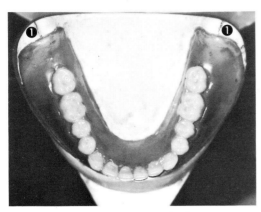

FIG. 15-6. *Arrangement of the posterior mandibular teeth. Notice the relation of the buccal cusps and the central sulci with the guide line designating the crest of the posterior residual ridge (1). The distal of the cuspid is rotated in the direction of this point.*

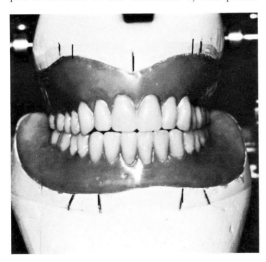

FIG. 15-7. *Arrangement of the posterior maxillary teeth. The lingual cusps are in contact in the fossae and marginal ridges of the mandibular posterior teeth, which are on a plane. This places the buccal cusps of the maxillary posterior teeth in a more lateral position than the buccal cusps of the mandibular posterior teeth (horizontal overlap).*

mandibular molars. The posterior occlusal plane is placed at half the vertical height of the retromolar pad when cusp form teeth are set on a plane. This position allows the molars to be elevated to the bottom of the upper third of the retromolar pad when the teeth are inclined for balanced occlusion. When noncusp teeth are set on a plane, the bottom of the upper third of the retromolar pad is used.

The maxillary posterior teeth are arranged in centric occlusion with the mandibular posterior teeth (Fig. 15-7). The buccal and the lingual cusp tips of the mandibular posterior teeth and the incisal edges of the mandibular anterior teeth are arranged on a plane. A flat metal plate is used as a guide. No attempt is made to arrange the teeth in balanced occlusion in eccentric positions or to develop compensating curves until all maxillomandibular records have been evaluated and the articulator has been adjusted.

Finally, the wax is contoured and smoothed to make it compatible with the lips, the cheeks, and the tongue (Fig. 15-8).

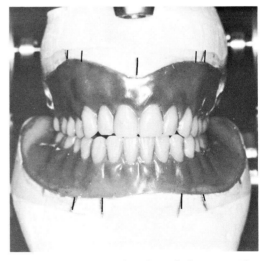

FIG. 15-8. *A completed trial denture. The wax is contoured, extended into the vestibule, and smoothed. The stability and retention of these trial dentures should be almost as adequate as that of the finished processed dentures.*

REFERENCES

1. Goyal, B. K., and Bhargava, K.: Arrangement of artificial teeth in abnormal jaw relations: Maxillary protrusion and wider upper arch. J. Prosth. Dent., *32*:107, 1974.

2. ———: Arrangement of artificial teeth in abnormal jaw relations: Mandibular protrusion and wider lower arch. J. Prosth. Dent., *32*:458, 1974.

3. Jordan, L. G.: Arrangement of anatomic-type artificial teeth into balanced occlusion. J. Prosth. Dent., *39*:484, 1978.

4. Roraff, A. R.: Arranging artificial teeth according to anatomic landmarks. J. Prosth. Dent., *38*:120, 1977.

Relating Inclinations of Teeth to Concepts of Occlusion

16

When discussing the inclinations of the teeth for complete dentures, one must consider the concepts of different occlusal schemes. The *neutrocentric concept* using noncusp form posterior teeth arranged on a plane and the *balanced occlusion* concept using cusp form posterior teeth arranged in balance in the centric and eccentric jaw positions are presented in depth.

The occlusal form will be decided by the type of occlusion to be developed. If the teeth are to be balanced in the centric and eccentric positions, a cusp form tooth is indicated. If the posterior teeth are to be arranged on a plane and balanced in centric position only (when the condyles are in their superior terminal relation in the fossae), monoplane teeth are used. Patients have not experienced a deficiency in masticating with either form of tooth. Soreness and discomfort of the supporting tissues have not been appreciably different. The study of the bony support has not produced any difference either in quantity or quality. The many variables encountered in a study of osseous structures have made it impossible to evaluate definitely the loss of, or the maintenance of bone as related to the various tooth forms.

It should be understood that the concept of balanced occlusion is desired when using cusp or modified cusp form teeth and that nonbalanced occlusion in the eccentric positions is desired for monoplane cusp form teeth. There are basic differences in the philosophy of using these two entirely different occlusal forms and arrangements.

Balanced occlusion is based primarily on the premise that stability is provided mechanically to the denture bases on their basal seats. When the teeth are brought together at any relationship of the jaws, at least a tripod type of contacting of the teeth provides stability to the bases.

The neutrocentric arrangement of the teeth on a plane (flat) parallel with the bony support is based primarily on physiologic principles. Although neutrocentric is used to denote the contacting of the teeth, the concept of arranging the teeth flat does involve jaw relationships. The physiologic principles involve the influence of the somatic nervous system in the control of muscle movement and proprioception. The mechanism involves making contact of the teeth when the condyles are in a comfortable, stable position in the fossae and the denture bases are stable and comfortably seated on the basal seats. The arrangement of teeth on a flat plane does not provide stability to the denture bases when the teeth contact with the jaws eccentrically related. When the teeth contact on unstable bases, the condyles are not in a stable position. When either the condyles or the denture bases are unstable, the result is discomfort, either excessive pressure or pain or both. The somatic nervous system—the receptors in and around the joints, in the periosteum, and in the mucosa of the lips, tongue, and cheeks—notifies the central nervous system of the discomfort. It is notifying the central nervous system to modify the muscle pattern until comfort is established. When this occurs, the muscle is programmed to make a jaw closure to tooth contact when the condyles are terminally related in the fossae. DeVan stated this thusly, "the patient will become a chopper, not a chewer or grinder."[5]

The results of arranging monoplane teeth in any other manner than that described in the neutrocentric concept should not be compared with other tooth forms or concepts. Arranging monoplane teeth in balanced occlusion provides a long inclined plane, a long cusp, and would be expected to produce different results.

A failure to discuss here in detail techniques for arranging artificial teeth in accordance with other concepts is not to say that other concepts are incapable of producing acceptable results. There is no scientific proof that teeth arranged in accordance with any concept will be acceptable in every situation. Clinical results are the criteria used today in evaluating the acceptability of complete dentures. One must maintain an open mind in each phase of denture procedure.

The concept of *spherical* occlusion involves the positioning of the teeth with anteroposterior and mediolateral inclines in harmony with a spherical surface.

The concept of *organic occlusion* calls for altering the shape of the cusps of the teeth to provide prosthetic teeth that have cusps suitable for the individual patient. The ridge and groove directions of the posterior teeth are determined as a result of the movements of the condyles. The cusp height, fossa depth of posterior teeth, and the proper concavity of the lingual surfaces of the maxillary anterior teeth are determined as a result of mandibular movements. The cusp-fossa contact relation is developed when the jaws are in centric relation.

As defined by Stuart, centric relation of the mandible occurs "when both condyles are firmly seated in their most posterior positions in the glenoid fossae. The jaws may be said to be in centric closure when this position of the condyles exists and the teeth are brought together. . . . The mandible is not in centric position if only one condyle is in its fossa; both must be in place."[25a]

When the mandible is moved in a protrusive direction, the incisors cause separation of the posterior teeth. When the mandible is moved in a lateral direction, the cuspids cause separation of the posterior teeth. The posterior teeth are altered by grinding and inclined to provide a lack of contact on the working and balancing side in eccentric mandibular movements. The cusps are related to a cusp-fossa centric relation in which the cusp can enter the fossae and escape without lateral or sagittal interferences. An articulator capable of receiving and reproducing pantograms in three planes is recommended to develop the organic concept of occlusion.

Neutrocentric Concept

The *neutrocentric* concept of occlusion maintains that the anteroposterior plane of occlusion should be parallel with the plane of the denture foundation and not dictated by the horizontal condylar guidances. A plane is a flat, level surface. When teeth are arranged on a plane, they are not inclined to form compensating curves. In a mediolateral direction the teeth are set flat with no medial or lateral inclination (Fig. 16-1).

The term *neutrocentric* is not used in connection with the relationship of the maxillae and mandible, but to denote a concept of occlusion that eliminates any anteroposterior or mediolateral inclines of the teeth and directs the forces of occlusion to the posterior teeth. The posterior teeth are placed in as mediolateral a relation in reference to the residual ridge as the tongue function will allow. The patient is instructed to avoid incising with the anterior teeth; therefore, there is no need to be concerned with the sagittal condylar incline. Be-

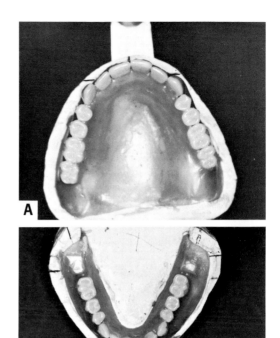

FIG. 16-2. *Occlusal view of trial dentures arranged for neutrocentric occlusion.* **A.** *Maxillary.* **B.** *Mandibular. Notice that the anteroposterior and mediolateral inclines have been eliminated for the posterior teeth.*

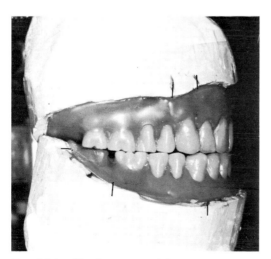

FIG. 16-1. *Teeth arranged for neutrocentric concept of occlusion.*

cause the form of the posterior tooth is devoid of cusp, there is no projection above or below the occlusal plane (Fig. 16-2). When incising is avoided and no cusps project above or below the occlusal plane, the horizontal condylar guidances of the articulator may be set at zero. Since the teeth are not arranged for balancing contacts when the jaws are eccentrically located, the lateral condylar guidances of the articulator also may be set at zero. The condylar elements of the articulator may be secured to function in the opening and closing movements. To direct force toward the center of the support and to reduce the frictional forces, the buccolingual width of the teeth is reduced. In addition, the number of teeth is reduced to direct the forces in the molar and bicuspid area of support and to refrain from placing a tooth on the ridge incline in the second molar area (Fig. 16-3).

Balanced Occlusion

The concept of *centralizing the working occlusal surfaces* requires bringing the occlusal surfaces toward the center of the denture foundation to their ideal positions for favorable leverage (Fig. 16-4). In the anteroposterior direction the center of the basal seat is in the area of the bicuspids and the first molars. This is the area where food is masticated. These working occlusal units ideally consist of the lingual halves of the two maxillary bicuspids and the first molar and their corresponding mandibular teeth. Most favorable leverage is obtained when the occlusal working surfaces are placed to the lingual sides of the ridge crests. The second molars are not always placed in the arrangement; if they are, they are placed out of occlusion. Depending upon the patient's maxillomandibular relation records, the working occlusal unit may consist of the distal half of the second bicuspid and the first molar or just the first molar.

In centric occlusion only the working occlusal units are in contact. The first bicuspids, the cuspids, and the incisors have at least 1 millimeter clearance when the teeth are in centric occlusion. In the mediolateral direction the buccal surfaces of the posterior teeth that extend over the lateral half of the residual alveolar ridge are ground to have at least 1 millimeter clearance with their antagonists. The upper and lower incisal units meet only when the mandibular

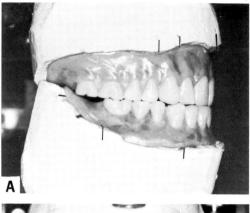

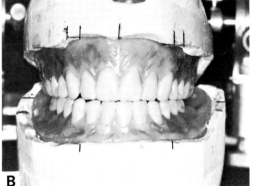

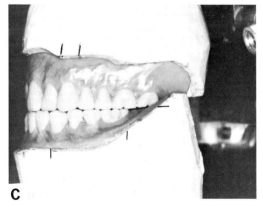

FIG. 16-3. *Inclinations of teeth for neutrocentric occlusion.* **A.** *Teeth arranged on a plane.* **B.** *Anterior teeth for slightly protruded mandible arranged with incisal edges end to end.* **C.** *Mandibular posterior teeth on a plane parallel with mean denture base. The maxillary second molar is not inclined for protrusive balance but is placed to support the cheek. Note the reduction in the number of mandibular posterior teeth.*

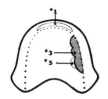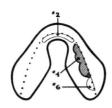

FIG. 16-4. *Diagram to show arrangement of the upper and lower occlusal units to centralize the working occlusal surfaces: maxillary (1) and mandibular (2) incisal units; maxillary (3) and mandibular (4) occlusal units placed to the lingual sides of the ridge crests; upper first molar (5) inclined for bilateral balance in lateral occlusion; lower second molar (6) inclined for protrusive balance. (From Nagle and Sears: Denture Prosthetics, 2nd ed. St. Louis, The C. V. Mosby Company, 1962.)*

teeth are protruded, and the protrusive balancing unit functions only when the upper and lower incisal units contact. The lingual surface of the maxillary first molar provides bilateral balance in lateral occlusion of the teeth. If the maxillary working occlusal units must be placed on the labial side of the crest, the lingual surface of the first molar helps to balance the upper denture. The mandibular second molar may likewise be used to obtain bilateral balance.

The inclinations of teeth can be arranged on a Class II, Type 3 articulator to provide bilateral (Fig. 16-5) and protrusive (Fig. 16-6) *balanced occlusion*. The number and exact positions of contact developed on the articulator may or may not be reproduced in the exact number or position in the mouth. The resiliency and displaceability of the supporting tissues, the methods and materials used in making maxillomandibular relation records, and the inability of the articulator to receive and duplicate records of the eccentric mandibular movements account for the discrepancies. Although it is not an exact

duplication, sufficient simultaneous contacts will take place in the three areas of the arches to exert a stabilizing force sufficient to prevent dislodging the denture. When a cusp form posterior tooth is used, it is necessary to develop balanced occlusion. If premature tooth contacts occur in gliding occlusion, they are evaluated in the mouth and removed by grinding the offending tooth or teeth.

To incline the teeth to develop a balanced occlusion one needs an adjustable articulator with some additional features. It should (1) receive a kinematic face-bow transfer, (2) adjust to individual intercondylar distance, (3) have an adjustable guide table, and (4) have the condylar elements in the mandibular bow and the condylar guides attached to the maxillary bow (Arcon principle).

To adjust the articulator requires (1) a centric relation record, (see page 273) and (2) an eccentric protrusive record (see page 285). Right and left lateral relation records are desirable if the articulator is capable of accurately accepting and being adjusted to the records. If the articulator will not receive the lateral records and is a tracking or Hanau type of instrument, use the formula suggested by Hanau to adjust the lateral condylar guidance:

$$L = \frac{H}{8} + 12.$$

The maxillary cast is transferred from the patient to the articulator with a face-bow. When the actual hinge axis is located, use the kinematic face-bow. When the arbitrary points of location of the hinge axis are used, use the Snow type of face-bow. When the Bergstrom or Whip Mix articulators are used, a special face-bow using the external auditory meatus as point of orientation for the opening axis is used. When the casts have been properly

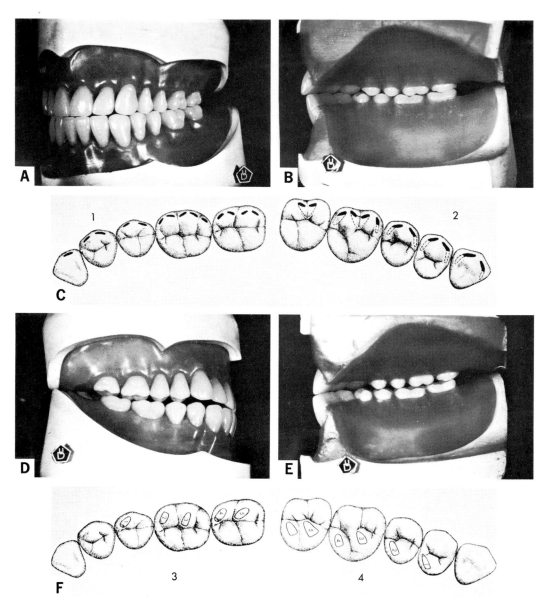

Fig. 16-5. *Teeth inclined for bilateral balanced occlusion. Buccal (**A**) and lingual (**B**) views of the teeth inclined to make occlusal contacts on the working side. (Courtesy of the Universal Dental Company, Philadelphia, Pennsylvania.)* **C.** *The dark areas designate the contact areas of the tips of the mandibular buccal cusps on the working side (1) and the tips of the maxillary buccal cusps (2). The guiding inclines are within the broken lines, as illustrated on the lingual inclines of the buccal cusps of the maxillary teeth (2). (From Ramfjord and Ash: Occlusion. Philadelphia, W. B. Saunders Company, 1966.) Buccal (**D**) and lingual (**E**) views of the teeth inclined to make occlusal contacts on the balancing side. (Courtesy of the Universal Dental Company, Philadelphia, Pennsylvania.)* **F.** *The numbered areas on the buccal cusps of the mandibular teeth (3) make contact with the areas of like numbers on the lingual cusps of the maxillary teeth (4). (From Ramfjord and Ash: Occlusion. Philadelphia, W. B. Saunders Company, 1966.)*

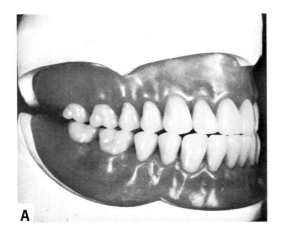

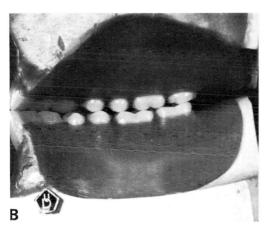

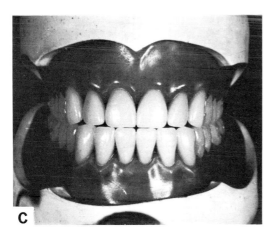

FIG. 16-6. *Teeth inclined for protrusive balance.* **A.** *Buccal view. Note the incline relations of the cusps.* **B.** *Lingual view. Note the tip relations of the cusps.* **C.** *Frontal view. Note the relations of the incisal edges.*

mounted on the articulator, the antero-posterior and mediolateral positions of the teeth are determined (page 255). Vertical positions of the incisal edges of the anterior teeth and the occlusal surfaces of the posterior teeth are established on a plane from the lower lip line to the bottom of the top third of the retromolar pad. This position on the retromolar pad is used to allow the mandibular molars space to be inclined in a vertical direction when the teeth are altered for balance and not to exceed the top of the pad (page 323). The maxillary and mandibular anterior teeth are positioned for esthetics (page 327), and the posterior teeth are positioned in centric occlusion on the plane for the trial denture (Fig. 16-7). When the accuracy of the centric relation record has been verified, the vertical dimension of occlusion has been determined, and the positions of the teeth have been accepted for esthetic purposes, the protrusive relation record is made and the articulator is adjusted for condylar guidance.

To balance the occlusion, the teeth are inclined to harmonize with the three controlling end factors, the right and left condylar inclinations and the incisal guidance (Fig. 16-8). Condyle paths are peculiar to each individual, and the dentist has no control over horizontal or lateral inclinations. The dentist can in no way modify the condyle path. When the condylar inclinations have been registered and the articulator has been set, it is not the right of the dentist to increase or decrease the articulator settings.

The *sagittal* incisal guide angle is the angle formed with the horizontal plane by drawing a line in the sagittal plane between incisal edges of the maxillary and mandibular central incisors when the teeth are in centric occlusion. The term *incisal guidance* refers to the in-

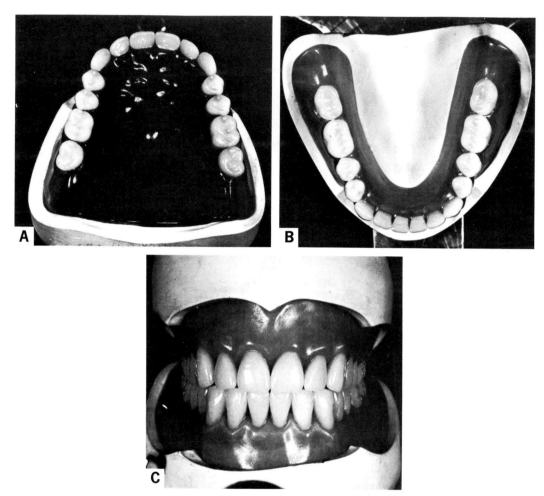

FIG. 16-7. A. *Occlusal view of the maxillary trial denture, showing the anterior teeth positioned for esthetics and the posterior teeth arranged in harmony with the mandibular posterior teeth.* **B.** *Occlusal view of the mandibular trial denture with the anterior teeth positioned to direct a vertical force toward the crest of the residual ridge. The central sulci of the posterior teeth are positioned over the crest of the posterior residual ridge.* **C.** *Frontal view of the completed arrangement of teeth for the trial denture. The mandibular teeth are on a plane. The wax is contoured and smooth. (Courtesy of the Universal Dental Company, Philadelphia, Pennsylvania.)*

fluence on mandibular movements of the lingual surfaces of the maxillary anterior teeth. The incisal guidance may be expressed in degrees from the horizontal plane (Fig. 16-9).

The *lateral* incisal guide angle may be defined as the steepest angle formed with the horizontal plane by drawing a line between the incisal edges of the maxillary and mandibular incisors and cuspids of both the right and left segments when the teeth are in centric occlusion. In complete denture construction the dentist has control over the

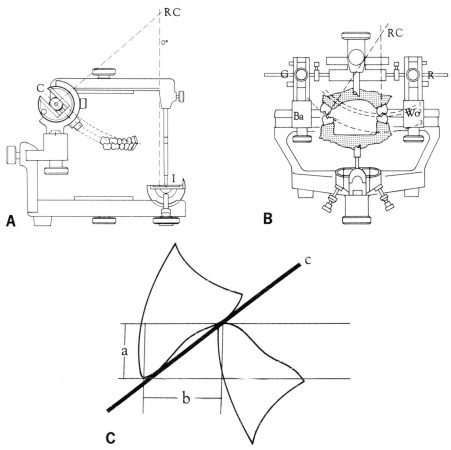

Fig. 16-8. *Schematic representation of controlling end factors.* **A.** *The teeth must be inclined in harmony with the anteroposterior compensating curve. The condyle paths are fixed. The incisal guidance can be controlled within the limits of esthetic acceptance. Condylar guide (C); incisal guide table (I); rotational center (RC).* **B.** *The teeth must be inclined in harmony with the mediolateral compensating curve. The curve is steeper on the balancing side (Ba) than on the working side (Wo). The gliding condyle (G); the rotating condyle (R); rotational center (RC).* **C.** *Diagram of the sagittal incisal guide angle: vertical overlap (a); horizontal overlap (b); incisal guide angle (c). (Suggested by Swenson's Complete Dentures. 5th ed. St. Louis, The C. V. Mosby Company, 1964.)*

incisal guidance. The decision to use this control depends upon the shape, fullness, and relationship of the residual ridges, the vertical interarch space, and the esthetic requirements of the patient.

When all other factors are acceptable, the esthetic requirements of the patient are frequently the factor the dentist

must consider. The patient's desire to have the artificial anterior teeth placed in the same positions occupied by the clinical crowns of the natural teeth may present a compromising situation. When the natural teeth are related with a steep vertical overlap without compensating horizontal overlap, this relationship may

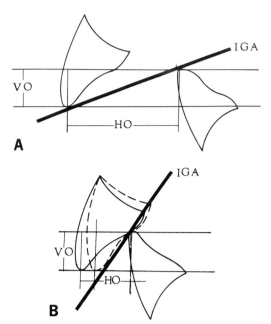

FIG. 16-9. *The amount of horizontal (HO) and vertical (VO) overlap determines the sagittal incisal guide angle (IGA). **A.** The sagittal incisal guide angle is less when the horizontal overlap is increased by separating the teeth in an anteroposterior direction. The reverse is true when the horizontal overlap is decreased. **B.** The sagittal incisal guide angle is less when the horizontal overlap is increased by inclining the incisal edge of the maxillary anterior teeth in an anterior direction. The reverse is true when the incisal edges of the maxillary anterior teeth are inclined in a distal direction. (Suggested by Swenson's Complete Dentures. 5th ed. St. Louis, The C. V. Mosby Company, 1964.)*

or may not be physiologically tolerated. This situation appears to be tolerated in some mouths, for undoubtedly the mandibular movements have accommodated to the tooth positions.

If the artificial teeth are placed in this relationship, protrusive balanced occlusion would not be possible unless a very steep anteroposterior and mediolateral pitch of the posterior teeth is provided. This positioning of teeth for complete dentures is not desirable. It is desirable to arrange the anterior teeth with a vertical and horizontal overlap with an incisal guide angle of near zero degrees. This positioning of the teeth reduces the inclines in a mediolateral and anteroposterior direction. Forces directed at inclines are more dislodging than forces directed at right angles to the support. It appears that the steeper the incline, the more dislodging the force.

When the vertical incisal position of the maxillary anterior teeth is esthetically acceptable, the vertical occlusal position of the mandibular teeth has been evaluated for esthetic and functional positions, and the condylar guidances have been determined by a protrusive record, one must decide whether to balance the teeth in bilateral and protrusive mandibular positions or to balance the teeth in a bilateral position with no balance in the protrusive position. A deviation from protrusive and bilateral balanced occlusion is not in accord with the concept of balanced occlusion. It is a compromise. When (1) the maxillary cast is mounted on the articulator with a face-bow transfer, (2) the mandibular cast is mounted with a centric relation record at the acceptable vertical dimension of occlusion, (3) a protrusive relation record has been made and the horizontal and lateral condylar guidances have been adjusted, and (4) the vertical position of the maxillary anterior teeth has been accepted for esthetic positions, the inclines of the teeth are arranged in harmony with the anteroposterior and mediolateral dictates of the end-controlling factors. When the teeth are inclined to harmonize with their dictates, the mediolateral and anteroposterior compensating curves are developed (Fig. 16-8).

To establish *balanced gliding occlusion* during the travel of the condyles along their paths necessitates an accurate reproduction of the curvature of the paths. Pantograms and individually contoured condylar guide paths are used to reproduce the condyle paths.

REFERENCES

1. Beck, H. O.: Occlusal concepts in complete dentures. J. Prosth. Dent., *30*:515, 1973.
1a. Becker, C. M., Swoope, C. C., and Guckes, A. D.: Lingualized occlusion for removable prosthodontics. J. Prosth. Dent., *38*:601, 1977.
1b. Christensen, F. T.: Cusp angulation for complete dentures. J. Prosth. Dent., *8*:910, 1958.
2. ———: The effect of Bonwill's triangle on complete dentures. J. Prosth. Dent., *9*:791, 1959.
3. ———: The compensating curve for complete dentures. J. Prosth. Dent., *10*:637, 1960.
4. ———: The effect of incisal guidance on cusp angulation in prosthetic occlusion. J. Prosth. Dent., *11*:48, 1961.
5. De Van, M. M.: Synopsis, stability in full denture construction. Penn. Dent. J., *22*:8, 1955.
5a. Elkins, W. E.: Gold occlusal surfaces and organic occlusion in denture construction. J. Prosth. Dent., *30*:94, 1973.
6. Ford, W. B.: Technic and occlusal form designed to produce stability in dentures. J.A.D.A., *54*:212, 1957.
7. Frahm, F. W.: Incisal guidance—its influence in compensation and balance. J.A.D.A., *13*:771, 1926.
8. Gillis, R. R.: Setting up the full dentures producing a balanced articulation. J.A.D.A., *17*:228, 1930.
8a. Gronas, D. G., and Stout, C. J.: Lineal occlusion concepts for complete dentures. J. Prosth. Dent., *32*:122, 1974.
9. Gysi, A.: Resiliency and the like in its effect on the facet angulations of artificial teeth. Dent. Dig., *36*:623, 1930.
10. Hall, W. A.: Orientation of the plane of occlusion in complete removable dentures. J. North Carolina Dent. Soc., *37*:98, 1954.
11. Hardy, I. R.: Technique for the use of non-anatomic acrylic posterior teeth. Dent. Dig., *48*:562, 1942.
11a. Javid, N. S., and Porter, M. R.: The importance of the Hanau formula in construction of complete dentures. J. Prosth. Dent., *34*:397, 1975.
11b. Jordan, L. G.: Arrangement of anatomic-type artificial teeth into balanced occlusion. J. Prosth. Dent., *39*:484, 1978.
11c. Koyama, M., Inaba, S., and Yokoyama, K.: Quest for ideal occlusal patterns for complete dentures. J. Prosth. Dent., *35*:620, 1976.
11d. Levin, B.: Review of artificial posterior tooth forms including a preliminary report on a new posterior tooth. J. Prosth. Dent., *38*:3, 1977.
11e. ———: A reevaluation of Hanau's laws of articulation and the Hanau Quint. J. Prosth. Dent., *39*:254, 1978.
12. McNamara, D. C.: Occlusal adjustment for a physiologically balanced occlusion. J. Prosth. Dent., *38*:284, 1977.
12a. Mehringer, E. J.: Function of steep cusps in mastication with complete dentures. J. Prosth. Dent., *30*:367, 1973.
12b. Mjor, P. S.: The effect of the end controlling guidances of the articulation on cusp inclination. J. Prosth. Dent., *15*:1055, 1965.
13. Needles, J. W.: The mechanics of spherical articulation. J.A.D.A., *9*:866, 1922.
14. ———: Practical uses of the curve of Spee. J.A.D.A., *10*:918, 1923.
15. Perkins, G. T.: Equalization of pressure by symmetrical setup. J. Prosth. Dent., *3*:155, 1953.
16. Pleasure, M. A.: Occlusion of cuspless teeth for balance and comfort. J. Prosth. Dent., *5*:305, 1955.
17. Porter, C. G.: The cuspless centralized occlusal pattern. J. Prosth. Dent., *5*:313, 1955.
18. Schlosser, R. O.: Arrangement of teeth in artificial dentures in accordance with accepted laws of articulation. J.A.D.A., *16*:1258, 1929.
19. Schuyler, C. H.: Full denture service as influenced by our understanding of tooth selection and articulation. J. Prosth. Dent., *2*:730, 1952.
20. ———: The function and importance of incisal guidance in oral rehabilitation. J. Prosth. Dent., *13*:1011, 1963.

21. Sears, V. H.: Balanced occlusion. J.A.D.A., *12*:1448, 1925.

22. ———: Scientific management of factors in bilateral prosthetic occlusion. J.A.D.A., *37*:542, 1948.

23. Shanahan, T. E., Jr.: The individual occlusal curvature and occlusion. J. Prosth. Dent., *8*:230, 1958.

24. Standard, S. G.: Establishing plane of occlusion in complete denture construction. J.A.D.A., *54*:845, 1957.

25. Stansbery, C. J.: Balanced occlusion in relation to lost vertical dimension. J.A.D.A., *25*:228, 1938.

25a. Stuart, C. E.: Articulation of human teeth. *In* McCollum and Stuart's *A Research Report*. South Pasadena, Calif., Scientific Press. 1955, p. 91.

26. Trapozzano, V. R.: Test of balanced and nonbalanced occlusion. J. Prosth. Dent., *10*:476, 1960.

27. ———: Laws of articulation. J. Prosth. Dent., *13*:34, 1963; Boucher, C. O.: Discussion of "laws of articulation." J. Prosth. Dent., *13*:45, 1963.

28. Villa, A. H.: Curved occlusal planes are contraindicated. J. Prosth. Dent., *9*:797, 1959.

29. ———: Technique for arranging posterior teeth. J. Prosth. Dent., *9*:803, 1959.

30. ———: A technique for the use of nonanatomic posterior teeth. J. Prosth. Dent., *12*:298, 1962.

31. Weinberg, L. A.: The occlusal plane and cuspal inclination in relation to incisal-condylar guidance for protrusive excursions. J. Prosth. Dent., *9*:607, 1959.

32. Woelfel, J. B., Winter, C. M., and Igarashi, T.: Five-year cephalometric study of mandibular ridge resorption with different posterior occlusal forms—Part I. J. Prosth. Dent., *36*:602, 1976.

Laboratory Procedures

17

Laboratory procedures are seldom performed by dentists. However, every dentist should know the requirements of the finished denture. This knowledge will enable him to evaluate the laboratory procedures and the finished denture.

Wax Contouring

Although the tissue sides of the denture bases are created in the impressions, the polished surfaces are developed by contouring the wax. The polished surfaces will be in contact with the oral tissues almost as intimately as the tissue side. Therefore, tissue tolerance, stability, and retention of the denture are greatly affected by the polished surface—its contours and finish (Fig. 17-1).

REQUIREMENTS

The requirements of the polished surfaces are as follows:

1. They should duplicate the covered soft tissue as accurately as possible—realistic, *not exaggerated* (Fig. 17-2).

2. The borders, both labial and buccal, should fill the vestibule.

3. Notches should be provided to accommodate the mucous membrane attachments (frenum), both in size and direction.

4. The contour of denture flanges should be compatible with the drape of the cheeks and lips.

5. The contour of the lingual flanges should be compatible with the tongue. This does not mean providing a trench in the flange to *trap* the tongue (Fig. 17-3).

6. The palatal section of the maxillary denture should be nearly a reproduction of the patient's palate, *rugae* included (Fig. 17-4). However, this is not suggested for a denture wearer if the palate was not reproduced in the denture initially. If he has become accustomed to a slick palate, don't make this change.

PROCEDURE

1. Contour wax carefully to prevent movement of the teeth.

2. Avoid a bulky wax-up. The additional bulk of acrylic resin may contribute to porosity and dimensional processing error.

3. Place strips of baseplate wax along the facial surface of the trial denture so that they extend from the gingival third of the teeth to the edge of the cast. With a hot spatula, lute the strips to the underlying wax at ¼ inch intervals, and melt the wax into contact with the necks of the teeth. After the wax has cooled, carve the interdental papillae to resemble the natural papillae. They vary with the age of the patient. Develop the

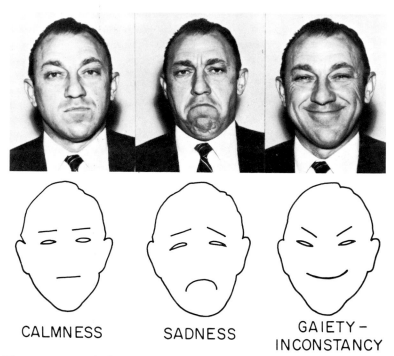

CALMNESS   SADNESS   GAIETY - INCONSTANCY

Fig. 17-1. *The positions of the teeth and the contour of the polished surfaces must be compatible with the surrounding oral environment. The muscles of facial expression should be uninhibited. The patient should be able to express calmness, sadness, gaiety, or any other emotion without restraint from dentures. (From Mosher, H. D.: Laryngoscope, 61:1–38, 1951.)*

margin by carving at a 45° angle to the neck of the tooth. The posterior area should have a marked fullness. The posterior tissues are rounded, devoid of groove and stippling. The festoons or ledges around the teeth are not contoured as roots of the teeth (Fig. 17-2B).

4. Wax the lingual flange of the mandibular denture thickly enough to fill all depressions and to slope down from the

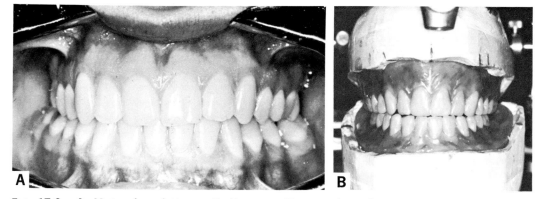

Fig. 17-2. A. *Natural oral tissue.* **B.** *Denture. To reproduce the natural contours so that the denture feels and looks natural, one must know the topography of the hard and soft tissues.*

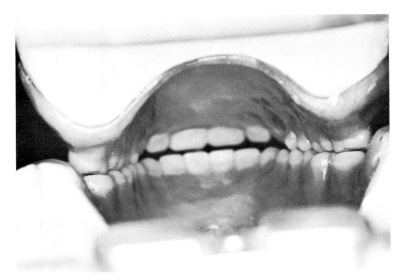

FIG. 17-3. *The contour of the palate and the lingual flanges should accommodate the tongue in repose and in function.*

necks of the teeth and inward toward the tongue. The slope of the flange should be free from undercuts and very slightly concave at or near the lower border.

5. Contour the wax around the necks of the maxillary posterior artificial teeth to form part of the clinical crowns and to make these teeth more natural in size and more compatible to the tongue

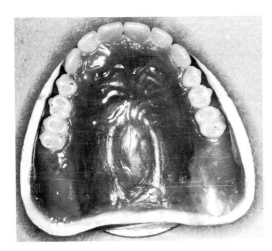

FIG. 17-4. *The palatal contours can be duplicated.*

(Fig. 17-3). As manufactured, these artificial teeth are short on the palatal side.

6. After the wax has been contoured, smooth it by flaming and then polish it with wet cotton. Oils are not recommended (Fig. 17-2B).

Flasking of Dentures

Flasking is the process of investing the cast with the waxed denture in a flask to make a sectional mold used to form the acrylic resin denture base. The following instructions apply to both the maxillary and the mandibular denture unless otherwise specified.

PROCEDURE

1. Soak the cast and mounting in water a few minutes. Separate the cast from the plaster articulator mounting. Save the plaster mounting, as it will be used to reposition the cast on the articulator after the dentures are processed. Adapt a layer of tinfoil to the base of the casts, slightly overlapping the edges (Fig. 17-5). This procedure, which takes very little effort and time, will insure

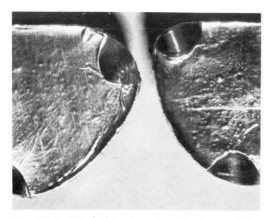

FIG. 17-5. *Tinfoil is placed on the base of the cast before flasking.*

clean removal from the investment. Apply liquid soap to the cast to act as a separator.

2. Invest the lower half of the flask first.

a. Center the cast in the lower half of the flask (Fig. 17-6A,B).

b. Use a mixture of half diluted plaster and half Hydrocal for this investment.

c. Remove any undercuts in the investment. Undercuts will prevent the separation of the upper ring from the lower portions of the flask after they boil out.

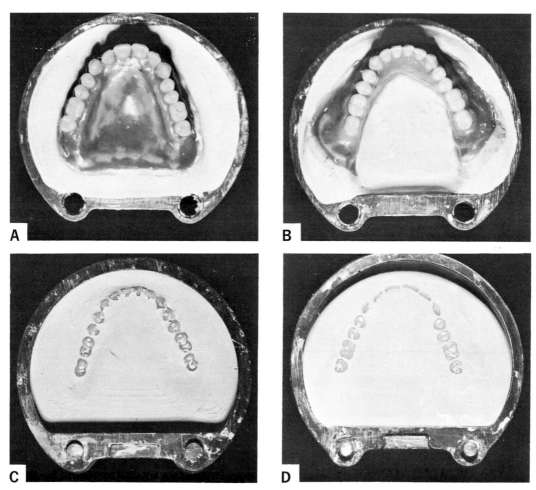

FIG. 17-6.   A, B. *The maxillary and the mandibular waxed dentures are centered and invested in the lower half of the flask in a mix of half plaster and half Hydrocal.* **C, D.** *The upper half of the flask is seated. A mix of half Hydrocal and half plaster is poured. Note that the occlusal surfaces of the anterior teeth are exposed.*

d. Allow the investment to set.

3. Proceed then with the second investment.

a. Apply a separating medium (liquid soap) to the investment in the lower half of the flask.

b. Position the ring portion of the flask. Carefully pour a second mix of half plaster and half Hydrocal over the teeth, and bring the stone to the occlusal surfaces of the invested teeth, leaving exposed the occlusal surfaces of the posterior and the incisal edges of the anterior teeth (Fig. 17-6C,D).

4. Make the final investment.

a. Apply a separating medium (liquid soap) to the ring portion of the investment.

b. Complete the investment with a mix of Hydrocal. Hydrocal resists more pressure than a mixture of Hydrocal and plaster.

c. Fill the ring with the mix, place the top of the flask in position, and secure the cast in the flask press.

Preparation of Mold

WAX ELIMINATION

After the flasking, let the stone completely set; place the flask on a ladle and lower it into boiling water for *five* minutes. This will soften the waxed denture base, which can then be easily removed from the mold when the flask is opened. After five minutes, remove the flask from the boiling water and gently open it. Do not force it open, but insert an instrument between the upper and lower halves and gently separate them.

Remove the semisolid pieces of the waxed denture base. All the teeth should remain in the top half of the flask. If any of them have been pulled loose from the mold, set them aside temporarily. Using hot water and a ladle, flush out all the remaining wax and any residue that may be present. Saturate

a piece of cotton with wax solvent and apply it around the teeth, scrubbing all the wax residue from the stone. As soon as possible, flush the mold with clean hot water to which a detergent has been added. The detergent will flush out the wax residue from areas that cannot be reached with the wax solvent. Immediately after using the detergent solution, flush the mold with clean hot water to remove all traces of the detergent solution.

It is essential to remove all wax residue. Acrylic resin will not adhere to a surface coated with wax (Fig. 17-7).

Stand the flask on its side and allow it to drain. If any teeth were pulled loose, clean them thoroughly with wax solvent and plain hot water. After the mold and the teeth have dried, carefully cement any loose teeth back in their correct positions with clear household cement.

While the flask is drying and cooling off, outline a relief over the incisive papilla. The tinfoil used to create the relief may be held in position with a small amount of household cement (Fig. 17-8). Although auxiliary personnel may place and cement the relief, the dentist himself should determine the need for relief areas and should be responsible for outlining them.

APPLICATION OF
TINFOIL SUBSTITUTE

Hardened plaster or stone is absorbent. The surface of the mold must therefore be made nonabsorbent, or liquid acrylic resin will soak into the stone during processing. If liquid acrylic resin penetrates the mold surface, the finished denture base will have a crust of acrylic resin and plaster or stone that will have to be removed during finishing. The result is an improperly contoured, and hence an unesthetic and a poorly fitting, denture base. This absorption of liquid resin may be pre-

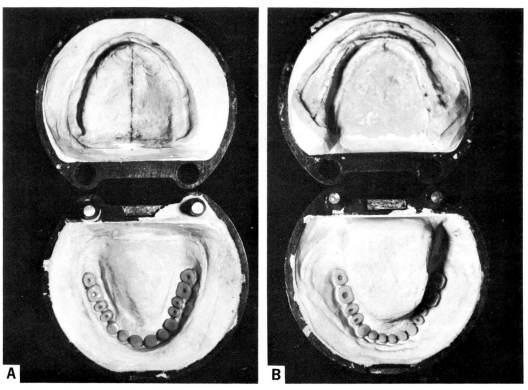

FIG. 17-7. *The flasks have been opened, the residue of wax has been removed, and the teeth are firmly seated in their matrices.* **A.** *Maxillary.* **B.** *Mandibular.*

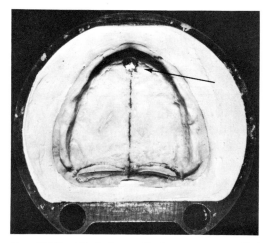

FIG. 17-8. *Tinfoil applied to create relief over the incisal papilla. The arrow designates the relief area.*

vented by applying a separating medium to the surface of the mold.

Many authorities consider that tinfoil is the best separating medium.[17,25a] The process of tinfoiling, however, is tedious and time-consuming unless a technician has had extensive practical experience with it.

An alternative method of preventing the absorption of liquid resin by the mold surface is the use of liquid tinfoil (alginate compound) substitute that can be painted on the mold to seal the pores of the investment. Present day tinfoil substitutes can be used successfully if all the wax residue is carefully cleaned from the pores of the plaster or stone and the tinfoil substitute is carefully applied to seal all the pores of the stone or plaster.

If tinfoil was applied to the waxed denture after it was half flasked, the upper section of the flask is ready for packing. If tinfoil was not applied, two coats of tinfoil substitute must be painted on the mold. Using an inlay brush, apply the liquid around the teeth and over the surface of the plaster or stone. *Do not paint the cast side of the flask at this time.* If the tinfoil substitute is applied as soon as possible after the wax elimination and drying process and while the mold is still warm, the liquid will dry quickly and adhere to the plaster or stone. Allow the first coat to dry; then apply the second coat in the same manner, and allow it to dry. This procedure should produce a smooth and shiny mold surface.

If the cast side of the flask is coated with one of the tinfoil substitutes, apply it after packing the flask and a trial closure, but before the final closure.

Preparing and Packing Acrylic Resin

Observe strict cleanliness in handling and packing acrylic resin denture base material to avoid introducing foreign matter that may change the color of the material as well as its physical properties. Never touch the material with bare hands. The oil on the hands can contaminate the material.

MIXING THE ACRYLIC RESIN

Measure and mix the polymer and monomer according to the manufacturer's directions. Usually 10 cc of monomer and 30 cc of polymer will be enough to pack an average-sized denture. First, pour the momomer into a clean porcelain jar; then add the polymer. Stir with a clean spatula until the monomer and polymer are thoroughly combined.

Place the lid on the jar and allow the mixture to stand; then open the jar, and

test the material with a spatula. When it is doughy but not sticky, the material is ready for packing. If too little time is allowed for the monomer to soften the polymer completely before the acrylic resin is packed, there will be fine pinholes on the surface of the polished denture.

PACKING THE ACRYLIC RESIN

Pack the material in the upper half of the flask, being sure to press it well into the area around the teeth. Use the index finger covered with cellophane. To avoid trapping air between the material and the mold, pack in one direction. Use enough material to insure overpacking on the first closure.

Place two pieces of wet cellophane between the folds of a towel to remove the excess water; then place the cellophane over the acrylic resin. Put the lower half of the flask in position, and press the flask together, using hand pressure. Place the flask in a bench press, and close it very slowly to give the acrylic resin plenty of time to flow. Finger pressure is adequate until the final closure.

Remove the flask from the press, open the flask carefully, and trim off the excess acrylic resin with a sharp Roach carver or scalpel. Add a small amount of acrylic resin in three or four places, using new cellophane, close the flask, and return it to the press. Close the press slowly, and again remove any excess material as before. Test pack until all excess material has been removed, and the metal edges of the parts of the flask are in complete contact.

Apply a tinfoil substitute to the lower part of the mold that contains the cast. Two coats are sufficient. Allow the first coat to dry before applying the second coat. Assemble the upper and lower halves of the flask and place them in the processing press. Secure the press with positive pressure to insure that the metal edges of the flask are flush together.

Processing of Dentures

The processing or polymerization of acrylic resin is the conversion of the monomer to the polymer when a mixture of the two is subjected to heat. Polymerization can also be induced by chemical activators such as those in the acrylic resins used for repairs.

The amount of heat must be controlled while processing acrylic resin, as the reaction is exothermic and becomes very rapid at temperatures between 140° and 160°F. Once polymerization has begun, the temperature of the resin may be considerably higher than the temperature of the water bath. For this reason, the temperature of the water should be maintained at, or below, 160°F for at least 1½ hours so that the exothermic heat can be conducted away from the resin into the investing material. The time required for the temperature of the resin to drop to the temperature of the water bath depends on the type and size of the flask, the amount of resin in the mold, and the temperature of the flask when packed.

The boiling point of the monomer is 212°F. If the heat is not controlled, the exothermic reaction will cause the monomer in the thick bulky sections of the denture to boil during the curing process and result in areas of porosity.

SLOW PROCESSING

If a long, slow cure in water is used, 9 hours at a constant 160°F is considered adequate for the average denture. If boiling also is desired in the slow cure, the temperature should be held at 160°F for nine hours and then raised to 212°F for thirty minutes.

Deflasking of Dentures

REMOVING THE MOLD

After the acrylic resin of a denture base has been processed, the flask should be cooled slowly to room temperature before the denture is deflasked. Remove the cover and put the flask, with its open end up, into the ejector deflasking press. Place the metal plate of the press on the stone and, using minimum pressure, eject the mold from the upper half of the flask. Invert the lower half of the flask, put it into the press, and place the metal plate used in ejecting the mold from the lower half of the flask over the knockout plug in the bottom. Using minimum pressure, slowly force the mold out of the lower half of the flask.

REMOVING THE DENTURE AND CAST

With a saw, cut the outer walls of the stone from top to bottom in the right and left cuspid areas and at the right and left distal ends. With a plaster knife, gently pry the sectioned plaster away from the facial surfaces of the teeth. If reasonable care is used, the teeth will not fracture because the plaster and stone in the lingual or the palatal section of the mold will support the teeth against the force used in fracturing the plaster when the outer sections are cut away. After removing the outer sections of stone from the denture, trim the stone away from the lingual surfaces of the teeth before attempting to remove the inner section of plaster and stone. This procedure will reduce the likelihood of breaking the teeth and will also prevent lifting the denture from the cast when the remaining plaster is removed. Remove the thin layer of plaster and tinfoil from the flat surface of the cast.

During deflasking be careful to preserve the cast; also, do not lift or remove the dentures from the casts. Clean all

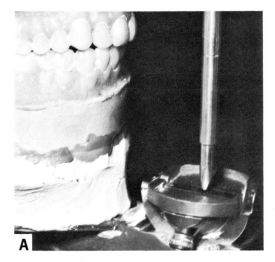

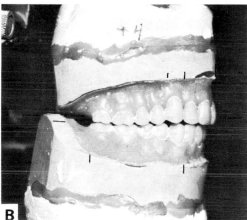

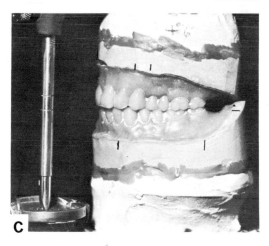

A

B

C

plaster and bubbles from the exposed acrylic resin and from around the teeth. Scrub the denture and cast thoroughly before starting the laboratory remount.

Laboratory Remount Procedure

Before removing the deflasked dentures from the cast, remove the investing Hydrocal from the teeth, the denture, and the cast. Remount the cast on the articulator so that any change in contact relation of the occlusal surfaces that may have occurred during processing may be noted and corrected.

Reposition the stone casts on the original plaster mountings. Attach the mountings to the articulator; lock the condylar elements in centric relation, and close the articulator. If the incisal pin does not touch the incisal guide table when the articulator is closed, the occlusal vertical dimension has been altered and must be re-established (Fig. 17-9A).

To re-establish the occlusal vertical dimension, lock the upper arm of the articulator so that only a hinge movement will be possible. Check the occlusion by first opening and closing the articulator and then by loosening the locks on the condylar elements and moving the dentures laterally (Fig. 17-9B). Relock the condylar elements before grinding. The interceptive occlusal contacts are found by lightly tapping the teeth together on interposed silk ribbon, dental tape, carbon paper, or articulating paper. Since smearing of the indicating color of articulating paper may cause false markings, which make

FIG. 17-9. *Remounted casts.* **A.** *Incisal guide pin 1.5 mm above incisal guide table.* **B.** *Alteration in occlusal relations.* **C.** *Vertical* dimension re-established by selective grinding of the teeth. The incisal guide pin rests on the incisal guide table.

determination of the initial interceptive occlusal contact more difficult, ribbon, tape, or carbon paper is preferred in selective grinding procedures.

If the cusp is high in both centric and eccentric positions, reduce the cusp. If the cusp is high in centric position only, deepen the fossa. The vertical dimension is re-established when the incisal pin again touches the incisal guide table (Fig. 17-9C). The final refinement of eccentric occlusion is reserved until new records are obtained from the patient at the time of denture insertion and used to remount the denture.

After the occlusal vertical dimension has been re-established, prepare a plaster index of the occlusal surface of the maxillary denture on the lower arm of the articulator to which is attached a remount platform (Fig. 17-10). Save this plaster index until the maxillary denture has been finished and polished. The use of this record makes a repetition of the face-bow transfer unnecessary when the dentures are remounted at the insertion appointment.

Recovering the Complete Denture from the Cast

With a saw, cut the base of the cast partly through in several directions. These cuts should be made gradually and inspected closely to avoid sawing the borders of the denture. The lingual flange of the mandibular denture and the palatal area of the maxillary denture may vary greatly in height and contour; therefore, the depth of the saw cuts must vary accordingly.

Insert a plaster knife into the cuts and gently separate the sections of stone so that they may be removed individually. Removing the cast in sections will help to prevent the fracture of dentures with undercuts.

A machine using ground walnut hulls and air pressure or an ultrasonic machine may be used to remove any stone that continues to adhere to the tissue surface of the dentures or to clean investment from the necks of the teeth. A compressed-air gun is helpful if used properly.

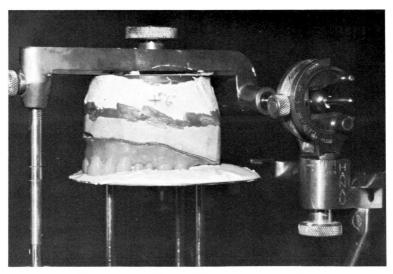

FIG. 17-10. *The remount jig and the plaster record.*

Finishing the Complete Denture

The finishing of dentures consists of perfecting the final form of the denture by removing any flash of acrylic resin at the denture border (Fig. 17-11), any flash and stone remaining around the teeth, and any nodules of acrylic resin on the surfaces of the denture base resulting from processing. The flash is the acrylic resin that was forced out between the halves of the flask by the pressure applied during the processing procedure. If the denture was packed carefully, there will be a minimum of flash.

Take care to preserve the border and contour of the denture during the finishing process. If the impression was correctly boxed and the trial denture was carefully waxed, the outline of the denture can be determined easily. Moreover, if the trial denture was carefully wax contoured into the form desired in the finished denture, little finishing will be necessary.

To remove the flash of acrylic resin from the denture border, press the denture base lightly against a slowly revolving arbor band. Carefully remove any flash and any remaining stone from around the necks of the teeth with a small sharp pick that can be made by sharpening a broken stainless steel explorer or excavator. Inspect the denture for any nodules of acrylic resin, and if any are present, carefully remove them with small stones or with acrylic carbide burs that are made for denture finishing. Air bubbles or particles of foreign matter entrapped just under the surface of the stone mold create small voids. Pressure applied during the packing procedure causes the acrylic resin to break through into the voids and to appear on the surface of the processed denture as nodules.

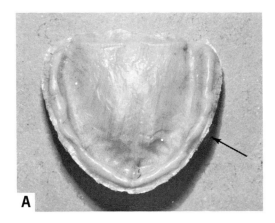

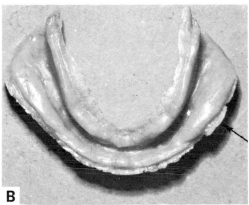

FIG. 17-11. *A minimum of flash. Arrows point to flash that must be removed.* **A.** *Maxillary denture.* **B.** *Mandibular denture.*

Polishing the Complete Denture

The mucosa lining the lips, cheeks, and floor of the mouth and the mucosa covering the tongue are not usually recorded in the impression; however, they are in contact with the dentures. Since the mucosa covering the dorsum and sides of the tongue is a specialized tissue capable of detecting minute particle size, the non-tissue surface of the tongue side of the denture base should be polished. The lining mucosa of the floor of the mouth is thin and fragile, whereas that covering the muscles of the cheeks, lips, and underside of the tongue is usually

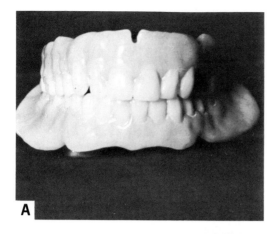

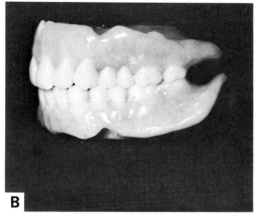

FIG. 17-12. *The finished dentures.* **A.** *Frontal view.* **B.** *Lateral view.*

highly elastic and immovably attached to the fascia of the muscle. Both are easily abraded. To avoid abrasion one must polish smooth the contacting denture surfaces.

The polishing of dentures consists of making a denture or a casting smooth and glossy without changing its contour. To develop a high gloss on acrylic resin or metal, remove all scratches and rough areas. Use a series of progressively finer abrasives to produce a mirror-like surface on the material being polished. A special wheel and brush should be assigned for use with each of the polishing agents and should never be used interchangeably.

Either a felt cone or a small brush wheel may be needed for polishing some areas where access is difficult. Use a brush wheel and powdered pumice to polish around the necks of the teeth and the interproximal spaces. Constantly change the angle of the brush wheel to reach into the interproximal spaces and to prevent the removal of excessive contour and staining from the facial surfaces. Remove the fine scratches left by the pumice with a rag wheel and tripoli, which should be used as carefully as pumice. Finally, using very light pressure, polish the denture with wet whiting and a rag wheel. The completed denture should have a high gloss, compatible contour, and a natural appearance (Fig. 17-12). It is easier to keep a glossy surface clean.

Plaster Cast for Denture Remount Procedures

When the dentures are finished and polished, make plaster remount casts and mount the maxillary cast on the articulator in the original face-bow transfer position (Fig. 17-13). Accurate plaster remount casts save chair time at the appointment for the insertion of dentures.

PREPARATION OF REMOUNT CAST

1. Eliminate all undercuts on the tissue side of the denture with wet pumice.

2. Fill the tissue side of the dentures with soft plaster, including the borders.

3. When the plaster has set, remove the cast from the dentures and with a gentle stream of water remove the pumice from the cast and dentures.

4. Trim the cast neatly, preserving the borders.

5. Reseat the dentures on the casts and check for accurate seating.

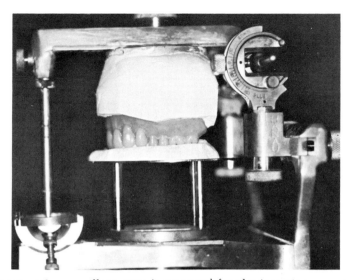

Fig. 17-13. *The maxillary cast is mounted for the insertion appointment.*

6. Place the maxillary teeth in the plaster remount index and attach the maxillary cast to the upper member of the articulator (Fig. 17-13). This procedure orients the maxillary cast in the same relations with the opening axis of the articulator as in the original facebow transfer position. The mandibular cast will be attached to the articulator at the time of denture insertion.

REFERENCES

1. Becker, C. M., Smith, D. E., and Nicholls, J. I.: Comparison of denture-base processing techniques. Part I—Material characteristics. J. Prosth. Dent., *37*:330, 1977.
1a. ———: Comparison of denture-base processing techniques. Part II—Dimensional changes due to processing. J. Prosth. Dent., *37*:450, 1977.
1b. Bell, D. H.: Clinical evaluation of a resilient denture liner. J. Prosth. Dent., *23*:394, 1970.
1c. Blanchard, C. H.: Transferring facial surfaces from the impression to the denture. J. Prosth. Dent., *4*:621, 1954.
2. Campbell, R. L.: Effects of water sorption on retention of acrylic resin denture bases. J.A.D.A., *52*:448, 1956.

2a. Choudhary, S. C., Craig, J. F., and Suls, F. J.: Characterizing denture base for non-caucasian patients. J. Prosth. Dent., *33*:73, 1975.
2b. Ciujon, S., Huget, E. F., and De Simon, L. B.: Modification of the fluid resin technique. J.A.D.A., *85*:109, 1972.
2c. Crum, R. J., Loiselle, R. J., and Rooney, G. E., Jr.: Clinical use of a resilient mandibular denture. J.A.D.A., *83*:1093, 1971.
3. Docking, A. R.: Plaster and stone. Dent. Clin. N. Amer., November, 1958, p. 727.
4. Everett, A. E.: Simulation of gum recession in artificial dentures. Int. Dent. J., *3*:210, 1952.
5. Fairhurst, C. W., and Ryge, G.: Effect of tin-foil substitute on the strength of denture base resins. J. Prosth. Dent., *5*:508, 1955.
6. Fish, E. W.: Principles of full denture prosthesis. 3rd ed. London, John Bale and Sons, Curnow, Ltd., 1937.
6a. Grant, A. A., and Atkinson, H. F.: Comparison between dimensional accuracy of denture produced with pour-type resin and with heat processed materials. J. Prosth. Dent., *26*:296, 1971.
7. Gruenwald, A. H., Paffenbarger, G. C., and Dickson, G.: The effect of molding processes on some properties of denture resins. J.A.D.A., *44*:269, 1952.

8. Johnson, H. B.: Technique for packing and staining complete or partial denture bases. J. Prosth. Dent., 6:154, 1956.

9. Jordan, L. G.: Are prominent rugae and glossy tongue surfaces on artificial dentures to be desired? J. Prosth. Dent., 4:52, 1954.

9a. Koehne, C. L., and Morrow, R. M.: Construction of denture teeth with gold occlusal surfaces. J. Prosth. Dent., 23:449, 1970.

9b. Kraut, R. A.: A comparison of denture base accuracy. J.A.D.A., 83:1376, 1971.

10. Kyes, F. M.: Laboratory's role in successful dentures. J. Prosth. Dent., 1:196, 1951.

10a. Lang, B. R.: The use of gold in construction of mandibular denture bases. J. Prosth. Dent., 32:398, 1974.

11. Mahler, D. B.: Change of articulation after processing of complete dentures. (Abst.) J. Dent. Res., 30:500, 1951.

12. ———: Inarticulation of complete dentures processed by the compression molding technique. J. Prosth. Dent., 1:551, 1951.

12a. McGivney, G. P.: Comparison of adoption of different mandibular denture bases. J. Prosth. Dent., 30:126, 1973.

12b. Means, C. R., Rupp, N. W., and Paffenbarger, G. C.: Clinical evaluation of two types of resilient liners on dentures. J.A.D.A., 83:1376, 1971.

13. Mirza, F. D.: Dimensional stability of acrylic resin dentures, clinical evaluation. J. Prosth. Dent., 11:848, 1961.

13a. Moffa, J. P., Jenkins, W. A., and Weaver, R. G.: Silane bonding of porcelain denture teeth to acrylic resin denture bases. J. Prosth. Dent., 33:620, 1975.

13b. Morrow, R. M., Matvias, F. M., Windeler, A. S., and Fuchs, R. J.: Bonding of plastic teeth to two heat-curing denture base resins. J. Prosth. Dent., 39:565, 1978.

13c. Mutti, N. M., and Pazzini, L. I.: Horizontal fit of flasks as a factor in complete denture disarticulation. J. Prosth. Dent., 32:448, 1974.

14. Payne, S. H.: Denture base materials and refitting dentures. J.A.D.A., 49:562, 1954.

15. Peyton, F. A., Shiere, H. B., and Delgado, V. P.: Some comparisons of self-curing and heat-curing denture resins. J. Prosth. Dent., 3:332, 1953.

16. ———: and Anthony, D. H.: Evaluation of dentures processed by different techniques. J. Prosth. Dent., 13:269, 1963.

17. ———et al.: *Restorative Dental Materials: Manipulation and Processing of Denture Base Plastics.* 2nd ed. St. Louis, The C. V. Mosby Company, 1964, pp. 438–455.

18. Proctor, W. J.: Characterization of dentures. J. Prosth. Dent., 3:339, 1953.

19. Pryor, W. J.: Internal strains in denture base materials. J.A.D.A., 30:1382, 1943.

20. ———: Methods of producing more lifelike dentures, including the preparation and processing of acrylic resins. J.A.D.A., 28:894, 1941.

21. Rayliens, N. H.: The polished surface of complete dentures. J. Prosth. Dent., 13:236, 1963.

21a. Renner, R. P., and Blakeslee, R. W.: Basic wax contouring for complete dentures. J. Prosth. Dent., 40:343, 1978.

21b. Rosenthal, R. L., and Kemper, J. T.: The "Blow-wax" technique for stippling dentures. J. Prosth. Dent., 32:344, 1974.

22. Schiesser, F. J.: The neutral zone and polished surfaces in complete dentures. J. Prosth. Dent., 14:854, 1964.

23. Schuyler, C., Fredrich, E. G., and Vaughn, H. C., Jr.: Processing acrylic dentures: compression and injection method. U. S. Navy Med. Bul., 43:297, 1944.

24. Shippee, R. W.: Control of increased vertical dimension of compression-molded dentures. J. Prosth. Dent., 11:1080, 1961.

25. Skinner, E. W., and Jones, P. M.: Dimensional stability of self-curing denture base acrylic resins. J.A.D.A., 51:426, 1955.

25a. ——— and Philips, R. W.: *The Science of Dental Materials,* 5th ed. Philadelphia, W. B. Saunders Company, 1965, p. 187.

26. Sweeney, W. T.: Acrylic resins in prosthetic dentistry. Dent. Clin. N. Amer., November, 1958, p. 593.

27. ———: Denture base material, acrylic resins. J.A.D.A., 26:1863, 1939.

28. ———, Paffenbarger, G. C., and Beall, J. R.: Acrylic resins for dentures. J.A.D.A., 29:7, 1942.

28a. Vig, R. G.: Method of reducing the shifting of teeth in denture processing. J. Prosth. Dent., *33*:80, 1975.

29. Walker, T. J., and Orsinger, W. O.: Palate reproduction by the hydrocolloid-resin method. J. Prosth. Dent., *4*:52, 1954.

29a. Welker, W. A., Kramer, D. C., and Mercer, R. W.: A technique for finishing and polishing denture bases. J. Prosth. Dent., *39*:240, 1978.

30. Woelfel, J. B., Paffenbarger, G. C., and Sweeney, W. T.: Dimensional change occurring in dentures during processing. J.A.D.A., *61*:413, 1960.

31. ———: Some physical properties of organic denture base materials. J.A.D.A., *67*:489, 1963.

32. Winkler, S., et al.: Processing changes in complete dentures constructed from pour resins. J.A.D.A., *82*:349, 1971.

33. Wormley, J. H., and Brunton, D. A.: Weighted mandibular dentures. J. Prosth. Dent., *32*:101, 1974.

34. Zakhari, K. N.: Relationship of investing medium to occlusal changes and vertical opening during denture construction. J. Prosth. Dent., *36*:501, 1976.

Denture Insertion

18

After the dentist has educated the patient in proper denture acceptance and has carefully carried out each procedure in denture construction, both dentist and patient anticipate with pleasure the appointment for the insertion of the dentures.

Before the insertion appointment inspect the dentures to determine (1) that the polished surfaces are smooth and devoid of scratches, (2) that no imperfections on the tissue surface remain, and (3) that the borders are round with no sharp angles in the border areas. In addition, be sure (1) that the accurate maxillary remount cast is properly attached to the articulator and (2) that an accurate mandibular cast is prepared for the patient remount.

The Insertion Procedures

Patients receiving their first complete denture are familiar with neither the physiologic requirements of dentures nor with the use and care of the dentures. How one can fabricate a prosthesis as intricate as a complete denture, insert it, and instruct the patient "to go use it" is beyond comprehension. The procedures during the insertion appointment should be precise and carried out in an orderly manner.

REVIEWING INSTRUCTIONS

The first step at the insertion appointment is to review with the patient the instructions that were given to him during the diagnostic phase (page 93). The patient has had an opportunity to study these instructions, and this review allows the dentist to discuss any that the patient does not understand.

EVALUATING TISSUE SIDE

The second step is evaluation of the tissue side of the denture base for undercut areas and accuracy of tissue contact. Each denture should be evaluated individually. Before inserting the denture, paint the entire tissue side of the denture base with a thin coat of pressure disclosing paste (Fig. 18-1). Insert and remove the denture. When tissue undercuts are present, the paste will be dragged from the denture base in the area of tissue contact (Fig. 18-2). Repeat this procedure to be positive of the area. It may also be advisable to have the patient insert and remove the denture, as the method of inserting and the path of insertion may vary with two individuals. When the undercut area is positively established, relieve the denture by grinding with an acrylic bur. Repeat the procedure until adequate relief is assured. Smooth the altered surface with a burlew wheel revolving

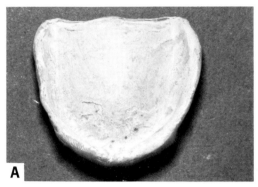

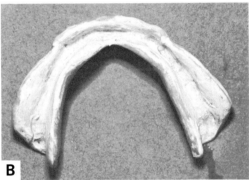

FIG. 18-1. *The tissue side of the dentures has been painted with a thin coat of pressure disclosing paste. A thick uneven application will result in false information, even though the impression may have been accurate.* **A.** *Maxillary.* **B.** *Mandibular.*

at a slow rate to prevent heating the acrylic resin. Relieving the tissue side of the denture base in tissue or bone undercut areas prevents stripping the soft tissue covering from the underlying bone. When vascular tissue is removed from the bone, the exposed bone will undergo necrosis. This is not desirable because it results in unnecessary bone loss and is painful to the patient.

Areas of exostosis or areas of bone covered with tissue that is not displaceable, such as the midpalatal suture, often appear as pressure areas even when the denture is seated with very little pressure (Fig. 18-3). When these areas appear in the pressure disclosing paste, they are relieved by grinding.

The altered area is not smoothed until the denture is subjected to the pressure of occlusion and one can see that no further relief is required. When the dentures have a positively stabilized seat, it is advisable not to relieve any pressure areas until occlusal harmony is obtained. When tooth contact occurs prior to occlusal correction or evaluation, the patient's applying pressure to the teeth or denture with his fingers, or the dentist's applying pressure with his fingers can reflect as a pressure area by displacing the indicator paste. Under these circumstances the displaced paste does not necessarily reflect a pressure

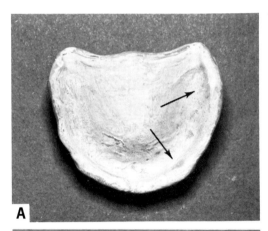

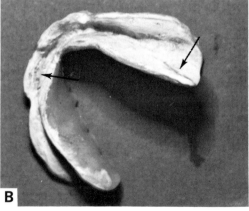

FIG. 18-2. *The arrows point to areas of the denture from which the paste has been removed. This removal usually indicates an undercut area.* **A.** *Maxillary.* **B.** *Mandibular.*

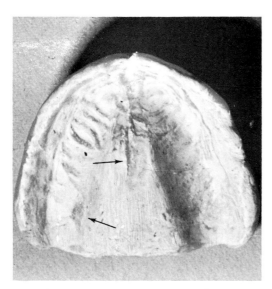

FIG. 18-3. *Tissue surface of maxillary denture. The areas indicated by arrows appear to be pressure spots. These areas should be thoroughly investigated and relieved until they no longer reflect in the paste.*

area which exists when the tooth contacts have been harmonized and the dentures are in function.

EVALUATING BORDERS

The third step is to evaluate the borders and the contour of the polished surfaces in the mouth to determine if (1) the border extensions and contour are compatible with the available spaces in the vestibules, (2) the borders are properly relieved to accommodate the frenum attachments and the reflection of the tissues in the hamular notch area, and (3) the dentures are stable during speech and swallowing.

Apply disclosing wax to the borders of the maxillary denture (Fig. 18-4) in the same manner as the impression compound was applied during the border refining procedures (page 194). Instruct the patient to open the jaws as in yawning, push the lower jaw forward, and move the lower jaw from right to left. Disclosing wax is more displaceable

than softened impression compound; therefore slight overextensions that might be developed with compound can be determined. Relieve any existing overextensions by grinding; polish the relieved area. Apply disclosing wax to the remaining borders of the maxillary denture and instruct the patient to smile, speak, laugh, and swallow. Relieve any overextended areas by grinding, and polish the relieved surface.

Apply disclosing wax to the mandibular denture borders (Fig. 18-5) in the same manner as the impression compound was applied in the border refining procedures (page 194). Instruct the patient to repeat the same movements that were made in border refining (page 194). Relieve by grinding any overextended areas and polish the

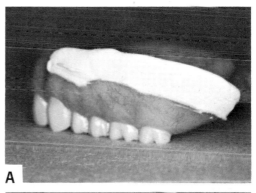

A

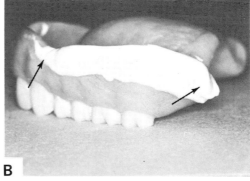

B

FIG. 18-4. **A.** *Disclosing wax has been applied to the denture border. Evaluate one area at a time.* **B.** *The arrows designate areas that may be slightly overextended.*

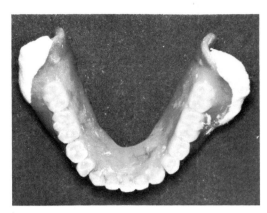

FIG. 18-5. *If the disclosing wax is applied bilaterally to the mandibular denture, the paste will indicate if the denture is not centered.*

relieved surface. Reapply disclosing wax to the borders, and instruct the patient to smile, speak, laugh, and swallow. Relieve any overextended areas by grinding and polish the relieved surface.

CORRECTING OCCLUSION

The fourth step in the insertion procedures is the occlusal correction. Occlusal harmony in complete dentures is necessary if the dentures are to be comfortable, to function efficiently, and to preserve the supporting structures. It is difficult to see occlusal discrepancies intraorally with complete dentures. The resiliency of the supporting soft tissues and the displaceability of the tissues in varying degrees tend to disguise premature occlusal contacts. The tissues permit the dentures to shift; as a result, after the first interceptive occlusal contact the remaining teeth appear to make satisfactory contacts. Patients are seldom aware of faulty occlusion in complete dentures; yet they always seem to notice an improvement after the fault has been corrected. The eye cannot be relied upon to observe occlusal discrepancies, and the patient cannot be depended upon to diagnose

occlusal faults. It is the responsibility of the dentist to find and correct these occlusal discrepancies and permit the patient to depart free of occlusal disharmony.

One must assume that there are occlusal faults in all complete dentures until he proves otherwise. Occlusal faults can be determined by obtaining an interocclusal record from the patient and remounting the dentures on an articulator. These faults can be corrected by careful selective grinding procedures. Remounting the dentures on the articulator and selective grinding procedures should be carried out at the time of placement of the dentures. Postponing this important step will lead to (1) a deformation of the underlying soft tissues, (2) discomfort, and (3) destruction of the supporting bone. Later the occlusal errors may be concealed and impossible to locate and correct because of distorted and swollen tissues.

Occlusal disharmony in the completed dentures may result from (1) undetected errors in registering jaw relations, (2) errors in mounting casts on the articulator, (3) differences in tissue adaptation between the processed denture bases and the record bases that were used in recording maxillomandibular relations, and (4) changes in the supporting structures since the impressions were made. This is particularly true if the patient is using other dentures.

Clinical Errors

The laboratory remount procedure will not correct for clinical errors in recording maxillomandibular relation records and in mounting the cast on the articulator.

ERRORS IN REGISTERING
JAW RELATIONS

Errors in registering maxillomandibular relations may be the result of one or more factors.

1. Record bases that do not fit accurately.

2. A shifting of the record bases over displaceable tissues.

3. Excessive pressure exerted by the patient during the registering of maxillomandibular relations.

4. Unequal distribution of stress during the registering of maxillomandibular relations.

5. Record bases placed on soft tissues that have been deformed by ill-fitting dentures.

6. Patients not registering centric relation because of systemic factors, such as muscle spasm, abnormalities of the temporomandibular joints, and impairment of muscle tonus, or because of the failure of mental, aged, or senile patients to understand instructions—factors beyond the control of the dentist.

ERRORS IN MOUNTING CASTS

Errors in mounting casts on the articulator may be caused by:

1. Record bases that are not properly seated and secured to casts during mounting procedures.

2. Occlusion rims not being definitely locked or keyed for correct orientation during the mounting on the articulator.

3. Interference of casts in the posterior region during mounting.

4. Articulator not maintaining horizontal and vertical relationship of casts.

5. Inaccuracies introduced by changes in the plaster used to mount the casts.

Correcting Occlusal Disharmony

There are many acceptable intraoral methods for correcting occlusal disharmony. However, the intraoral methods are more accurate if the uneven contacting of the teeth has been first corrected with laboratory remount and patient remount procedures. Some of the intraoral methods follow.

ARTICULATING PAPER

Articulating paper alone will not give as accurate an indication of premature contacts as some other methods. The resiliency of the supporting tissues allows the dentures to shift; therefore, the paper markings are frequently false and misleading. The denture bases can move from the basal seat causing the teeth in the opposite side of the arch or the opposite end of the arch to contact prematurely and produce an incorrect marking. To place articulating paper on one side of the arch may induce the patient to close to or away from that side. Articulating paper should be placed on both arches, a procedure sometimes difficult to do accurately (Fig. 18-6).

CENTRAL-BEARING DEVICES

Some operators use one type of central-bearing device, the correlator, to correct occlusion in the mouth. The central-bearing pin works on a spring. As the patient closes his mouth, the pin

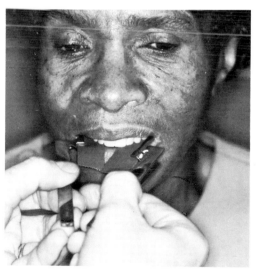

FIG. 18-6. *The articulating paper in holders designed for this procedure is placed bilaterally between the occlusal surfaces of the teeth.*

in the mandibular mounting contacts a metal plate in the vault of the maxillary denture. Thus, by holding the maxillary denture up and the mandibular denture down, the pin creates a tension before the teeth contact. If a premature contact is made by one tooth, the dentures do not shift because the spring holds the other teeth apart. The interceptive occlusal contacts are located with articulat-

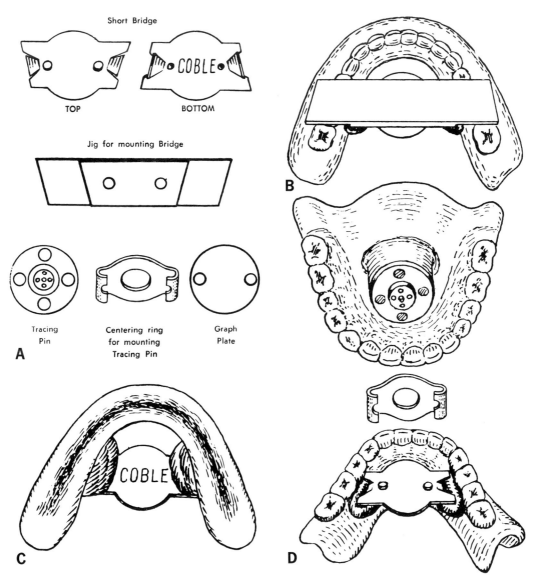

FIG. 18-7. **A.** *The parts of the Coble apparatus: short bridge, jig, tracing pin, centering ring, and graph plate.* **B.** *Jig and bridge mounted on the occlusal surfaces of the lower denture. Note that they are centered opposite mesial of first molar and bicuspid.* **C.** *Inverted view of mounted bridge, showing bridge fastened to denture with stick compound.* **D.** *View of the separated dentures with centering ring removed from tracing pin, which has been fastened to upper denture by softened compound seared to the palate and cooled. (Courtesy of the Coble Denture Research Co., Inc.)*

ing ribbon. The central-bearing device can be mounted on dentures in three to four minutes and will serve to disprove the theory that occlusion can be corrected by having the patient close down on a piece of articulating paper alone.

Another type of central-bearing device, the Coble device, has a central-bearing pin without a spring. Like the correlator, it requires careful control of the patient throughout the procedure (Fig. 18-7).

OCCLUSAL WAX

Adhesive green wax is placed on the occlusal surfaces of the mandibular denture. Points of penetration that occur upon closing with the jaws in centric relation may be marked with a lead pencil and relieved where indicated (Fig. 18-8). With this method one may also locate points of interference during functional movements. One disadvantage of this method is that shifting of the dentures over resilient supporting tissues in eccentric jaw positions will give false markings. This is an excellent method for correcting occlusion in the centric position.

ABRASIVE PASTE

The use of abrasive paste in the mouth has many disadvantages. The shifting

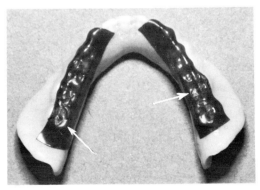

FIG. 18-8. *The arrows indicate points of premature tooth contacts. The adhesive green wax is less than a millimeter thick.*

of the base as a result of premature contact may result in altering the occlusion so that centric occlusion does not correspond to centric relation. Cusps that maintain the occlusal vertical dimension may be destroyed. Abrasive paste is not selective.

PATIENT REMOUNT AND SELECTIVE GRINDING

The patient remount method is to remount the dentures on an articulator by means of interocclusal records made in the patient's mouth. This is by far the most accurate procedure. It has the following advantages:

1. It reduces patient participation.
2. It permits the dentist to see better what he is doing.
3. It provides a stable working foundation; bases are not shifting on resilient tissues.
4. The absence of saliva makes possible more accurate markings with the articulating paper or tape.
5. Corrections can be made away from the patient, thus preventing occasional objections when patients see their dentures being ground.

To carry out a patient remount procedure, orient the mandibular denture to the maxillary denture by means of an interocclusal record with the jaws in centric relation.

1. Place two thicknesses (approximately 1½ millimeters) of passive type wax on the occlusal surfaces of the mandibular teeth. Soften with a flame from alcohol torch or immerse in water at 130°F.
2. Carry to the mouth and have the patient close into the wax when the jaws are in centric relation. Closure must be short of tooth-to-tooth contact. The wax record is not acceptable if the teeth penetrate to make contact. Chill with cold air and remove.
3. Do not return wax record to mouth,

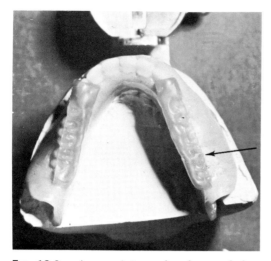

FIG. 18-9. *A wax interocclusal record that is attached to the mandibular posterior teeth. The arrow indicates the area of wax that is trimmed to allow better visibility as the maxillary teeth are seated in the record.*

as it may be distorted by the patient. Trim the wax so that only slight indentations remain, and expose the facial side so that the seating of the maxillary denture can be visually checked (Fig. 18-9).

After properly orienting the mandibular denture to the maxillary denture by means of the interocclusal record, secure with sticky wax. Seat the mandibular cast in the denture and attach to the mandibular member of the articulator with plaster.

To check what has been recorded to be the patient's centric occlusion, make another wax interocclusal record. Replace the dentures on the articulator. With the condylar elements freed, place the teeth in the indentations in the wax record. The condylar elements should rest against the stops (Fig. 18-10). Re-

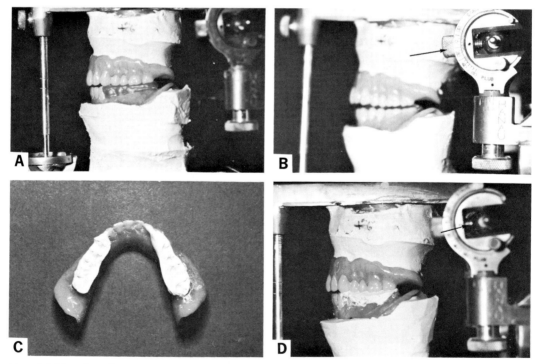

FIG. 18-10. A. *The dentures are mounted on the articulator with the maxillary teeth accurately seated in the indentations in the interocclusal wax record that is attached to the mandibular posterior teeth.* **B.** *The arrow points to the condylar element, which must be against the centric stop.* **C.** *Plaster is used to make an interocclusal check record.* **D.** *The articulator receives this record. The condylar element is against the centric stop.*

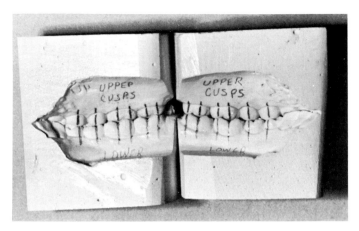

FIG. 18-11. *This lingual view of the bisected articulated plaster casts demonstrates the desired cusps fossae relations of the posterior teeth in centric occlusion. (Courtesy of J. Marvin Reynolds, Department of Restorative Dentistry and Director of Curriculum in Occlusion, Virginia Commonwealth University School of Dentistry.)*

peat the procedure until three consecutive records are accepted. When the accuracy of the articulator mountings is verified, occlusal disharmony when the jaws are in centric relation or in eccentric relation can be corrected by selective grinding procedures.

When *cusp form* posterior teeth are used and balanced occlusion is desired, it is best to have an even distribution of tooth contacts of the posterior teeth. Develop the contacts bilaterally. This involves a cusp fossae marginal ridge relation of maximum intercuspation when the jaws are in terminal hinge position (Fig. 18-11). When the teeth move to and from centric and eccentric positions, they move in the approximate directions indicated in Figure 18-12.

An articulator that travels in a straight path does not travel the same path as the condyles in the fossae. It has been generally accepted that the error is so negligible that the resiliency of the supporting tissues accommodates for the error. There is no scientific proof that this assumption is correct, and this may not be true in all situations. Undoubtedly this error is tolerated by the majority of patients.

When the jaws are moving to and from centric and eccentric positions, within the functional range of the teeth in gliding occlusion, the teeth can be altered to maintain harmonious contact on the articulator. This harmonious contact from fossae to cusp tips will not be repeated in the mouth unless the condyle path is straight and flat.

When the teeth are altered to make maximum intercuspation when the jaws are in centric relation, balanced centric occlusion is achieved (Fig. 18-13). One can expect this maximum intercuspation to be repeated in the mouth.

When the teeth are altered by selective grinding to make simultaneous cusp tip to cusp tip contact on both sides of the arch when the jaws are in a right or left lateral position, balanced occlusion in a static eccentric position exists. Some of these static contacts may be repeated in the mouth. When the mandible is in a straight protruded relation with the maxillae and the posterior teeth are altered to make cusp contacts at the same time the anterior teeth make incisal edge to incisal edge contact, *balanced occlusion in protrusion* exists (Fig. 18-14). One may expect this

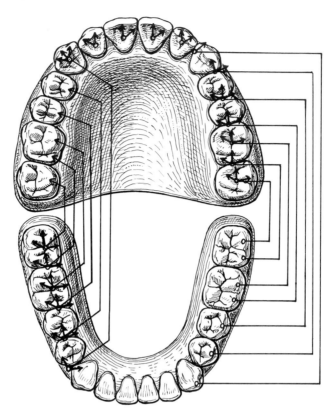

FIG. 18-12. *A diagrammatic illustration with lines that connect from the cusp or point on one denture to the fossa on which it rests in centric relation on the opposing denture. Three arrows denote the direction in which this point or cusp travels in the working side movement, the balancing side movement, and the protrusive movement. (Courtesy of Dr. C. H. Schuyler, from* Swenson's Complete Dentures. *5th ed. St. Louis, The C. V. Mosby Company, 1964.)*

static occlusal and incisal edge relation to exist in the mouth when the mandible is protruded to the same forward position.

When teeth are arranged and the anteroposterior horizontal relations of the jaws are even (considered normally related), the buccal cusps of the mandibular posterior teeth and the lingual cusps of the maxillary posterior teeth maintain the vertical dimension of jaw separation by contact in the fossae and on the marginal ridges of their antagonists. When the horizontal position of the mandible is in a more forward position than the maxillae or in a situation where the mandible is larger in a lateral direction than the maxillae, the posterior teeth are frequently arranged in a reverse relation (Fig. 18-15). The buccal cusp tips of the maxillary posterior teeth and the lingual cusp tips of the mandibular posterior teeth maintain the vertical dimension of jaw separation. After the occlusal surfaces of the teeth have been altered by grinding to achieve balanced occlusions with the jaws in centric relation, the cusps that maintain the vertical dimension of jaw separation are *not* altered.

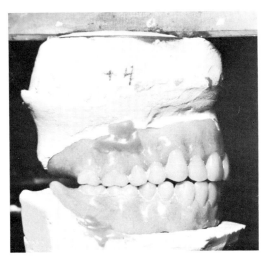

FIG. 18-13. *The teeth have been altered by selective grinding to produce maximum intercuspation.*

Selective Grinding Procedures

The displaceability of the basal seat mucosa must be considered when the teeth are altered by selective grinding

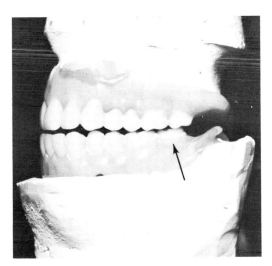

FIG. 18-14. *The arrow indicates excessive tooth contact in the molar area when the articulator moved to a straight protrusive position. Selective grinding procedures are needed to produce balanced occlusion in the eccentric positions.*

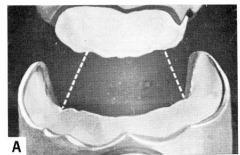

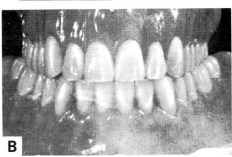

FIG. 18-15. A. *The disproportion of the maxillary and the mandibular arches necessitates a change in the tooth positions.* **B.** *The posterior teeth are arranged in reverse relation. The lingual cusps of the mandibular posterior teeth occlude in the central fossae of the maxillary teeth. (From Boucher: Swenson's Complete Dentures. 5th ed. St. Louis, The C. V. Mosby Company, 1964.)*

procedures. Hanau described this factor as *realeff*, derived from *resiliency* and *like effect*, and pointed out that "dentures built on the Hanau articulator Model H articulate in the mouth with a component of over-protrusion within a range." He described the effect by saying "that the teeth have a tendency to find premature contact of the distal inclines of the lower cusps with the mesial inclines of the upper cusps."

When the impressions for complete dentures are made and the relations of the jaws are recorded, the basal mucosa is at or near an undisplaced position. The casts are related on the articulator with the jaw relation record that was made at centric or terminal relation at the vertical dimension of occlusion. Maximum intercuspation or posterior tooth contact is developed at that given amount of jaw separation. When the dentures are inserted in the patient's mouth and the force of jaw closure is exerted on the teeth, the mucosa under the maxillary denture is displaced in a superior direction at the same time the mucosa under the mandibular denture is displaced in an inferior direction. When the denture bases follow this tissue displacement, the jaws come closer together and the vertical dimension of jaw separation is changed. As the jaws come closer together, the mandible is slightly more forward in relation to the maxillae. This change in maxillomandibular relation would result in the distal inclines of the mandibular posterior cusps having a tendency to find premature contact with the mesial inclines of the maxillary cusps. This would occur regardless of the articulation upon which the denture was constructed if the jaw relation records were made with a passive recording material such as plaster, softened wax, or impression compound. The more displaceable the tissue the more the tendency for premature contact.

The "correction technique" described by Hanau requires multiple remount procedures using first "unstrained" jaw relation records and then "strained" jaw relation records made with the jaws in terminal relation. An "unstrained" record is recorded with a passive material necessitating no undue force that would displace the mucosa. Selective grinding is accomplished first with this "unstrained" mounting. The mandibular cast is then remounted with "strained" jaw relation records that are made with a resistant recording material necessitating the jaws to be closed with a force that displaces the supporting tissue.

Selective grinding procedures using this technique of remounting will result in an area of freedom of occlusion with the jaws in terminal relation. This area of freedom of occlusion may be referred to as *long centric* or *short protrusive* occlusion.

In the first step cusp form teeth are altered by selective grinding to obtain balanced occlusion when the jaws are in centric relation. Occlusal balance in a lateral direction is obtained by having all of the posterior teeth and the cuspids in contact on the working side and in posterior contact *only* on the balancing side. In the protrusive balance the anterior teeth should make incisal edge contact at the same time that the tips of the buccal and lingual cusps of the posterior teeth contact.

The techniques are as follows:

1. Adjust the horizontal and lateral condylar inclinations of the articulator to the settings dictated by the protrusive interocclusal maxillomandibular relation record.

2. Release the horizontal condylar elements to allow freedom of the articulator movements in the eccentric positions.

3. Raise the incisal guide pin from the guide table and secure it above the height of the table.

4. Evaluate the areas of tooth contact in the centric and eccentric positions prior to selection of the point or area to be reduced or altered.

5. With the condylar elements against the centric relation stops, close the articulator until the posterior teeth are in contact. The anterior teeth should not be in contact. Examine the lingual cusps of the maxillary posterior teeth and the buccal cusps of the mandibular posterior teeth. Premature contact appears when the remainder of the teeth fail to make maximum intercuspation. Record the area or areas of premature con-

tact. The contacts may be in varying amounts and may involve more than one cusp or tooth. These varying situations make necessary critical evaluation prior to grinding procedures in the centric position; however, further evaluation in the eccentric positions is necessary before one starts any grinding.

6. Secure the right condylar element in the centric position and place the lingual cusps of the maxillary posterior teeth in balancing relation with the buccal cusps of the mandibular posterior teeth. This procedure also places the buccal and lingual cusps of the maxillary and mandibular posterior teeth and the cuspids in their working position on the opposite side. The teeth are placed in these positions and not shifted from the centric to the eccentric position with the teeth in contact. This procedure often results in breaking or chipping teeth.

When the teeth on the balancing side are not in the correct relation, the error appears on either the balancing or working side. If the balancing contact is excessive, the working side teeth will not be in contact. If the working side contact is excessive, the excess prevents contact on the balancing side (Fig. 18-16).

If the teeth on the working side are too long, there will be no contact on the balancing side. If a single tooth is high on the working side, there will be contact neither on the balancing side nor on the working side.

7. Record the premature contacts. Repeat the procedure with the left side as the working side and record the premature contacts.

Use articulating tape to mark the areas of premature contact for selective grinding. When using tape, exercise care to prevent the tape from wrinkling or doubling, as this will result in an error in marking. Place the tape on the occlu-

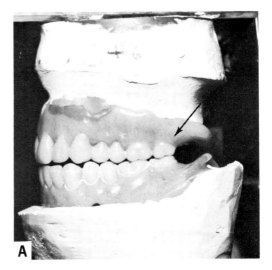

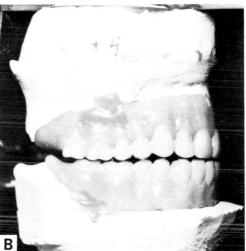

FIG. 18-16. *Excessive molar contact on the working side (arrow) prevents teeth from making contacts on the balancing side.* **A.** *Working side.* **B.** *Balancing side.*

sal surfaces and the incisal edges of all the mandibular teeth. When the teeth are brought together, this position assures that the same force is exerted on all the teeth.

8. Return the incisal guide pin to the table and use the following grinding procedures to ensure balanced occlu-

sion in the centric and eccentric position.

a. If the cusp is high in centric and eccentric position, reduce the cusp.

b. If the cusp is high in centric and *not* in the eccentric position, deepen the fossae or the marginal ridges. After all interceptive contacts have been removed in the centric and eccentric positions, (1) *do not* reduce the maxillary lingual cusp or the mandibular buccal cusp and (2) do not deepen the fossa or marginal ridge of any tooth.

9. When one wishes to refine the teeth to retain contact when the articulator is being moved to and from centric and eccentric position—balanced gliding occlusion—use the following selective grinding procedures:

On the working side reduce the inner inclines of (a) the buccal cusps of the maxillary teeth and (b) the lingual cusps of the mandibular teeth.

On the balancing side reduce the inner inclines of the mandibular buccal cusps. To achieve balance in protrusive excursion reduce the distal inclines of the maxillary cusps and the mesial inclines of the mandibular cusps.

10. After completing the selective grinding procedures to establish and maintain the desired occlusion (a) refine the occlusal anatomy, using the mounted inverted cone points and (b) polish all the ground surfaces with wet powdered pumice on a wet rag wheel.

When noncusp form posterior teeth are used and selective grinding procedures are instituted, the occlusal surfaces of the posterior teeth are altered to make harmonious contact on the right side and on the left side when the jaws are in centric relation (Fig. 18-17).

1. Secure the horizontal condylar elements on the articulator against the centric relation stops.

2. Place articulating tape over the occlusal surfaces and incisal edges of all of the mandibular teeth.

3. Tap the teeth together to record the contacting areas.

4. Using a mounted wheel, grind the occlusal surfaces of the teeth until simultaneous even contacting areas on the right and left are developed. Do not allow the anterior teeth to make contact. Develop small areas of contact uniformly dispersed over the occlusal surfaces of the distal of the first bicuspid, the second bicuspid, the first molar, and the mesial of the second molar (Fig. 18-18).

5. Polish all altered surfaces with wet pumice on a wet rag wheel.

6. Exercise care to maintain the occlu-

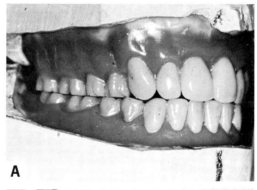

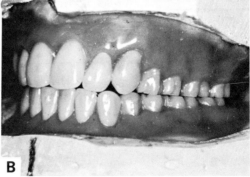

FIG. 18-17. *The noncusp form posterior teeth are arranged to make maximum planned contact in the centric position. The anterior teeth are not in contact.*

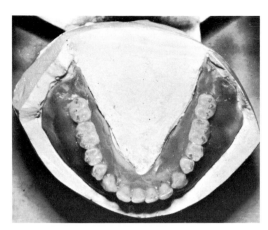

FIG. 18-18. *Articulating tape was used to demonstrate posterior tooth contact.*

sal surfaces of the mandibular arch on a plane.

7. When using porcelain teeth in one arch to oppose acrylic resin teeth in the opposite arch, do all grinding of the occlusal surfaces on the acrylic resin teeth.

REFERENCES

1. Boone, M. E.: Masticatory forces accurately identified. J.A.D.A., *81*:1338, 1970.

1a. Fish, E. W.: *Principles of Full Denture Prosthesis*, 3rd ed. London, John Bale and Sons, Curnow Ltd., 1937.

2. Gehl, D. H.: Denture insertion adjustment and maintenance. Bull. Greater Milwaukee Dent. Ass., *23*:53, 1957.

2a. Holt, J. E.: Research on remounting procedures. J. Prosth. Dent., *38*:338, 1977.

3. Hooper, B. L.: Instructions for the edentulous patient. J.A.D.A., *19*:205, 1932.

4. Jankelson, B.: Adjustment of dentures at time of insertion to compensate for tissue change. J.A.D.A., *64*:521, 1962.

5. Naylor, J. C.: What the patient should know about complete dentures. J. Prosth. Dent., *9*:832, 1959.

6. Perry, C.: Printed literature for denture patients. J.A.D.A., *64*:552, 1962.

7. Rayliens, N. H.: The polished surface of complete dentures. J. Prosth. Dent., *13*:236, 1963.

8. Sears, V. H.: Information for denture patients. Dent. Dig., *34*:643, 1928.

9. ———: Occlusal refinements on completed dentures. J.A.D.A., *59*:1250, 1959.

10. Schlosser, R. O.: Checking completed dentures for adaptation and retention and establishing balanced articulation. J.A.D.A., *15*:1717, 1928.

11. Schuyler, C. H.: Fundamental principles in the correction of occlusal disharmony, natural and artificial. J.A.D.A., *22*:1193, 1935.

12. Sussman, B. A.: Insertion of a full upper and lower denture. J. Ontario Dent. Ass. *34*:16, 1957.

13. Young, H. A.: Denture insertion. J.A.D.A., *61*:505, 1962.

Treating Problems
Associated with Denture Use

19

A complaint is an utterance of pain, discomfort, or dissatisfaction. Patients have expressed their distaste for the use of the word. When asked about their *complaint,* they readily assure the dentist that they are not complaining or finding fault. It is for this reason that I suggest the use of the word *problem,* which is defined as "a situation proposed for solution or consideration."

It requires patience on the part of the patient and patience, skill, and experience on the part of the dentist to correct the many problems associated with the use of dentures. The dentist also needs thorough knowledge of anatomy, physiology, pathology, and psychology. He must be capable of differentiating between normal and abnormal tissue responses. He must distinguish between a physical disorder that is aggravated by the psychic and emotional processes of a patient and one that is solely physical. When the dentist has knowledge of the basic sciences and skill and experience to investigate these problems, he will readily see that in the majority of instances they are real and not psychosomatic. He will exercise patience in helping the patient solve his problem and will not accuse the patient of finding fault.

Review of Denture Requirements

A basis must be established to determine when a complete denture has failed to serve the purpose for which it was made or the reason for the problem. It is time to recall the requirements of a complete denture:

1. Compatibility with the surrounding oral environment.
2. Restoration of masticatory efficiency within realistic limits.
3. Harmony with the functions of speech, respiration, and deglutition.
4. Esthetic acceptability.
5. Preservation of the supporting tissues.

Incompatibility

Even though it is not living tissue, a denture is compatible when it is accepted as having actual being with the oral environment. The chemical composition of the denture material should be inert. The artificial teeth should be placed in positions that do not produce trauma when they are brought together. The forces of occlusion should be directed toward the most acceptable support. The arrangement of the teeth should be such that when they make contact they are in harmony with mandibular positions and movements. When the mandible is at physiologic rest position, sufficient interocclusal distance must exist to allow full contraction of the elevator muscles of the mandible before the occlusal surfaces of the posterior teeth make maximum contact. The artificial teeth should be placed to give support to the lips and cheeks and be compatible with the actions of not only the lips and cheeks but also the tongue. The denture bases should cover the basal seat areas to achieve a "snowshoe" effect of maximum support. The soft tissues that are supported by bone should be recorded in their undisplaced form to assure even contact with the tissue side of the denture bases and to minimize the pressure to the underlying bone.

Problems with Mastication

Artificial replacement of parts of the body cannot be expected to be as functionally efficient as the natural normal healthy organ. Inability to perform certain masticatory acts such as chewing hard or sticky food or biting with the front teeth does not mean that the dentures are a failure. Denture wearers who experience problems in eating may need further instruction (Chapter 3). The patient must be made to realize that the problem can be solved if he will face reality.

Disharmony

Compatibility and harmony overlap somewhat. Harmony of complete dentures is concerned with the nonmasticatory acts of speech, respiration, and deglutition. In addition to being compatible with the oral environment, the denture bases must be accurately adapted to the supporting tissues, the polished surfaces properly contoured, and the artificial teeth placed in positions to allow enunciating, breathing, and swallowing to take place in a normal manner. Rough unpolished surfaces can irritate oral tissues and through the somatic nervous system interfere with normal function. Overextended borders are not compatible with normal function.

Dissatisfaction with Esthetics

Mental and emotional responses to the appearance of dentures vary. What is acceptable to one person may be unacceptable to another. If the patient complains that the artificial teeth do not look natural, check the arrangement, form, size, and hue of the teeth (Chapters 12, 13, and 14). It is through experience that one learns that, regardless of age or sex, esthetics is an important factor in denture acceptance. The contour of the denture bases must allow the facial expressions to be normal. When anatomic landmarks are used as guides in placing the teeth, contouring the body of the denture, and extending the denture flanges, normal action of the muscles of facial expression is possible. Most patients will advise the dentist when the denture fails to meet this requirement. Some, however, may relate other problems that cannot be demonstrated when, in fact, they do not like the appearance.

Deterioration of Supporting Tissues

Problems involving the soft tissues and/or bony support are particularly serious. Preservation of the supporting structures is one of the greatest challenges for the dentist and his patient, for loss of denture support usually results in denture failure. In treating these structures the dentist must be guided by his knowledge of their physiology (Chapter 1).

Soft Tissue Considerations

The soft tissues available to support dentures can be divided into three types: (1) mucosa with a tightly attached submucosa; (2) mucosa with a loosely attached submucosa, and (3) mucosa with a differentiated submucosa.

Oral mucosa with a tightly attached submucosa is the masticatory mucosa, which covers the crest and slopes of the residual ridges and the anterior third of the hard palate in the rugae area. The stratified squamous epithelium is highly keratinized, and the submucosa is firmly attached. The ability to produce keratin and the mode of attachment of the submucosa are considered desirable properties to resist pressure and the frictional impact of the denture bases (Fig. 19-1).

Oral mucosa with a loosely attached submucosa is located in the vestibular fornix and the soft palate distal to the palatine bones. The stratified squamous epithelium is not keratinized, and the submucosa allows movement of the mucosa between the denture and the base. Oral mucosa with a loosely attached submucosa is not considered desirable to resist stress but is desirable to form a seal with the borders of the dentures (Fig. 19-1).

Oral mucosa with a differentiated submucosa is located in the posterior two thirds of the hard palate, except for the palatine raphe, and in the retromolar pad. The irregular compartments in the palate contain adipose tissue and glands. The anterior spaces contain more adipose tissue, and the posterior spaces contain more glands. The retromolar pad contains fat, gland, loose connective tissue, and muscle fibers. Oral mucosa with a differentiated submucosa is not considered stress-bearing tissue (Fig. 19-1).

The mucosa that has a transitional submucosa is located in and near the junctions of the three different types of submucosa on the slopes of the residual ridges near the vestibules, in the palate, and distal to the retromolar papilla. The predominating characteristic determines the stress-bearing potential of the mucosa in the transitional zones (Fig. 19-1).

The soft tissues that contact but do not support the denture bases may be classified into two types: (1) the lining mucosa and (2) the specialized mucosa (Fig. 19-2).

The lining mucosa covers the cheeks, the lips, the under surface of the tongue, and the floor of the mouth. This mucosa has a thin epithelium and is lightly or not at all cornified. The lining mucosa that covers the muscles of the cheek, lip, and tongue is usually highly elastic and immovably attached to the fascia of the muscle. The lining mucosa of the floor of the mouth is very thin, mobile, and displaceable.

The specialized mucosa covers the dorsal surface of the tongue. The surface is rough and irregular, and the epithelial covering is cornified. The papillae are (1) the filiform, (2) the fungiform, and (3) the circumvallate. The papillae project on the surface of the tongue and help to produce the rough irregular surface. The taste buds are located in some of the papillae.

The histologic differences and the relations of the oral mucosa to the dentures account for the differences in tissue response to injury. Injuries to oral tissues occur principally in three areas: (1) the tissues that support and resist stress, (2) the tissues that act to form a seal with the denture borders, and (3) the tissues that contact the polished surfaces and the teeth.

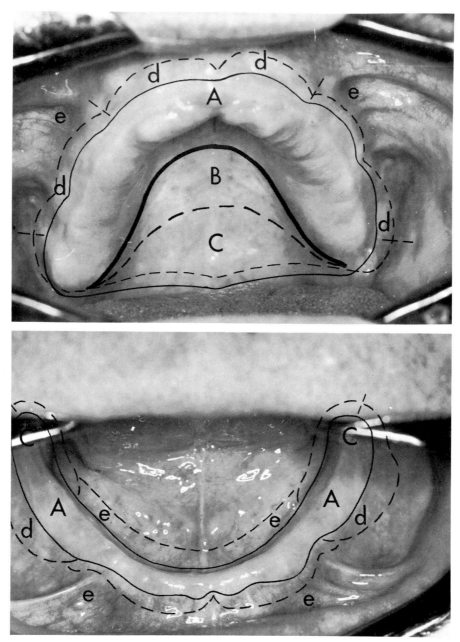

FIG. 19-1. *The soft tissues that support the dentures: tightly attached submucosa (A); differentiated submucosa (B and C); transitional submucosa (d); loosely attached submucosa (e).*

STRESS-BEARING MUCOSA

The signs and symptoms of traumatic injury to the stress-bearing mucosa follow:

1. Traumatic lesions of the stress-bearing mucosa of the palate and the crest and slopes of the residual ridges are usually the result of imperfections in or on the surface of the tissue side of the denture base, pressure areas on

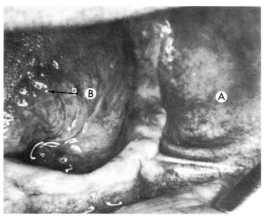
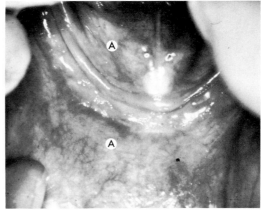

FIG. 19-2.   *Lining mucosa (A). Specialized mucosa (B).*

the tissue side of the denture that were developed either in the impression procedures or as a result of damage to the master cast, and disharmony in occlusion in either the centric or the eccentric jaw positions. Lesions occurring in the mucosa that covers the palate and the crest of the residual ridges are small, well circumscribed, and indurated. The presence of excessive keratin often causes the area to be white.

2. Lesions that appear punched out and the surrounding mucosa hyperemic are usually the result of imperfections in the denture base, trauma from food particles, or an injury produced when the dentures were not in the mouth.

3. Lesions that are hyperemic and painful to the pressure of closure are usually a result of pressure directed toward an area of exostosis, a sharp spur of bone, or a foreign body (Fig. 19-3).

4. Occasionally severe irritation and a detaching of the overlying mucosa occurs. This is encountered over the mylohyoid ridge, the cuspid eminences, the alveolar tubercles, and areas of exostosis. This is usually produced by the denture flange during the insertion and removal of the denture or from

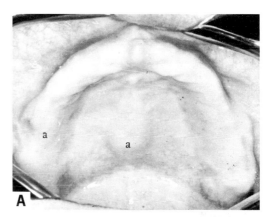
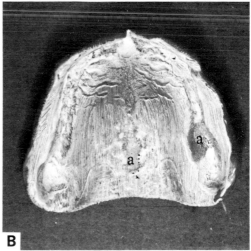

FIG. 19-3.   *Pressure areas can be demonstrated with pressure disclosing paste.* **A.** *Pressure areas (a).* **B.** *The extent of the pressure areas (a) is disclosed.*

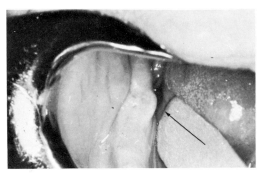

FIG. 19-4. *Horizontal projections will drag pressure disclosing paste from the denture flange. Note the projection of the lingual tuberosity at the arrow point.*

excessive friction when the denture moves during function (Fig. 19-4).

5. Hyperemic, painful, and detached areas of epithelium that develop on the slope of the residual ridges are usually the result of disharmony of occlusion when the teeth are making unbalanced contact in eccentric jaw positions. This is a horizontal torquing or shearing force.

BASAL SEAT MUCOSA

Two problems associated with the basal seat mucosa are hypertrophy and inflammation.

Inflammatory reactions of the mucosa covering the basal seat are usually the result of the following:

1. Some patients do not remove their dentures to allow the tissues to rest. The constant pressure of the dentures retards the normal blood supply, which oxygenates the tissues and removes the waste products (Fig. 19-5A).

2. A generalized hyperemia of the crest and slopes of the residual ridges accompanied by pain in the muscles attached to the mandible, the production of hyperkeratin, and a looseness of the dentures are often the result of insufficient interocclusal distance.

3. In certain circumstances it appears

that the tightly attached submucosa becomes loose in some areas. Loosely attached submucosa constitutes a poor seat for a complete denture. This condition usually occurs on the lingual surface of the mandibular residual ridge. The dentures glide upon the mucosa as a result of lack of stability. The friction of the underlying bone against the undersurface of the mucosa produces the inflammation. This deep-seated inflammation is not always readily visible to the dentist.

4. In some situations the submucosa of the lingual of the mandible in the molar and in the anterior regions appears to become detached from the periosteum. This produces a very pain-

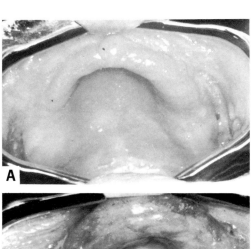

FIG. 19-5. *Inflammatory reactions.* **A.** *Generalized hyperemia and edema in a patient who never removed his dentures for tissue rest.* **B.** *Localized hyperemia and edema in a patient with a complete maxillary denture opposed by natural mandibular anterior teeth and a removable partial denture.*

ful inflammatory condition. It is a vexing problem that is not always satisfactorily resolved.

5. A complete denture opposite natural teeth or a partial denture may cause localized hyperemia and edema (Fig. 19-5B).

6. Poor oral hygiene can result in inflammatory reactions.

7. An unbalanced diet and avitaminosis contribute to inflammatory conditions in all age groups. Unsupervised crash diets, alcoholism, and senility may lead to malnutrition, which is reflected in the inability of the oral mucosa to resist the pressure of dentures (Fig. 19-6).

8. Endocrine gland disturbances and parafunction resulting from neurosis can cause inflammation of the oral mucosa.

9. Systemic debilitating diseases contribute to poor tissue tone and poor tissue resistance to the stress of dentures (Fig. 19-6).

10. Allergic reactions of the supporting tissues to denture base materials appear to occur more fictionally than really. In thirty years of observing patients with acrylic resin dentures, the author has never seen a single patient with an acute or inflammatory tissue condition who demonstrated a positive reaction to patch tests. This is not to be interpreted that a patient cannot develop a sensitivity to methyl methacrylate resin, for in this same period two patients, both prosthetic laboratory technicians, developed a sensitivity. However, neither used either partial or complete dentures.

Hypertrophy, an abnormal increase in the size of the oral mucosa that is considered stress bearing, is unusual. However, in the midpalatal suture area, particularly when a relief is placed in the tissue side of the denture base, hypertrophy of the mucosa does occur. Small nodules, which are defined as

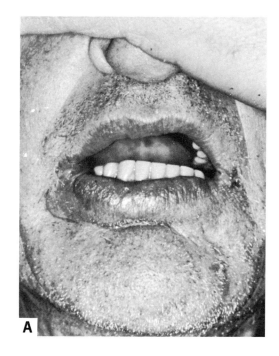

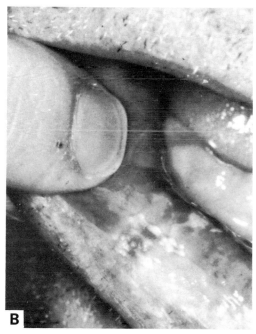

FIG. 19-6. **A.** *Commissural cheilosis characteristic of riboflavin deficiency.* **B.** *Benign lip lesion. Poor oral hygiene, unbalanced diet, and a debilitating systemic disease contribute to these tissue reactions.*

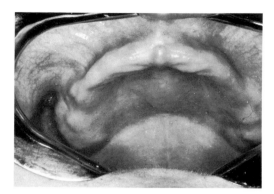

Fig. 19-7. *The incisal papilla is slightly enlarged. The mucosa is smooth, shiny, and hyperemic. The patient's problem is pain.*

"papilloma-like hypertrophy," develop throughout the area.

The incisal papilla of the basal seat mucosa is another area that becomes enlarged, hyperemic, and painful. When the cause is not removed or corrected, the tissue becomes pendulous (Fig. 19-7).

TRANSITIONAL SUBMUCOSA

Hypertrophy can also occur in the areas of transitional submucosa, such as border extensions. The lesions occurring in the border extension areas are usually slitlike fissures. The fissures vary in length and depth, are painful, and often become ulcerated. These lesions result primarily from overextension of the border but can result from sharp or unpolished borders. The lesions can occur in any border area; however, they are most frequently encountered in these areas in the order named: (1) frenum attachments, (2) the retromylohyoid space, (3) the retromolar pad, (4) the masseter groove, (5) the hamular notch, (6) the vestibular fornix, (7) the floor of the mouth, and (8) the soft palate.

Signs and symptoms of traumatic lesions can also occur in the areas of loosely attached submucosa and specialized mucosa.

LINING MUCOSA

Abrasions appearing on the mucosa of the cheeks and lips are frequently the result of (1) cheek biting, (2) rough margins on the teeth, or (3) unpolished denture bases (Fig. 19-8).

SPECIALIZED MUCOSA

Ulcerations and other lesions appearing on the margins and apex of the tongue are results of (1) tongue biting often caused by improper placement of the teeth either in a horizontal or vertical position, (2) an unpolished denture base or a too pronounced rugae area, and (3) rough margins on the teeth.

One frequently sees hypertrophy at the junction of the tightly and loosely attached submucosa. The initial trauma may be a result of disharmony of occlusion in the eccentric jaw positions. This is especially true when the forces of occlusion are directed toward the anterior residual ridges in biting. The bone loss results in a loose denture, and a loose denture produces more trauma (Fig. 19-9). Hypertrophy in the labial flange areas often occurs following the insertion of an immediate complete denture when the occlusion and denture bases have not been altered to meet the changes taking place in the

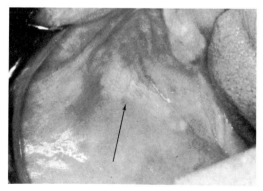

Fig. 19-8. *Abrasions resulting from a rough denture border. The arrow is directed to the damaged area.*

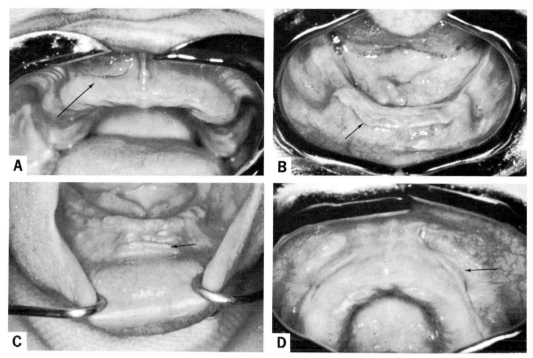

FIG. 19-9. *Hypertrophy.* **A, B,** *and* **C.** *The arrows point to the fibrous tissue in which hypertrophy was not reversible and had to be treated with surgical procedures.* **D.** *A reversible situation. Tissue recovery procedures were successful, and surgical procedures were not necessary.*

basal seat. In many instances the enlarged tissues contain bands or bundles of fibrous tissue, fibrous hyperplasia. The fibrous tissue, which acts as a foreign body between the hard denture base and the bone, then aggravates the condition. Hypertrophy in the flange areas is usually painless until the condition has advanced. Advanced hypertrophy that contains fibrous tissue is not reversible; it will not disappear when the cause is removed.

Problems Involving Bone

The loss of bone, which is a constant problem with denture users, was discussed in Chapter 1. The alveolar residual ridge is the major bony support for the denture base to resist torquing and horizontal forces. On the basis of statis-

tical calculations Jozefowicz concluded that wearing dentures enhances the atrophy of the residual ridges.[9a] In the presence of excessive and/or rapid loss of these ridges it is not always easy to determine the cause. The dentures may be the source, but they should not be classified as failures until extensive diagnostic procedures have been completed.

Isolated spinous processes may develop on the surface of the bone. The soft tissue covering is caught between the hard denture base and the spine of bone with resulting discomfort and pain.

The crest of the residual ridge often becomes pendulous; then it is pinched between the knife edge of bone and the denture base.

Bone growth on the surface, exostosis, results in a thinning of the overlying mucosa. These areas of bony growth act as fulcrum and pressure points.

The mylohyoid ridge is frequently sharp and/or prominent. When sharp, it acts like a knife-edge ridge; when prominent, it makes an undercut area.

Rarely encountered in senile patients is a condition that has been defined as a bone sore mouth. These unfortunate patients demonstrate no soft tissue damage but express a feeling of constant soreness and the desire to remove the dentures whenever possible. They also express the same feeling regarding the bone of the foot and the bridge of the nose. The desire to remove the glasses and shoes is as demanding as the desire to remove the dentures.

Treatment Procedures

Dentures that are essentially satisfactory can be ruined by indiscriminately altering the denture base or the teeth. To determine the etiology, the dentist must conduct these procedures in a systematic manner.

1. Examine each denture for stability and retention with the mouth at rest and with the mouth in function. To check functional stability and retention, instruct the patient to speak, laugh, yawn, wipe the lips with the tip of the tongue, and swallow.

2. Check the dentures for indications of undercut areas. Apply pressure disclosing paste to the tissue side of either the maxillary or the mandibular denture. Instruct the patient to insert and remove the denture. An undercut appears when the paste is removed from the denture as if it were dragged from the surface. When it has been definitely established that an undercut exists and that the denture is abusing the mucosa, alter the tissue side of the denture base by grinding with an acrylic bur.

It is better to grind too little than too much, since tissue contact with the denture must be maintained. Smooth and polish all ground areas. Repeat the procedure with the other denture.

3. Apply pressure disclosing paste to the entire tissue side of the maxillary denture. Instruct the patient to insert both dentures and tap the teeth together with the jaws in centric relation. Instruct the patient to exercise care when inserting the maxillary denture and not to apply finger pressure to the denture. It is possible to displace the paste and produce an area which appears as a pressure area or fulcrum point when pressure is applied with the fingers. When the teeth have been tapped to place, an area of displaced paste on the tissue side of the denture is a sign of pressure. It is best to repeat the procedure. The pressure area may result from premature tooth contact or an imperfection of the denture base. The cause must be determined before institution of corrective measures. Repeat the procedures for the mandibular denture.

4. To determine if the pressure area is produced by faulty occlusion, institute patient remount procedures (page 381). When occlusion causes the pressure, adjust the occlusion (page 379). When the denture base causes the pressure, relieve the denture base by grinding with an acrylic bur; then smooth and polish. It is possible that both denture base and occlusion may need correction.

5. When occlusal disharmony causes lesions, inflammatory areas, or hypertrophy of the mucosa on the slopes of the ridges, refine the occlusion. When the problem results from loose and ill-fitting dentures, either remake or rebase the dentures.

6. When a generalized inflammatory condition exists or hyperkeratosis is

present in the stress-bearing mucosa, evaluate the interocclusal distance (page 264). If the interocclusal distance is not adequate, alter the teeth to provide adequate space.

7. When traumatic lesions are present in the denture border areas, apply disclosing wax to the borders of one denture at a time in the same manner that impression compound was applied during the border refining procedures (page 377). Instruct the patient to speak, swallow, laugh, yawn, wipe the lips with the tip of the tongue, and place the tip of the tongue in the buccal and labial vestibular spaces. If the disclosing wax is moved from the border of the denture, overextension is indicated. At times the overextension is so limited that disclosing wax is not accurate. When this is so, the lesion can be touched with indelible coloring material to mark the contacting area of the denture border. Remove the overextended area by grinding with an acrylic bur. Smooth the ground surface with a Burlew wheel and wet pumice on a wet rag wheel.

8. Hypertrophy of the mucosa which does not include fibrous hyperplasia is usually reversible and will resolve when the source of the trauma is removed. Because fibrous hyperplasia is not reversible, surgical procedures are necessary for removal.

9. When abrasions and ulcerations of the tongue and cheek occur, the vertical and horizontal positions of the teeth must be evaluated. A loss of muscle tonus allows the cheek to sag, and the result may be cheek biting. Tongue biting can occur in patients who have diseases of the nervous system, such as epilepsy.

10. Surgical procedures or systemic therapy usually resolves problems involving bone.

Other signs and symptoms of denture problems which do not necessarily result in traumatic lesions, inflammatory reactions, hypertrophy, fibrous hyperplasia, or result from bone include:

PROBLEMS WITH MAXILLARY DENTURE

1. Dislodgment during functions is a result of (a) overfilled buccal vestibule, (b) overextension in the hamular notch area, (c) inadequate notches for frenum attachments, (d) excessively thick denture base over the distobuccal alveolar tubercle area leaving insufficient space for the forward and medial movement of the anterior border of the coronoid process, (e) placing the maxillary anterior teeth too far in an anterior direction, (f) placing the maxillary posterior teeth too far in a buccal direction, (g) placing the posterior palatal seal too far in a superior direction causing overdisplacement of soft palate tissues, or (h) lack of occlusal harmony. When the teeth do not make harmonious contact, the seal between the tissues and the denture base is often broken. The result is loss of stability and retention.

2. Dislodgment when the jaws are at rest is a result of (a) underfilled buccal vestibule, (b) inadequate border seal, (c) excessive saliva, or (d) xerostomia

When the maxillary denture slowly loses retention, the consistency of the saliva, excessive saliva, or the lack of saliva is usually involved.

When the drop or loosening of the denture is sudden, the cause is usually mechanical. As an example, when the wearer smokes or whistles, the contraction at the modiolus dislodges the denture if the denture flange is not contoured properly.

PROBLEMS WITH MANDIBULAR DENTURE

1. Dislodgment during function is the result of (a) overextension in the masseter groove area, (b) extending in

a lateral direction beyond the external oblique line, (c) overextension of the lingual flanges, (d) placing the occlusal plane too high, causing dislodgment when the tongue tries to handle the bolus of food, (e) underextension of the lingual flanges causing the border to become the playground for the tongue, (f) improper contour of the polished surface, or (g) overextension in the retromolar pad area, causing contact between the denture base that covers the alveolar tubercle and the denture base that covers the retromolar pad when the mandible is protruded. This contact dislodges the mandibular denture in the anterior section.

Clicking

A clicking noise when the teeth contact during functional movements is a result of insufficient interocclusal distance, a dropping of the maxillary denture, or a vertical displacement of the mandibular denture.

Treatments for "clicking" teeth are as follows:

1. When the dentures are loose, correct the stability and retention by rebasing or remaking the dentures.

2. If the dentures are not loose, if sufficient interocclusal distance exists, and if the teeth are porcelain, replace the porcelain teeth with acrylic resin teeth.

3. When the interocclusal distance is not sufficient, alter the occlusal surfaces of the teeth with remount procedures to provide adequate space.

Commissural Cheilitis

Commissural cheilitis, inflammation of the angles of the mouth, is frequently attributed to excessive interocclusal distance. However, placing the maxillary posterior teeth too far in a lateral direction eliminates the buccal corri-

dor. When the crowns of the teeth are against the cheeks, the saliva collects at the necks of the teeth and makes its escape in the area of the cuspids. Commissural cheilitis often develops when these conditions exist.

When commissural cheilitis is considered the result of excessive interocclusal distance or the improper placement of the teeth, it is advisable to construct new dentures.

Gagging and Vomiting

Patients who develop a gagging or vomiting problem with dentures are frequently difficult to treat, and the difficulty is primarily one of determining the cause. Some patients have a hypersensitive gagging reflex evident prior to and during the denture construction. The insertion or removal of complete dentures may elicit gagging. However, occasionally a patient develops a gagging problem after denture insertion.

Vomiting and gagging can result from chemical irritants, toxic materials ingested with food, specific drugs, severe pain, strong emotional situations, or mild stimulation of the pharynx or fauces. Vomiting is a protective involuntary reflex present at birth. The protective action of the vomiting reflex is associated primarily with the maintenance of a patent airway and the removal of noxious stimuli from the gastrointestinal tract.

Swallowing results from the stimulation of the afferent fibers of the fifth, ninth, and tenth cranial nerves. Stimulation of the swallowing receptors can result in a series of uncoordinated and spasmodic movements of the swallowing muscles. The uncoordinated and spasmodic movements are referred to as gagging. Stimulation of the sensitive areas in the posterior pharyngeal wall, the soft palate, the uvula, the fauces, or the posterior dorsal surface of the tongue can produce gagging. The stimulating impulse may result from tactile, visual, acoustic, olfactory, or psychic stimuli.

A complete denture patient may develop a gagging or vomiting problem as a result of (1) loose dentures, (2) poor occlusion, (3) incorrect contour of the dentures, particularly in the posterior area of the palate and the retromylo-hyoid space, (4) underextended denture borders, (5) placing the maxillary teeth too far in a palatal direction and the mandibular teeth too far in a lingual direction so that the dorsum of the tongue is forced into the pharynx during the act of swallowing, (6) an increased vertical dimension of occlusion, and (7) psychogenic factors. Patients may refuse to swallow for fear the dentures will dislodge and strangle them. As a result of not swallowing, the saliva accumulates and triggers the gagging reflex.

The treatment for gagging is as follows:

1. Determine the cause when possible.

2. Remove all biological and mechanical factors that may contribute to the problem.

3. Prescribe a combination of hyoscine, hyoscyamine, and atropine with a sedative during the initial period of denture use. Certain drugs act as selective depressors of the parasympathetic portion of the autonomic nervous system. Among these drugs are the sedatives, the antihistamines, parasympatholytics, and the central nervous system depressants.

4. Consider referring the patient for psychiatric help. Pursue all other etiologic factors prior to psychiatric referral unless the patient has been or is under active psychiatric treatment.

Burning Tongue and Palate

The burning sensation which some patients experience in the anterior third of the palate may result from pressure on the nasopalatine area. Relief of the denture over the incisive papilla is usually effective.

Burning tongue and burning palate are often associated with climacteric, a critical period of life, occurring in women at the termination of the reproductive period, and characterized by endocrine, somatic, and psychic changes and ultimate menopause. A corresponding period occurs in men and is called male climacteric. It is extremely difficult to determine what produces the burning sensation.

Corrective procedures are instituted as follows:

1. Instruct patient in good oral hygiene. Recommend cleaning the tongue with gauze, not a brush.

2. Avoid hot spicy foods and caustic mouth washes.

3. For vitamin deficiency prescribe vitamins A and B_{12} for three months; discontinue for one month and re-evaluate.

4 Prescribe a mild tranquilizer.

5. When this condition is severe and persists, refer the patient to an oral surgeon for possible surgical intervention.

6. When the condition is persistent and is complicated with other problems that may be associated with psychic changes, refer the patient for psychiatric consultation.

REFERENCES

1. Bartels, H. A.: Significance of yeastlike organisms in denture sore mouths. J. Orthodont. Oral Surg., *23*:90, 1937.

1a. Bauman, R.: Chairside modification of dentures for tissue conditioning materials. J. Prosth. Dent., *40*:225, 1978.

1b. Bell, D. H., Jr.: Problems in complete denture treatment. J. Prosth. Dent., *19*:550, 1968.

1c. Berg, H., Carlsson, G. E., and Helkimo, M.: Changes in shape of posterior parts of upper jaws after extraction of teeth and prosthetic treatment. J. Prosth. Dent., *34:*262, 1975.

2. Caselli, O. J.: Treatment of temporomandibular joint disturbances caused by chronic partial subluxation. J. Prosth. Dent., *9:*98, 1959.

3. Cohn, L. R.: Denture sore mouth. New York Dent. J., *15:*158, 1949.

4. Collett, H. A.: Oral conditions associated with dentures. J. Prosth. Dent., *8:*591, 1958.

4a. Desjardins, R. P., and Tolman, D. E.: Etiology and management of hypermobile mucosa overlying the residual alveolar ridge. J. Prosth. Dent., *32:*619, 1974.

5. Earnshaw, R., and Smith, D. C.: Angular stomatitis and artificial dentures. (Abst.) New York J. Dent., *25:*305, 1955.

5a. Enlow, D. H., Bianco, H. J., and Eklund, S.: The remodeling of the edentulous mandible. J. Prosth. Dent., *36:*685, 1976.

6. Fisher, A. A.: Allergic sensitization of the skin and oral mucosa to acrylic denture materials. J.A.M.A., *156:*238, 1954.

7. ———, and Rashid, P. J.: Inflammatory papillary hyperplasia of the palatal mucosa. Oral Surg., *5:*191, 1952.

8. Frölich, E., and Masshoff, W.: Alteration in the mucous glands caused by complete upper dentures. Dent. Abst., *1:*549, 1956.

9. Hall, R. E.: Tissue atrophy resulting from compression of tissues for the retention of dentures. J. Nat. Dent. Ass., *8:*919, 1921.

9a. Harris, W. T., and Mack, J. F.: Conditioning dentures for problem patients. J. Prosth. Dent., *34:*141, 1975.

9b. Jozefowicz, W.: The influence of wearing dentures on residual ridges: a comparative study. J. Prosth. Dent., *24:*137, 1970.

10. Kapur, K., and Shklar, G.: The effect of complete dentures on alveolar mucosa. J. Prosth. Dent., *13:*1030, 1963.

11. Kennedy, C. A., Jr.: Trouble shooting in full denture construction. J. Prosth. Dent., *3:*660, 1953.

12. Kimball, H. D.: Factors to be considered in the control and elimination of chronic tissue soreness beneath dentures. J. Prosth. Dent., *4:*298, 1954.

12a. Klingler, S. M., and Lord, J. L.: Effect of common agents on intermediary temporary soft reline materials. J. Prosth. Dent., *30:*749, 1973.

12b. Koper, A.: Difficult denture birds. J. Prosth. Dent., *17:*532, 1967.

12c. Kouats, J. T.: Clinical evaluation of the gagging denture patient. J. Prosth. Dent., *25:*613, 1971.

13. Kuck, M.: Irritations of the oral mucosa caused by the addition of coloring matter to acrylic denture materials. Dent. Abst., *2:*635, 1951.

14. Lam, R. V.: Contour changes of the alveolar processes following extractions. J. Prosth. Dent., *10:*25, 1960.

15. Lambson, G. O.: Papillary hyperplasia of the palate. J. Prosth. Dent., *16:*636, 1966.

15a. ———, and Anderson, R. R.: Palatal papillary hyperplasia. J. Prosth. Dent., *18:*528, 1967.

16. Landa, J. S.: The torus palatinus and its management in full denture construction. J. Prosth. Dent., *1:*236, 1951.

17. ———: Trouble shooting in complete denture prosthesis, part I. Oral mucosa and border extension. J. Prosth. Dent., *9:* 978, 1959.

18. ———: Trouble shooting in complete denture prosthesis, part II. Lesions of the oral mucosa and their correction. J. Prosth. Dent., *10:*42, 1960.

19. ———: Trouble shooting in complete denture prosthesis, part III. Traumatic injuries. J. Prosth. Dent., *10:*263, 1960.

20. ———: Trouble shooting in complete denture prosthesis, part IV. Proper adjustment procedures. J. Prosth. Dent., *10:*490, 1960.

21. ———: Trouble shooting in complete denture prosthesis, part V. Local and systemic involvements. J. Prosth. Dent., *10:*682, 1960.

22. ———: Trouble shooting in complete denture prosthesis, part VI. Factors of oral hygiene, chemicotoxicity, nutrition, allergy, and conductivity. J. Prosth. Dent., *10:*887, 1960.

23. ———: Trouble shooting in complete denture prosthesis, part VII. Mucosal irritation. J. Prosth. Dent., *10:*1022, 1960.

24. ———: Trouble shooting in complete denture prosthesis, part VIII. Interference with anatomic structures. J. Prosth. Dent., *11:*79, 1961.

25. ———: Trouble shooting in complete

denture prosthesis, part IX. Salivation, stomatopyrosis, and glossoporosis. J. Prosth. Dent., 11:244, 1961.

26. ———: Trouble shooting in complete denture prosthesis, part X. Nerve impingement and the radiolucent lower anterior ridge. J. Prosth. Dent., 11:440, 1961.

26a. Loue, W. D., Goska, F. A., and Mixson, R. J.: The etiology of mucosal inflammation associated with dentures. J. Prosth. Dent., 18:515, 1967.

26b. Lytle, R. B., Atwood, D. A., and Beck, H. O.: Minimum standards of adequate prosthodontic service. J. Prosth. Dent., 19:108, 1968.

27. Mann, A. W.: Diet and nutrition in the edentulous patient. Dent. Clin. N. Amer., March, 1957, p. 285.

27a. McCarthy, J. A., and Moser, J. B.: Mechanical properties of tissue conditioners—Part I. J. Prosth. Dent., 40:89, 1978.

27b. ———: Mechanical properties of tissue conditioners—Part II. J. Prosth. Dent., 40:334, 1978.

27c. Means, A. C., and Flenniken, I. E.: Gagging—a problem in prosthetic dentistry. J. Prosth. Dent., 23:614, 1970.

28. Mehringer, E. J.: The saliva as it is related to the wearing of dentures. J. Prosth. Dent., 4:312, 1954.

28a. Meyer, F. S.: Dentures, causes of failures and remedies. J. Prosth. Dent., 1:672, 1951.

28b. Michman, J., and Langer, A.: Clinical and electromyographic observations during adjustment to complete dentures. J. Prosth. Dent., 19:252, 1968.

28c. ———: Postinsertion changes in complete dentures. J. Prosth. Dent., 34:125, 1975.

29. Miller, R. H., Jr.: Mucosal edema: a new syndrome. J. Prosth. Dent., 9:743, 1959.

29a. Moghadam, B. K., and Scandrett, F. R.: A technique for adding the posterior palatal seal. J. Prosth. Dent., 32:443, 1974.

29b. Morstad, A. T., and Peterson, A. D.: Postinsertion denture problems. J. Prosth. Dent., 19:126, 1968.

29c. Murrell, G. A.: The management of difficult lower dentures. J. Prosth. Dent., 32:243, 1974.

30. Nagle, R. J.: Postinsertion problems in complete denture prosthesis. J.A.D.A., 57:183, 1958.

31. Nyquist, G.: Study of denture sore mouth. An investigation of traumatic, allergic, and toxic lesions of the oral mucosa arising from the use of full dentures. Acta Odont. Scand., Supp. 9., 10:11, 1952.

32. ———: Influence of denture hygiene and the bacterial flora on the condition of the oral mucosa in full denture cases. Acta Odont. Scand., 11:24, 1953.

32a. Pietrokovski, J.: The bony residual ridge in man. J. Prosth. Dent., 34:456, 1975.

32b. Pudwill, M. L., and Wentz, F. M.: Microscopic anatomy of edentulous residual alveolar ridges. J. Prosth. Dent., 34:448, 1975.

32c. Ritchie, G. M., et al.: The etiology, exfoliatine cytology, and treatment of denture stomatitis. J. Prosth. Dent., 22:185, 1969.

33. Robinson, H. B. G.: Diagnosis of lesions associated with dentures. J. Prosth. Dent., 7:338, 1957.

34. Schmitz, J. F.: A clinical study of inflammatory papillary hyperplasia. J. Prosth. Dent., 14:1034, 1964.

35. Shanahan, T. F. J.: Paresthesia due to lower denture pressure. J.A.D.A., 67:10, 1963.

35a. Sharp, G. S.: Treatment for low tolerance to dentures: Supplemental report. J. Prosth. Dent., 17:222, 1967.

35b. Sharry, J. J.: Denture failures related to occlusion. Dent. Clin. N. Amer., 16:119, 1972.

35c. Sheppard, I. M., Schwartz, L. R., and Sheppard, S. M.: Oral status of edentulous and complete denture wearing patients. J.A.D.A., 83:614, 1971.

36. Siegel, B.: Paresthesia of the lower right lip resulting from pressure of the full lower denture on the mental nerve and foramen. J.A.D.A., 45:40, 1952.

36a. Silverman, M. M.: The whistle and swish sound in denture patients. J. Prosth. Dent., 17:144, 1967.

36b. Simpson, H. E.: Experimental investigation into the healing of extraction wounds in Macacus rhesus monkeys. J. Oral Surg., 18:391, 1960.

36c. ———: Effects of suturing extraction wounds in Macacus rhesus monkeys. J. Oral Surg., 18:461, 1960.

36d. ———: Healing of surgical extraction

wounds in Macacus rhesus monkeys. J. Oral Surg., *19*:227, 1961.

36e. Singer, I. L.: The marble technique: a method for treating the "hopeless gagger" for complete dentures. J. Prosth. Dent., *29*:146, 1973.

37. Spies, T. D.: Vitamins and avitaminosis. *In* Duncan, G. G.: *Disease of Metabolism.* Philadelphia, W. B. Saunders Co., 1947.

38. Stansbery, C. J.: Tissue changes under dentures. J.A.D.A., *15*:349, 1928.

39. Stout, C. J.: Construction of new dentures for old denture wearers. Dent. Clin. N. Amer., November, 1964, p. 749.

39a. Stysiak, Z. D.: Allergy as a cause of denture sore mouth. J. Prosth. Dent., *25*:16, 1971.

40. Syrop, H. M.: Allergic problems related to dentistry. Ann. of Allerg., *15*:603, 1957.

40a. Thompson, J. C.: The load factor in complete denture intolerance. J. Prosth. Dent., *25*:4, 1971.

40b. Turrell, A. J. W.: Vertical dimension as it relates to the etiology of angular cheilosis.

41. Van Huysen, G., Fly, W., and Leonard, L.: Artificial denture and the oral mucosa. J. Prosth. Dent., *4*:446, 1954.

42. Vilter, R. W.: Sore tongue and sore mouth. In McBryde, C. M.: *Signs and Symptoms.* Philadelphia, J. B. Lippincott, 1947.

42a. Welker, W. A.: Prosthodontic treatment of abused oral tissues. J. Prosth. Dent., *37*:259, 1977.

42b. Wendt, D. C.: The degenerative denture ridge—care and treatment. J. Prosth. Dent., *32*:477, 1974.

42c. Winkler, S., Ortman, H. R., and Ryczek, M. T.: Improving the retention of complete dentures. J. Prosth. Dent., *34*:11, 1975.

43. Woods, V.: Management of postinsertion problems. Dent. Clin. N. Amer. November, 1964, p. 742.

44. Wright, W. H.: The importance of tissue changes under artificial dentures. J.A.D.A., *16*:1027, 1929.

45. ——: Morphological changes in the mucous membrane covering the edentulous areas of the alveolar process in the human mouth. J. Dent. Res., *13*:159, 1933.

Treating Abused Tissues

20

Abuse of the tissues supporting dentures (discussed in Chapter 19) deforms these soft tissues and destroys bone (Fig. 20-1.) When the bone has resorbed and the tissues are deformed so much that minor procedures no longer will make the dentures acceptable, the dentures must be rebased or remade.

The severity of the injury to the tissues is not always in proportion to the accuracy of the denture or to the disharmony of occlusion with mandibular movements. Pathologic conditions of the supporting tissues frequently result from systemic diseases. The treatment of the systemic factors is often a joint endeavor between dentist and physician. The ideal situation is to eliminate or control the systemic condition before refitting the old dentures or constructing new dentures. In the treatment of systemic diseases, debilitating in nature, dentures are frequently desirable, and the treatment plan must be altered from the ideal. Fortunately, this situation is the exception, not the rule.

The treatment of local factors, occlusal disharmony, inaccurate denture bases, and other mechanical factors that result in tissue abuse are the responsibility of the *dentist* and the *patient*. The extent of the abuse, the dentist's willingness to educate the patient in all factors involved in the treatment, and the patient's willingness to follow instructions govern the treatment plan. There appears to be a close relationship between failure to follow instructions in the use and care of dentures and extensiveness of abused tissues. Although this correlation is not always significant, it is better to base the treatment plan on the rule and not on the exceptions. The dentist must recognize also that certain results are the exception and must investigate the biologic factor in these cases. The investigation and study of exceptional reactions may lead to better techniques and procedures.

Regardless of the extent of tissue abuse, the first step is to educate the patient in his responsibility in the treatment plan. The treatment may be extensive, time-consuming, and expensive and may require surgery. In many situations, removing the dentures until the tissues recover is essential for an early recovery. Often failure to remove the dentures complicates the treatment. When continued use of the dentures is the primary etiologic factor, removing the dentures assures recovery. However, this approach, though ideal, is not always possible. The most favorable prognosis results when the abused soft tissues are allowed to recover to a normal, healthy condition before impressions for a rebase or for a new denture are made.

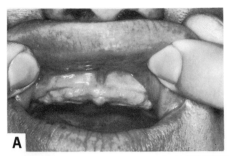

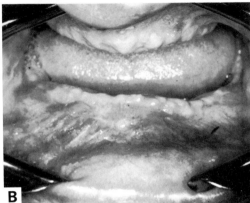

FIG. 20-1. *The soft tissues in the anterior sections of the maxillary and mandibular arches evidence changes of abuse.* **A.** *In the maxillary arch note the folding of the mucous membrane at the junction of the tightly and loosely attached submucosa. This indicates the beginning of hypertrophic changes that are commonly referred to as "epulis fissuratum."* **B.** *In the mandibular arch note the hyperemia in the labial vestibule and the irregular contour of the mucosa over the crest of the residual ridge—signs of injury.*

If the patient cannot or will not cooperate in the prescribed program or cannot afford an extensive treatment plan, a rebase or new denture may be no more than a temporary expedient. Temporary treatments often result in further soft tissue abuse and hard tissue destruction. The dentist may exercise the same prerogative as a physician in declining to accept patients who do not cooperate in the prescribed treatment. Without the cooperation of the patient, attempts to treat conditions that affect his health and well-being are usually unsuccessful. Many dentists do not continue to treat uncooperative patients, but this decision should not be made until every effort has been made to educate the patient. Fortunately most patients will accept their responsibility once they understand all the factors involved.

Tissue Recovery Routines

The first step, therefore, in treating abused tissue is to advise the patient of the treatment plan and to spell out his responsibility in the treatment (pages 92–97). For some persons extent of abuse, occupation, social obligations, or related conditions that do not permit removal of the dentures all the time may complicate the treatment. The complications and the extensive treatment plan should be explained to the patient both verbally and in writing so that he knows what to expect. The treatment plan may include any or all of the following procedures.

1. Surgical removal of hypertrophied tissue, pendulous tissue, or fibrous hyperplasia; alterations of the bony support; repositioning of the sulci. Before surgery, institute a tissue recovery program, a procedure that often reduces the extensiveness of the surgery.

2. The correction of occlusal disharmony by patient remount procedures (pages 381–385).

3. Correcting pressure areas in the tissue surface of the dentures or stabilizing the dentures. This procedure frequently requires a chairside reline. The use of a lining material requires not only accurate adaptation of the liner but also maintenance of the correct interocclusal space and harmonizing the occlusion with the mandibular movements. The lining material must have ready flow, quick set, and consistency hard enough to allow patient remount procedures.

4. Massage of the soft tissues two or three times a day to stimulate the blood supply and aid recovery. Instruct the patient to dissolve one-half teaspoon of table salt in a half glass of warm water and vigorously swirl the solution against the tissues by inflating and deflating the cheeks.

5. The removal of the dentures from the mouth for at least eight out of twenty-four hours. Patients usually agree to this program, since it can be accomplished during sleeping hours. However, instructing the patient to remove the dentures day and night meets with disapproval in many instances. When a patient properly understands the treatment plan, he usually accepts readily. Inform him that his health is involved, that the tissues are treated to promote his comfort, and that preservation of the support for his dentures is essential to continued successful denture use. When the old dentures are suitable for rebasing procedures and the tissues have returned to an acceptable healthy condition (Fig. 20-2A,B) with a program of occlusal correction, tissue rest at night, tissue massage, and minor corrections of the denture base, carry out rebase procedures (page 412). With this procedure the dentures may be serviceable for an indefinite period, or the tissues can be maintained in a healthy condition during the construction of new dentures.

It is not always mandatory for recovery of tissues to remove the dentures from the mouth continuously before making new dentures or a rebase. When the tissue abuse is extensive and the patient cannot leave the dentures out of the mouth for tissue recovery, it is advisable to institute the following plan of treatment.

1. Establish a tissue recovery routine that includes leaving the dentures out of the mouth at least eight out of twenty-four hours, making occlusal corrections, relieving pressure areas in the existing dentures, reducing any overextended borders, and allowing as much tissue recovery as possible.

2. Institute surgical procedures if necessary (page 137). At times the existing dentures can be used as a satisfactory surgical splint, but this is not often the rule, and the denture must be carefully evaluated. Remember that the dentures may be the sole cause of the tissue condition; temporary alterations with compound, wax, or other materials may be unsatisfactory.

3. When the surgical procedures have been completed or when no surgical procedures are needed, institute a tissue recovery program that includes chairside reline procedures (page 388).

Tissue Conditioners

The most expedient and yet the most effective method for treating abused basal tissues is for the patient to remove the dentures from the mouth for an extended period of time. For most patients, however, social and economic considerations preclude this simple but direct approach. The need to accomplish rehabilitation of abused tissues without the continuous removal of patients' dentures has led to the development and widespread acceptance of tissue-conditioning materials. These substances are soft elastomers that function as short-term reline materials by restoring the fit and stability of a denture base. They are composed of a powder, usually polyethylmethacrylate, and a liquid consisting of an aromatic ester-ethyl alcohol mixture. The exact compositions and proportions vary with different names and are considered to be trade secrets. Obviously, the manufacturers' instructions should be closely followed.

Tissue-conditioning materials are formulated to be soft, resilient, and to flow under pressure. These properties enable

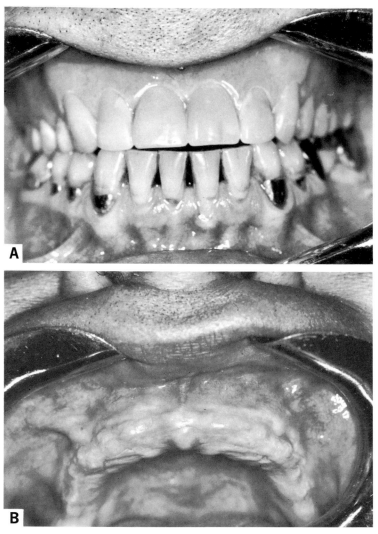

FIG. 20-2. A. *These denture teeth had not been altered appreciably and were considered suitable for rebase procedures.* **B.** *This enlarged tissue contained no bands of fibrous tissue, and the condition was reversible. The patient removed the denture for one week, and the tissues then appeared healthy.*

the material to readily adapt to the basal mucosa and the basal denture surface to form an intervening cushion. Consequently, the transmission of masticatory forces to the supporting mucosa are equalized, thereby eliminating isolated pressure spots typical of a loose, ill-fitting denture. As long as the material remains soft and resilient, it will have a rehabilitating or conditioning effect on basal mucosa that is traumatized, irritated, deformed, or abused. The rehabilitating effect, however, is limited to tissue changes that are reversible, such as tissue displacement, abrasion, ulceration, swelling due to edema, and a reduction in the inflammatory response. Irreversible changes, such as tissue overgrowth due to hyperplasia and/or hypertrophy, are not directly affected.

Paradoxically, although the primary indication for tissue conditioners is the treatment of abused mucosa, the materials themselves are sometimes abused by their ease of application. While they temporarily correct the basal surface of a denture base, they provide little relief from gross occlusal disharmonies and denture borders that are improperly extended. Unfortunately many mandibular complete dentures fall into the category of "ridge runners" and are characterized by underextended borders, especially in the buccal shelf and retromolar and retromylohyoid areas. In these cases the supporting basal mucosa is overloaded due to the limited surface area available for the dissipation of masticatory forces. On the other hand, it is not uncommon for denture borders that initially were properly established to become overextended with the passage of time. This is a direct consequence of "settling" of the denture base subsequent to osseous resorption of the residual ridge and occurs frequently with immediate dentures. By direct extension and pressure necrosis, overextended borders can bring about the ulceration, clefting, and hyperplasia of the vestibular mucosa—a pathological condition commonly termed *epulis fissuratum.*

A basic tenet of maxillomandibular relationships is that a centric relation record is valid only at the vertical dimension of occlusion at which it is made. Unless there is a fortuitous coincidence of the patient's terminal hinge axis and the arbitrary axis established with a face-bow, any change in the vertical dimension of occlusion will cause a subsequent change in the centric relation record. Occlusal wear of the posterior teeth and osseous resorption of both residual ridges normally occur concomitantly and effect a reduction in the occlusal vertical dimension. As the vertical dimension of occlusion changes, so does

the centric relationship between the denture bases, thereby initiating occlusal discrepancies. Once established, occlusal discrepancies between opposing denture teeth cause the bases to shift bodily or skid, resulting in additional irritation to the supporting mucosa. Potentially, the most serious tooth discrepancies occur when the opposing anterior teeth come into contact. Heavy anterior contacts should never be established nor condoned, since they frequently traumatize the anterior edentulous ridges, especially the mandibular anterior ridge which has been shown to have the greatest susceptibility to resorption.

In recapitulation, it needs to be reemphasized that occlusal disharmonies and improperly extended borders should be corrected before initiating a tissueconditioning program. Failure to heed this admonition will seriously compromise any treatment plan designed to rehabilitate abused basal mucosa.

If the recovery of inflamed, compressed, deformed, and displaced basal tissue is to be achieved, the "physiologic cushion" formed by tissue-conditioning material must be present in an adequate and fairly uniform thickness. The minimal acceptable thickness of most tissue-conditioning materials is about 1.5 mm. After placement of the material and removal from the mouth, areas that are too thin will appear as translucent spots with the color of the denture base showing through. These areas are potential pressure spots. As such they should be reduced with an acrylic bur followed by placement of additional material to the relieved areas. The denture is reinserted and the patient instructed to close lightly into centric relation. The new material will normally flow and blend with the initial material. The procedure is repeated as many times as necessary until a uniform layer is developed.

One of the inherent problems of tissue conditioners is that their effectiveness in alleviating reversible tissue changes is normally limited to three to four days. The liquid portion of the mixture contains a plasticizer which controls the resiliency and flow of the material. Unfortunately, the flushing action of saliva causes the plasticizer to leach out. Histological studies have demonstrated that the critical limit is reached after three or four days. At this time the material begins to manifest a loss of resiliency and after three to four weeks it gradually changes into a rigid liner. Accordingly, the material should be removed and replaced every three to four days. The total number of treatments required will depend on the severity of the abused mucosa and the rapidity of a favorable tissue response. Again, the composition and proportions of commercially available tissue conditioners vary along with their physical properties and therefore the manufacturer's directions should be carefully scrutinized and adhered to.

The first step in treating abused oral tissue is to apprise the patient of the etiologic factors and the need for a healthy basal mucosa. Once patients thoroughly comprehend the cause-and-effect relationship between a loose, ill-fitting denture and abused basal mucosa, their motivation and cooperation are visibly enhanced. The treatment plan for tissue recovery may include any or all of the following procedures:

1. Complete tissue rest can be effected only by removing the dentures for a continuous and extended period of time. This will vary from several days to several weeks. The unmatched effectiveness of this simple but direct method lies in the immediate and total elimination of all the contributing factors developed by a loose, ill-fitting denture.

2. The reduction of sharp and overextended denture borders as manifested by tissue hyperplasia and/or hypertrophy and the formation of artifical clefts and fissures in the vestibular mucosa.

3. The available basal surface area should be increased when the denture borders are severely underextended, i.e., lower "ridge runners." Ultimately, this becomes a critical consideration in mandibular residual ridges characterized by extreme resorption. Stick modeling compound is used to border mold and extend the peripheries to within normal physiologic limits, and the newly extended denture base is relined with a tissue conditioner.

4. Occlusal disharmonies are corrected by patient remount procedures (pages 381–385).

5. Treatment with a tissue conditioner is instituted. The patient should be advised to avoid heavy or sustained masticatory pressures with either the anterior or posterior teeth, and since many patients clench their dentures while sleeping, the dentures should not be worn during this time. Finally, during cleansing, the surface of the liner should not be brushed but rinsed with warm water.

6. And last but not least, nutritional deficiencies and systemic disabilities are identified and corrected in order to increase the physiologic tolerances of the supporting mucoperiosteum.

Rebase and Reline Procedures

To *rebase* a denture is a process of making an impression in an existing denture and replacing the denture base material without changing the occlusal relations of the teeth. The purpose is to make the tissue surface of the denture fit the existing position of the tissues.

To *reline* a denture is a process of *resurfacing* the tissue side of a denture to make it fit more accurately.

Analysis of these definitions shows

that the terms are not synonomous. To *replace* is to take the place of or to provide a substitute and equivalent for the denture base. To *resurface* is to put a new or different surface on the tissue side of the denture. To accomplish either of these procedures without changing the occlusal relations of the teeth, without encroaching on the interocclusal space, or without displacing the supporting tissues from their rest position is difficult. It is possible to rebase or reline dentures with an acceptable result, but the procedures are not simple. The procedures must be precise, for there are many places where uncorrectable errors can occur.

When the dentures are to be worn for an indefinite period, the tissue surfaces should be adapted by *rebase* procedures. When the dentures are to be used temporarily or during the treatment of abused tissues, the tissue side should be fitted by *reline* procedures.

The following entities must be understood and evaluated before either replacing the denture base material (rebasing) or resurfacing the tissue side of the denture base (relining).

1. Impressions made with the jaws closed and the teeth in contact cannot be expected to record the tissues in rest position. The patient cannot be expected to determine the degree of pressure that will distort the tissues. Pressure that is considered light by one patient may be considered heavy by another and vice versa; therefore, to instruct a patient to close and maintain closure with light pressure may introduce displacement of the tissues beyond acceptance.

2. Impressions made with the teeth contacting may produce an inaccurate impression with resulting disharmony of occlusion beyond correction. The mandible can move and shift the denture on its base before the recording material is set. A premature tooth contact can cause the patient to shift the

mandible to a more comfortable tooth contact and this too can shift the denture on its base before the impression or lining material can set.

3. Dentures that cannot be stabilized by border refining procedures or dentures in which occlusal disharmony is beyond correction are not suitable for reline or rebase procedures.

4. In order to guarantee a minimum of pressure when adapting relining material or making an impression for rebasing, do not allow the teeth to contact during the flow or set phase. Remount the dentures to reestablish an acceptable interocclusal distance and harmonize the occlusion with jaw movements.

5. Allow abused tissues to recover to a normal state before making the impressions for a rebase.

6. A reline is possible as a chairside procedure. The material is self-activated and may set hard or in varying degrees of softness. It should set hard enough to allow pouring of a remount cast without distortion. Correct occlusal errors and reestablish adequate interocclusal space with an articulator and patient remount procedures.

7. When both the maxillary and mandibular denture need rebase or reline procedures, handle the maxillary denture first, make occlusal corrections, allow an adjustment period, and then proceed with the mandibular denture. Occasionally, when the availability of the patient makes time a controlling factor, this procedure must be altered. In these situations make the maxillary impression for rebase or reline prior to making the impression or relining the mandibular denture. Before proceeding with the mandibular denture, correct the resulting occlusal errors, using intraoral methods (page 378).

The reason for making the impression or reline of the maxillary denture first is that it is easier to stabilize the mandibular denture in the original antero-posterior position. The patient is not allowed to keep the teeth in contact when the impression material or the reline is flowing; however, the relations of the teeth are used as a guide in the procedure.

Chairside Procedures for Reline or Rebase Impression

When patients have abused tissues and the dentures need to be made to fit by rebasing or new dentures are to be made, chairside reline procedures may be a part of the treatment plan. When the tissue abuse is extensive, the reline procedures may be repeated until the tissue response is considered satisfactory. For this reason the relining material must be simple to use, compatible with the tissues, free flowing, and easy to remove from the dentures.

When the abuse of the tissues is minimal and the dentures are to be made to fit by rebasing, chairside reline procedures are not necessary.

The chairside reline or rebase procedures are essentially the same. In one, the reline material is used and in the other an impression material is used. The occlusion is corrected in both procedures; therefore, they both are considered in the following:

1. Instruct the patient in the use and care of dentures (pages 92–97).

2. Instruct the patient to leave the dentures out of the mouth at least eight out of twenty-four hours, preferably at night, for four or five days. Before a morning appointment he should remove the dentures for forty-eight to seventy-two consecutive hours, depending on the extent of abuse. This appointment can be arranged following a weekend for the patients who must leave the dentures in during the weekdays.

3. Reduce the borders of the maxillary denture approximately 2 mm below the vestibular spaces and frenum attachments and refine with impression compound (a) the distobuccal flanges and the posterior palatal seal area, a bilateral procedure, (b) one buccal flange and then the opposite one, and (c) one side of the labial vestibule and then the opposite side (Fig. 20-3). Refinement of the borders may not be necessary for the treatment reline; however, no borders should remain overextended. When border refining is necessary, check the relations of the teeth to assure that the bases have not shifted during the process.

4. Relieve the tissue side of the maxillary denture base in all areas covering stress-bearing mucosa. (Fig. 20-4).

a. Palpate the mucosal covering over the slopes of and crest of the basal seat and palate.

b. Record the approximate displacement of tissues in millimeters.

c. Relieve the denture base with an acrylic bur.

d. Provide escape holes in the palatal area by the procedure used for a maxillary individualized impression tray (Fig. 20-4B).

5. Mix the relining or impression material according to the manufacturer's instructions. The instructions will vary, and it is essential to carry them out correctly in order to obtain the most satisfactory results.

6. Load the denture with the mixed material. It is important to apply an even coating of 2 or 3 mm to the entire tissue surface, including the borders. Excessive material is not desirable and should be avoided.

7. Seat the denture with an antero-posterior path of insertion. Seat the labial flange in the labial vestibule first, and then seat the posterior of the den-

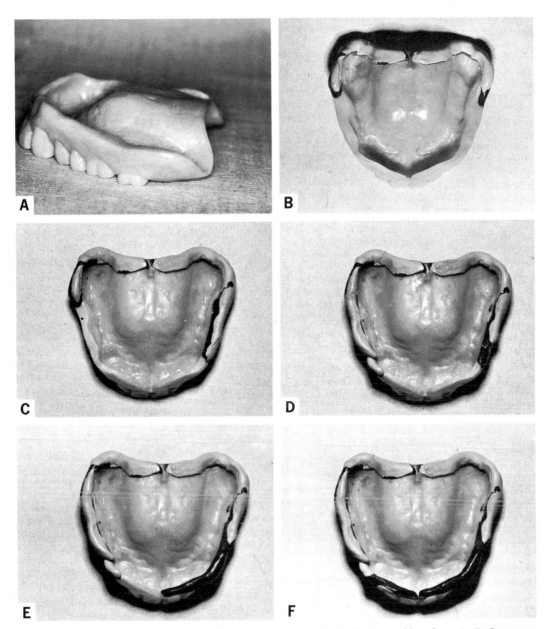

FIG. 20-3. *Steps in reducing and refining the borders.* **A.** *Reduction of borders.* **B.** *Refinement of distobuccal flange and posterior palatal seal area.* **C.** *Refinement of right buccal flange.* **D.** *Refinement of left buccal flange.* **E.** *Refinement of right labial vestibule.* **F.** *Refinement of left labial vestibule.*

ture with a superior and slight posterior motion. Do not use excessive pressure.

8. When the denture is seated, instruct the patient to close the jaw until tooth contact is made. It may be necessary to stabilize the maxillary denture with one hand and guide the mandible to centric relation with the other. When you are sure that the teeth are in the

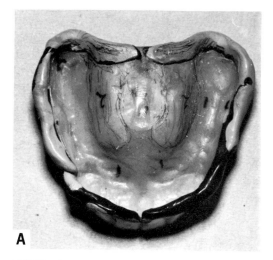

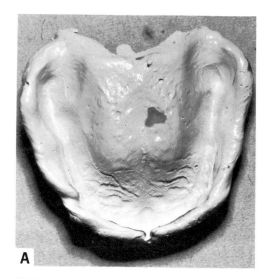

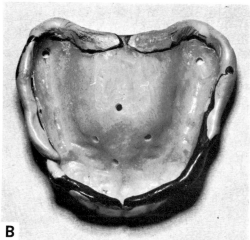

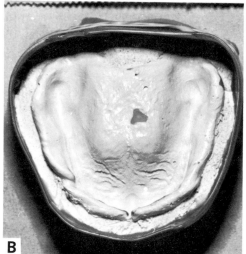

FIG. 20-4. *Relief of tissue side.* **A.** *Displacement of tissue recorded.* **B.** *Denture base that has been relieved by an acrylic bur. Note escape holes.*

correct anteroposterior relation, support the denture with the middle and index fingers in the bicuspid area. Instruct the patient to open the jaws to a relaxed position, to protrude and retrace the lips as in grinning, to swallow, and to relax

FIG. 20-5. **A.** *Refined impression for rebase.* **B.** *Impression beaded and boxed.* **C.** *Hydrocal poured in boxed impression. Note rubber bands securing wax.*

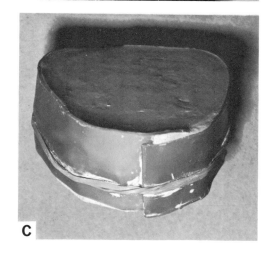

the jaws. Avoid pressure when inserting the denture.

9. Allow the material to set. Remove the impression, bead, box, and pour the cast in Hydrocal (Fig. 20-5):

a. Place the refined impression in a mixture of half dental plaster and half pumice to form a beading or shoulder.

b. Cut a sheet of baseplate wax in half lengthwise and place it around the set plaster and pumice mixture.

c. Secure the wax with rubber bands and pour Hydrocal into the boxed impression.

The above procedures result in a fitted maxillary denture base and in most instances some occlusal disharmony.

10. After the denture base material has been removed and replaced with processed acrylic resin (rebased), remount procedures are done:

a. Eliminate any undercuts in the denture base with wet pumice and make an accurate remount cast of dental plaster (Fig. 20-6).

b. Make an accurate cast of the opposing arch.

c. Make a facebow transfer of the maxillary cast (Fig. 20-7). Transfer the face-bow and attached fork and record to the articulator. Support the fork and record prior to seating the denture in the record. Place the denture teeth in the wax record and secure them by melting the wax to the teeth with a hot spatula.

d. Relate the mandibular cast (or denture) to the maxillary denture with an interocclusal maxillomandibular relation record with the mandible in centric relation (Fig. 20-8). The mandible is elevated to make a record in the passive wax, but the teeth are not allowed to penetrate through the wax. To complete the articulator mounting procedures, attach the mandibular cast to the articulator with plaster.

e. Using selective grinding proce-

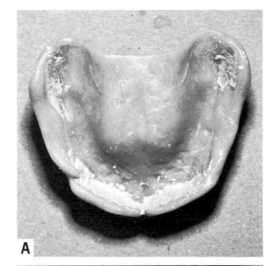

A

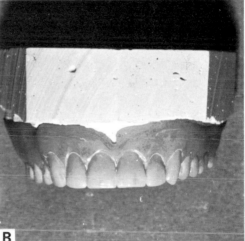

B

FIG. 20-6. **A.** *Pumice placed in the undercuts in maxillary denture base.* **B.** *Plaster remount cast.*

dures (page 385), return the teeth to an acceptable occlusal relation at the correct vertical dimension of occlusion (Fig. 20-9).

When both dentures are relined or impressions are made for rebasing at the same appointment, correct any gross occlusal disharmony with occlusal indicator wax; then make the mandibular impression in the following manner:

1. Allow the maxillary denture to remain in the stable fitted position.

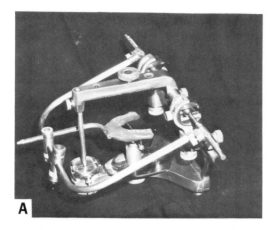

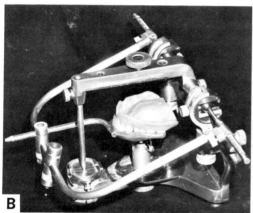

FIG. 20-7. *Mounting the maxillary cast with a face-bow transfer.* **A.** *Face-bow with attached fork and record transferred to the articulator. Note that fork and record are supported.* **B.** *Denture teeth placed in the wax record.*

2. Remove the mandibular denture, dry the teeth, and apply occlusal indicator wax (page 381).

3. Insert the mandibular denture and instruct the patient to chop the teeth together with the jaws in centric relation. Reduce the premature or heavy contacting areas until an even contact of the posterior teeth is assured.

To reline or make the rebase impression for the mandibular denture use the following procedures:

1. Reduce and refine the borders

with impression compound if the denture is for rebase (Fig. 20-10). Remove any overextended border if the denture is for reline. Check the positions of the teeth to assure that the dentures have not been shifted in the base.

2. Palpate the mucosal covering of the residual ridge to determine areas of displaceable tissue. Relieve the tissue side of the denture that covers the crest and slopes of the residual ridge by grinding

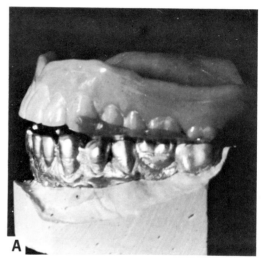

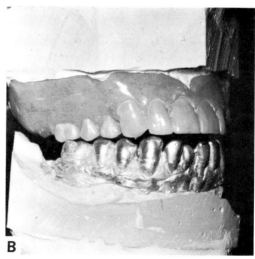

FIG. 20-8. *Mandibular cast mounted with wax interocclusal record.* **A.** *Teeth related.* **B.** *Cast attached to articulator with plaster.*

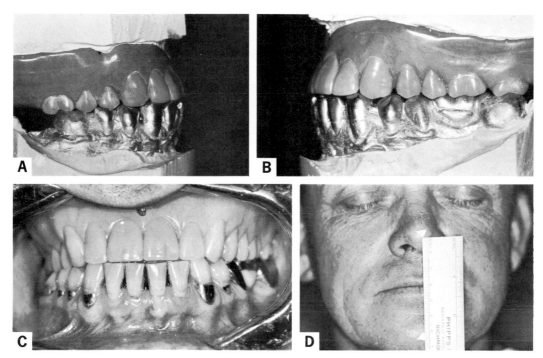

FIG. 20-9. *Evaluation of occlusion after refinement with selective grinding procedures.* **A.** *Occlusal harmony as viewed from the right.* **B.** *Occlusal harmony as viewed from the left.* **C.** *Denture inserted.* **D.** *Verification of vertical dimension of occlusion to assure that an acceptable interocclusal distance has been established.*

to a depth of approximately 2 mm with an acrylic bur (Fig. 20-11A). This provides space for the displaced tissues to return to rest position. Place escape holes when excessively displaceable or pendulous tissue is present to allow space for adequate flow of the recording material and allow the tissue to return to rest.

3. Make the final impression. Mix the reliner or impression material according to the manufacturer's instructions and apply an even layer approximately 3 mm thick over the entire surface and borders. The denture base should not be visible over the crest or slopes of the residual ridge; however, the border refined areas may show through the impression material.

4. Seat the denture, guide the patient to centric jaw relation, and instruct the

patient to close until the posterior teeth make contact. Observe the anteroposterior relation of the teeth to ascertain that the dentures have not been shifted on their bases.

5. Instruct the patient to open the jaws in a relaxed position, support the denture with the index fingers, and allow the lining or impression material to flow.

6. As the material is in the process of setting, instruct the patient to smile, protrude the lips, and retract the lips as in grinning. These movements help refine the border areas. Adequate notches for the frenum are placed after the liner is set.

7. Bead the refined impression by placing it in a mixture of half dental plaster and half coarse pumice, box with baseplate wax, and then pour the impression with Hydrocal (Fig. 20-11C,D).

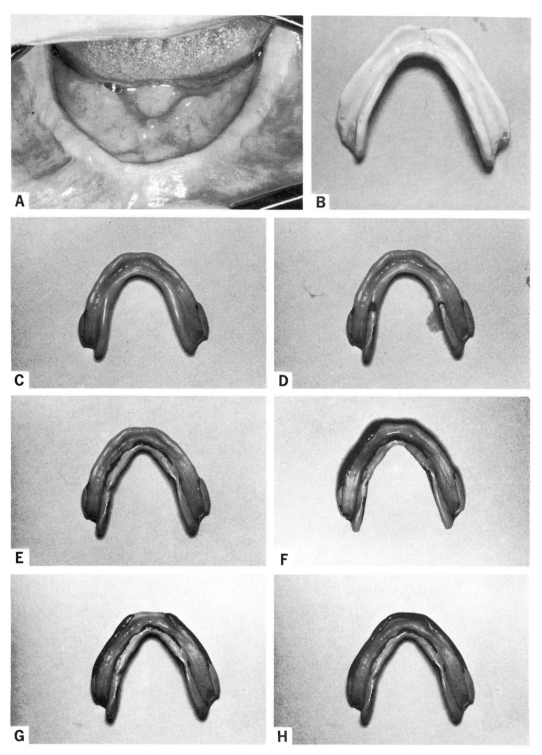

Fig. 20-10. *Steps in border refining to rebase a mandibular denture.* **A.** *Tissue recovery.* **B.** *Reduction of borders above tissue reflections in the vestibular space and frenum attachments.* **C** *and* **D.** *Refinement of borders in masseter groove, buccal shelf, and distobuccal flange areas bilaterally.* **E.** *Border refining in the lingual sulcus.* **F.** *Border refining of buccal and labial flange on one side.* **G.** *Border refining of other buccal and labial flanges.* **H.** *Completed borders.*

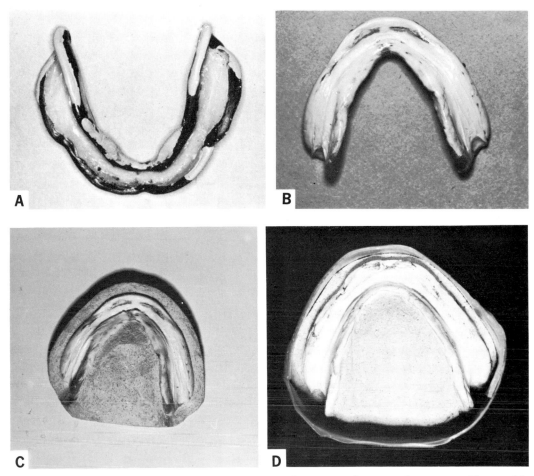

FIG. 20-11. *Mandibular denture base refined with zinc oxide-eugenol paste.* **A.** *Tissue side covering crest and slopes of residual ridge relieved by grinding with acrylic bur.* **B.** *Final impression. Note that the denture base is not visible over the crest and slopes of the residual ridge but that a few border refined areas show through the impression material.* **C.** *Refined impression placed in mixture of half dental plaster and half coarse pumice to form beading or shoulder.* **D.** *Hydrocal poured in impression boxed with baseplate wax.*

In the rebase impression the material of choice is the zinc oxide-eugenol paste.* For the reline material the silicone rubbers and zinc oxide-eugenol paste can be used; however, remount procedures are difficult. The self-activated soft liners that set hard enough to allow remount procedures are preferable.

In many instances less chair time

*Peyton, Anthony, Asgar, Charbeneau, Craig, and Myers: *Restorative Dental Materials,* 2nd ed. St. Louis, The C. V. Mosby Company, 1964, p. 178.

is required to make new dentures than to carry out the procedures necessary for an accurate rebase. Abused tissues resulting from dentures that lack stability and retention or from dentures in which the occlusal relations of the teeth are not in harmony with mandibular movements will recover more rapidly to a normal condition if the dentures are discarded and complete tissue recovery is allowed. This is not always possible, and treatment plans can be formulated to give satisfactory results; however,

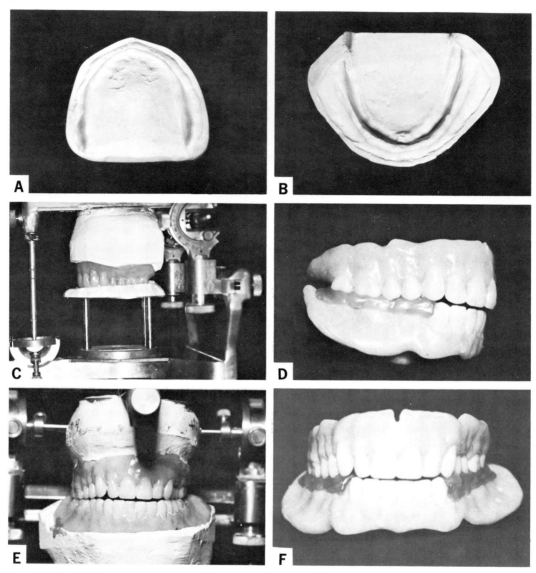

Fɪɢ. 20-12. *Patient remount procedures. **A** and **B.** Maxillary and mandibular plaster remount casts. **C.** Denture teeth in plaster remount record with plaster cast attached to the articulator. **D.** Interocclusal wax record with mandible in its most protruded position. **E.** Mandibular teeth seated in mandibular cast and mounted by attaching cast to the articulator with plaster. **F.** Interocclusal wax check record to verify original mounting.*

the patient must also compromise in some of his desires if the treatment is to be considered successful.

Accurate casts and patient remount procedures are mandatory for either rebase or reline procedures. (Fig. 20-12).

1. Place the denture teeth in the plas-ter remount record. Place the plaster cast in the denture and attach the cast to the articulator.

2. Make an interocclusal wax record. The mandible should be in its most re-truded relation to the maxillae when the latter are elevated to make the interoc-

clusal mounting record (Fig. 20-12D).

3. Seat the mandibular cast in the mandibular denture. The maxillary denture is placed on the mounted maxillary cast, and the mounting is completed by attaching the mandibular cast to the articulator with plaster.

4. Make multiple interocclusal wax check records to verify the original mounting before adjusting the occlusion. Failure to refine the occlusion and establish the acceptable interocclusal distance with wax check records will result in denture failure.

REFERENCES

1. Boos, R. H.: Preparation and conditioning of patients for prosthetic treatment. J. Prosth. Dent., 9:4, 1959.
1a. Boucher, C. O.: The relining of complete dentures. J. Prosth. Dent., 30:521, 1973.
2. Brauer, G. M., et al.: Denture reliners—direct, hard, self-curing resins. J.A.D.A., 59:270, 1959.
3. Christie, D. R.: Relining acrylic dentures without distortion. J. Canad. Dent. Ass., 17:374, 1951.
4. Craig, R. G., and Gibbons, P.: Properties of resilient denture liners. J.A.D.A., 63:382, 1961.
5. Geiger, E. C. K.: A relining technique in activated acrylic resin for complete dentures. Dent. Clin. N. Amer., November, 1964, p. 705.
6. Gillis, R. R.: A relining technique for mandibular dentures. J. Prosth. Dent., 10:405, 1960.
7. Hansen, J. N.: Rebasing and relining complete dentures: a technique. Dent. Clin. N. Amer., November, 1964, p. 693.
8. Hardy, I. R.: Rebasing the maxillary denture. Dent. Dig., 68:402, 1962.
9. Harris, E.: A plea for more research on denture base materials. J. Prosth. Dent., 11:673, 1961.
10. Harris, L. W.: Progress report on immediate permanent relines. J. Prosth. Dent., 3:178, 1953.
11. Hickey, J. C., and Stromberg, W.R.: Preparation of the mouth for complete dentures. J. Prosth. Dent., 14:611, 1964.
12. Jaffe, V. N.: Cold-cured acrylic resins for intraoral correction of full dentures. J.A.D.A., 47:441, 1953.
12a. Knoblanch, K. R., and Reynik, R. J.: Analysis of a clinical evaluation of materials used intraorally. J. Prosth. Dent., 29:244, 1973.
13. Lammie, G. A., and Storer, R.: A preliminary report on resilient denture plastics. J. Prosth. Dent., 8:411, 1958.
13a. Levin, B.: A reliable reline-rebase technique. J. Prosth. Dent., 36:219, 1976.
14. Lytle, R. B.: Complete denture construction based on a study of the deformation of the underlying soft tissues. J. Prosth. Dent., 9:539, 1959, and J. South Calif. State Dent. Ass., 1959.
15. Means, C. R.: A study of the use of home reliners in dentures. J. Prosth. Dent., 14:623, 1964..
16. ———: A report of a user of home reliner materials. J. Prosth. Dent., 14:935, 1964.
17. ———: The home reliner materials: the significance of the problem. J. Prosth. Dent., 14:1086, 1964.
18. Orlean, B.: Hornification of gums. J.A.D.A., 17:1977, 1930.
19. Ostrem, C. T.: Relining complete dentures. J. Prosth. Dent., 11:204, 1961.
20. Robinson, J. E.: Clinical experiments and experiences with silicone rubber in dental prosthetics. J. Prosth. Dent., 13:669, 1963.
20a. Schannon, J. L.: Use of the remount jig as aid in relining upper dentures. J. Prosth. Dent., 34:393, 1975.
20b. Terrell, W. N.: Relines, rebases, or transfers and repairs. J. Prosth. Dent., 1:244, 1951.
21. Travaglini, E. A., Gibbons, P., and Craig, R. G.: Resilient liners for dentures. J. Prosth. Dent., 10:664, 1960.
22. Uccellani, E. L.: Evaluating the mucous membranes of the edentulous mouth. J. Prosth. Dent., 15:295, 1965.
22a. Ward, J. E.: Effect of time lapse between mixing and loading on the flow of tissue conditioning materials. J. Prosth. Dent., 40:499, 1978.
23. Wiland, L.: Dentures, inclined planes and traumatic occlusion. J. Prosth. Dent., 14:892, 1964.

24. Woelfel, J. B., Kreider, J. A., and Berg, T., Jr.: Deformed lower ridge caused by the relining of a denture by a patient. J.A.D.A., 64:763, 1962.

25. Wright, W. H.: Morphological changes in the mucous membrane covering the edentulous areas of the alveolar process in the human mouth. J. Dent. Res., 13:159, 1933.

Immediate Complete Dentures

21

The purpose of this chapter is to consider the factors involved for patients for whom complete dentures are contemplated and to describe diagnostic procedures for determining if the natural teeth may be replaced immediately after extraction. Also included in these considerations are factors that are deemed favorable for the use of immediate complete dentures, their advantages and disadvantages, and predictions as to the course and outcome of the treatment plan.

Definition

An immediate complete denture is a dental prosthesis constructed to replace the lost dentition and associated structures of the maxillae and/or mandible and inserted immediately following removal of the remaining teeth. An immediate complete denture may replace one tooth or all sixteen teeth in either the maxillary or the mandibular arch or in both arches. It is not easy to compare the outcome of a treatment procedure with a basis as variable as that presented by these different situations. Hospitalized patients present a different basis on which to consider a diagnosis, treatment procedure, or prognosis than do patients receiving treatment in the office of the dentist. The additional professional as-

sistance, the facilities, and the *assured* availability of the hospitalized patients present a more favorably controlled situation, particularly for the preoperative and postoperative procedures. Multiple extractions may be a routine procedure under favorable conditions but can present an unfavorable prognosis under less favorable conditions. It is desirable to select a treatment plan which, when all factors are analyzed, can be expected to produce a favorable result.

Requirements

Patients vary greatly in what they want, expect, and demand. A prosthesis is not living tissue, but it must be an accepted part of a system composed of living tissue. It must be physiologic and be tolerated by the patient. To attain the maximum degree of success, the following requirements should be satisfied: (1) compatibility with the surrounding oral environment, (2) restoration of masticatory efficiency within limits, (3) harmony with the functions of speech, respiration, and deglutition, (4) esthetic acceptabil-

Parts of this chapter were included in an article by C. M. Heartwell, Jr., and F. W. Salisbury, which was published in the Journal of Prosthetic Dentistry (July-August, 1965), and are reprinted by permission of the publisher, The C. V. Mosby Company.

ity, and (5) preservation of the remaining tissues. It is a challenge to the dentist to accomplish the requirements in immediate denture service. To accomplish these requirements, it is mandatory that each patient be analyzed and evaluated on an individual basis. Any deviation to satisfy one requirement at the expense of another should be carefully considered, and the patient should be apprised of the possible effects. A patient cannot be expected to accept his rightful responsibilities in any dental service unless he is properly informed and educated by the dentist.

Advantages

The advantages of an immediate complete denture include the following:

1. The denture acts as a bandage or splint to help control bleeding, to protect against trauma from the tongue, food, or teeth if present in the opposing arch, to keep mouth fluids and particles of food from entering the tooth sockets, and to protect the blood clot and thus promote rapid healing.

2. Patients seem to regain adequate function in speech, deglutition, and mastication much sooner than when the lips, tongue, and cheeks have gone unsupported for a time.

3. Many patients are not as reluctant to have diseased teeth removed if they can have them replaced immediately. They do not have to meet their families in an edentulous state, and they can carry on social and business activities without embarrassment. In many instances it is a financial necessity for the patient to continue his or her business with a minimum of interruption.

4. There is less difficulty in making the polished surface of the dentures compatible with the surrounding structures. The tongue, lips, and cheeks have not altered their positions because of lack of tooth support.

5. Patients afforded immediate complete denture service rarely relinquish their dentures.

6. The natural teeth aid in establishing the vertical dimension of occlusion and in positioning the artificial replacements.

When the advantages of immediate complete dentures are considered, it must be understood that most patients are primarily concerned with esthetics and eating. The dentist is aware of the many other possible advantages, but he must thoroughly evaluate these before they are applied to all individuals. The recorded advantages of the immediate complete denture must be compared with the advantages of a complete denture inserted after all the teeth have been extracted and healing has been completed. This is not the only treatment plan that can be offered. Additive dentures or surgical splints are advisable in many situations.

Although an immediate denture does act as a bandage or splint, a surgical splint (Fig. 21-1) will also act as a splint and bandage to protect the unhealed sockets from the forces of occlusion. When it is a financial necessity for the patient to continue business activities,

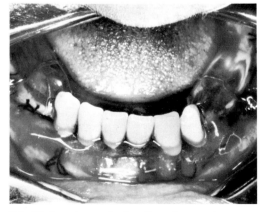

FIG. 21-1. *A surgical splint does not necessarily require the replacement of teeth.*

a treatment plan that requires hospitalization may offset the advantage of a complete immediate denture. This can include patients who require multiple extractions, extensive surgical procedures, and a general anesthetic. For the patient who refuses to carry out the instructions regarding tissue rest the advantages could become serious disadvantages (Fig. 21-2).

The remaining natural teeth can *aid* in determining the vertical dimension of occlusion; however, the vertical dimension of occlusion in the remaining dentition is not necessarily the vertical dimension of occlusion that should be reproduced in the dentures. The continuous eruption of the teeth has not necessarily been in harmony with the attrition of the tooth surfaces, and an increase in the interocclusal distance could result. The attrition of tooth surfaces, however, is not always a criterion for increasing the interocclusal distance because the alveolar process and/or teeth can extrude or migrate and maintain the physiologically accepted interocclusal distance. The appearance of overclosure (too small an occlusal vertical dimension) does not always indicate the need for an increase in the inter occlusal distance because disharmony

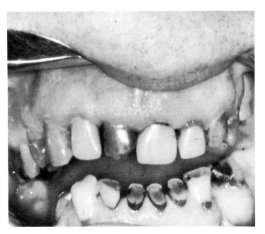

FIG. 21-3. *The vertical dimension of occlusion must be evaluated carefully, even in situations of excessive loss of tooth structures.*

between the centric relation and the centric occlusion may produce this appearance. The contacts of the remaining teeth can be used as a guide in establishing the vertical dimension of occlusion, but to accept their occlusion as being correct *could* be an error. An increase in the interocclusal distance is potentially damaging to the temporomandibular joints. An encroachment on the interocclusal distance will result in bone loss until the proper interocclusal distance is restored. The maintenance of the correct vertical dimension of occlusion is an essential factor in physiologic acceptability of any denture (Fig. 21-3).

The remaining teeth *aid* in positioning the artificial teeth, but reproduction of their positions is *not* always desirable. In many immediate denture patients, the centric relation and centric occlusion are not in harmony. If the artificial teeth are placed in the same positions as the natural teeth, balanced occlusion in the centric or eccentric jaw positions will not be possible, and the positions of the teeth on their movable bases will not be physiologically acceptable to the support. If a cusp form of posterior tooth is

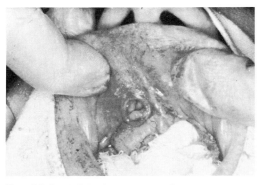

FIG. 21-2. *The damage to the tissues was painless and was unnoticed by the patient. The tissues were not allowed to rest.*

used, balanced occlusion in all jaw positions is important in complete dentures and is even more important in immediate complete dentures because the new bone is in the process of being produced in the alveoli. Bone is plastic in nature, and it can be molded. However, the shock of forces exerted through teeth not in harmony with mandibular movements induces osteoclastic action. If cuspless posterior teeth are used, balanced occlusion in the centric position is imperative because a lack of balanced occlusion will induce unfavorable bone reaction.

Although anatomy and physiology must receive consideration in the arrangement of artificial teeth, the mechanical factors must also receive consideration. Natural teeth are fixed in bone, except for movement within the limits of their periodontal attachments. The artificial substitutes are attached to a movable base resting on soft tissue that can be displaced. The displacement of this tissue varies in the same individual. The natural teeth are capable of acting singly or as a unit, but artificial teeth must act as a unit. The presence of wear facets on natural teeth often indicates that there is a disharmony

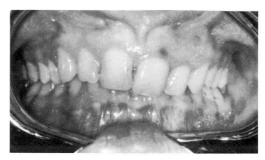

FIG. 21-5. *Steep vertical overlap.*

between centric relation and centric occlusion (Fig. 21-4). To record the jaw position in centric relation with the remaining teeth contacting in centric occlusion can perpetuate an error. A steep vertical overlap without a compensating horizontal overlap, either anteriorly or posteriorly, is a potentially damaging situation. The steep vertical overlap anteriorly (Fig. 21-5) is of particular concern, since the labial cortical layer of bone is thin (Fig. 21-6). Orban stated that "there is very little, if any, spongy bone in the region of the anterior teeth. The cortical bone is usually fused with

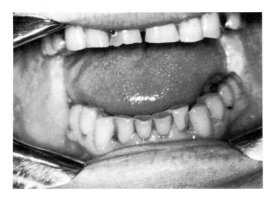

FIG. 21-4. *The use of wear facets like these to articulate casts can lead to errors in maximum intercuspation and centric relation.*

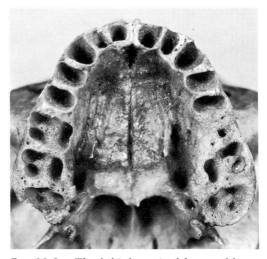

FIG. 21-6. *The labial cortical layer of bone from the second bicuspid to the second bicuspid is thin.*

the alveolar bone proper.* This is particularly true in the cuspid regions.

The positions of the anterior teeth are not always compatible with esthetics (Fig. 21-7). Therefore, it would not be desirable esthetically to duplicate these positions for every patient.

The buccal shelf area in the mandibular arch is bordered externally by the external oblique line and internally by the slope of the residual ridge. The bone is very dense, since the resultant forces of the elevator muscles are directed to this area, and the trabeculation of the bone is arranged to resist these forces.

*Orban, B.: *Oral Histology and Embryology.* 3rd. ed. St. Louis, The C. V. Mosby Company, 1953, p. 200.

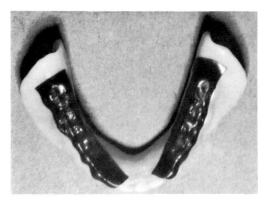

FIG. 21-8. *The maximum forces of occlusion should be directed in the area of the buccal shelf as shown in this wax record.*

The buccal shelf is designated as the primary stress-bearing area, since its density, its mucosal covering, and its relation to the direction of the closure of the jaws are favorable for resisting the occlusal forces. Regardless of the positions formerly occupied by the natural posterior teeth, this information should be used in the arrangement of the artificial teeth (Fig. 21-8).

Disadvantages

Although the advantages of immediate complete dentures exceed the disadvantages, they are not of such magnitude that the technical procedures can be abused. The primary disadvantages follow:

1. The immediate denture does not replace the stimulation that was supplied to the bone by the natural teeth.

2. The procedures are precise and time-consuming and require more appointments, particularly during the adjustment phase.

3. The resorption of bone and the shrinkage of unhealed soft tissue are greater and faster than the changes of healed tissue. These changes require new impressions to keep the denture

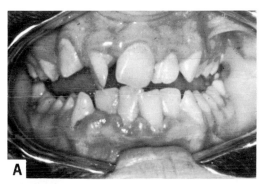

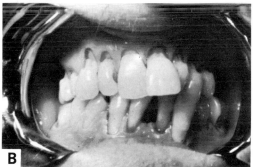

FIG. 21-7. *Perpetuating the positions of these teeth may not be acceptable.* **A.** *It is not advisable to have four teeth contact when the mandible is in terminal relation to the maxillae.* **B.** *The loss of bone support to these natural teeth may be attributed to the locked-in occlusion.*

base adapted to the basal seat. The re-mounting of the dentures to refine the occlusion is necessary whenever the denture base is altered. These procedures are expensive.

4. There is no opportunity to observe the anterior teeth at the try-in appointment; therefore, the esthetic result cannot be evaluated until the dentures are inserted.

When the disadvantages are considered, it must be remembered that the requirements of the prosthesis are demanding. The preservation of the remaining tissues becomes a greater challenge to the dentist as life expectancy increases.

The belief that the forces applied by any denture replace the stimulation supplied to the bone by the natural teeth and that these forces stimulate bone building is not only subject to question but has been denied by many investigators. This information is of particular significance with immediate complete dentures because the forces are applied while the bone is undergoing reformation and changes in internal structure to meet the change in direction and magnitude of forces applied against it. Osteoclastic action accompanies this change in structure in healed bone. This osteoclastic action may be of greater magnitude in unhealed bone.

Lytle* demonstrated the reparative change of bone between the buccal and lingual cortical plates in a young patient when a slight extension of the denture base was allowed to remain in an incompletely healed socket. He further demonstrated the degenerative change that occurred when pressure was reapplied (Fig. 21-9). These clinical findings are very significant. The forces from the denture were exerted on an area where

there is an absence of periosteal bone. The force applied by a denture against the bone in the space between the cortical plates may induce osteoclastic action. What happens when the labial cortical plate is removed or diminished and the forces applied through a denture are directed against the unsupported medullary bone or weakened cortical bone?

Clinical observations do not always substantiate some of the statements about the resorption or atrophy of residual alveolar ridges. The stresses exerted by dentures, even those that are considered to be well constructed, are so variable that it is impossible to render a definite prognosis. Likewise, clinical observation does not show that rapid and extensive loss of the residual ridge occurs as a result of atrophy of disuse following the removal of all teeth (Fig. 21-10). Just because atrophy has been rapid after the removal of a single tooth (as compared with the adjacent alveolar bone), it does not necessarily follow that the loss of all the teeth will result in the same rapid changes. The stimuli applied to the mucosa in the completely edentulous mouth are quite different from those applied to an isolated edentulous region with adjacent teeth present. The atrophy is proportional to the extent of the disuse. It is unfortunate that the study of cadavers, most of which are those of aged individuals from a financially underprivileged group, cannot give the answer to these perplexing problems.*

Campbell's investigation with institutionalized patients is very enlightening.† It revealed much more loss of bone by the denture patient than by the nondenture patient, particularly in the mandibular arch. If these findings are verified

*Lytle, R. B.: Complete denture construction based on a study of the deformation of the underlying soft tissues. J. Prosth. Dent., 9:539, 1959.

*Pendleton, E. C.: The reaction of human jaws to prosthetic dentures. J.A.D.A., 27:671, 1940.

†Campbell, R. L.: A comparative study of the resorption of the alveolar ridges in denture-wearers and nondenture-wearers. J.A.D.A., 60:143, 1960.

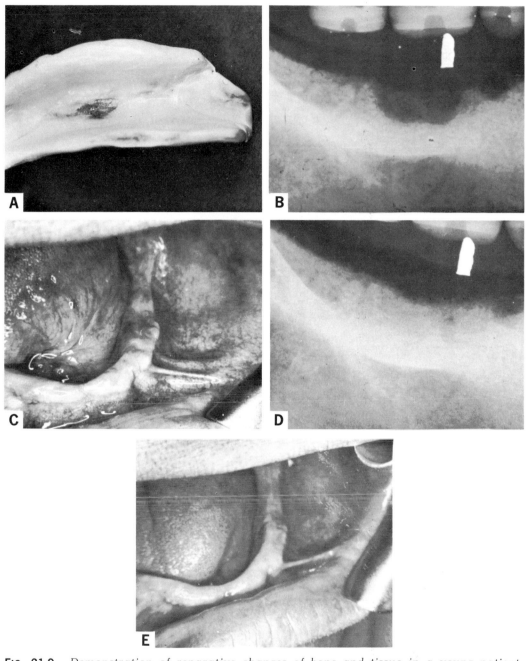

FIG. 21-9. *Demonstration of reparative changes of bone and tissue in a young patient.*
A. *The pressure spot is demonstrated with pressure indicator paste.* **B.** *The roentgenogram discloses the radiolucent area of the bone.* **C.** *The damaged area is visible on the residual ridge.* **D.** *Tissue rest from the pressure of the denture allowed the bone to recover.* **E.** *The soft tissues returned to a healthy state. (From Lytle, R. B.: Complete denture construction based on a study of the deformation of the underlying soft tissues. J. Prosth. Dent., 9:539, 1959.)*

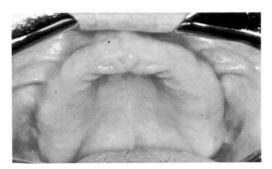

Fig. 21-10. *This edentulous ridge is in a healthy state. Resorption appears minimal. The patient has been completely edentulous for 16 years and has never had complete dentures or removable partial dentures.*

by further investigation, part of the answer may be in the placement of the mandibular artificial teeth. The forces are directed toward the crest of the ridge, particularly the anterior ridge. Furthermore, when a patient is at physiologic rest position, the forces are released to the maxillary arch, whereas the mandibular denture will still be exerting a force due to gravity. These forces are not intermittent but continuous.

Forces applied to bone that is covered with vascular tissue will inevitably result in resorption.*

Diagnosis and Treatment Planning

Diagnosis and treatment planning are so closely related that they are considered together. *Diagnosis* has been defined as the determination of the nature, location, and cause of disease.† This definition does not include the complete investigation that should be conducted prior to formulating a treatment plan for the partially edentulous patient. The investigation must also in-

*Weinman, J. P., and Sicher, H.: *Bone and Bones.* 2nd ed. St. Louis, The C. V. Mosby Company, 1955, pp. 333 and 137.

†Webster's *New World Dictionary.* College Edition.

clude the nonpathologic, the normal and abnormal conditions, the expectations of the patient, and the evaluation of the patient's reactions to the instructions that are so pertinent to denture acceptance. These factors must be evaluated by dentists who use the more recent knowledge of anatomy, physiology, and psychology. To recommend the removal of the remaining teeth with a subsequent healing period, the use of additive dentures, transitional dentures, or the retention of all the teeth is a diagnostic challenge.

Treatment planning is a consideration of all diagnostic findings that have a bearing on the preoperative treatment, impression making, maxillomandibular relation records, the occlusion to be developed, the surgical procedures, and the postinsertion treatment. In formulating a treatment plan, the requirements of the prosthesis must be met. It does not necessarily follow that patients who are to have the remaining teeth extracted present conditions which contribute to a favorable prognosis for an immediate complete denture. Neither does it follow that all patients who present conditions which contribute to an unfavorable prognosis will be denied this treatment.

DIAGNOSTIC PROCEDURES

The diagnostic findings are determined by investigating the local oral conditions, the patient's mental attitude, systemic status, and past dental history.

It is advisable to divide the diagnostic procedures into two phases: (1) patient examination, and (2) consultation interview. The examination of the patient should include findings of local and systemic origin, roentgenographic study, accurately articulated study cast, visual and digital examination, and an appraisal of any existing prosthesis and all anatomic entities that influence the procedures incident to the construction of dentures. In the consultation interview the patient's mental attitude is appraised and his expectations and wants, past dental history, and existing systemic conditions of which he is aware are determined. In addition to the information that the dentist receives from the patient, the dentist must advise the patient what to expect from dentures and must outline the responsibilities of the patient in the use and care of dentures (see Chapter 3). When the treatment plan is decided, other specific instructions may be necessary.

In the diagnostic procedures it is often necessary to seek professional assistance from the medical diagnostician before a treatment plan can be made.

In the first phase the local factors are evaluated by roentgenographic study, accurately articulated study casts, and visual and digital examination. The local factors of particular significance in complete immediate denture treatment are (1) the condition of the teeth to be extracted (Fig. 21-11), (2) the positions of the teeth (Fig. 21-12A), (3) the presence of foreign bodies (Fig. 21-12B), (4) the presence of bony or tissue undercuts that must be reduced or eliminated (Fig. 21-12C), (5) exostosis (Fig. 21-12D), (6) bone loss adjacent to the remaining teeth (Fig. 21-13), and (7) muscle coordination.

The significance of the positions of the teeth, particularly the maxillary anterior teeth, and diseases that affect the neuromuscular coordination have been discussed (Chapter 4).

The prognosis is unfavorable for patients who have extensive bone loss of a chronic nature adjacent to the remaining teeth. Such patients will have a rapidly changing support for the dentures. These changes will be reflected in the occlusal relations, and unless these relations are kept in harmony, bone loss will result. To keep this harmony requires additional appointments for remounting to correct occlusal disharmony and for refitting the denture base to the ever changing support. The resorption of bone as a result of the surgical removal of soft tissue and the placing of sutures is not fully understood. Until further investigation it appears advisable to minimize the surgical removal of soft tissue in the presence of extensive chronic bone loss.

The conditions of the teeth, such as endodontically treated roots, multiroots, ankylosed roots, hypercementosis, hooked or curved roots, embedded or impacted, and badly decayed clinical crowns, may require extensive surgery. Tissue or bony undercuts, foreign bodies, cystic areas, or exostoses that require extensive surgical procedures at the time of insertion of the denture may result in conditions unfavorable to a good prognosis.

Lack of muscular coordination can result from systemic factors; however, there are local factors that may make maxillomandibular relation records extremely difficult or almost impossible to obtain. Among these factors are slowness in understanding instructions, language differences, and senility.

The first procedure in the consultation interview is to determine the patient's mental attitude (Chapter 4). The best patient for immediate dentures is the *philosophical type*. His motivation for dentures is the maintenance of health and appearance and he accepts replacement of natural teeth that cannot be saved as a normal procedure. This patient overcomes conflicts and organizes his time and habits in an orderly manner. He also eliminates frustrations and learns to adjust rapidly. The philosophic patient will listen to and carry out instructions in an intelligent manner. His mental attitude contributes to a favorable prognosis for the immediate denture.

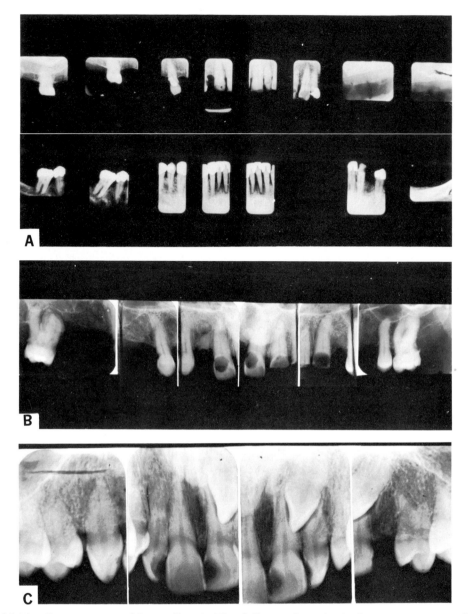

FIG. 21-11. *Roentgenographic studies.* **A.** *The full mouth periapical roentgenograms do not reveal any unerupted teeth, foreign bodies, fractures, or cystic areas.* **B.** *The roots of the maxillary anterior teeth are conical in shape, normal in size, and straight.* **C.** *This roentgenogram reveals an unerupted cuspid—a more complicated surgical problem than extraction of an erupted tooth.*

The *exacting* patients, on the other hand, can be very demanding. They like each step in the procedure explained to them. The mental attitude of these patients can contribute to a favorable prognosis if they are intelligent and understanding. If they lack intelligence or do not understand readily, extra hours

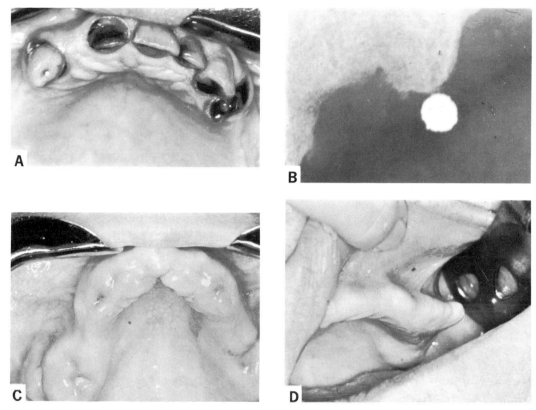

FIG. 21-12.   Other local factors. **A.** The positions of these teeth are acceptable for duplication. **B.** The round foreign body revealed in this roentgenogram is in the soft tissue and should not present a surgical problem. **C.** These opposing undercuts would not be tolerated. **D.** Bony growths like this must be removed.

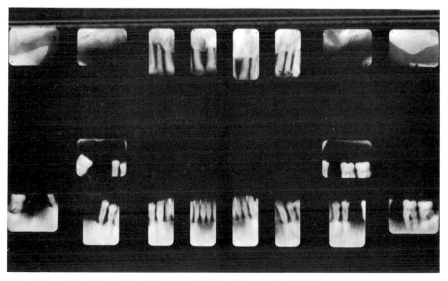

FIG. 21-13.   Extensive bone loss is revealed by the periapical roentgenograms.

spent prior to treatment in sufficient patient education for complete understanding is the best beginning in the treatment plan. The positioning of the artificial teeth as related to the former positions of the natural teeth is more apt to be a major issue with the exacting type of patient, and there should be a thorough understanding in this phase of the procedure. When these patients are properly instructed their mental attitude contributes to a favorable prognosis.

The *indifferent* patient presents an unfavorable mental attitude for dentures inserted after extractions and healing and a much more unfavorable prognosis for acceptance of the immediate complete denture. Since he is uninterested and lacking in motivation, he will pay no attention to instructions, will not cooperate, and may blame the dentist for poor oral health. Many young patients are indifferent to the consequences of not following advice in the use and care of their dentures; they attempt feats with their dentures that are impossible to perform with natural teeth. They fail to return for postinsertion procedures, and as a result develop inflammatory hyperplasia. With this patient the additive denture is the treatment of choice. This treatment plan may stimulate the patient to denture acceptance when other approaches fail.

The *hysterical type* is emotionally unstable, excitable, excessively anxious, and hypertensive. For these patients the treatment plan may include the retention of condemned teeth by whatever means are possible. Professional assistance by the psychiatrist is often advisable prior to and during treatment. The additive type denture may aid until a more favorable mental attitude exists.

SYSTEMIC STATUS

When patients are completely edentulous and the supporting tissues for a denture are completely healed, the systemic condition of the patient has definite influences on the treatment plan and

SIGNS AND SYMPTOMS MANIFEST IN MENOPAUSE* (CLIMACTERIC)
(AGE GROUP 40-55 YEARS)

ORAL	METABOLIC	PSYCHOSOMATIC	NEUROGENIC
Desquamative Stomatitis	Osteoporosis	Frigidity or Aphanisis	Paresthesia
Aphthosis (Canker Sores)	Enuresis	Restless Sleep	Globus Hystericus (Lump in Throat)
Herpes Labiales (Fever Blisters)	Muscle & Joint Pain	Melancholia	Tachycardia
Taste Aberrations (Bitterness-Metallic-Saltiness)	Regressive Skin Changes	Irritability	Abnormal Muscular Contractions (Cramps-Spasms)
Xerostomia	Atrophic Vaginitis	Malaise-Headaches	Hidrosis
Burning Tongue	Hyperpigmentation	Cancerphobia	Vasomotor Instability (Hot Flushes)

* These findings are not necessarily exclusive to menopause - other concomitant degenerative systemic diseases compatible for this age group should also be considered.

FIG. 21-14. *Signs and symptoms manifest in menopause. (Prepared by Harold Syrop, D.D.S., Department of Diagnosis, Virginia Commonwealth University School of Dentistry.)*

prognosis. When teeth are present, the basis for a treatment plan is different, and the evaluation of the systemic status must vary.

For the partially edentulous patients any systemic complication that adversely affects the formation of the essential components of healing and of tissue regeneration, both soft and hard, will offer a poor prognosis for the immediate complete denture.

Systemic conditions affecting the basal seat include the following:

1. Necrosis, osteoporosis, and xerostomia in patients with poorly controlled diabetes.

2. Poor clotting mechanism in patients with cardiovascular and cerebrovascular diseases. A good blood clot influences good bone healing.

3. Mucosal disorders, psychogenic symptoms of burning tongue or palate, and carcinophobia in patients undergoing natural menopause (Fig. 21-14).

4. Mucosal disorders, such as desquamative stomatitis, developing after surgical menopause (Fig. 21-15A).

5. Keratotic lesions, hyperkeratosis, and dyskeratosis (Fig. 21-15B), resulting from vitamin A and B deficiency, hyperestrogenism, hypercholesterolemia, and a past history of syphilis.

6. Dermatologic diseases like psoriasis (rare), pemphigoid lesions that ulcerate easily and stand limited pressure, and erosive lichen planus (Fig. 21-15C).

7. Collagen disorders—arthritis affecting the hands, which are so essential in manipulating the denture, scleroderma, lupus erythematosus—and disorders requiring steroid therapy.

8. Osteoporosis occurring as a result of bone matrix defects, as in malnutrition resulting from colitis, diabetes, and hyperthyroidism.

9. Defects in the osteoblast.

10. Ovarian agenesis or atrophy and lack of estrogen and androgen.

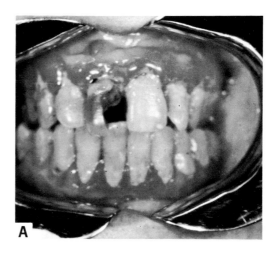

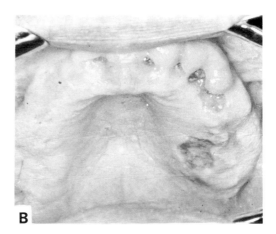

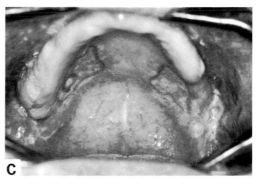

FIG. 21-15. *Examples of systemic conditions affecting the basal seat.* **A.** *Desquamative stomatitis associated with poor oral hygiene.* **B.** *Dyskeratosis that was confirmed by biopsy.* **C.** *Erosive lichen planus.*

11. Poor synthesis of the bone matrix in senility and vitamin deficiency of the alcoholic.

12. Adult rickets caused by poor absorption of calcium and phosphorous in patients with digestive disorders.

13. Hyperthryoidism.

14. Fibrous dysplasia involving the jaws.

Some of the other diseases resulting in conditions that offer an unfavorable prognosis for the immediate denture include diseases of the *nervous system*, Bell's palsy, Melkersson's syndrome, tic douloureux, Parkinson's disease; alcoholism; bronchial asthma; and vascular disorders, such as purpura or capillary fragility. Loss of bodily functions and memory in senility likewise affects the prognosis, as does recent irradiation therapy.

When the healing processes are understood and the insertion and postinsertion procedures of the complete immediate denture are evaluated, it is readily understood why other treatment plans often offer a more favorable prognosis.

PAST DENTAL HISTORY

The prosthodontic experiences of partially edentulous patients are important, but dental experiences related to the missing natural teeth are also essential information. Hemorrhagic tendencies, excessive swelling, excessive postoperative pain, or an allergic reaction to local anesthetics when the teeth were extracted must be evaluated.

The insertion procedures are influenced by the anesthetic used. Sensitivity to local anesthetics may necessitate the use of a general anesthetic. It is difficult to check occlusion by remount procedures when the patient has undergone surgery under a general anesthetic. Hemorrhagic tendencies may indicate the use of a surgical splint as a bandage. Patients prone to excessive swelling

after extractions may present problems in occlusal correction during the postoperative phase (Fig. 21-16).

SURGICAL PREPARATION

The surgical preparation of the mouth for immediate dentures is referred to as alveolotomy, alveolectomy, and alveoloplasty. When vulcanized rubber was the denture base material and porcelain the only type of artificial tooth available, it was almost mandatory for esthetic purposes to sacrifice a part or all of the labial cortical plate from first bicuspid to first bicuspid. This is no longer true. The available denture base materials can be "characterized," and the acrylic resin teeth can be contoured to become part of the denture base. The use of a combination of these materials makes possible the fabrication of dentures that will be esthetically acceptable. If the blood clot, the young connective tissue, the fibrillar

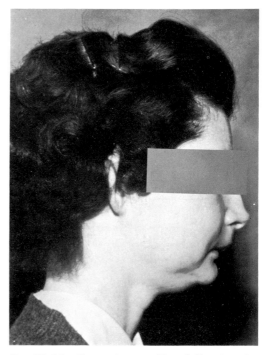

Fig. 21-16. *Extensive swelling following the extraction of teeth.*

bone, and finally the mature cancellous bone, which successively occupy the alveoli, are protected by undisturbed cortical bone and its periosteal covering, a good residual ridge can be expected. The preservation of what remains loses its significance when what could have remained has been surgically removed. Wolff's law postulates that all changes in the function of bone are attended by definite alterations in its internal structure. The law also pertains to changes in the direction of the force and its magnitude. There is an accompanying osteolysis when these forces are applied by a denture to healed bone. To apply these additional forces to unhealed bone that has been subjected to the trauma of extraction, the reflecting of the periosteum and removal of cortical bone in toto or part could be accompanied by very rapid and excessive resorption. This is the opposite to the desires of dentists.

The results of Simpson's investiga-tions into the healing of extraction wounds, the effects of suturing extrac-tion wounds, and the removal of tips of the alveolar crest should receive serious consideration in the surgical prepara-tion for dentures.*

It is possible that overenthusiasm for a smoothly contoured residual alveolar ridge is responsible for excessive resorp-tion. A more sound procedure would be to advise patients who must have extensive surgical intervention to forego the use of immediate dentures until coarse fibrillar bone or immature bone has occupied the alveoli. Perhaps it would be better to follow the procedure

*Simpson, H. E.: Experimental investigation into the healing of extraction wounds in *Macacus rhesus* monkeys. J. Oral Surg., 18:391, 1960.

———: Effects of suturing extraction wounds in *Macacus rhesus* monkeys. J. Oral Surg., 18:461, 1960.

———: Healing of surgical extraction wounds in *Macacus rhesus* monkeys. J. Oral Surg., 19:227, 1961.

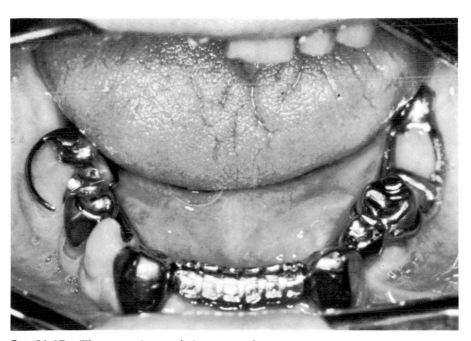

FIG. 21-17.   *The opposing arch is prepared.*

advocated by Pound.* Insertion of immediate dentures is discouraged, and the patient is educated to accept a transitional service or to use the additive denture as advocated by DeVan and Payne.†

When all the factors involved in complete immediate denture service are evaluated and found favorable, a complete denture may be inserted immediately after the extraction of the remaining anterior maxillary teeth. In certain situations this procedure may include the single-rooted first bicuspids. The posterior teeth are removed, necessary surgical treatment of the posterior arch is performed, and a six to eight weeks' healing period is usually allowed. The mandibular teeth are restored or the completely or partially edentulous mandibular arch is prepared for the construction of a removable prosthesis to oppose the immediate maxillary denture (Fig. 21-17).

*Pound, E.: Preparatory dentures: a protective philosophy. J. Prosth. Dent., 15:5, 1965.

†DeVan, M. M.: The transition from natural to artificial teeth. J. Prosth. Dent., 11:677, 1961; Payne, H. S.: A transitional denture. J. Prosth. Dent., 14:221, 1964.

REFERENCES

The references for this chapter appear at the end of Chapter 22 (pages 468–469).

Immediate Complete Denture Construction Procedures

22

When the anterior maxillary teeth are to be replaced by an immediate complete maxillary denture, the treatment plan must be systematically recorded and followed. A treatment plan is a sequence of procedures that are particular ways of accomplishing something or a series of steps followed in a regular definite order to accomplish something. Dental literature usually focuses attention on *how* to accomplish something and *what* materials to use but seldom explains *why* the procedures and the materials were selected.

This chapter will discuss the *how*, the *what*, and the *why* of the preparatory, the insertion, and the postinsertion treatment necessary for the fabrication of an immediate complete maxillary denture that will fulfill the requirements for successful complete denture service. (See page 425). The complete denture described is for a patient with removable partial mandibular denture and gold occlusal coverage on the mandibular teeth (Fig. 21-17, page 439).

Preparatory Treatment

The first step is to review the instructions given to the patient during consultation and diagnostic evaluation.

(See chapters 3 and 4.) This review allows the patient the opportunity to have clarified any instructions not clearly understood.

The second step is to record any information deemed useful during the treatment phase. Intraoral and extraoral color slides should be made. The intraoral pictures focus attention on the anterior teeth and on the mucosa covering the residual ridges. These aid in the selection of anterior teeth and the tinting of the denture base for esthetic acceptability.

Extraoral photographs include full face (Fig. 22-1A) and profile (Fig. 22-1B) pictures with the jaws at rest and with the remaining teeth in maximum occlusion. These photographs can be enlarged to life size. The facial topography is a guide to (1) the positioning of the teeth, (2) the establishing of the dimensions of maxillomandibular relationships in the three dimensions of vertical, anteroposterior, and mediolateral, and (3) the contouring of the polished surface of the denture base. The existing vertical dimension of occlusion is recorded by measuring between landmarks on the upper and the lower halves of the face. These landmarks, such as tattoo points, skin imperfections, or scars, must re-

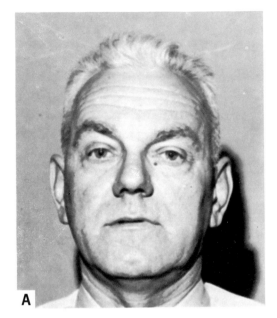

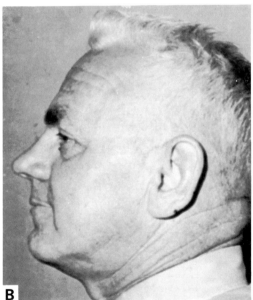

FIG. 22-1. *Extraoral photographs to evaluate maxillomandibular relations and esthetic results.* **A.** *Full face with jaws at rest.* **B.** *Profile with teeth in occlusion.*

treatment procedures and are recorded at the time of the face-bow registration.

The third step is to establish training exercises for the patient in protruding and retruding the mandible and in closing the mandible when it is in centric relationship to the maxillae. The patient is instructed to place the index fingers on the dentist's lower jaw buccally to the first molars with the tips of the thumbs resting lightly at the sides of the chin point. The dentist then protrudes and retrudes with the jaws apart. The patient recognizes these movements and also recognizes the feeling when the mandibular condyles reach their most retruded positions in the fossae. After repeating these movements several times, the dentist closes into occlusion when the mandible is in the most retruded position. The patient is now instructed to repeat the procedure, placing his fingers and thumbs on his own jaw. When the dentist is satisfied that the patient understands, he seats the patient in a comfortable upright position in the dental chair. The dentist places his index fingers intraorally to the buccal side of the mandibular molars with the thumb tips resting lightly on the sides of the chin point and instructs the patient to repeat the protruding and retruding exercise. When the patient is in the most retruded position, he is instructed to open and close but to stop closing before the teeth touch. The patient is instructed to repeat these exercises at least three times daily, and at each subsequent appointment the dentist repeats the training. These conditioning exercises prepare the patient for the recording of maxillomandibular relationships during the treatment phase.

Treatment

The procedures in the treatment plan include the preliminary impression, the final impression, the record of the maxil-

main until treatment is terminated. If the kinematic axes of rotation are desired, they are located and recorded on the skin by tattooing. The arbitrary hinge axis locations are used in the subsequent

lomandibular relations, the try-in, and the insertion itself.

PRELIMINARY IMPRESSIONS

The objective of the preliminary impression is to record the basal seat of the denture and the adjacent anatomic landmarks. An ideal impression material is accurate, it incorporates a minimum of tissue displacement over the stress-bearing areas and hard palate, and it is not complicated. It does not require elaborate equipment nor does it consume excessive time. Displacement in the vestibular fornix and border seal areas is not critical, as these areas are redeveloped with low-fusing impression compound during the border refining procedures. The irreversible hydrocolloid impression materials (alginates) have suitable properties to accomplish the desired objectives.

PRELIMINARY IMPRESSION TECHNIQUE. The patient is seated in a comfortable upright position, head supported at the occiput by the head rest. The head is tilted in a slightly flexed position. The back rest is under the scapula, and the patient is instructed to place both feet flat on the base of the foot rest. This positioning keeps the patient from tiring, permits the tissues to be recorded in the position that will usually support the denture, and does not interfere with the breathing or swallowing activities.

Select a slightly oversized perforated impression tray. Stock impression trays can be contoured more accurately with utility or carding wax. Apply the wax over the distobuccal flanges and extend on the tissue side of the tray across the posterior palatal seal (Fig. 22-2). The wax is not applied to make a larger tray. That over the distobuccal flanges will hold the cheeks laterally and allow the impression material to flow into the buccal vestibules and the hamular notch areas. The wax in the posterior palatal seal area

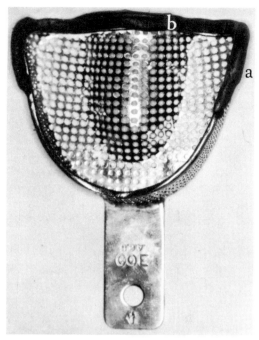

FIG. 22-2. *Stock impression tray contoured with utility or carding wax to hold the cheek laterally (a) and to retain the impression material in intimate contact with the palate (b).*

holds the impression material in intimate contact with the soft palate as the patient places the tip of the tongue against the lingual of the mandibular teeth. If the patient has a high palate, add wax in the vault of the tray to assure a more even thickness of the impression material.

Mix the irreversible hydrocolloid impression material according to the manufacturer's directions. Instruct the patient to rinse the mouth with an astringent type mouth wash to reduce the viscosity of saliva. Meanwhile, load the tray from the sides to avoid trapping air. Wipe the posterior area of the palate with surgical gauze to remove glandular secretions. Place a small amount of impression material in the vault of the palate to avoid trapping air. Insert the loaded impression tray into the mouth, center it, and then seat it. As the tray is seated anteriorly and then posteriorly, quietly instruct the patient to keep his eyes open, breathe slowly through the nose, start counting silently, and to raise a finger when he reaches a hundred and fifty. This occupation of mind allows little time for the thought of gagging. The impression material is held firmly in place until set, usually three minutes. Remove the impression with one quick pull. Do not tease from place. Wash the impression with cold tap water; inspect the tissue and border surfaces for accuracy (Fig. 22-3). Dry the tissue surface with a gentle stream of air and pour immediately with Hydrocal. Since drying of the impression material may alter the surface of the cast, the

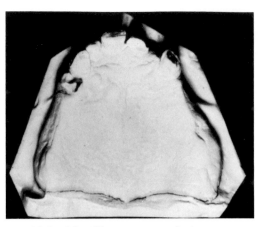

FIG. 22-4. *Maxillary cast made in an accurate impression. Note the extension of the hamular notches, the reproduction of minute detail of the soft tissues, and the positions and imperfections in the teeth.*

poured impression is placed in a humidor with 100 per cent humidity or after the initial set is wrapped in a wet towel. This prevents the drying of the impression material. The cast is separated forty-five to sixty minutes after pouring (Fig. 22-4).

FINAL IMPRESSION

The final impression is the impression used to make the master cast, which must be an accurate replica of the basal seat area. Accurate impressions are difficult to make unless an accurate impression tray is used. A self-curing acrylic resin tray made by the sprinkle on technique is suitable for making the final impression, as it is rigid and stable.

IMPRESSION TRAY CONSTRUCTION. The outline for the tray is drawn on the preliminary cast (Fig. 22-5) with an indelible pencil as follows: A line is drawn transversely across the posterior border connecting the pterygoid hamulus points, (A & A') in such a manner that the connecting line passes posterior to the fovea palatina (B). This line follows the curved contour of the posterior

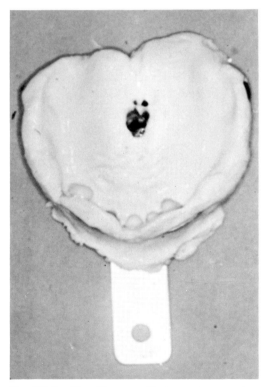

FIG. 22-3. *Maxillary preliminary impression made with irreversible hydrocolloid. The excess of carding wax in the vault will not allow space for the impression material to flow.*

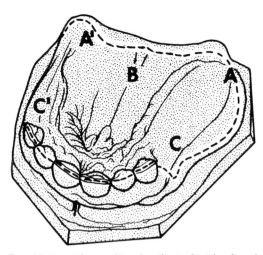

FIG. 22-5. *The outline for the individualized impression tray. The hamular notches at* **A** *and* **A'** *are included in the tray. The fovea palatina at* **B** *are anatomic guides at or near the posterior nasal spine in the midline of the palate. The tray is not allowed to engage undercuts at the distopalatal line angle of the cuspids,* **C** *and* **C'.**

surface of the palatine bone. A line outlining the mucobuccal fold is drawn from the distobuccal termination of the hamular notches to the distal of the cuspids (C & C'). This line follows the junction of the tightly and loosely attached submucosa or the point where the loosely attached submucosa begins to reflect from the lateral surface of the residual ridge. This outline includes notches for the buccal frenum attachments. The line from points C & C' is extended to follow the distopalatal line angle of the cuspids onto the incisal edges of all the remaining teeth.

The tray will have a positive stop on the incisal edges but does not extend onto the labial surfaces. A wax platform approximately 3 mm thick is formed below the mucobuccal fold outline and adjacent to the line on the distal side of the cuspids and labial to the line on the incised edges of the teeth. Flow a thin coat of wax into the interproximal spaces and into any defects present in the palatal surfaces of the teeth (Fig. 22-6Aa). A separating medium of alginate compound applied to the outlined surface of the dried cast is allowed to dry. Wet one third of the cast with monomer. Sprinkle enough polymer on the wet surface to absorb completely the liquid monomer. Repeat this procedure until the desired thickness of 3 or 4 mm is reached, then start another segment. When sufficient acrylic resin has been sprinkled on, the cast is allowed to set for at least ten minutes and is then placed in warm water in a pressure cooker under 120 pounds of pressure for twenty minutes to hasten polymerization

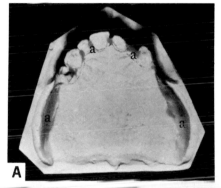

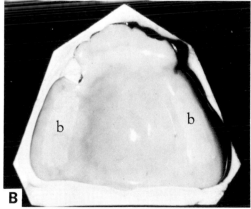

FIG. 22-6. **A.** *Undercuts* (a) *are altered with wax before a separating medium is applied.* **B.** *The ridge crest and slopes* (b) *are left rough.*

and eliminate excess monomer. The cast is removed from the tray by "shell blasting," cutting, or severing the cast, not by prying the tray from the cast. Smooth and polish the palate and the borders. Allow the ridge crest area to remain rough (Fig. 22-6Bb).

Apply sticky wax to the rough ridge crest and attach impression compound occlusal ramps to the sticky wax. The occlusal ramps are made to approximate the height and width of teeth and are positioned to occupy the space which later will be occupied by the teeth (Fig.

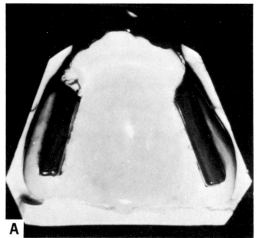

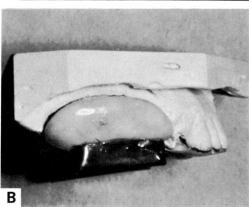

FIG. 22-7. *Compound occlusion rims are placed in the approximate positions that will be occupied by the teeth.* **A.** *Occlusal view.* **B.** *Buccal view.*

22-7). The ramps (1) act as handles for manipulating the tray, (2) provide a convenient bilateral rest for finger support to the tray when the final impression material is flowing and setting, (3) substitute for the teeth in supporting the cheeks during border refining movements, and (4) assure positive seating of the impression of the posterior segment of the arch when making the irreversible hydrocolloid impression of the anterior segment of the arch.

When the impression trays are tested in the mouth for proper extension and adaptation, check definite areas.

1. After the tray has been seated, instruct the patient to open wide as in yawning. If the tray is displaced, look for overextension in the hamular notches or in the areas of the modiolus.

2. While the patient's jaws are separated, tell the patient to thrust the lower jaw forward and to move the jaw from right to left. If this action results in unseating the tray on either or both sides, there is not sufficient space between the alveolar tubercle and the anterior border of the ramus of the mandible; therefore, reduce the thickness of the tray.

3. Inspect the distobuccal flange area with the patient's cheeks relaxed to assure that the flanges are extended to 2 or 3 mm shy of the vestibule. The cheeks should be gently moved in an anteroposterior direction to see if sufficient space has been provided to accommodate the buccal frenum. The posterior extension of the tray is the same as the extension for the completed denture.

4. Determine the posterior palatal seal created in the soft palate distal to its junction with the hard palate by (1) palpating with a blunt instrument or (2) closing the patient's nostrils with the fingers and instructing the patient to exhale through his nose. The soft palate reflects inferiorly at or near the junction of the

aponeurosis and the distal of the palatine bone. Observe the activity of the palatal musculature when the patient says "ah" in a normal moderate manner. The anterior point of reflection or movement superiorly is termed the *vibrating line*. A second less active vibrating line is sometimes seen distal to the fovea. The fovea palatina are very small orifices situated distal to the hard palate in the area of the posterior palatine spinous process. The anterior vibrating line is near the junction of the bone and aponeurosis, whereas the distal vibration line is near the junction of the aponeurosis and palatal muscles. In the majority of instances, gradually sloping soft palates have more passive muscle action than the soft palates which drop abruptly toward the throat. If the musculature is very active when the patient says "ah," the posterior seal extension distally is limited and the vertical height must be increased; however, if the musculature is passive, the seal can be extended for considerable distance posteriorly and can be reduced vertically.

Next remove the palatal secretions with gauze and outline the posterior seal area with a color transfer applicator* (Fig. 22-8A). The outline is transferred to the tissue side of the tray, and the tray is altered to accommodate the extension (Fig. 22-8B,C). Frequently, when the attachment of the aponeurosis at the midline to the posterior palatal spine is like a cord (D, in Fig. 22-8A), a seal is not indicated over this cord, but at times relief is needed in the denture base. The posterior palatal seal is developed to maintain contact between the denture base and the movable soft palate during speech and swallowing and is not developed to allow the patient to bite on the anterior teeth.

*Great Plains Dental Products Company, Cunningham, Kansas 67035.

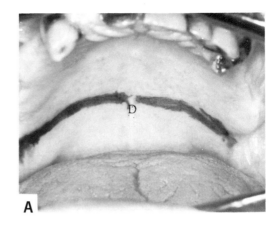

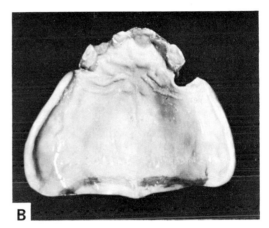

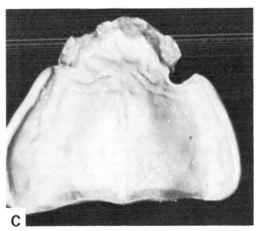

FIG. 22-8. A. *The posterior palatal seal area is outlined. The cordlike attachment of the aponeurosis to the posterior nasal spine is at D.* **B.** *The palatal seal outline is transferred to the impression tray.* **C.** *The altered tray.*

FINAL IMPRESSION TECHNIQUE. The final impression technique is divided into two procedures: (1) border refining the denture seal area and (2) refining the entire denture-bearing area.

Border refining is done to form a seal in the soft palate with the mucosa that has a loosely attached submucosa. The intimate contact between the borders of the denture and the mucosa in the vestibular fornix furnishes additional retention to the denture. This contact is achieved by first applying low-fusing impression compound to the superior surface of the buccal flange and by extending the compound from distal to the buccal frenum to cover the distobuccal and lateral surface of the tray, the hamular notches, and the posterior palatal seal area.

Apply the material bilaterally and in sufficient quantity to remain plastic enough to flow when seated in the mouth (Fig. 22-9A). Soften the compound with an open flame, exercising care not to overheat the material, temper it in a water bath at 113° to 120°F, and seat in the mouth (Fig. 22-9B). Tell the patient to open the jaws wide as in yawning, thrust the lower jaw forward, and move the jaw to the right and to the left. Repeat this procedure until the desired contour is developed and tissue contact is assured. This often requires the use of another impression compound that will flow at a lower temperature than that which was applied initially, utilizing the first as part of the tray (Fig. 22-9C). Low fusing impression compound is used because it is plastic at a temperature that will not cause discomfort to the patient. It will harden completely at, or slightly above, mouth temperature. When it is hard, it should withstand trimming with a sharp knife without flaking and withdrawal from the mouth without being deformed or fractured. Whenever possible, compound should

be softened with dry heat. When a direct flame is applied, the compound should not be allowed to boil or ignite so that important constituents are volatilized.

Placing the impression material bilaterally assures proper centering of the impression tray. The combined action of opening, protruding the mandible, and moving it to the right and to the left forces the impression material into the hamular notches, provides space in the impression for the reflection of the tissue over the pterygomandibular ligament, and determines the available space for the denture base between the anterior borders of the ramus of the mandible and the lateral borders of the alveolar tubercles.

Placing compound across the posterior palatal seal area maintains intimate contact of the impression with the tissues of the soft palate but does not displace the soft palate.

The unrefined buccal flanges are refined unilaterally (Fig. 22-9E,F,G) as the tray is already centered, and softened compound is easier to manipulate through the lips on one flange at a time than on both flanges. When the compound is softened, tempered, and seated, the relaxed cheek is manually moved in an anteroposterior direction to develop the contour necessary to accommodate the buccal frenum (Fig. 22-9D,F). The refined borders should fill the vestibule.

The final border refining is performed by having the patient first protrude the lips then retreat the lips and cheeks while the softened material is held firmly in place or by having the patient suck against the finger (Fig. 22-9H).

TECHNIQUE FOR REFINING. The refining of the entire denture base allows recording of the tissues as nearly as possible in their rest position. Intimate contact between the tissues and the denture sur-

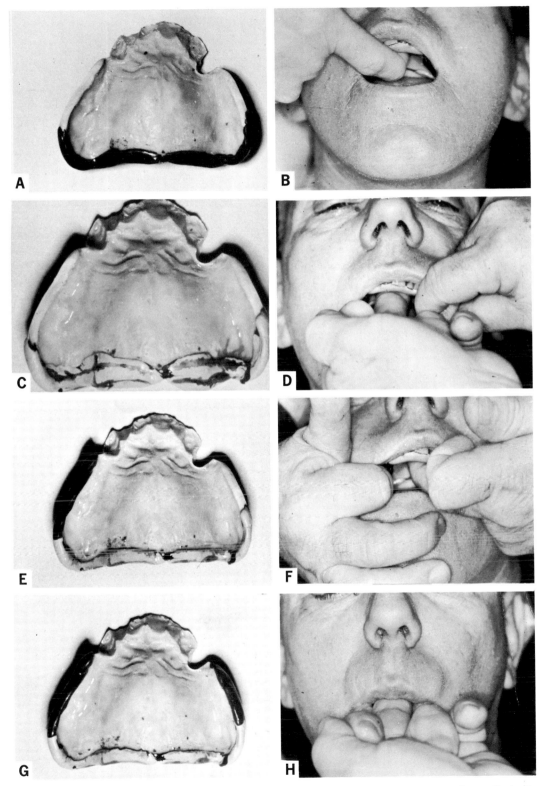

FIG. 22-9. *Border refining procedures.* **A.** *Low-fusing impression compound applied.* **B.** *Seating the tray.* **C.** *Additional applications of compound.* **D.** *Manual manipulation.* **E.** *Refining the right buccal flange.* **F.** *Manual manipulation.* **G.** *Refining left buccal flange.* **H.** *Holding impression in place.*

face assures stability to the finished denture. When tissues are displaced in an impression, pressure is exerted by the denture base in the same area, and bone, which is covered by vascular tissue, will resorb as a result of continuous pressure. When a plastic impression material is placed in an impression tray and seated in the mouth, the movable tissues are displaced. To allow the tissues to rebound to their undistorted position, the impression tray is relieved and escape holes are placed in selected areas.

Zinc oxide and eugenol impression paste is the material of choice for this refining procedure. This material, which is carried to the mouth in a plastic state in which it has a ready flow, has a controlled setting. Only a minimum time should take place between the flow and the setting. Pastes that set rapidly are superior to the slower setting materials in reproducing minute detail, since prolonged setting may result in unavoidable movement of the tray by the patient or dentist and subsequent distortion in the impression while the material is still soft. When zinc oxide and eugenol paste impression material sets, it is firm and resists distortion when it is withdrawn from the mouth. There is no significant dimensional change after setting, and the impression can be easily separated from the stone cast. Separating media are unnecessary.

The denture-bearing tissues are palpated with a ball burnisher to determine the areas of displaceable tissue and the extent of the displaceability (Fig. 22-10A). The depths of the displaceable areas are recorded on the tissue side of the tray; then with an acrylic bur the tray is relieved to the required depths (Fig. 22-10B,C). To avoid trapping air in the vault, holes approximately the size of a #8 round bur are placed in the rugae area and posterior palatal seal area (Fig. 22-10D). Apply petrolatum or cold cream to the patient's cheeks, lips, and chin to keep the impression material from sticking. Mix the impression material according to the manufacturer's directions, and when it is sufficiently spatulated, place it in the tray.

While the material is spatulating, instruct the patient to wash the mouth with an astringent type mouth wash. Wipe the vault and soft palate with gauze, and seat the loaded impression tray with positive pressure (Fig. 22-10E). Have the patient flex his head forward and instruct him to breathe slowly through the nose. Watch holes in the rugae and the posterior seal area, and when the impression material flows through the holes and over the distal of the impression tray, release all pressure and use the index and middle fingers to support the tray bilaterally in the areas of the first bicuspids. Support the impression tray until the impression material has set and the excess is removed.

Choose a perforated impression tray that will accommodate the anterior teeth and extend far enough posteriorly to cover the occlusion rims. Spatulate irreversible hydrocolloid impression material (alginate), fill the tray, place impression material to fill the labial vestibule, and insert and seat the loaded tray (Fig. 22-10F) posteriorly and then anteriorly. This seating sequence assures that the posterior impression will not be displaced. Allow the irreversible hydrocolloid to set for three to four minutes before removing from the mouth (Fig. 22-10G). The anterior and posterior impressions usually are removed together (Fig. 22-10H). However, failure to do so does not necessarily require another impression because the occlusion rims act as guides in the proper positioning of the posterior impression.

Wash the impression with tap water,

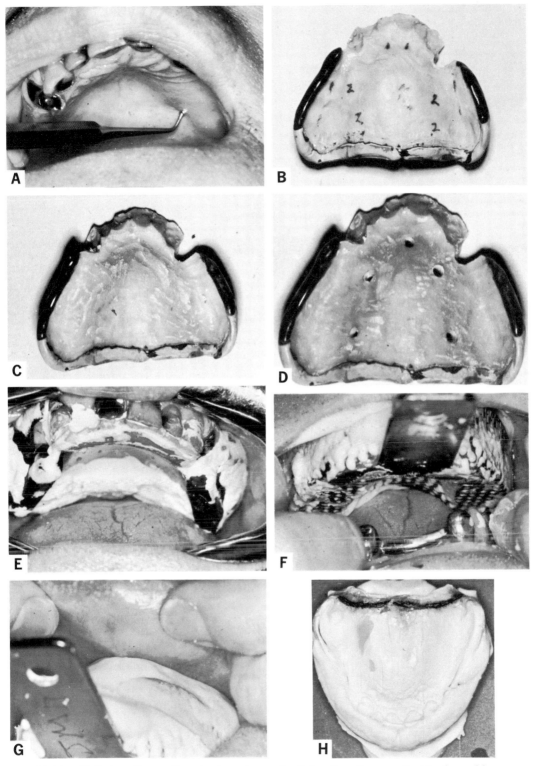

FIG. 22-10. *Refining the entire denture base.* **A.** *Palpating tissues.* **B.** *Displaceable areas recorded.* **C.** *Tray relieved.* **D.** *Holes in vault placed.* **E.** *Zinc oxide-eugenol impression paste in place.* **F.** *Index and middle fingers supporting the tray.* **G.** *Upper lip reflected to break seal between the impression and the tissue.* **H.** *Final impression with irreversible hydrocolloid.*

remove the excess water with air and pour immediately in dental stone. Place the poured impression in a humidor of 100 per cent humidity and allow to set for forty-five to sixty minutes. Then the cast is separated and trimmed, and re-mount indices are placed in the base of the cast.

RECORD BASE

A stabilized record base or baseplate is "a temporary form representing the base of a denture."* It is used to record maxillomandibular relations and to ar-range teeth. After the posterior teeth have been arranged, they are returned to the mouth on the same record base used to record the maxillomandibular rela-tions. Centric relation and centric occlu-sion are verified, and when required, eccentric jaw relations are recorded. The record base must be rigid, fit accurately, and be stable in the mouth, and the borders should be developed in the same manner as the borders of the finished denture. All surfaces that contact the lips, cheeks, and tongue should be smooth, rounded, and polished. The crest and buccal slopes should be kept thin to provide space for tooth arrange-ment but should be allowed to remain rough for better wax attachment. The more comfortable and compatible the record base is to the surrounding tissues, the more normal will be the jaw move-ments. A record base of self-curing methylmethacrylate resin made by the sprinkle on technique is acceptable.

TECHNIQUE.   Alter undercuts on the cast by flowing wax from above and into the undercut (Fig. 22-11). Apply a sep-arating medium of alginate compound and allow to dry. Use the sprinkle on technique previously described (page

Glossary of Prosthodontic Terms.

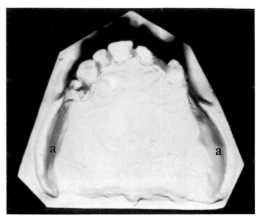

FIG. 22-11.   *Undercuts (a) are altered to avoid damaging the cast.*

445). Extend the record base anteriorly to the remaining teeth. Gain rigidity by adding resin in the palate and to the borders. Before complete polymeriza-tion lift, but do not remove, the base from the cast, and reseat immediately until polymerization is completed. Re-move from the cast and smooth and polish the borders. Smooth and polish the inferior palatal surface. *Do not* pol-ish the crest of the residual ridge (Fig. 22-12A).

Occlusion rims are occluding surfaces built on the record base where later will be the artificial teeth (Fig. 22-12B). Hard baseplate wax is used, since it is easy to manage in making maxillomandibular relation records, a good medium for at-taching the teeth to the record base, a good color for the try-in procedures, and does not distort when contacting lower fusing waxes.

The final contouring of the occlusion rims is done during the making of maxil-lomandibular relation records. The con-touring of the posterior buccal surface begins just distal to the cuspids. Slant the wax slightly toward the palate to create an acceptable space between the cheeks and the rim. This space, the

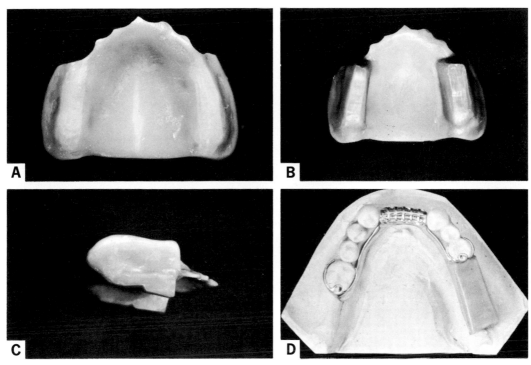

FIG. 22-12. **A.** *The record base is polished.* **B.** *Occlusion rims of hard baseplate wax are adapted.* **C.** *A notch is placed in the occlusion rims. This is accomplished at the chairside appointment.* **D.** *Occlusion rims are adapted to the mandibular removable partial denture frame.*

buccal corridor, is visible when the patient speaks or smiles. Establish the vertical length at the first molar area one quarter of an inch below the orifice of Stensen's duct. Make the anteroposterior contour of the occluding surface to coincide with a line drawn from the inferior border of the ala of the nose to the superior border of the tragus of the ear, Camper's line. This distal extension terminates slightly anterior to the alveolar tubercle. Make a half V-shaped notch buccopalatally in the first molar area to help reseat the occlusion rim in the wax on the face-bow fork and the centric occlusion records (Fig. 22-12C). The occlusion rim for the mandibular arch is attached to the free end distal extension of the removable partial denture frame (Fig. 22-12D).

MAXILLOMANDIBULAR RELATION RECORDS

As has been pointed out in Chapter 11, vertical dimension refers to the length of the face and is maintained by either the occlusion of the teeth or the balanced tonic contraction of the muscles attached to the mandible. It is a postural position and is determined when the patient is standing or sitting with the head in a comfortable upright position. The vertical dimension of physiologic rest position is important, as it is a measurable position and a place from which to start the vertical components in the recording of maxillomandibular relations. It is generally conceded that the teeth are not in contact when the jaws are in their rest position and that an interocclusal space must exist or pathologic conditions will develop. In the strictest sense there is no precise scientific method for recording the exact vertical dimension of physiologic rest position. Therefore, any method that aids in this determination is useful, and it is advisable to use several of the following methods and compare the results.

1. *Facial Measurements.* Measuring between a point on the nose and a point on the chin can be accomplished by placing a triangular-shaped piece of adhesive tape on the tip of the nose and another piece on the point of the chin (Fig. 22-13). Place the maxillary record base and contoured occlusion rim in the mouth. Have the patient stand, focusing his sight on some object that places his head in an upright comfortable position. Instruct the patient to wet the lips with the tongue, to swallow, and relax. When the mandible is observed to drop to rest, the distance between the points of tape

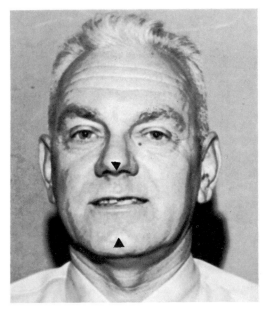

FIG. 22-13. *The triangles of adhesive tape provide points for making facial measurements.*

is recorded. The occlusion rims and the teeth should not be in contact.

2. *Tactile Sense.* Ask the patient about the contacting of the teeth and occlusion rim. If the patient feels that the contact is premature during closure or if he has to close excessively for contact, there is insufficient or excessive interocclusal space. If the patient feels that there is contact at the correct amount of closure, there is adequate but not excessive interocclusal space.

3. *Phonetics.* The use of phonetics is more valuable after the teeth have been arranged for the try-in and the wax has been contoured properly. Instruct the patient to say "three thirty-three." There should be space between the anterior teeth to allow for the thrust of the tip of the tongue. Have the patient repeat the word "Emma." There should be no contacting of teeth. When the patient says "fifty-five," the incisal edge of the maxillary central incisors should contact the vermilion border of the lower lip at the junction of the rough and smooth mucosa without tooth interference posteriorly. When *Mississippi* is pronounced, there should be no contacting of teeth.

4. *Facial Expression.* A protruded mandible seen in profile may indicate excessive interocclusal space. If the chin looks too close to the nose in a full face view, there may be excessive interocclusal space. Compressed lips, without strain, indicate overclosure. If the smooth mucosa is overly exposed or if the chin is strained to allow lip contact, the jaws are being kept too far apart. The mentolabial sulcus is obliterated when the jaws are too far apart and deeply furrowed when they are too close together. The nasolabial sulcus curves backwards excessively in overclosure

and is made excessively straight in over opening. When the patient's facial expression appears relaxed, request that the jaws be closed to contact. If no closure is possible, no interocclusal distance exists. If closure is possible, some interocclusal distance does exist, and this can be measured.

FACE-BOW TRANSFER. The face-bow is used to record the relationship of the maxillae to the temporomandibular joint and to orient the maxillary cast with the opening axis of the articulator in this same relationship. Errors in occlusion resulting from failure to use the face-bow may be small. However, no error should be incorporated that can be eliminated or reduced. It is extremely difficult to make all maxillomandibular relation records at precisely the same degree of acceptable jaw separation in the construction of conventional complete dentures. In the construction of the complete immediate denture in situations where teeth are present in both arches, the centric occlusion record is made at a slightly more open maxillomandibular relation than exists with the teeth in contact. This is done to eliminate any guiding influence by the contacting of the teeth. When the existing vertical dimension of occlusion is maintained, the articulator is closed from the recorded position to the existing position. Unless a face-bow transfer is made, the altering of the vertical dimension produces an error in occlusion.

When an arbitrary face-bow is used, the opening axis of the jaw is located by placing a marker 12 mm anterior to the tragus of the ear on a line drawn from the outer canthus of the eye to the middle of the tragus of the ear. This point is usually located in the second vertical wrinkle in the skin anterior to the tragus (Fig. 22-14).

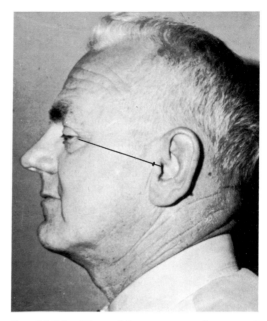

FIG. 22-14. *The arbitrary point of terminal hinge axis.*

Soften a sheet of baseplate wax, fold it, shape it like the prongs of the face-bow fork, and attach it to both surfaces of the fork. The wax-coated prongs are placed between the jaws, and the patient is instructed to close firmly into the wax. The stem of the fork should extend forward and parallel to the sagittal plane. As previously stated, this record is made to orient the cast in the articulator and this method of closure is not to be confused with the recording of maxillomandibular relationship. The patient is not uncomfortable in this closure, the maxillary record base is supported firmly in place, the fork is stable, and the patient's hands are not in the way (Fig. 22-15A).

The registration is completed by attaching the bow to the stem of the bite fork and placing the inner ends of the right and left condylar rods symmetrically over the axis markers. After the bow is tightened in position, the whole assembly is removed from the patient

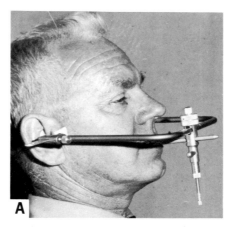

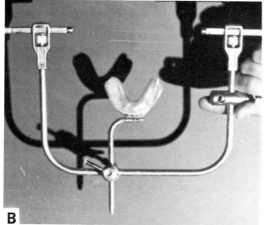

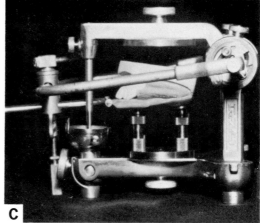

FIG. 22-15. *The face-bow transfer.* **A.** *The face bow has been centered over the arbitrary hinge axis points with the front of the bow parallel to the pupils of the eyes and has been secured to the stem of the bite fork.* **B.** *The face-bow record has been removed from the mouth for inspection.* **C.** *The face-bow is centered on the articulator. The face-bow transfer record is elevated to the correct incisal height and is supported before the cast and record bases are seated.*

and is assembled symmetrically on the articulator (Fig. 22-15B). The face-bow is raised or lowered until the incisal edge is level with the groove on the incisal pin. The groove also serves as a third point of reference for the arranging of teeth. If the axis orbital indicator is used, the relation of the maxillary cast on the articulator to the Frankfort horizontal plane will be the same as the relation to the maxillae. Support the bite fork and bow adequately prior to seating the cast and occlusion rim in the wax record

(Fig. 22-15C). Failure to support the assembly adequately often results in a posterior inferior displacement of the mounting. To assume better retention, soak the base of the cast in water for ten to fifteen minutes before attaching it to the upper member of the articulator with plaster. Allow the plaster to set thoroughly before removing the face-bow assembly and support.

TENTATIVE CENTRIC OCCLUSION AND CENTRIC RELATION. The existing vertical dimension of occlusion is not necessarily the vertical dimension to be reproduced in the denture. The maximum contacts of the remaining teeth may not be in harmony with centric relation. Therefore, the maxillomandibular relationship is recorded with the teeth out of contact. The recording medium should introduce a minimum of resistance to closure, harden rapidly, and be rigid after it is hard.

The maxillomandibular relationship is recorded with a wax that is passive when softened. Reduce the occlusion rims vertically until a clearance of 3 to 5 mm exists between the rim and the opposing posterior teeth. Seat the patient in a comfortable position with head upright. Have him practice the training exercises of protruding, retruding, and closing the jaws until the exercise is effortless. Shape softened wax into a roll approximately two thirds the diameter of a lead pencil and attach to the occluding surface of the occlusion rim. When the complete immediate denture is opposed by a removable partial denture or natural teeth, the passive wax is placed on the maxillary occlusion rims. When it is opposed by a complete denture, the wax is placed on the mandibular occlusion rims. While the wax is soft, shape it into a cone with the base adjacent to the hard wax (Fig. 22-16A). Soften the wax with an open flame or in 130°F water. After seating the record base in the mouth and placing the index fingers in the areas of the first molar, instruct the patient to retrude the jaw and close. Closure is stopped prior to tooth contact (Fig. 22-16B). The contact is broken after the wax has hardened, and the record is removed from the mouth and allowed to bench harden further before it is inspected.

Examine the record to see if a definite repositioning index was recorded (Fig. 22-16C). Reinsert the record and observe

carefully for accuracy in the anteroposterior relation. Remember that wax is easily distorted. With the record in centric occlusion, measure the vertical dimension of the face. When the vertical dimension of occlusion is less than the vertical dimension of physiologic rest position, the difference is considered the amount of interocclusal distance as measured between points on the upper and lower half of the face. The records made with occlusion rims are considered tentative records to be verified after the teeth have been arranged and the wax has been contoured and smoothed in order to be compatible with the surrounding oral environment.

Soak the mandibular cast in water ten to fifteen minutes. Place the articulator in the mounting jig. Put the tentative centric relation record on the maxillary cast. Place the mandibular cast into the record and seal the wax to the cast with a hot spatula. Attach the mandibular cast to the lower member of the articulator with plaster (Fig. 22-16D).

ARRANGING THE POSTERIOR TEETH FOR TRY-IN. For this particular patient the relationship of the jaws, the form of the occlusal surfaces of the mandibular posterior teeth, and the coordination of the neuromuscular controls of mandibular movements indicate a cusp form posterior tooth arranged in balanced occlusion. Another patient may require different treatment. Acrylic resin teeth are used to oppose the gold occlusal coverage of the mandibular teeth. It has been observed clinically that gold opposing acrylic resin does not abrade excessively. The posterior teeth should be arranged on a plane in centric occlusion without altering the occlusal surfaces. After the teeth have been arranged, wax is applied to the teeth and record base. Then it is contoured and smoothed

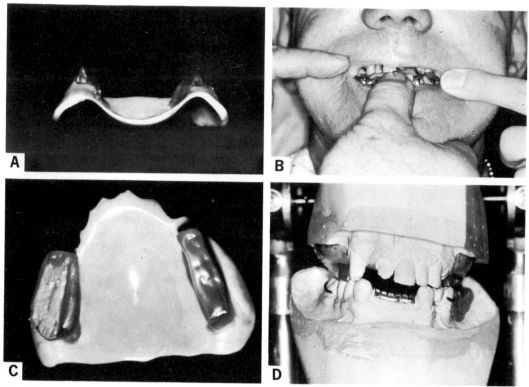

FIG. 22-16. *Recording maxillomandibular relationship.* **A.** *Cone-shaped wax attached to occlusion rim.* **B.** *Rehearsing the patient prior to making jaw relation record.* **C.** *A definite record in the wax.* **D.** *Mounted cast.*

for compatibility with the oral tissues during the try-in procedure.

TRY-IN AND VERIFICATION OF MAXILLO-MANDIBULAR RECORDS. The tentative relation records of centric relation and centric occlusion are verified at this time by an interocclusal check record. This record is an imprint in a wax recording media to verify the positions of the articulated casts.

The patient is seated comfortably in the same position as that required for the tentative record. Soften two thicknesses of a passive wax and place over the occlusal surfaces of the maxillary posterior teeth. Resoften the wax in a water bath at 138°F or with a controlled open flame and immediately seat the record

base in the mouth. Instruct the patient to retrude the lower jaw and close until the first contact is felt. The properly trained patient, provided the neuromuscular controls are coordinated, will need very little guidance for this procedure. Allow the wax to harden before removing the record from the mouth. Inspect the record to make sure the teeth did not penetrate the wax and contact opposing teeth (Fig. 22-17). Remove any excess wax with a sharp instrument.

Release the condylar elements of the articulator and assemble the check record on the articulator. Discrepancies between the check record and the tentative mounting, if present, are found by observing the positions of the condylar

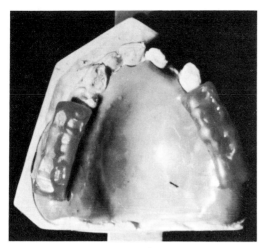

FIG. 22-17. *An interocclusal check record.*

elements in relation to their stops. The condylar elements will not be against the centric stop if there is a discrepancy (Fig. 22-18). Any discrepancy or lack of discrepancy is noted and the check record is repeated until three records verify the discrepancy or the lack of it. If the check records fail to agree with the original mounting, make a new maxillomandibular relation record. Detach the mandibular cast and remount it with the new record. When a remounting is necessary, new check records must be made and repeated.

PROTRUSIVE RELATION RECORD. A protrusive relation record is made to establish a point of reference in the condyle path and to adjust the horizontal and lateral condylar inclinations of the articulator. The condyle path is not recorded in a protrusive record, nor do the condyles travel in a straight path as on the adjustable articulator. However, there must be some adaptability to slight changes in the temporomandibular

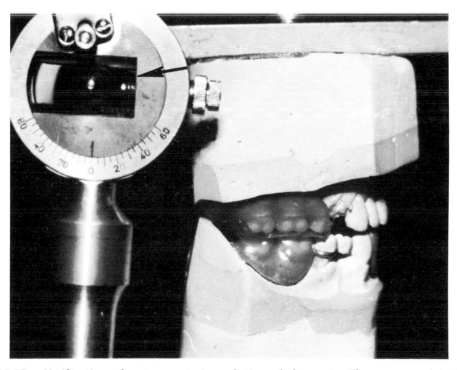

FIG. 22-18. *Verification of anteroposterior relation of the casts. The arrow points to the condylar element against the centric stop.*

joints; otherwise few dentures could be tolerated.

Ask the patient to protrude the chin until the incisal edges of the maxillary anterior teeth are opposite the incisal edges of the mandibular teeth and then to close straight to contact the teeth. When the patient is trained in these movements, four layers of passive wax are softened and shaped to conform to the occlusal surfaces and incisal edges of the mandibular arch. The passive wax is contoured in a vertical direction higher over the posterior teeth than over the anterior teeth to assure simultaneous contacting in the anterior and posterior regions. The patient protrudes and closes the lower jaw. The closure is stopped prior to tooth contact. The record is allowed to harden before it is removed and placed on the cast. The horizontal condylar guides are adjusted (Fig. 22-19) and then the lateral settings are adjusted, using the Hanau formula:

$$L = \frac{H}{8} + 12$$

POSTERIOR PALATAL SEAL.   The posterior palatal seal area is outlined in the same manner as that used when the impression tray was corrected for posterior extension. The indelible marking is transferred by the record base to the cast, and the cast is altered in this area by scraping (Fig. 22-20). This procedure must be accomplished by the dentist and not assigned to auxiliary personnel.

Using a ball burnisher, palpate the soft tissue covering of the denture-bearing areas. When the resiliency of the tissues over the primary and secondary stress-bearing areas is the same as the resiliency of the tissues across the palate and on the slopes of the ridges, no relief is required. If the resiliency is not the same, areas having no resilient

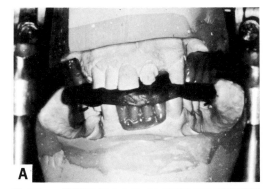

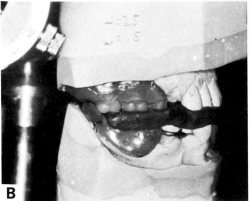

FIG. 22-19.   **A.** *A protrusive interocclusal jaw relation record in wax.* **B.** *The protrusive record is used to adjust the horizontal and lateral condylar guides.*

tissue are outlined with the color transfer applicator and transferred to the cast. Add an extra thickness of wax over the recorded areas to provide extra thickness of denture base material so that the reliefs, when necessary, can be made in the finished denture.

The incisive papilla area is relieved by placing one thickness 0.002 inch tinfoil over the entire incisive papilla (Fig. 22-20). Any additional relief in this area is accomplished at the insertion appointment. The pad of fibrous connective tissue protecting the nasopalatine nerve and blood vessels may not be sufficient protection in the presence of dentures.

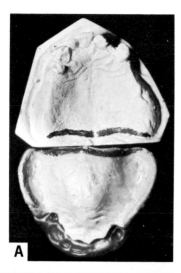

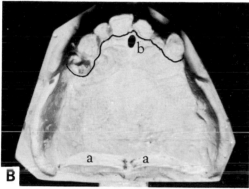

FIG. 22-20. **A.** *The posterior palatal seal area outlined.* **B.** *The cast is altered by scraping to the determined length and depth (a). The incisive papilla is marked (b) for the placing of relief material.*

SELECTING AND ARRANGING ANTERIOR TEETH

In the majority of instances the form, size, and shape of the natural teeth are the best guides in the selection of the anterior teeth. The characteristics of the natural teeth and the desires of the patient determine the use of personalized or characterized teeth. Acrylic resin is usually the material of choice for artificial teeth in immediate dentures because it can be contoured to become a part of

the denture base without destroying their retention in the denture base material.

The arrangement of the anterior teeth is primarily associated with esthetics. A steep vertical overlap anteriorly without a compensating horizontal overlap is a potentially damaging situation and makes it mandatory to place very steep cusp with a steep cusp inclination to provide balanced occlusion in protrusive and lateral eccentric jaw positions. This arrangement of teeth is difficult to keep in balanced occlusion but is of particular importance in immediate denture insertion, as the thin cortical plate of bone is unsupported during the initial stages of healing of the extraction sites. To meet the esthetic requirements it is not always possible to have protrusive balance. In these situations compromises must be made. The horizontal overlap may be increased to help provide a better balanced occlusion. The cuspids can be slightly shortened to provide balance in the lateral positions. Although the positions of the remaining natural teeth may not be compatible with the desired esthetic result, duplicating their positions may not be functionally acceptable in the denture. The functional, as well as the esthetic, results must be considered. Artificial teeth act as a unit, since they are attached to the same movable base. Natural teeth act individually. This difference must be considered in harmonizing the artificial teeth with mandibular movements.

The arrangement of artificial teeth is a systematic procedure. The procedures in arranging the anterior teeth are dictated by the individual circumstances. If the positions of the natural teeth are to be reproduced exactly, remove one tooth at a time from the cast. This procedure allows the adjoining tooth to act as a guide. If positions of natural teeth

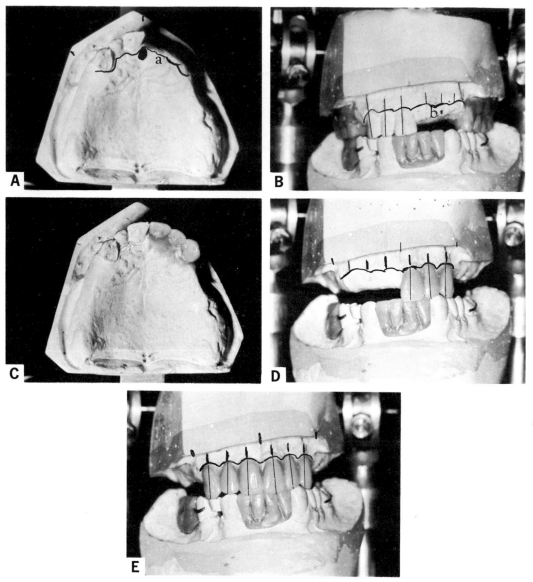

FIG. 22-21. *Guide lines on the cast are aids to arranging teeth and contouring the cast.*
A. *Occlusal view. The left central, lateral, and cuspid teeth have been removed, and the cast has been contoured to the palatal guide line* **(a)**. **B.** *Anterior view. The left central, lateral, and cuspid teeth have been removed, and the cast has been contoured to the labial guide line* **(b)**. **C.** *Left anterior teeth arranged.* **D.** *Right anterior teeth removed from the cast.* **E.** *Anterior teeth replaced.*

are not to be reproduced, remove the cuspid, the lateral, and the central teeth from one side of the cast (Fig. 22-21A,B,C). As a guide, retain the teeth on the side which is more acceptable. Guide lines

on the labial and palatal surfaces of the cast aid in contouring the cast from cuspid to cuspid (Fig. 22-21A,B,D,E). Place the labial line approximately 3 mm superiorly from the gingiva, and place the palatal line approximately 2 millimeters palatally from the gingiva (Fig. 22-21Aa Bb). Surgical procedures to remove alveolar bone are not anticipated for this patient, but when a tooth is extracted, a collapse of the free gingival tissue occurs, and the contouring of the cast by scraping between these lines is an attempt to compensate for this collapse. Anterior labial thickness of wax allows for relief on the tissue side when necessary at the time of insertion (Fig. 22-22).

CORRECTING FOR
PROCESSING ERROR

After the denture is processed and removed from the flask, it is repositioned on the articulator, an aid in eliminating any processing error. Use the remount indices in the base of the cast to orient the denture accurately for this procedure. Seal the cast to the plaster mounting on the articulator with sticky wax and analyze the occlusion. If occlusal disharmony exists, the change is usually reflected in the position of the incisal

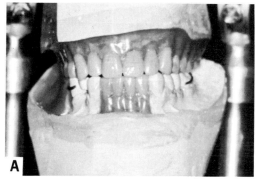

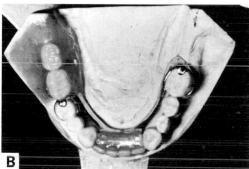

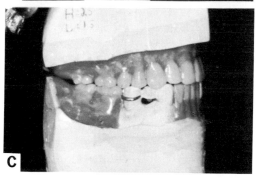

FIG. 22-22. *The wax is contoured.* **A.** *Anterior view of both arches.* **B.** *Occlusal view of mandibular arch.* **C.** *Buccal view of right side.*

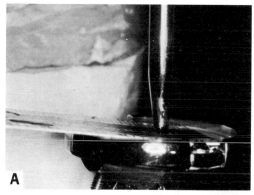

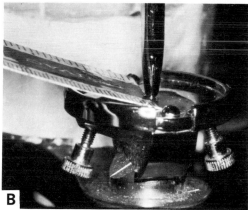

FIG. 22-23. *Correcting processing error on an articulator.* **A.** *The incisal pin is elevated from the table, reflecting occlusal disharmony.* **B.** *Interocclusal distance is restored. The incisal pin has returned to the table.*

guide pin in relation to the incisal guide table. Elevation of the incisal guide pin above the guide table indicates an increase in the vertical dimension of occlusion with an accompanying decrease in interocclusal distance (Fig. 22-23A). The occlusal surfaces of the teeth must be altered by selective grinding until the guide pin is returned to the table, indicating that the vertical dimension of occlusion has been returned to its recorded position (Fig. 22-23B).

PLASTER REMOUNT INDEX

After the processing error has been corrected, attach the plaster remount index platform to the lower member of the articulator. Place a thin mix of quick-setting plaster on the platform and close the upper articulator member until the guide pin is flush on the guide table (Fig. 22-24). The incisal edges and occlusal surfaces of the teeth should extend into the soft plaster deep enough to reposition the denture. Allow the plaster to harden before removing the denture. This remounting index saves time at the insertion appointment, since it eliminates the necessity of another face-bow transfer at the time of remounting the den-

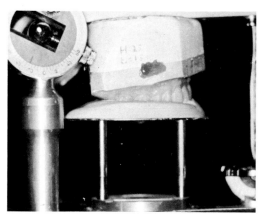

Fig. 22-24. *Articulator with plaster remount index platform attached and the plaster remount made.*

tures with new maxillomandibular relation records. Only a centric relation record is required for remounting the maxillary cast.

PREPARATION FOR THE INSERTION APPOINTMENT

Remove the stone cast from the denture and prepare the denture for polishing. Reduce the labial flange vertically to the area of the junction of the firmly and loosely attached mucosa. Reduce the undercut areas on the tissue side of the labial flange, particularly over the cuspid eminences. The superior and posterior path of insertion allows some undercut in the labial area of the arch which will not be damaging during the insertion or removal of the denture. Allow a slight excess in thickness of the labial flange to remain and remove this after the tissue side has been adjusted at insertion. Any prominences or concavities resulting from the removal of the teeth from the cast are removed, and the denture is smoothed with a round or blunt-nosed acrylic bur. The posterior palatal seal area is rounded superiorly to present a rounded polished surface when contacted by the dorsum of the tongue. Round and polish the borders for comfort in the mouth.

Block out all undercuts in the denture with wet pumice and make an accurate plaster cast for remounting. Position the teeth in the remounting plaster matrix and attach the cast to the upper member of the articulator with plaster. The denture is removed from the plaster cast, and the pumice is removed from the denture and the cast.

SURGICAL PROCEDURES AND INSERTION

Before surgery, the acrylic resin teeth should have been contoured to become a part of the natural appearing denture resin base, and the path of insertion should have been determined. At the insertion appointment, seat and adjust the mandibular removable partial denture before taking the patient to surgery. Make an irreversible hydrocolloid (alginate) impression with the removable partial denture in place. Remove the partial denture from its impression and pour a plaster cast.

If the maxillary frenum attachments are acceptable, no surgical procedures other than the removal of the teeth need be anticipated. A satisfactory residual ridge can be expected if the blood clot, the young connective tissue, the fibrillar bone, and finally the mature bone that successively occupy the alveoli are protected by undisturbed cortical bone and its periosteal covering.

Anesthetize the teeth, using a local anesthetic with infraorbital block and palatal infiltration. In the removal of the teeth, try to preserve as much of the bony and soft tissue as possible. Avoid reflections, tears, and avulsions of the soft tissues (Fig. 22-25). Denuding of the alveolar process often results in necrosis and extrusion. The excessive osteoclastic action, which is clinically noted after removing the tips of the alveolar crest,

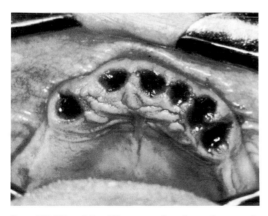

FIG. 22-25. *Maxillary arch after the teeth have been removed. Observe the absence of reflection, tears, or avulsions of the soft tissues.*

suturing, and reflecting the periosteum, is best avoided by *not* performing these procedures unless absolutely necessary. The eventual loss of the alveolar ridge is inevitable; therefore, all possible precautions should be exercised to retain it as long as possible.

The dentist who is responsible for the prosthodontic treatment inserts the denture, and if any surgical alterations are required, they are done immediately. The denture is removed, and the patient is instructed to close against sterile gauze until the cessation of bleeding. The tissue side of the denture is washed, dried, and painted with an even coating of a pressure disclosing material. The denture is inserted, removed, and examined for any indications that the flanges have passed over an undercut. Pressure disclosing material being dragged from the surface of the denture shows such pressure areas. Particular attention should be directed to the cuspid eminence and alveolar tubercle areas (Fig. 22-26Aa). If the disclosing paste has been removed, the denture base is relieved in the area by grinding, and the procedure is repeated until the pressure is relieved (Fig. 22-26Bb). The altered areas are smoothed and again the tissue side of the denture is painted with a thin, even covering of disclosing paste. After instruction in the correct procedures, the patient is allowed to insert and remove the denture. Reinspect the flange surfaces and reduce any vertical overextension of the labial flange. Observe the frenum attachments to see if adequate space has been provided in the denture base for their action. Reduce any excessive thickness of the labial flange.

REMOUNT PROCEDURE AT INSERTION. After the surfaces have been smoothed, apply two thicknesses of passive wax to the occlusal surfaces of the posterior

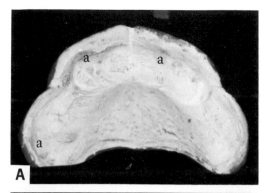

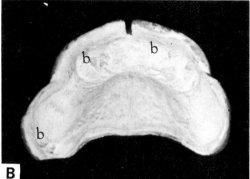

FIG. 22-26. **A.** *Undercut areas* (a) *where the pressure relief cream has been dragged from the denture.* **B.** *The tissue side of the denture base has been relieved by grinding pressure areas* (b) *with an acrylic bur.*

teeth and make a centric interocclusal record. The mandibular cast is seated in the centric occlusal record and is attached to the lower member of the articulator with plaster (Fig. 22-27). Remove the undercut areas on the clasped teeth to facilitate removal of the partial denture from the cast. Verify the accuracy of the articulated cast with repeated check records. Correct any discrepancies in occlusion by selective grinding procedures. It is undesirable to have maloccluding teeth at any time and particularly during the organization of the blood clot.

Instruct the patient not to remove the maxillary denture until the next appointment. Unless contraindicated, an anal-

gesic is prescribed. The application of an ice pack is especially indicated if the patient has had swelling following previous extractions.

Postinsertion Treatment

It is imperative to see the patient the day after insertion. Seat the patient in a comfortable upright position. Make a centric occlusal record as before. This check record is used to evaluate the recordings and mounting of the previous appointment (Fig. 22-27). Follow the same procedures for occlusal correction and relieving of undercuts as in the insertion phase (Fig. 22-28). Apply

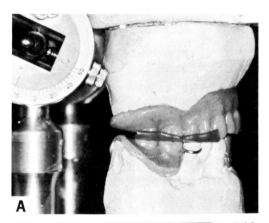

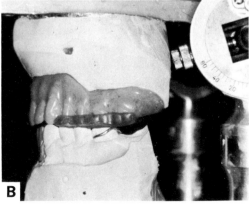

FIG. 22-27. *The casts mounted for occlusal evaluation.* **A.** *Right lateral view.* **B.** *Left lateral view.*

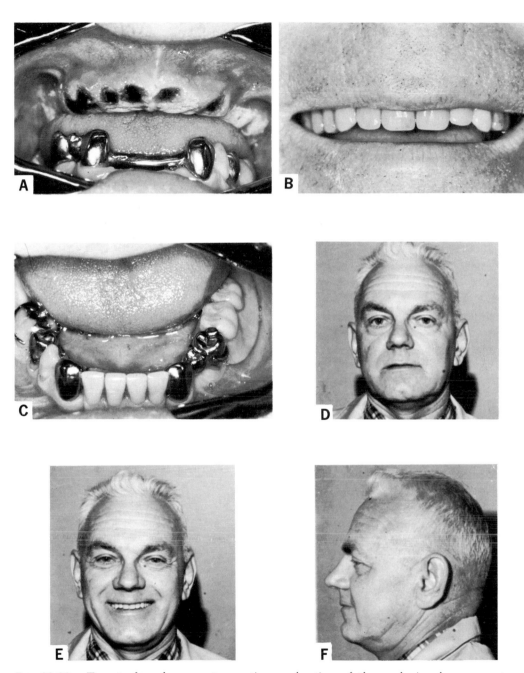

Fig. 22-28. *Twenty-four hour postoperative evaluation of the occlusion by remount procedures (Fig. 22-27) and the following:* **A.** *The soft tissues are evaluated.* **B.** *Phonetics are checked.* **C.** *The removable partial denture is evaluated for retention.* **D.** *The vertical dimension of occlusion is evaluated.* **E, F.** *The esthetics are evaluated.*

a thin, even coat of pressure disclosing material to the tissue surface of the denture to determine the presence of pressure areas over the basal rest. Insert the denture and have the patient tap the teeth together with the jaws in terminal position. Borders are best analyzed by using disclosing wax. Apply disclosing wax in a manner similar to that for applying impression compound for border refining.

Instruct the patient to open wide, protrude, and swing the mandible to the right and to the left. The disclosing wax will be removed from the denture flanges if the flanges have been over-contoured during the wax-up stage or overextended in the impression procedures. Apply disclosing wax in the buccal frenum attachment areas and have the patient protrude and retrude the lips. The base of the frenum attachment should be visible in the notch that was provided for its action, and the labial vestibule should be filled. When these procedures are finished, observe the tissues for irritation. When satisfied that all areas have been checked, ask the patient to relate his experience with the dentures. This sequence of procedures convinces the patient that he will be treated to relieve any problem without his having to ask the dentist. When the patient says that "the areas of discomfort have been corrected," the patient assures the dentist that he has confidence in his professional abilities.

These same procedures are repeated two days later. The patient is advised to remove the dentures at night, to use the knife and fork for biting, to take small mouthfuls of food, and to return whenever problems occur. The atrophy or resorption of bone after removal of the natural teeth is reason enough to minimize the forces directed to the bone to maintain an adequate blood supply.

The changing of the tissues of the basal seat area following the insertion of an immediate complete denture necessitates the refitting of the denture base within the first six months, either by rebasing or remaking the denture. Place the patient on a one-month recall schedule until these changes take place.

REFERENCES

1. Appleby, R. C., and Kirchoff, W. F.: Immediate maxillary denture impression. J. Prosth. Dent., 5:443, 1955.
1a. Aseltine, L. F.: Preparation of the mouth for immediate dentures. J. Prosth. Dent., 1:151, 1951.
2. Bennett, C. C.: Characterized immediate dentures. J. Prosth. Dent., 11:648, 1961.
2a. Bolouri, A.: Double-custom tray procedure for immediate dentures. J. Prosth. Dent., 37:344, 1977.
3. Brigante, R. F.: Instant dentition: preferential procedures for single-phase extractions. Dent. Clin. N. Amer., March, 1966, p. 195.
4. Bruce, R. W.: Immediate denture service designed to preserve oral structures. J. Prosth. Dent., 16:811, 1966.
4a. Burgoyne, J. R.: Alveoplasty in preparation for the immediate denture insertion. J. Prosth. Dent., 1:254, 1951.
5. Colter, S. W., and Budill, E. J.: Intravenous anesthesia (Pentothal Sodium) as an adjunct to immediate denture service. J. Prosth. Dent., 3:358, 1952.
5a. Cupero, H. M.: Impression technique for complete maxillary denture. J. Prosth. Dent., 39:108, 1978.
5b. Demer, W. J.: Minimizing problems in placement of immediate dentures. J. Prosth. Dent., 27:275, 1972.
6. DeVan, M. M.: The transition from natural to artificial teeth. J. Prosth. Dent., 11:677, 1961; and J. Tenn. Dent. Ass., 41:197, 1961.
7. Disick, D.: Emergency temporary denture. J. Prosth. Dent., 7:590, 1957.
8. Freese, A. S.: Simplified impression for immediate complete dentures. J.A.D.A., 54:240, 1957.
9. Geiger, E. C. K.: Duplication of the esthetics of an existing immediate denture. J. Prosth. Dent., 5:179, 1955.

10. Geiler, C. W.: Immediate denture prosthesis: tooth arrangement and esthetics. J.A.D.A., 35:185, 1947.
11. Gimson, A. P.: Immediate dentures: alveolar ridge trauma from socketed anteriors. Brit. Dent. J., 98:387, 1955.
12. Harris, H. L.: An immediate full denture technic. J.A.D.A., 22:1656, 1935.
13. Heartwell, C. M., Jr., and Salisbury, F. W.: Immediate complete dentures: an evaluation. J. Prosth. Dent. 15:615, 1965.
14. Hughes, F. C.: Immediate denture service: advantages, disadvantages, and technical procedures. J.A.D.A., 34:30, 1947.
15. ———: Transition from natural to prosthetic dentures. J. Prosth. Dent., 1:145, 1951.
15a. Javid, N., Tanaka, H., and Porter, M.: Split-tray impression technique for immediate upper dentures. J. Prosth. Dent., 32:348, 1974.
15b. ——— and Porter, M. R.: The construction of transitional immediate dentures. J. Prosth. Dent., 30:210, 1973.
16. Jerhi, F. C.: Trimming the cast in the construction of immediate dentures. J. Prosth. Dent., 16:1047, 1966.
17. Kelly, E. K.: Follow-up treatment for immediate denture patients. J. Prosth. Dent., 17:16, 1967.
18. Klein, I. E.: Immediate denture prosthesis. J. Prosth. Dent., 10:14, 1960.
18a. Lam, R. V.: Contour changes of the alveolar processes following extraction. J. Prosth. Dent., 10:25, 1960.
19. Maison, W. G.: Preparation of the mouth and casts for immediate dentures. J. Prosth. Dent., 3:66, 1953.
19a. McCartney, J. W.: The transitional immediate complete denture. J. Prosth. Dent., 40:593, 1978.
19b. McFee, C. E., and Meier, E. A.: A technique for enhancing cosmetics in immediate dentures. J. Prosth. Dent., 31:585, 1974.
19c. Michael, C. G., and Barsoum, W. M.: Comparing ridge resorption with various surgical techniques in immediate dentures. J. Prosth. Dent., 35:142, 1976.
20. Passamonti, G.: Immediate denture prosthesis. Dent. Clin. N. Amer., November, 1964, p. 781.
21. Payne, H. S.: A transitional denture. J. Prosth. Dent., 14:221, 1964.
22. Pound, E.: An all-inclusive immediate denture technic. J.A.D.A., 67:16, 1963.
23. ———: Preparatory dentures: a protective philosophy. J. Prosth. Dent., 15:5, 1965.
23a. ———: Controlled immediate dentures. J. Prosth. Dent., 24:243, 1970.
24. Schlosser, R. O.: Advantages of conservative procedure in complete immediate denture prosthesis. J. Canad. Dent. Ass., 14:611, 1948.
25. Schweitzer, J. M.: Treatment plan for a difficult immediate denture case. Dent. Dig., 52:550, 1946.
26. Sears, V. H.: Immediate denture restoration. J.A.D.A., 10:644, 1923.
27. Swenson, M. G.: Improving immediate dentures in general practice. J.A.D.A., 47:550, 1953.
27a. Swoope, C. C., Depew, T. E., Wisman, L. J., and Wands, D. H.: Interim Dentures. J. Prosth. Dent., 32:604, 1974.
27b. Terrell, W. H.: Immediate restorations by complete dentures. J. Prosth. Dent., 1:495, 1951.
28. Tillman, E. J.: Immediate dentures and psychic trauma. J. Prosth. Dent., 14:1040, 1964.
28a. Walsh, J. F., Walsh, T., and Griffiths, R.: An immediate denture technique to reproduce labial alveolar contour. J. Prosth. Dent., 37:222, 1977.
29. Waltz, M. E.: Considerate postoperative care for immediate denture patients. J. Prosth. Dent., 16:822, 1966.
30. Wictorin, L.: An evaluation of bone surgery in patients with immediate dentures. J. Prosth. Dent., 21:6, 1969.

The Single Complete Denture

23

The primary consideration for continued denture success with a single conventional complete denture is the preservation of that which remains. Under certain conditions the decision to advise its use is a difficult task. The diagnostic procedures are time-consuming but should not be neglected. Many variable factors must be evaluated if the treatment is to achieve success.

The single complete denture should not be confused with the tooth-supported complete denture (Chapter 24), which conforms to a different philosophy. A generalization of the overall philosophy of the single complete denture will be presented, but no attempt will be made to analyze all of the different factors that may be involved in the decision to provide this treatment. After considering the diagnostic entities that were discussed in Chapter 4, the dentist must evaluate the individual problems presented by the variable considerations. The monetary factors and the availability of the patient are not discussed. Although the availability of the patient (time factor) and his ability to pay (monetary factor) may influence the treatment plan, they are not considerations in the diagnostic evaluation procedures. One must remember that each situation presents individual problems. Similar appearing conditions do

not always dictate the same treatment plan.

A single complete denture may be desirable when it is to oppose any one of the following:

1. Natural teeth that are sufficient in number not to necessitate a fixed or removable partial denture.

2. A partially edentulous arch in which the missing teeth have been or will be replaced by a fixed partial denture.

3. A partially edentulous arch in which the missing teeth have been or will be replaced by a removable partial denture.

4. An existing complete denture.

In the first three situations the maxillary arch is usually the edentulous arch. Among the reasons for this occurrence is that a maxillary complete denture is more stable, easier to retain in position, and tolerated better by patients than a mandibular denture. Therefore, many are less reluctant to allow the loss of the maxillary teeth and at times insist upon their removal. To retain the mandibular teeth, some dentists have sacrificed restorable maxillary teeth. This is not a philosophy to which one should subscribe. Dentists are becoming more aware of the desirability of retaining the natural teeth in both arches to help preserve the residual alveolar ridges.

Mandibular Denture to Oppose Natural Maxillary Teeth

Although the mandibular arch is seldom the edentulous one, this condition does occur. It usually happens as a result of either surgical or accidental trauma. An example of surgical trauma is the removal of the mandibular teeth for persons who are to undergo irradiation therapy for a tumor. The teeth may have been quite serviceable; however, because of their periodontal condition or their closeness to the site of irradiation, they are condemned. The mandibular teeth may be lost as a result of a fall, vehicle accident, or gunshot. The beautiful young girl who was in a motor vehicle accident and lost her mandibular teeth is a candidate for sympathy. Frequently the remaining maxillary teeth and periodontium are free of disease and the teeth are cosmetically attractive. The teeth may or may not be supporting a fixed or removable prosthetic restoration; however, the situations are comparable.

In these situations it is necessary to consider the total patient. Three factors in particular must be carefully evaluated: preservation of the residual alveolar ridge, necessity for retaining maxillary teeth, and mental trauma. When all factors have been evaluated and it is decided to prescribe a complete mandibular denture, the patient should be well educated to the possible consequences. If this is done seriously and sincerely, the treated patient will understand the consequences and help to minimize them.

PRESERVATION OF THE RESIDUAL ALVEOLAR RIDGE

For the continued satisfactory use of a mandibular denture the residual alveolar ridge must be preserved in the mandibular arch. Research has shown that the force of jaw closure with natural teeth is greater than that with complete dentures. It is known that the greater the force the more the pressure, and pressure is a contributing factor to bone resorption. It is not known how much force is exerted when natural teeth in one arch are opposed by a complete denture. Undoubtedly this will vary; however, one cannot guess that the force will be minimal and tolerated with no deterioration of the bone (Fig. 23-1).

The mandible is the movable member of the stomatognathic system; therefore, it is more difficult to stabilize the mandibular denture. Another factor involved

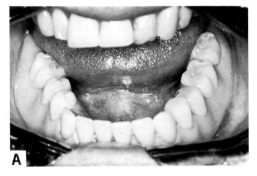

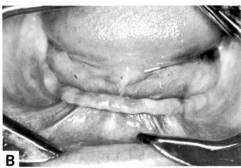

FIG. 23-1. A. *Complete mandibular denture opposing natural maxillary teeth. The patient, a 36-year-old male in good health, lost his mandibular teeth as a result of trauma in an automobile accident.* **B.** *The mandibular residual ridge after using the denture for less than 12 months. Note the pendulous tissue covering the anterior residual ridge.*

in stabilizing the mandibular denture is its proximity to the tongue, one of the most active muscles in the body, which in its activity may displace the denture. This denture movement increases the pressure and stress on the mucosa and bone. This is detrimental to comfort for the patient and to preservation of the support.

Another factor is the minimal availability of mucosa with tightly attached submucosa for mandibular denture support. The more concentrated the stress, the more damage to the supporting structures results.

If the single factor dictating the prescription of a complete mandibular denture is preservation of the residual ridge, then such a prescription should never be made. However, in a health service the use of *never* is dubious philosophy. The fact that one person has done well with a complete denture in the mandibular arch opposing natural teeth only proves that there are exceptions to all rules and should not influence one to prescribe this treatment. The young patient who insists on this treatment must know that there may come a time in middle life when not being able to tolerate dentures as a result of support loss will be a disastrous situation (Fig. 23-2).

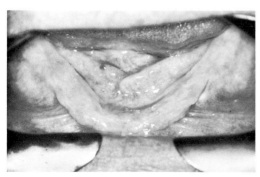

FIG. 23-2. *Abused tissue and loss of residual alveolar ridge in a patient who used a complete mandibular denture opposed by natural maxillary teeth for 14 years. At the age of 50 she has a severe denture problem.*

NECESSITY FOR RETAINING MAXILLARY TEETH

The maxillary dentition may be needed to retain a prosthesis (Fig. 23-3). This situation is usually associated with congenital defects, such as cleft palate, or a stoma resulting from surgical or accidental trauma. The primary considerations for these patients is the ability to speak clearly enough to be understood and to swallow food and fluids without their passing into the nasal cavity.

MENTAL TRAUMA

The loss of teeth is such a traumatic mental experience for some persons that

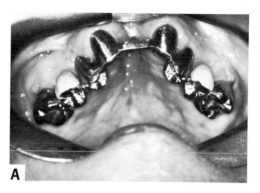

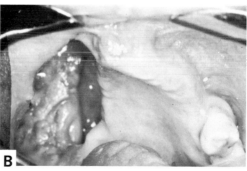

FIG. 23-3. **A.** *Natural maxillary teeth retained and prepared for an overlay removable partial denture opposite a complete mandibular denture. The anterior teeth will support the veneer anterior teeth, the palatal section will obturate an anterior cleft, and a speech bulb will be attached posteriorly.* **B.** *Two molars retained to provide retention for a maxillary prosthesis opposite a complete mandibular denture.*

they become depressed. Their depression may lead to more complicated psychologic problems. If this mental state exists when the patient loses the mandibular teeth, removal of the remaining maxillary teeth may be more than he or she can endure mentally. It must be remembered that the face is the most exposed part of the body, and it is usually the first part of the body that the individual scrutinizes each morning and is usually the first part of the body that others see. Change in the appearance of the face is a factor that all dentists must consider when treating the total patient.

Even though the potential for the destruction of the mandibular residual ridge is great, the necessity for retaining maxillary teeth for retentive purposes and the mental trauma created by the loss of the mandibular teeth may be the deciding factors for prescribing a complete mandibular denture to oppose natural teeth in the maxillary arch (Fig. 23-4). With patient education, and at times psychiatric help, the problem may be resolved in a different manner at a later date.

Single Complete Maxillary Denture to Oppose Natural Mandibular Teeth

More frequently encountered than the singular mandibular denture is the single maxillary denture. The diagnostic procedures should determine that there are sufficient teeth in the mandibular arch, periodontal health is acceptable, and there are no missing teeth to be replaced. The number of mandibular teeth considered sufficient should include the first molars in jaws that have a Class I or Class III relation. In Class II related jaws the anterior teeth and premolars bilaterally may suffice. When these conditions are met, it would appear that one could proceed; however, there may be problems to consider.

The result of inadequate diagnostic evaluation, dental hygiene, and denture care and insufficient mandibular posterior occlusion is illustrated in Figure 23-5. The patient, a 52-year-old woman, had the time and money for treatment and was in good systemic condition. During the initial visit she reported that her teeth contacted when she talked and her jaws were always tired. These symptoms suggest a lack of interocclusal distance or free-way space. She further reported a burning sensation in her pal-

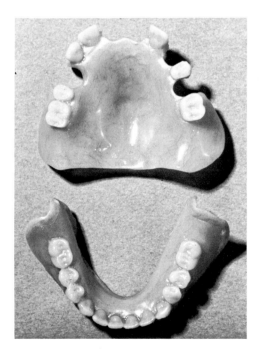

FIG. 23-4. *Complete mandibular and transitional maxillary dentures constructed to avoid further mental trauma for a patient who was receiving radiation therapy for cancer of the nasal pharynx. His mandibular teeth were a poor risk for retention.*

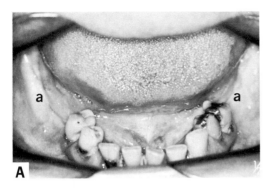

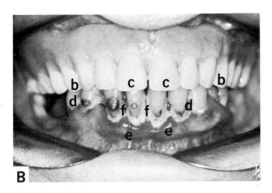

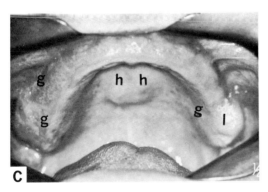

ate and discomfort, although the dentures had been relined four times during the 18 months she had been attempting to use them. The radiographic examination was essentially negative.

When cusp form posterior teeth are used, balanced occlusion enhances the stability and retention of the dentures. Balanced occlusion should be provided when the jaws are in terminal relation and/or in eccentric relation and the teeth are brought together. It has also been established that the teeth must be positioned to conform with the dictates of the incisal and condylar guidances if they are to provide balanced occlusion.

The occlusal forms of the natural teeth usually act as the guide in selecting the occlusal form for the maxillary posterior teeth. In most situations this would be a cusp tooth (Fig. 23-6). However, if the natural teeth are abraded and are not restored prior to treatment, the monoplane form may be the choice for the occlusal surfaces of posterior teeth.

One of the five requirements of a denture is its esthetic acceptability (Chapter 14). Sometimes the positions of the mandibular anterior teeth will not allow the maxillary anterior teeth to be positioned in an esthetically acceptable manner or for balanced occlusion. This problem may be resolved as follows:

1. Reposition the natural teeth with orthodontic procedures.

2. Alter the clinical crowns of the teeth by grinding or with restorations.

FIG. 23-5. A. *Occlusal view of partially edentulous mandibular arch. The molars (a) have been removed from both sides of the arch. The residual alveolar ridge appears adequate to support a prosthesis, and the mucosa are healthy, firm, pink, and stippled.* **B.** *Anterior view of occlusion. Teeth of the maxillary denture are in maximum intercuspation with mandibular premolars (b). The anterior teeth (c) are in contact, and the Class I related jaws are approximately 9 mm anterior to terminal relation. Note the carious lesions at the necks of the teeth (d), irritation of the gingiva (e), and the gross detritus and calculus.* **C.** *Maxillary arch. The mucosa (g) is irritated and hyperemic, there is evidence of lack of palatal relief over the torus palatinus (h), and a collection of detritus is visible in the left molar area (l).*

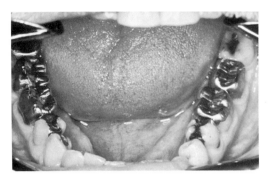

FIG. 23-6. *Mandibular natural teeth prepared to oppose a complete maxillary denture with cusp teeth. Occlusal surfaces of the restored molars follow the forms of the natural teeth.*

3. Accept balanced occlusion with the jaws in terminal relation and not in the eccentric positions.

The mandibular posterior teeth may be malposed or missing, and the forces of occlusion to the maxillary teeth lacking. Abused mucosa over the maxillary residual alveolar ridge is frequently encountered when a complete single denture opposes malpositioned natural teeth (Fig. 23-7). The mandibular teeth should then be altered either by selective grind-

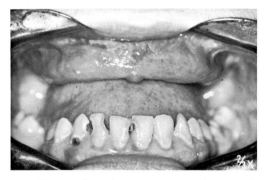

FIG. 23-7. *Abused mucosa over the maxillary residual alveolar ridge after use of a single complete denture opposite malpositioned natural teeth. The missing mandibular first molar, caries, and poor oral hygiene all contribute to a poor prognosis for denture success.*

ing procedures or by placing restorations.

An irregular occlusal plane, picket fence arrangement, is objectionable. In this situation the functional occlusion and esthetics are unacceptable. This irregularity must be altered by grinding or by placing restorations.

When the occlusal surfaces of the natural teeth, the food tables, are considered to be too large in the buccolingual dimension, they can be altered by removing some but not all of the enamel from both the buccal and lingual surfaces. After the grinding, the enamel should be polished with flower of pumice in a rubber cup.

When the incisal edges and/or occlu-

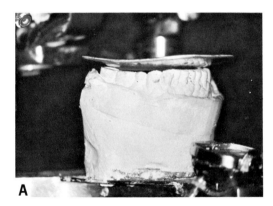

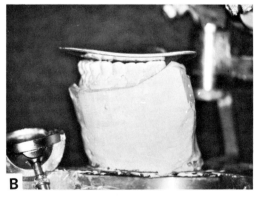

FIG. 23-8. *Metal template in place.* **A.** *Right side.* **B.** *Left side. The template and altered cast can be used as guides for altering the teeth by selective grinding.*

sal surfaces of the natural teeth are altered, either by grinding or restorations, an occlusal template can be used to provide a more favorable occlusal plane to which artificial teeth can be arranged (Fig. 23-8). This procedure is best accomplished by making accurate stone casts of the edentulous maxillary arch and the dentulous mandibular arch and mounting them on an articulator in the same relation that will be used during denture construction and setting of the maxillary teeth. The occlusal surfaces of both the artificial teeth and the natural teeth are altered. Casts can be spray painted with flat enamel, then the altered areas become unpainted, making it easier to see altered areas. The altered areas of the mandibular stone teeth are used as a guide when making the tooth alterations orally. The metal template is sterilized and used as a guide in the oral procedures.

Another problem, usually with patients who have neglected their dental care, is the prior loss of all maxillary posterior teeth and remaining anterior maxillary teeth that are not restorable. For some unexplainable reason the mandibular teeth have not been lost and are restorable. The mandibular arch will then present two planes of occlusion, an anterior plane from canine to canine and a much higher posterior plane. The mandibular posterior teeth have extruded, and not only is the occlusal plane objectionable but interridge tooth space is at a premium. To prepare this mouth to receive a single complete maxillary denture requires extensive restorative procedures in the mandibular arch and possible surgery in the maxillary arch.

To proceed with complete maxillary denture procedures without first preparing the environment into which the artificial teeth will be placed is to invite trouble. So many factors contribute to the decision to suggest a treatment involving a compromise that such a plan will not be outlined. When natural mandibular teeth are properly prepared, however, a complete maxillary denture can be prescribed and used with success (Fig. 23-9).

Complete Maxillary Denture to Oppose a Partially Edentulous Mandibular Arch with Fixed Prosthesis

When a complete maxillary denture is to oppose a partially edentulous mandibular arch in which the missing teeth have been or will be replaced, the problems presented are usually in the diag-

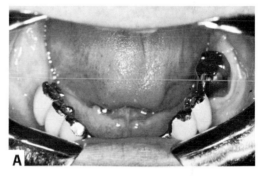

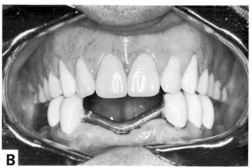

FIG. 23-9. **A.** *Occlusal view of restorative procedures for mandibular posterior teeth to oppose a maxillary complete denture.* **B.** *Anterior view of the complete maxillary denture in place prior to placing the mandibular partial denture.*

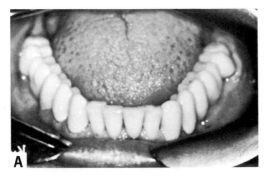

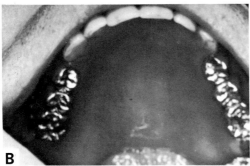

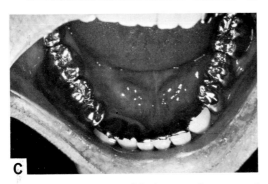

FIG. 23-10. **A.** *Mandibular teeth restored with porcelain crowns. The teeth support fixed partial dentures.* **B.** *Maxillary complete denture with anterior teeth characterized in acrylic resin and posterior teeth with gold occlusal surfaces to oppose gold occlusal surfaces.* **C.** *Mandibular teeth with gold occlusal surfaces on the restored and replaced posterior teeth.*

nostic procedures related to the existing restorations. At that time it must be determined if the fixed restorations are acceptable, if they can be made acceptable, or if they must be rejected.

When the restorations are acceptable, one must then decide what occlusal concept will be pursued. It must be remembered that the teeth in the single complete denture are on a movable base and even though they function against natural teeth they will function as a unit. The same principles of occlusion that apply to complete dentures apply to the single complete denture (Chapter 7).

Another consideration is the material composition of the artificial teeth to be used to complete the denture (Fig. 23-10). When the occlusal surfaces of the teeth and fixed prosthesis are made of porcelain, the artificial teeth of choice are porcelain or acrylic resin. When the occlusal surfaces are mixed enamel and gold or gold alone, the occlusal surfaces of the artificial teeth are preferably gold; however, acrylic resin teeth are acceptable.

After the fixed prosthesis and restorative procedures have been completed, there should be no complications to prescribing the complete maxillary denture. The procedures are planned and made to conform to acceptable dental treatment.

Complete Maxillary Denture to Oppose a Partially Edentulous Arch and a Removable Partial Denture

The most frequently encountered situation for a single complete denture is opposite a partially edentulous arch in which the missing teeth have been or will be replaced with a removable partial denture. As with the mandibular arch with a fixed prosthesis, there should be no other diagnostic complications, and no contraindications for using a complete denture to oppose a removable partial denture in the mandibular arch.

The remaining mandibular teeth should be in an acceptable state of dental health. When there is a removable partial denture, it must be evaluated critically. The partial denture must meet the requirements of an acceptable prosthesis. The occlusal plane, tooth arrangement for occlusion, esthetics, and the material composition of the teeth must be such that an accepted complete denture can be constructed to oppose it. Because of the considerable time and effort that will be expended in the procedures to supply a complete denture to oppose that which remains, it should not be embarrassing to condemn the existing prosthesis if it will not be suitable opposite a complete denture. When the removable partial denture is to be supplied, there should be no particular problem related to the complete denture construction, since the treatment plan is or should be formulated for both arches at the same time (Fig. 23-11).

Single Complete Denture to Oppose an Existing Complete Denture

The decision to construct a single complete denture against an existing complete denture can be approached in a systematic manner by answering and analyzing the following five questions:

1. How long has the existing denture been in use (Fig. 23-12)?

2. Was the denture an immediate insertion at the time of tooth removal?

The answers to these two questions have a direct relation to the extent of bone resorption one may expect to find. The loss of bone determines the accuracy of adaptation of the denture base to the basal seat and should be thoroughly investigated. The patient may not be experiencing a feeling of loss of retention and a cursory examination may

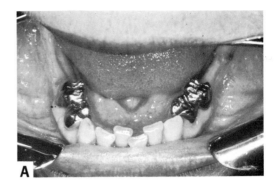

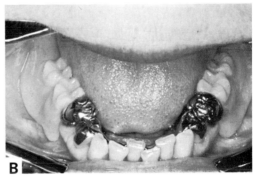

FIG. 23-11. **A.** *Mandibular partially edentulous arch prepared to support a removable partial denture.* **B,** *Partial denture with cusp anterior teeth to follow form of the natural teeth to oppose a complete maxillary denture.*

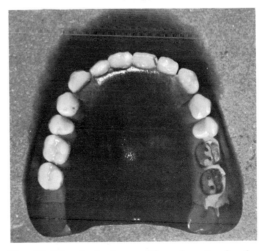

FIG. 23-12. *A denture with vulcanized rubber base and porcelain teeth that had been used for forty-three years.*

not divulge the necessary information because (1) the muscles of the lip, tongue, and cheeks may have adapted to retain the denture in place or (2) edema is not always accompanied by hyperemia. The first of these factors can be investigated by the use of pressure disclosing paste and disclosing wax in the same manner as when new dentures are checked for accuracy of adaptation and border extension (Chapter 18). The second may require that the denture be left out of the mouth for a period of twelve to twenty-four hours.

3. Does the denture meet the requirements of an acceptable denture? There are no shortcuts in determining the answer to this question. Some of the principles that are accepted as essential for denture acceptance may be difficult to analyze and may require an extensive examination unless the existing denture was constructed by the examiner. The examination is demanding and time-consuming. In addition to the accuracy of tissue adaptation and border extension, one must evaluate the tooth position, esthetic acceptance, condition of the polished surfaces, including contour and finish, and the occlusal plane (Fig. 23-13).

4. Has the denture opposed another complete denture, a partially edentulous arch that supported a removable partial

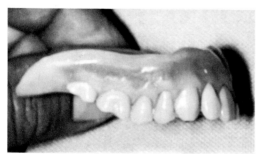

FIG. 23-13. *An existing denture with a posterior occlusal plane that may be undesirable opposite a single complete denture.*

denture, restored natural teeth, a fixed partial denture, or natural teeth in which no restorations have been placed? Each of these different situations influenced the arrangement, size, shape, form, and color of the teeth used in the existing denture. Therefore, the next consideration will be whether they can be satisfactorily matched to provide satisfactory results. Does the posterior tooth form coincide with the philosophy of the operator's concept of occlusion? If not, is there sufficient tooth remaining to allow selective grinding procedures for alterations (Fig. 23-14)? Sometimes the denture is unsatisfactory because the patient has attempted to alter it himself. If the denture teeth were made to oppose natural teeth, regardless of whether they supported a fixed or removable prosthesis, or if the remaining teeth have not been restored, it is difficult to duplicate the situation in the new denture.

5. Is the operator satisfied to institute complete denture procedures utilizing the existing denture? Rarely is this a satisfactory solution. A most serious consideration is the fact that the dentist assumes the responsibility for both dentures as soon as he accepts the patient for treatment of the single denture. Few old dentures fulfill the ideal requirements in all areas.

One type of dentures is defined as additive, transitional, or treatment dentures. These dentures evolve into complete dentures inserted at the time of the removal of the last teeth or tooth. This type of single complete denture has been used with success. However, it must be understood that within a period of six to eight months they will be replaced with a new denture.

The decision to make a single complete denture cannot be considered lightly. The procedure is not one that takes half as much time and effort as one would devote to complete dentures, even

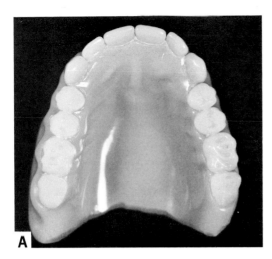

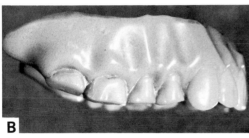

FIG. 23-14. A. *An old denture with wear or grinding of the occlusal surfaces of the teeth that is unsatisfactory for use against a new denture. The posterior palatal seal area appears to have been altered by the patient.* **B.** *A denture unfavorable for retention opposite a new mandibular complete denture because of the occlusal plane and alterations by grinding.*

though only one denture is involved instead of two. Careful observation and recording of all diagnostic information must be considered before a decision is reached to construct a single complete denture. It is also extremely important that just as much care be devoted to the fabrication of a single complete denture as to a pair of complete dentures.

REFERENCES

1. Bruce, R. W.: Complete dentures opposing natural teeth. J. Prosth. Dent., 26:448, 1971.
2. DeFurio, A., and Gehl, D. H.: Clinical study of the retention of maxillary complete dentures with different base materials. J. Prosth. Dent., 23:374, 1970.
3. Ellinger, C. W., Rayson, J. H., and Henderson, D.: Single complete dentures. J. Prosth. Dent., 26:4, 1971.
4. Faber, B. L.: Retention and stability of mandibular dentures. J. Prosth. Dent., 17:210, 1967.
5. Kelly, E.: Changes caused by a mandibular removable partial denture opposing a maxillary complete denture. J. Prosth. Dent., 27:140, 1972.
6. Kolb, H. R.: Variable denture—limiting structures of the edentulous mouth, Part I. J. Prosth. Dent., 16:194, 1966.
7. ———: Variable denture—limiting structures of the edentulous mouth, Part II. J. Prosth. Dent., 16:202, 1966.
8. Oursland, L. E.: Stabilizing mandibular dentures. J. Prosth. Dent., 16:13, 1966.
9. Rudd, K. D., Morrow, R. M., and Hall, W.: Occlusion and the single denture. J. Prosth. Dent., 30:4, 1973.
10. Shanahan, T. E. J.: The individual occlusal curvature and occlusion. J. Prosth. Dent., 8:230, 1958.
11. Sharry, J. J.: Textbook, *Complete Denture Prosthodontics*, 2nd ed. Englewood Cliffs, N. J., McGraw-Hill, 1968, p. 299.
12. Stansbury, G. B.: Single denture construction against a nonmodified natural dentition. J. Prosth. Dent., 1:692, 1951.
13. Sussman, B. A.: More successful complete upper dentures. J. Prosth. Dent., 10:37, 1960.
14. Tillman, E. J.: Removable partial upper and complete lower dentures. J. Prosth. Dent., 11:1098, 1961.
15. Tyson, K. W.: Physical factors in retention of complete upper dentures. J. Prosth. Dent., 18:90, 1967.
16. Vig, R. G.: A modified chew-in and functional impression technique. J. Prosth. Dent., 14:214, 1964.
17. Wallace, D. H.: The use of gold occlusal surfaces in complete and partial dentures. J. Prosth. Dent., 14:326, 1964.
18. Wright, C. R.: Evaluation of the factors necessary to develop stability in mandibular dentures. J. Prosth. Dent., 16:414, 1966.

Tooth-Supported Complete Denture

24

Some complete dentures, unlike conventional complete dentures, use one or more modified natural teeth for support and stability or for support, stability and retention (Fig. 24-1). The diagnosis, treatment plan, and clinical procedures for this type of denture involve knowledge and skill in several areas in dentistry. General practitioners, as well as specialists, should use this treatment.

The procedures apply to either the maxillary or the mandibular arch. The denture that provides support and stability is especially advantageous for the intact mandibular arch, whereas the denture that provides support, stability, and retention is particularly advantageous in certain situations in the maxillary arch.

Definitions

Overlay denture, overdenture, telescoped denture, and *biologic denture* are among the many terms used to define the tooth-supported complete denture. These terms may confuse or mislead the reader, for they are restricted in their meanings. *Overlay* is a term used to describe a removable partial denture that has a metal casting or an acrylic resin extension on or over the occlusal or incisal surfaces of natural teeth. An *over-*

denture is a denture that may be supported by soft tissue, bone, the root of a tooth, or a modified tooth. *Telescoped* is more commonly used in relation to optical instruments. It is true that the

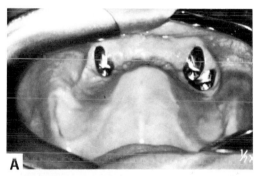
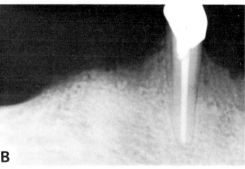

FIG. 24-1. A. *Natural teeth modified to support and stabilize a complete maxillary denture.* **B.** *Endodontically treated tooth that can be modified to support, stabilize, and retain a complete denture.*

male and female members of the attachment device slide one within the other telescopically. However, this is only one part of the total prosthesis. *Biologic* implies the desire to make the restoration biologically acceptable to the environment. However, even though the stimulation from the periodontal attachments is more conducive to biologic acceptance by the bone, it is questionable if the term *biologic denture* is scientifically descriptive.

A *tooth-supported complete denture* is a dental prosthesis that replaces the lost or missing natural dentition and associated structures of the maxillae and/or mandible and receives partial support and stability from one or more modified natural teeth.

Classification

The following classification of tooth-supported dentures is based on the method of abutment preparation along with contemporary clinical terminology. Essentially, there are three different abutment categories: (1) noncoping, (2) coping, and (3) attachments.

NONCOPING ABUTMENTS

Selected root abutments are reduced to a coronal height of 2 to 3 mm and then contoured to a convex or dome-shaped surface. Most teeth require endodontic therapy and in the final step are prepared conservatively to receive an amalgam or composite type restoration (Figs. 24-2A, 24-3A, 24-3B).

ABUTMENTS WITH COPINGS

Cast metal copings with a dome-shaped surface and a chamfer finish line at the gingival margin are fabricated and cemented. At either extreme there are two distinct types of copings: the short coping and the long coping.

Short cast copings are 2 to 3 mm long and normally require endodontic ther-

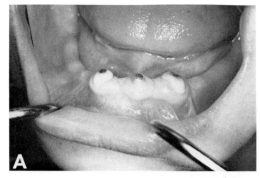

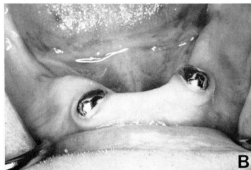

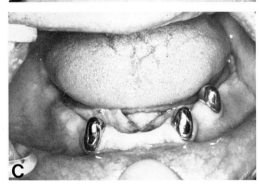

FIG. 24-2. **A.** *Noncoping abutments with amalgam restorations.* **B.** *Short cast gold abutment copings. Note accumulation of plaque and debris along the gingival margins. (Courtesy Dr. V. E. Urbanek, Medical College of Georgia.)* **C.** *Long cast gold abutment copings. (Courtesy Dr. R. H. Hill, Medical College of Georgia.)*

apy because the required coronal root reduction would expose the pulp. Attached to the cast coping is a post fitted to the canal. For this reason canals should be obturated with soft gutta percha-like material rather than with metal points (Fig. 24-2B).

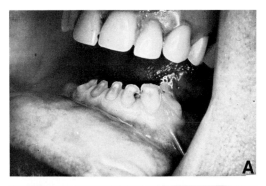

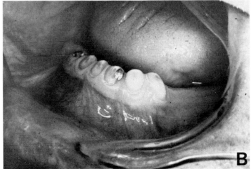

FIG. 24-3. **A.** *Extreme attrition of natural teeth in a sixty-five-year-old male patient by an opposing maxillary denture with porcelain denture teeth. The remaining teeth were vital with the exception of the right lateral incisor which required endodontic therapy. **B.** The distal carious lesion in the left lateral incisor was restored with amalgam after which all the teeth were "rounded off" to within 2 to 3 mm of the gingival margins. This was the extent of abutment preparation for a tooth-supported denture. (Courtesy Dr. V. E. Urbanek, Medical College of Georgia.)*

Long cast copings are normally 5 to 8 mm long. An attempt is made to circumvent endodontic therapy by a conservative reduction of coronal tooth structure. The end result is a long ellipsoidal-shaped coronal coping and a larger crown-root ratio (Fig. 24-2C). Consequently, long cast copings require a greater level of osseous support. And, not infrequently, endodontic therapy instead of being obviated is simply put off till a later time.

ABUTMENTS WITH ATTACHMENTS

Most attachments are secured to the abutment by a cast coping. The objective of any attachment is to improve fixation and/or retention of the denture base. And therein lies the problem. At this point it must be emphasized that there are two different schools of thought regarding clinical application of tooth-supported dentures. The old, traditional school has always advocated tooth abutments, but the available bone index and the periodontal supporting structures are so substantial that in many cases conventional artificial crowns, fixed prostheses, and removable partial prostheses can be used in place of the tooth-supported complete denture. The recent surge in tooth-supported dentures, however, occurred with the clinical disclosure that teeth in their terminal state—teeth normally treatment planned for extraction—could, under certain conditions, be salvaged to provide years of additional service. As long as the tooth-supported complete dentures remain functional, the resorption rate of the remaining residual ridge is significantly reduced.

Basically, what is required is a drastic reduction in the crown-root ratio and, where indicated, implementation of periodontal and endodontic therapy. In many cases the terminal roots have a minimum of 6 to 7 mm of intact alveolar bone. With proper consideration, such teeth can provide partial support for a denture base against forces acting in a tissue-ward direction (Fig. 24-4A, B, C, D). The considerable reduction in the crown-root ratio and the dome-shaped configuration of the root abutment, along with a careful adjustment of the contiguous denture base, facilitates an axial resolution of occlusal forces (Fig. 24-5). The physiologic objective is to provide for the tensile stimulation of as many of the oblique periodontal fibers as possible (Fig. 24-6A, 24-6B). Normally, the end

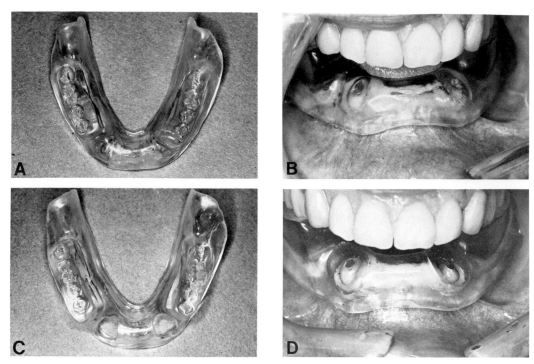

FIG. 24-4.   *Visual documentation depicting the variation in effect between a tooth-supported denture base and a conventional denture base on the basal mucosa during occlusal loading.* **A.** *Mandibular transparent tooth-supported denture base and posterior occlusion rims showing the imprints of the opposing teeth.* **B.** *Denture base in situ and in firm occlusal contact with the maxillary denture. Note the blanching of the supporting mucosa. Support against tissueward displacement is being provided by both abutments and the basal mucoperiosteum.* **C.** *The two circular openings in the transparent denture base denote complete removal of the abutment support areas.* **D.** *The original but modified denture base in situ and in firm occlusal contact with the maxillary denture. Note the intensification of blanching as compared to B. Under these conditions all of the tissueward forces are being transmitted to the underlying mucoperiosteum. (Courtesy Dr. V. E. Urbanek, Medical College of Georgia.)*

result is the deposition of more bundle bone followed by a concomitant decrease in abutment mobility. The crucial question when considering attachments is the adequacy of the remaining alveolar bone and periodontal support. However, when we increase the crown-root ratio, as we do with most attachments, and then torque or apply horizontal or vertical dislodging forces to root abutments in the terminal state, it then becomes totally unrealistic to expect a favorable prognosis. Unfortunately, it is necessary to clearly emphasize that the

use of stud and/or bar attachments with *terminal root abutments* is self-defeating.

Interestingly, until the past decade it was considered unthinkable to prepare a tooth-supported denture abutment without some type of cast coping with or without an attachment. The breakthrough occurred when clinical trial and error clearly demonstrated that under controlled conditions noncoping abutments can provide years of additional service.

In situ, the denture base protects the coronal portion of abutment teeth

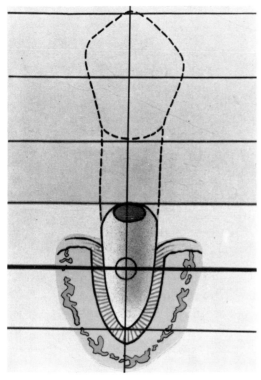

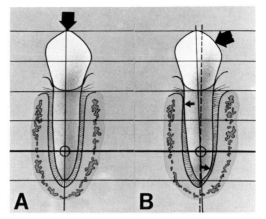

FIG. 24-5. *Schematic illustration of a "terminal" root abutment with a "dome-shaped" configuration of the coronal root surface. The rationale for the short, rounded coronal surface is to eliminate or minimize lateral occlusal stresses. Normally, the abutment surfaces of the denture base are relieved as are the areas adjacent to the collar of attached and marginal gingivae. During occlusal loading, displacement of the resilient mucosa allows the denture base to "bottom out" against the most coronal aspect of the abutment. As long as the remaining portion of the periodontal membrane remains viable, its proprioceptive input capability continues to contribute to the overall neuromuscular response. (Courtesy Dr. V. E. Urbanek, Medical College of Georgia.)*

FIG. 24-6. **A.** *Schematic illustration depicting the sequential transmission of axial occlusal forces to the main periodontal fiber group for resisting occlusal stresses—the oblique fibers. As these fibers run diagonally from cementum coronally into alveolar bone, they function as a suspensory "sling." While vertical occlusal forces are transmitted as pressure through the root, they are converted by the "stretching" of the oblique fibers into tensile stresses to the contiguous alveolar bone. Thus, in this sequence, occlusal pressure is converted and dissipated as tension. Histologically, tensile stimulation of alveolar bone results in an osteoblastic response.* **B.** *When transverse occlusal forces become predominant, an axis of rotation becomes established about two thirds of the way down the root. As a direct consequence only half of the available oblique fibers are "stretched," while the other half, indicated by the small arrows, are compressed. In these latter areas, occlusal pressure is transmitted directly to the alveolar bone as pressure per se. Histologically, direct pressure on alveolar bone is manifested by an osteoclastic response. (Courtesy Dr. V. E. Urbanek, Medical College of Georgia.)*

against the mechanical forces of mastication while biologic breakdown can be preempted through fluoride therapy and proper oral hygiene. However, as a consequence of denture base movement, some gradual attrition of abutments normally occurs over a period of months or years.

Having withstood the test of time, noncoping abutments have helped to popularize tooth-supported dentures by reducing the economic impact on the patient's pocketbook. And, from a pragmatic point of view, root abutments without cast copings are much more amenable to treatment, retreatment, and modification in contingency situations. Consequently they provide a greater degree of flexibility in formulating treatment plans, especially where immediate tooth-supported dentures are indicated. In the latter, extraction of teeth adjacent to selected root abutments is followed in time by a vertical reduction of alveolar bone and recession of the overlying mucosa. As these root abutments are often mobile and in their terminal state, the coronal portion should not exceed 2 to 3 mm in order to minimize leverage to lateral forces. If, however, cast copings are placed on abutments prior to extraction of adjacent teeth, one is eventually confronted with exposed gingival margins and an increased crown-root ratio. The only way to rectify such undesirable sequelae is to remake the coping. One should also bear in mind that normally 5 to 10 per cent of these abutments will require endodontic retreatment, the nature of which is not enhanced by the presence of a cast metal coping. Finally, cast copings, with plaque and debris accumulation along their gingival margins, have been known to mask recurrent root caries, thereby blocking early detection (Fig. 24-2B).

Whenever a root abutment is in the terminal state, the prognosis is guarded and, following proper treatment, only time will determine its capacity to survive. Consequently, many clinicians who routinely use cast copings prefer to wait six months to a year after denture insertion before fabricating metal copings, since time is now on the side of the operator. Furthermore, with autopolymer resins, it is a relatively straightforward procedure to modify an existing denture base to properly contact a modified root abutment. If at the onset, however, the remaining coronal portion of a root abutment is nonexistent or badly broken down, then a cast metal "build-up" may be the only available alternative.

SUBMERGED VITAL ROOTS

This additional abutment category is included because of current research and interest. The method is an innovative attempt to obviate some of the basic problems associated with the more conventional overdenture abutments. These include caries, gingivitis, periodontitis, and the need for endodontic therapy. In essence, selected vital roots are transected and reduced to 2 mm below the crestal bone and then covered by a mucoperiosteal flap. Published reports regarding the feasibility of this approach have been both discouraging[5b] and encouraging.[3E] The two major postoperative problems are the development of dehiscences over the retained roots and pulpal pathosis. Obviously the clinical use of submerged vital roots as overdenture abutments is still in an experimental stage and, therefore, at this time cannot be recommended.

Advantages

Using natural teeth to support a complete denture is not new in dentistry. Schweitzer relates that this approach in prosthodontics dates back to the 1800's.[9] Dentists have documented sufficient clinical data from patients in varying age groups to justify the routine use of this procedure.

When the remaining natural teeth are not sufficient in number, position, or stability to support either a fixed or a removable partial denture, the treatment plan does not have to include the removal of the teeth and construction of conventional complete dentures. This statement does *not* imply *nor* does it mean that all or some of the remaining natural teeth are suitable for the tooth-supported complete denture. It *does* mean that carefully evaluated teeth that can be salvaged by periodontal therapy and endodontic procedures to withstand the stress of attachment devices or copings are valuable to support, stabilize, and, in selected situations, help retain a complete denture.

In the construction of the tooth-supported dentures the procedures for modifying the retained dentition are added to those for assuring that a conventional complete denture is biologically acceptable to the supporting tissues (page 105). However, the use of teeth for denture support is not an infallible procedure, nor does their use negate the following of accepted procedures in denture construction. For some patients, though, carefully designed and fitted tooth-supported dentures have distinct advantages.

1. The roots of the teeth are present to provide tensile stimulation to the residual alveolar ridge. This type of stimulation is conducive to bone repair and maintenance. The physiology of the bone dictates that the use of a modified natural tooth or teeth to support a complete denture has more to offer for the preservation of the residual alveolar ridge than any other approach. The modified natural tooth, through the periodontal attachments, provides tensile stimulation conducive to bone repair and maintenance.

2. The modified teeth provide a definite vertical stop for the denture base. For example, a patient may have retained mandibular anterior teeth that oppose a complete maxillary denture. The mandibular posterior teeth may or may not have been replaced with a removable partial denture. More often than not there are extensive resorption of the maxillary anterior residual ridge and hypertrophy of the soft tissue covering. The soft tissue is of a spongy consistency and provides an unfavorable basal seat for stability and support to a

denture (Fig. 24-7A). The retention of several modified maxillary anterior teeth helps to prevent this situation (Fig. 24-7B,C).

3. Horizontal and torquing forces are minimized.

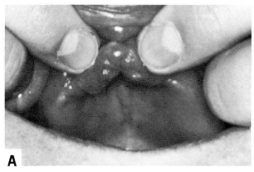

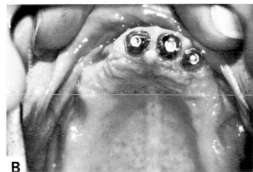

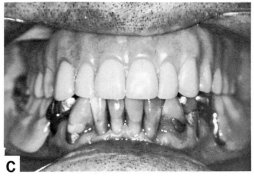

FIG. 24-7. A. *A mass of pendulous, hypertrophied tissue that would provide an unfavorable basal seat for a denture.* **B.** *Three maxillary anterior teeth prepared to give support and stability to a complete denture (26 months postinsertion).* **C.** *Tooth-supported complete denture opposed by natural mandibular anterior teeth.*

4. Stability and support are increased, and this reduces the forces of occlusion to the supporting tissues.

5. The psychologic advantage is subtle but real. To some persons the loss of all of the natural teeth is such a traumatic experience that many patients cannot or will not face it in a realistic manner. The retention of only one tooth frequently makes for a more favorable prognosis with these patients.

6. There are fewer postinsertion problems with the tooth-supported denture than with the conventional complete denture.

Indications

The tooth-supported complete denture should be considered for patients who face the loss of the remaining natural adult dentition. The younger the patient the greater the indication for this treatment, even though the prognosis for lengthy retention of the modified teeth may not be too favorable. This also applies to the geriatric patient who is mentally and physically able to undergo the additional treatment procedures. It should also be considered if the complete denture will be opposed by retained mandibular anterior teeth.

Attachments may be particularly indicated where retention is difficult to obtain or is of primary importance. Examples of this situation are (1) xerostomia or sialorrhea, (2) the absence of alveolar residual ridge in the edentulous areas, (3) loss of a maxilla or partial loss of a mandible, and (4) a congenital deformity, especially the cleft palate.

Contraindications

The expense, the time required, and the additional procedures are of concern. When a patient cannot economically afford or cannot or will not give the necessary time for the procedures, the treatment may be contraindicated.

Poor candidates also for the procedure are mentally and/or physically handicapped people for whom plaque control and good oral hygiene are difficult. They are poor prospects for most prosthodontic treatment; however, we should not deny them treatment.

More specific contraindications are the diagnostic findings related to the periodontic and endodontic procedures. Rarely is it found that teeth suitable for endodontic and/or periodontic therapy are unsuitable for copings or other forms of alteration to the abutments. The contraindications for using periodontically involved teeth as support are as follows:[*]

1. Class III mobility due to the loss of alveolar bone that cannot be corrected. Mobility cannot be corrected in the complete absence of bone. In doubtful situations, when the crown root ratio is unfavorable, the clinical crown should be reduced as much as possible, and the tooth should be taken out of function. Periodontal therapy is instituted and the tooth is evaluated further prior to endodontic treatment.

2. Soft tissue and osseous defects which are not correctable by surgery.

3. Patients who will not keep the retained teeth free of plaque. Good oral hygiene *must* be maintained to retain the modified natural teeth. (It is the responsibility of the dentist to educate the patient in this phase of personal oral hygiene.)

4. Failure to establish a sufficient zone of attached gingiva by mucogingival or grafting procedures.

[*]J. E. Kennedy, D.D.S., M.S., Associate Professor and Chairman, Department of Periodontics, Virginia Commonwealth University, School of Dentistry, W. M. Ormes, D.D.S., Associate Professor, Department of Periodontics, Virginia Commonwealth University, School of Dentistry.

5. Excessive reduction of the adjacent residual alveolar ridge as a result of elimination of osseous defects and the establishment of normal architecture.

The contraindications for endodontic treatment follow:*

1. Vertical fracture of the root or roots.

2. Mechanical perforation of the root.

3. Internal resorption that has perforated through the side of the root.

4. Broken instrument in the root canal.

5. Horizontal fracture of the root below the bony crest.

Treatment Planning

When it has been decided by diagnostic procedure that the remaining teeth are suitable for a tooth-supported complete denture, several factors must be considered in selecting the teeth to be retained.

1. The periodontal status. Ideally the teeth should present minimum mobility, have acceptable bone support, and be amenable to periodontal therapy. It should be considered that the clinical crown will be reduced and therefore the root-crown ratio will be more favorable for the reduction of any existing mobility. Do not condemn a tooth *only* on the basis of its mobility.

2. Acceptability of the tooth or teeth for endodontic treatment. There are two advantages to treating the abutment teeth endodontically: (a) the crown-root ratio can be made more favorable, and (b) the reduction of the clinical crown provides an interocclusal distance more favorable to placing the artificial tooth in an esthetically acceptable position and, at times, in a more favorable occlu-

sal relation to the opposing teeth. Endodontic treatment is mandatory when certain retentive attachments are used or if endosseous endodontic implants are contemplated.

3. The number and position of the teeth in the arch. Two teeth in each quadrant probably present an ideal situation in which stress is distributed over a rectangular area. The arrangement is typified by a cuspid or a first premolar and a second molar in each quadrant (Fig. 24-9A). The tripod is the next most favorable form for support and stability (Fig. 24-9B). The use of two teeth in each arch or one tooth in one arch has met with satisfactory results when the patient has been educated in what to expect from the treatment (Fig. 24-9C,D).

Morrow recommends that abutments should not be approximating because such "abutments are sometimes difficult for the patient to clean and marginal gingivitis frequently develops in the inter-proximal areas."* Approximating abutments may be unsatisfactory with certain types of attachments but suitable with other types.

Preparatory Treatment

The sequence and technical procedures of preparatory treatment are the same for all kinds of tooth-supported dentures. The only difference is in the design of the abutment teeth. Some are designed to offer minimal retention and others definite retention (Fig. 24-8).

The following sequence of treatment can be used as a general guide, but it may not be specifically applicable in all situations. The technical procedures, although not infallible, have been suc-

*T. P. Serene, D.D.S., Professor and Chairman, Department of Endodontics, Virginia Commonwealth University, School of Dentistry.

*Robert M. Morrow, Colonel, USAFDC, Paper presented to the Southeastern Academy of Prosthodontics, Richmond, Virginia, 1970.

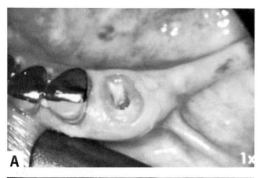

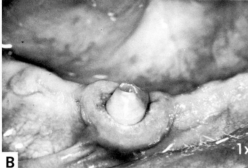

FIG. 24-8. A. *Root of a cuspid prepared for a Ceka attachment that will provide definite retention.* **B.** *Coping on this prepared cuspid to provide minimal retention.*

cessfully used by many prosthodontists.

1. Construct an immediate treatment claspless denture and make a cast from an irreversible hydrocolloid impression (Fig. 24-10). The purpose of this treatment prosthesis is to replace the missing and the hopelessly involved teeth for esthetic reasons and retain the jaw relations.

2. Remove the hopeless teeth and insert the removable prosthesis.

3. During the healing period institute the periodontic and endodontic treatment. The clinical crowns of the retained teeth may be reduced at this time. This may be particularly desirable if the mobility is such that the prognosis is questionable. The preparatory treatment phase varies with individuals; however, the preparation of retained teeth is not instituted until healing is satisfactory and the periodontic and endodontic treatment has been completed.

Preparation of the Retained Teeth

If the immediate treatment denture is to be retained in function until the complete denture is ready for insertion, make a full arch irreversible hydrocolloid impression with the prosthesis in place. Then place the impression, with the prosthesis in place, in a humidor until the preparations are completed. If the tissues have been abused by the treatment prosthesis, it may be desirable to remove the prosthesis during the final stages of construction. This part of the procedure must be understood by the patient *prior* to the appointment for tooth preparation.

TOOTH PREPARATION FOR
MINIMAL RETENTION

1. Remove sufficient tooth structure to provide favorable root-crown ratio to allow the insertion of the artificial replacement in an acceptable esthetic position and in a favorable occlusal relation with the teeth of the opposing arch (Fig. 24-11A).

2. Extend a chamfer type margin slightly beneath the free gingival margin (Fig. 24-1A).

3. Taper the preparation in the occlusogingival direction. The finished tooth with attached coping is the male member of the denture. The female member is a part of the denture base.

4. The occlusal and/or incisal surface must be of a dimension suitable to provide an area for the placing of a concavity in the coping to accommodate a cobalt chromium bearing (Fig. 24-11B). The radius of the concavity is slightly more than the radius of curvature of the bear-

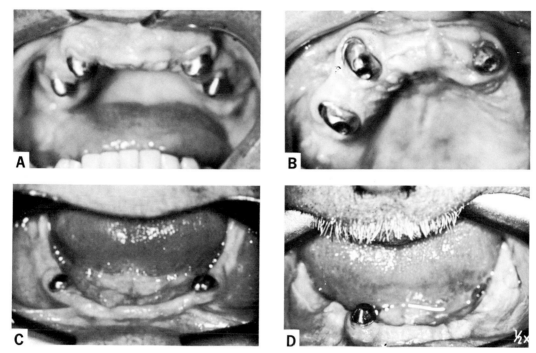

FIG. 24-9. A. *Ideal rectangular support provided by retention of two teeth in each maxilla (7 years postinsertion).* **B.** *Triangular or tripod support provided by retention of the second premolar and two cuspids.* **C.** *Support and stability provided by retention of second premolars (19 months postinsertion).* **D.** *One tooth retained (2 years postinsertion).*

ing. The bearing is a hemispherical-shaped casting of a pattern taken from the inside of the end of a #5 gelatin capsule* (Fig. 24-11C).

COPING FABRICATION
1. Make an accurate impression of the abutment and pour a die.
2. Carve the wax pattern (Fig. 24-12A). Place the concavity in the occlusal surface of the pattern, using a wax tool (Fig. 24-8B).
3. Cast the coping, using a hard type of class III gold.
4. Cement the polished coping to the tooth (Fig. 24-13).

---
* The technique for bearing construction and the waxing tool courtesy of Robert M. Morrow, Colonel, USAFDC.

5. Instruct the patient in home care of the abutment teeth.

IMPRESSION FOR THE DENTURE. The impression technique follows the same principles and procedures that are used in constructing a conventional complete denture (Chapter 6).

Preliminary Impression
1. Make an overextended irreversible hydrocolloid impression and pour into dental stone. Adapt the custom-made impression tray by applying one thickness of baseplate wax (1 to 2 mm) over the abutment teeth (Fig. 24-14).
2. Paint the cast with a tinfoil substitute as a separating medium.
3. Construct an impression tray of

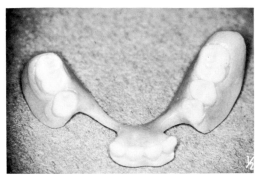

FIG. 24-10.   *Immediate claspless denture.
The patient for whom it was prepared was
not embarrassed by having to appear in
public without anterior teeth.*

activated acrylic resin using the "shake
on" technique (Fig. 24-14B).

Final Impression

1. Check the impression tray for accuracy.

2. Reduce the borders.

3. Refine the borders.

4. Alter the tray to provide space for
the impression material to flow and
allow the tissue to return to its undisplaced position.

5. Apply a thin layer of rubber base
adhesive to the refined borders and the
tissue side of the tray.

6. Make the refined impression. Mix
an impression material* with a ready
flow and quick set, according to the
manufacturer's instructions. Load the
tray and seat it to place with positive
pressure. Release the pressure in a manner similar to that in making a zinc oxide
and eugenol paste refined impression.

7. Box the impression and pour *immediately* (Fig. 24-14C).

RECORD BASES AND OCCLUSION RIMS.
The only difference in the construction
of the record bases for tooth-supported

*Micro-Seal, American Consolidated Manufac-
turing Company, Inc., 212 North 21 Street, Philadelphia, Pennsylvania 19103.

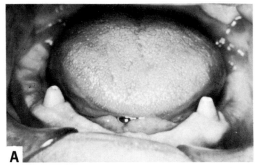

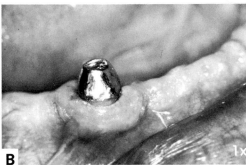

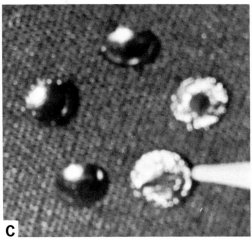

FIG. 24-11.   **A.** *Two mandibular premolars
properly prepared for a cast coping that will
provide support and stability for a complete
mandibular denture.* **B.** *Concavity in coping
of a retained tooth to accommodate a cobalt
chromium bearing.* **C.** *Bearings.*

dentures and conventional dentures
(Chapter 9) is the incorporation of the
metal bearing in the record base.

1. Apply one thickness of baseplate

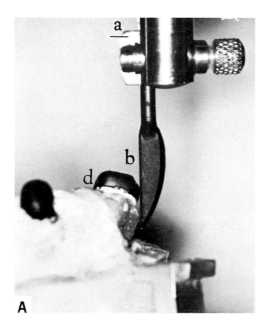

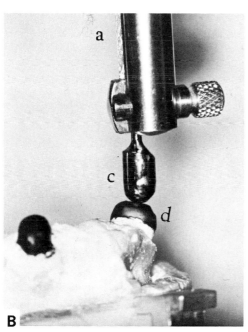

FIG. 24-12. *Coping fabrication with a surveyor: vertical arm of surveyor (a), wax carving instrument (b), wax tool of cobalt chromium alloy (c), and wax pattern for coping (d).* **A.** *Contouring copings in relation to each other.* **B.** *Placing the concavity for bearing contact.*

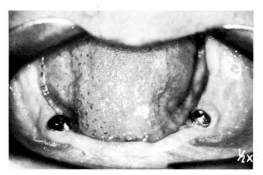

FIG. 24-13. *Cast copings cemented to the retention teeth.*

wax to the abutments, leaving the occlusal surface exposed.

2. Seat the bearing in the concavity and seal it to place with wax (Fig. 24-15A).

3. Eliminate any undercut areas with wax and construct a stable record base of activated acrylic resin using the "shake on" technique (page 240).

4. Attach wax occlusion rims to the record base (Fig. 24-15B).

RECORDING MAXILLOMANDIBULAR RELATIONS. A face-bow transfer is used to relate the maxillary cast to the articulator. The tentative records of the vertical dimension of occlusion with the mandible in terminal relation to the maxillae are made in the same manner as for conventional complete dentures (page 271). The jaw relations and arrangement of teeth for esthetics and phonetics are verified at the time of try-in.

TOOTH SELECTION. The posterior tooth form is determined by (1) the teeth in the opposing arch and (2) the concept of occlusion the dentist desires to use. The shade and material composition of the artificial teeth must be decided for each situation. It is understood that factors such as interridge space and mandibular muscle habits must also be considered.

1. The artificial teeth that are placed

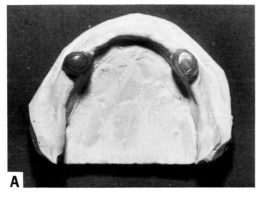

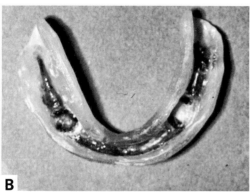

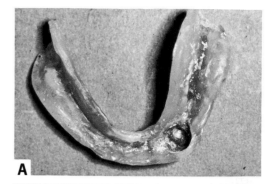

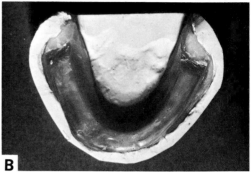

FIG. 24-15. **A.** *Record base for tooth-supported denture with metal bearing in its proper relation.* **B.** *Wax occlusion rim attached. Note the slight bulge in the right cuspid area.*

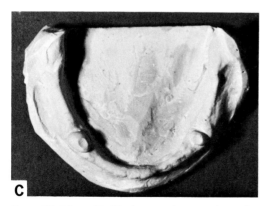

FIG. 24-14. *Preliminary impression for tooth-supported denture.* **A.** *Wax adapted over the abutment teeth.* **B.** *Impression tray prepared for the refined impression procedures.* **C.** *Cast separated after pouring and setting of stone.*

over the abutment teeth should be acrylic resin.

2. When the teeth in the opposing arch have gold occlusal surfaces, the occlusal surfaces of the artificial teeth should be either gold or acrylic resin, preferably gold.

3. If the teeth in the opposing arch have had the occlusal surfaces restored with porcelain, the artificial teeth preferably should be porcelain.

4. If the teeth in the opposing arch are natural teeth not restored with gold or porcelain, porcelain artificial teeth are preferred.

SETTING THE ARTIFICIAL TEETH. To set the acrylic resin tooth over the abutment requires (1) removing the acrylic resin record base to expose the abutment, (2) retrieving the metal bearing from the record base and repositioning it in the concavity by sealing the bearing to the abutment tooth, at the margins, with sticky wax, (3) hollowing the acrylic resin tooth with an acrylic bur until it is properly positioned and the occlusion is adjusted, (4) sealing the bearing to the acrylic resin tooth with sticky wax, (5) arranging the remainder of the teeth in maximum occlusion, and (6) contouring the wax for the try-in appointment.

TRYING IN THE TEETH. At this appointment perform the following procedures:

1. Verify the jaw relation records.

2. Make eccentric jaw relation records and adjust the articulator.

3. Assure esthetic acceptability by the patient.

4. Verify phonetic acceptability.

Laboratory Procedures

1. Contour the wax.

2. Flask the denture.

3. Eliminate the wax.

At this step the metal bearings are retrieved from the acrylic resin tooth, cleaned with boiling water, and dried. The cast is allowed to dry and the abutments, except the concavity, are painted with tinfoil substitute. The metal bearing is seated in the concavity and a coping of activated acrylic resin with cross-linked monomer is made, using the "shake on" technique (Fig. 24-16). The procedure assures the correct positioning of the bearing and allows trial packing of the heat-cured acrylic resin denture base.

4. Prepare the acrylic resin. While the dough is soft, the coping, with bearing, is held securely in place, and a small amount of the dough is pressed around the gingival surface of the coping.

5. When the dough is of proper consistency, the packing is completed in a manner similar to packing a removable partial denture (page 365). The acrylic resin is placed in both sides of the flask. Trial packing is possible when desired.

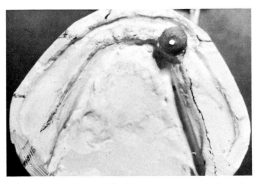

FIG. 24-16. *Metal bearing seated in the acrylic resin coping. Part of the sprue from the bearing extends through the coping to provide retention in the processed acrylic denture.*

After the denture has been processed (slow cure) for nine hours at 160°F the following procedures are performed:

1. The denture is recovered from the flask.

2. Remount procedures for processing errors are completed.

3. The dentures are recovered from the casts.

4. The dentures are finished and polished.

5. Remount casts are made.

6. The maxillary cast is attached to the articulator.

Denture Insertion

1. Review instructions in denture use and care and home care of the abutment teeth.

2. Use pressure disclosing paste to locate contacts between the female member in the denture base and the male abutments. There should be no contact except between the convex surface of the metal bearing and the concave bearing surface of the coping (Fig. 24-17).

3. Evaluate the tissue side of the denture base and the borders for pressure areas and overextension.

4. Perfect the occlusion by remount-

ing the dentures and selectively grinding the teeth.

5. Place the patient on a recall system. Individual response in home care and reactions to the dentures will dictate the frequency of office calls. As a rule, after the initial adjustment phase, the patients are seen once a month for the first six months and once every three months thereafter. This frequency of visits may not be necessary with all patients. However, this system has produced satisfactory results.

TOOTH PREPARATION TO PROVIDE RETENTION

In the definition of the tooth-supported denture a distinction is made between those that are designed to provide minimal retention and those prostheses designed to provide positive retention. Teeth with a clinical crown can be prepared to give positive retention when bars are attached to copings covering the prepared clinical crowns. However, the attachments now to be described use the endodontically treated root of the tooth and not the clinical crown.

Technical Procedures for B and D Anchor

Male Member

1. Prepare the clinical crown to the level of the gingiva (Fig. 24-18).

2. Make a root cap preparation. Open the root canal to the desired diameter and depth for retention and rigidity.

3. Make an individual impression of the root preparation and canal. Pour a stone die.

4. Fit a dowel with an acrylic knob attached into the canal in the die. This transfer dowel serves two purposes: (a) the knob is securely imbedded in the irreversible hydrocolloid impression, and (b) the extended dowel is used to position the die accurately for cast pouring.

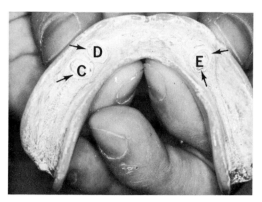

FIG. 24-17. *Evaluating contacts for tooth-supported denture. Note the displacement of pressure disclosing paste (arrows) where acrylic resin contacts the copings. The acrylic resin is relieved in these areas to provide freedom from coping contact until the bearings at C, D, and E are in positive contact.*

5. Make an irreversible hydrocolloid impression of the entire arch.

6. Fit the dies to the transfer dowels and pour the impression in dental stone.

7. Place remount indices in the base of the cast.

8. Cover the die with one thickness of baseplate wax prior to making a record base.

9. Make jaw relation records and at-

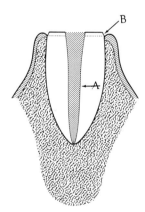

FIG. 24-18. *Root canal filled (A) and clinical crown prepared to the level of the gingiva (B).*

tach the casts to the articulator in the same manner as used for the construction of conventional complete dentures. The relationship of the opposing teeth is not only necessary for the arranging of the artificial teeth but is also useful in positioning the male member.

10. Place the male member as close to the center of the root as possible; however, sometimes a slight lingual position is more favorable for the esthetic positioning of the artificial tooth.

11. Wax the cap, post, and male member, invest in a flask, and cast in a hard gold alloy (Fig. 24-19).

12. Set all teeth and try them in.

Female Member. The female members are made of spring-hard clasp wire, 0.6 mm (0.024″) in diameter. Twin tubes are made by soldering two 3 mm long chrome alloy tubes having an inner lumen of 0.7 mm (0.028″) diameter. The tubes keep the springs in place in the denture base and allow slight movement in function.

1. Bend the clasp wire in the shape of a hairpin (Fig. 24-20).

2. Place the ends of the clasp wire in the twin tubes. This allows the clasp springs a little freedom to slide back and forth when functioning.

3. The hairpin-shaped wire must be fitted to reach the lingual surface of the lingual flange of the denture from the

Fig. 24-20. *Female attachment of B and C anchor. The twin tubes (A) are placed over the clasp wire (B) bent in the shape of a hairpin.*

buccal surface of its buccal flange (Fig. 24-21).

4. Place a 4 mm plaster cover over the anchor assembly and the immediate surrounding gingival area. According to Krogh-Paulsen, the marginal gingival of the supporting retainer teeth will be traumatized if relief is not provided in the tissue side of the denture.* Close the ends of the tubes with a little plaster to prevent acrylic resin from closing the tubes during the processing procedure.

5. Complete the wax up; invest the cast and denture in a flask and process the denture.

*W. Krogh-Paulsen, L.D.S., Dr. Med. Dent., Royal Dental College, Copenhagen, Denmark.

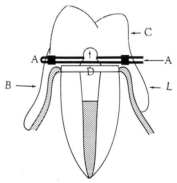

Fig. 24-21. *B and C anchor in place. The ends of the clasp wire (A) extend from the buccal flange of the denture (B) through the lingual flange (L). The clasp wire is over the male attachment (D) to provide retention. The acrylic resin artificial tooth (C) is prepared to allow the clasp wire (A) to snap over the male attachment (D).*

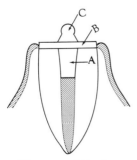

Fig. 24-19. *The post (A), the cap (B), and the male member (C) are cast in gold and cemented to place.*

6. Retrieve the cast and remount to correct any processing errors.

7. Make necessary records for remount procedures at the time of denture insertion.

8. Remove the cast from the denture. The male member will be attached to the female member. Remove the male member from the female and cement the cap and post to place in the retainer root.

9. Remove the spring clasp from the twin tubes. If the tubes are exposed on either the polished surfaces of the lingual or buccal flange, cover with activated acrylic resin and polish. ·

10. After the denture has been prepared for insertion and the remount procedures and selective grinding have been completed, replace the springs in the tubes. The denture is now ready for insertion.

THE CEKA-ANCHOR*. The Ceka-Anchor is an attachment that is placed upon and into the root of an endodontically treated tooth to provide stability, support, and retention. The roots should be kept as short as possible to provide extra working room when placing the artificial tooth.

The Ceka-Anchor (Fig. 24-22) is soldered on top of a post coping and is composed of a female member, space maintainer, male member with thread, base ring, and large space maintainer.

Technical Procedures

1. Make an accurate impression of the prepared root and canal.

2. Make a stone cast and wax the post and coping, making certain that the top of the coping is large enough to receive the base ring (Fig. 24-23). An undesirable undercut is created if the ring is larger than the coping.

3. Make an impression of the entire

*Ceka, U.S.A. Lielemans, 217 Hunter Lane, North Wales, Pa. 19454.

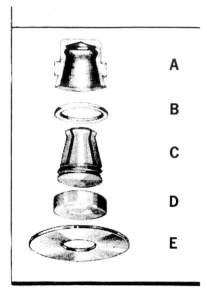

FIG. 24-22. *Ceka attachment: female ring closed on the top (A), space maintainer (B), male pin with outside thread (C), base ring closed at the bottom with dot of solder and inside thread (D), special space maintainers (E).*

arch with the copings in place and pour a master cast.

4. Make parallel the base rings on top of the copings, using mandrels.

5. Screw the base ring on the mandrel and grind the top of the coping to allow the base ring to seat flat.

6. Attach the base ring to the coping with sticky wax.

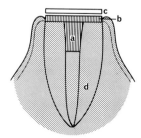

FIG. 24-23. *Cast for Ceka anchor. The post (a) and coping (b) are of wax in the stone die (d). The base ring (c) is used to assure that the coping (b) is large enough for the base ring. (Courtesy of Ceka, U.S.A. Lielmans, North Wales, Pa.)*

7. Remove the mandrel and assemble for soldering and embed in soldering investment.

8. Solder the base ring to the coping; the base rings are threaded to receive the male member (Fig. 24-24A).

9. Cement the post and copings to the tooth roots (Fig. 24-24B).

10. Place a filler into the threaded base rings and proceed with impression making, jaw relation records, try-in denture, processing, occlusal correction, and finishing.

11. Remove the filler from the threaded base ring and insert the male member (Fig. 24-24C).

12. Make holes in the denture base or acrylic resin tooth over the copings to allow seating of the denture (Fig. 24-25A).

13. Place the large spacer over the male member to rest on the copings.

14. Lubricate the coping, spacer, and male member with a silicone lubricant.

15. Snap the female closed member into place over the spring leaves of the male member (Fig. 24-25B).

16. Seat the denture with the fingers, *not by jaw closure!*

17. Secure the female member to the denture with activated acrylic resin by painting into the holes.

18. After the acrylic resin is polymerized, remove the denture and polish the added acrylic resin.

19. Remove the large spacer and insert the denture.

REFERENCES

1. Bergenholtz, A.: Radectomy of multi-rooted teeth. J.A.D.A., *85:*870, 1972.

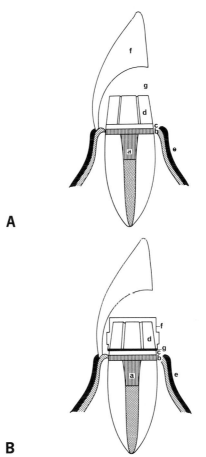

Fig. 24-25. **A.** *The lingual surface of the acrylic resin tooth (f) is removed at (g). The denture base (e) is seated in the mouth. The male member (d) is screwed into the base ring (c) which is soldered to the post (a) and coping (b).* **B.** *Completed assembly of the Ceka attachment: post (a), coping (b), base ring (c), male member (d), denture base (e), female member (f), and spacer (g).*

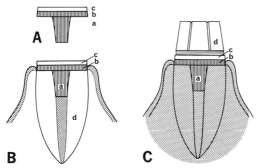

Fig. 24-24. **A.** *The post (a) and coping (b) have been cast and the base ring (c) soldered to the coping.* **B.** *The post (a), coping (b), and base ring (c) are cemented to the tooth root (d).* **C.** *The post (a), coping (b), and base ring (c) assembly will retain the threaded male member (d) when it is screwed into the base ring.*

1a. Brewer, A. A.: The tooth-supported denture. J. Prosth. Dent., *30*:703, 1973.

2. Brill, N.: Adaptation and the hybrid prosthesis. J. Prosth. Dent., *5*:811, 1955.

2a. Dodge, C. A.: Prevention of complete denture problems by use of "overdentures". J. Prosth. Dent., *30*:403, 1973.

3. Dolder, E. J.: The bar joint mandibular denture. J. Prosth. Dent., *11*:689, 1961.

3a. Fenton, A. H.: Interim overdentures. J. Prosth. Dent., *36*:4, 1976.

3b. ——— and Hahn, N.: Tissue response to overdentures. J. Prosth. Dent., *40*:492, 1978.

3c. Frantz, W. R.: The use of natural teeth in overlay dentures. J. Prosth. Dent., *34*:135, 1975.

3d. Garver, D. G., Fenster, R. K., Baker, R. D., and Johnson, D. L.: Vital root retention in humans. J. Prosth. Dent., *40*:23, 1978.

3e. Garver, D. G., Fenster, R. K., and Connole, P. W.: Vital root retention in humans: An interim report. J. Prosth. Dent., *41*:255, 1979.

3f. Guyer, S. E.: Selectively retained vital roots for partial support of overdentures: A patient report. J. Prosth. Dent., *33*:258, 1975.

3g. Immekus, J. E., and Aramany, M.: Adverse effects of resilient denture liners in overlay dentures. J. Prosth. Dent., *32*:178, 1974.

4. Kabcenell, J. L.: Tooth supported complete dentures. J. Prosth. Dent., *26*:251, 1971.

4a. Kay, W. D., and Abes, M. S.: Sensory perception in overdenture patients. J. Prosth. Dent., *35*:615, 1976.

4b. Kotwal, K. R.: Outline of standards for evaluating patients for overdentures. J. Prosth. Dent., *37*:141, 1977.

5. Loiselle, R. J., et al.: The physiologic basis for the overlay denture. J. Prosth. Dent., *28*:4, 1972.

5a. Lord, J. S., and Teel, S.: The overdenture: Patient selection, use of copings, and follow-up evaluation. J. Prosth. Dent., *32*:41, 1974.

5b. Masterson, M. P.: Retention of vital submerged roots under complete dentures: Report of 10 patients. J. Prosth. Dent., *41*:12, 1979.

5c. Marquardt, G. L.: Dolder bar joint mandibular overdenture: Technique for nonparallel abutment teeth. J. Prosth. Dent., *36*:101, 1976.

5d. Mensor, M. C.: Attachment fixation for overdentures. J. Prosth. Dent., *37*:366, 1977.

5e. ———: Attachment fixation of the overdenture—Part II. J. Prosth. Dent., *39*:16, 1978.

6. Miller, P. A., and Morrow, R. M.: Technique for constructing denture support bearings. J. Prosth. Dent., *23*:562, 1970.

7. Morrow, R. M., et al.: Tooth supported complete dentures: description and clinical evaluation of a simplified technique. J. Prosth. Dent., *22*:414, 1969.

7a. Morrow, R. M., Rudd, K. D., Birmingham, F. D., and Larkin, J. D.: Immediate interim tooth-supported complete dentures. J. Prosth. Dent., *30*:695, 1973.

7b. Pacer, F. J., and Bowman, D. C.: Occlusal force discrimination by denture patients. J. Prosth. Dent., *33*:602, 1975.

8. Powell, J. M., and Morrow, R. M.: Technique for constructing denture support bearings. J. Prosth. Dent., *25*:562, 1970.

8a. Quinlivan, J. T.: An attachment for overlay dentures. J. Prosth. Dent., *32*:256, 1974.

8b. Richard, G. E., Sarka, F. J., Arnold, R. M., and Knowles, K. I.: Hemisected molars for additional overdenture support. J. Prosth. Dent., *38*:16, 1977.

8c. Rissin, L., House, J. E., Manly, R. S., and Kapur, K. K.: Clinical comparison of the masticatory performance and electromyographic activity of patients with complete dentures, overdentures and natural teeth. J. Prosth. Dent., *39*:508, 1978.

9. Schweitzer, J. M., Schweitzer, R. D., and Schweitzer, J.: The telescoped complete denture: a research report at the clinical level. J. Prosth. Dent., *26*:357, 1971.

10. Stansbury, B. E.: A retentive attachment for overdentures. J. Prosth. Dent., *35*:228, 1976.

11. Thayer, H. H., and Caputo, A. A.: Effects of overdentures upon remaining oral structures. J. Prosth. Dent., *37*:374, 1977.

12. Toolson, L. B., and Smith, D. E.: A two year study of overdenture patients—Part I. J. Prosth. Dent., *40*:486, 1978.

13. White, J. T.: Abutment stress in overdentures. J. Prosth. Dent., *40*:13, 1978.

Bibliography

In a bibliography it is unfortunate that it is impossible to include references to all sources of information on a subject. The majority of the references have been selected from current periodicals and books on complete dentures and related sciences.

References applying primarily to the subject matter of a chapter are placed at the end of the chapter. Included in this section are general works on complete denture procedures or allied sciences.

The references are arranged alphabetically by author. Discussions of articles are listed with the articles. The originating author's name receives precedence.

Textbooks

Anthony, L. P.: *The American Textbook of Prosthetic Dentistry: In Contributions by Eminent Authorities.* 7th ed. Philadelphia, Lea & Febiger, 1942.

Archer, W. H.: *Oral Surgery.* 4th ed. Philadelphia, W. B. Saunders Company, 1966.

Boucher, C. O.: *Current Clinical Dental Terminology.* 2nd ed. St. Louis, The C. V. Mosby Co., 1974.

Cinotti, W. R., and Greiden, A.: *Applied Psychology in Dentistry.* 2nd ed. St. Louis, The C. V. Mosby Company, 1972.

Clark, J. W., et al.: *Diet and the Periodontal Patient.* Springfield, Ill., Charles C Thomas, 1970.

Colby, R. A., et. al: *Color Atlas of Oral Pathology.* 3rd ed. Philadelphia, J. B. Lippincott Company, 1971.

Copenhaver, W. M., and Johnson, D. D.: *Bailey's 16th Textbook of Histology.* ed. Baltimore, Williams & Wilkins, 1971.

Dental Technician, Prosthetic (Lab. Manual). Bureau of Naval Personnel. Navy Training Course Nav. Pers. 10685B. Washington, D. C., U. S. Government Printing Office, 1962.

Ferner, H. (Ed.): *Atlas of Topographical and Applied Human Anatomy.* Vol. 1. Head and Neck. Philadelphia, W. B. Saunders Company, 1963.

Fish, E. W.: *Principles of Full Denture Prosthesis.* 4th ed. London, John Bale & Sons, Curnow Ltd., 1948.

Frahm, F. W.: *The Principles and Technics of Full Denture Construction.* Brooklyn, Dental Items of Interest Publishing Company, 1934.

The Fundamentals of Radiography. 10th ed. Rochester, N. Y., Eastman Kodak Co., 1960.

Gehl, D. H., and Dresen, O. M.: *Complete Denture Prosthesis.* 4th ed. Philadelphia, W. B. Saunders Company, 1948.

Gorlin, R. J., and Goldman, H. M.: *Thoma's Oral Pathology.* Vol. II, 6th ed. St. Louis, The C. V. Mosby Company, 1970.

Gray's Anatomy of the Human Body. 29th ed. C. M. Goss, Ed. Philadelphia, Lea & Febiger, 1973.

Guyton, A. C.: *Physiology of the Human Body.* 5th ed. Philadelphia, W. B. Saunders Company, 1979.

Jersild, A. T.: *Child Psychology.* 4th ed. Englewood Cliffs, N. J., Prentice-Hall Inc., 1959.

Kakudo, Y.: *Occlusion, Mastication and Salivary Secretion.* Abstracts from Papers from the Department of Physiology and Oral Physiology, Osaka Dental University, Osaka, Japan, 1972.

Kerr, D. A., and Ash, M. J.: *Oral Pathology.* 4th ed. Philadelphia, Lea & Febiger, 1978.

Landy, C.: *Full Dentures.* St. Louis, The C. V. Mosby Company, 1958.

Lucia, V. O.: *Modern Gnathological Concepts.* St. Louis, The C. V. Mosby Company, 1961.

McCollum, B. B., and Stuart, C. E.: *Research Report on Gnathology,* South Pasadena, Scientific Press, 1955.

Nagle, R. J., and Sears, U. H.: *Denture Prosthetics.* 2nd ed. St. Louis, The C. V. Mosby Company, 1962.

Nichols, I. G.: *Prosthetic Dentistry.* St. Louis, The C. V. Mosby Company, 1930.

Nizel, A. E.: *The Science of Nutrition and Its Application in Clinical Dentistry.* 2nd ed. Philadelphia, W. B. Saunders Company, 1966.

Peyton, F. A., Anthony, D. H., Asgar, K., Charbeneau, G. T., Craig, R. G., and Myers, G. E.: *Restorative Dental Materials.* 2nd ed. St. Louis, The C. V. Mosby Company, 1964.

Posselt, U.: *Physiology of Occlusion and Rehabilitation.* Second Printing, Oxford, Blackwell Scientific Publications, 1966.

Ramfjord, S., and Ash, Mck.: *Occlusion.* Philadelphia, W. B. Saunders Company, 1966.

Schlosser, R. O.: *Complete Denture Prosthesis.* Philadelphia, W. B. Saunders Company, 1939.

————, and Gehl, D. H.: *Complete Denture Prosthesis.* 3rd ed. Philadelphia, W. B. Saunders Company, 1953.

Sears, V. H.: *Full Denture Procedures.* New York, The Macmillan Company, 1934.

Sharry, J. J.: *Complete Denture Prosthodontics.* New York, McGraw-Hill Book Company, 1962.

Sicher, H., and DuBrul, E. L.: *Oral Anatomy.* 6th ed. St. Louis, The C. V. Mosby Company, 1975.

Silverman, M. M.: *Occlusion in Prosthodontics and in the Natural Dentition.* Washington, D. C., Mutual Publishing Company, 1962.

————: *Oral Physiology.* St. Louis, The C. V. Mosby Company, 1961.

Skinner, E. W., and Phillips, R. W.: *The Science of Dental Materials.* 5th ed. Philadelphia, W. B. Saunders Company, 1962.

Sorensen, H., and Malm, M.: *Psychology for Living,* 6th ed. New York, McGraw-Hill Book Company, 1948.

Stedman's *Medical Dictionary.* 23rd ed. Baltimore, Williams & Wilkins, 1976.

Stuart, C. E., and Stallard, H.: *A Syllabus on Oral Rehabilitation and Occlusion.* Vol. 1. San Francisco, Postgraduate Education, School of Dentistry, U. of Cal. San Francisco Medical Center, 1959.

————: *A Syllabus on Oral Rehabilitation and Occlusion.* Vol. 11. San Francisco, Postgraduate Education, School of Dentistry, U. of Cal. San Francisco Medical Center, 1959.

U. S. Air Force Dental Laboratory Technicians Manual. No. 160-29. Washington, D. C., U. S. Government Printing Office, 1959.

Waite, D. E.: *Textbook of Practical Oral Surgery.* 2nd ed. Philadelphia, Lea & Febiger, 1978.

Wright, C. R., Swartz, W. H., and Godwin, W. C.: *Mandibular Stability: A New Concept.* Ann Arbor, The Overbeck Co., 1961.

X-Ray in Dentistry: Rochester, N. Y., Eastman Kodak Co., 1964.

Zegarelli, E. V., Kutscher, A. H., and Hyman, G. A.: *Diagnosis of Diseases of the Mouth.* 2nd ed., Philadelphia, Lea & Febiger, 1978.

Periodicals

Academy of Denture Prosthetics, 1959: Principles, concepts, and practices in prosthodontics. J. Prosth. Dent., *9:*528, 1959.

Academy of Denture Prosthetics, 1960: Principles, concepts, and practices in prosthodontics. J. Prosth. Dent., *10:*804, 1960.

Academy of Denture Prosthetics, 1963: Principles, concepts, and practices in prosthodontics. J. Prosth. Dent., *13:*283, 1963.

Academy of Denture Prosthetics: Principles, concepts, and practices in prosthodontics. J. Prosth. Dent., *19:*180, 1967.

Blanchard, C. H.: Some phases of our many-sided denture problem. J. Prosth. Dent., *1:*523, 1951.

Block, S.: Common factors in complete denture prosthetics. J. Prosth. Dent., *3:*736, 1953.

Bodine, R. L.: Essentials of a sound complete denture technique. J. Prosth. Dent., *14:*409, 1964.

Boos, R. H.: Complete denture technique, including preparation and conditioning. Dent. Clin. N. Amer. March, 1957, p. 215.

Boucher, C. O.: What knowledge, technical ability, and experience are essential to the graduating dental student in complete denture prosthesis? J. Ontario Dent. Assoc., *31*:12, 1954.

——: The current status of prosthodontics. J. Prosth. Dent., *10*:411, 1960.

——: Essentials of complete denture service. J. Prosth. Dent., *11*:445, 1961.

——: Trends in the practice and philosophy of prosthodontics in the United States. J. Prosth. Dent., *16*:873, 1966.

Brewer, A. A.: Treating complete denture patients. J. Prosth. Dent., *14*:1015, 1964.

Clark, W. D.: Ideas for problem upper dentures. J. Canad. Dent. Assoc., *22*:335, 1956.

DeVan, M. M.: Biological demands of complete dentures. J.A.D.A., *45*:524, 1952.

Edwards, L. F.: Some anatomic facts and fancies relative to the masticatory apparatus. J. Prosth. Dent., *5*:825, 1955.

Friedman, S.: Full dentures. New York J. Dent., *24*:74, 1954.

Geller, J. W.: Prosthetic dentistry. J. Prosth. Dent., *10*:33, 1960.

Gillis, R. R.: A denture technique applicable by the average dentist. J.A.D.A., *20*:304, 1933.

Hall, R. E.: Full denture construction. J.A.D.A., *16*:1157, 1929.

Hanau, R. L.: What are the physical requirements for and of prosthetic dentures? J.A.D.A., *10*:1044, 1923.

Hardy, I. R.: Realistic approach to the full denture problem from the standpoint of the general practitioner. New York J. Dent., *25*:242, 1955 (Abst.).

Hart, H. W.: Trends in the practice and philosophy of prosthodontics in Canada. J. Prosth. Dent., *16*:861, 1966.

Hickey, J. C., Boucher, C. O., and Woelfel, J. B.: Responsibility of the dentist in complete dentures. J. Prosth. Dent., *12*:637, 1962.

Hughes, F. C.: Elusive objectives in complete denture prosthesis. J. Prosth. Dent., *1*:543, 1951.

Jamieson, C. H.: Modern concept of complete dentures. J. Prosth. Dent., *6*:582. 1956.

Jones, P.: Realistic approach to complete denture construction. J. Prosth. Dent., *8*:220, 1958.

Kettlewell, N. L.: Factors concerning full dentures. J. Prosth. Dent., *4*:30, 1954.

Koper, A.: Why dentures fail. Dent. Clin. N. Amer., November, 1964, p. 721.

Kyes, F. M.: Pitfalls in full denture service. J.A.D.A., *43*:651, 1951.

Langer, A., Michman, J., and Seifert, I.: Factors influencing satisfaction with complete dentures in geriatric patients. J. Prosth. Dent., *11*:1019, 1961.

Martone, A.L.: Clinical applications of concepts of functional anatomy and speech science to complete denture prosthodontics. Part 7. Recording phases. J. Prosth. Dent., *13*:4, 1963.

——: Clinical applications of functional anatomy and speech science to complete denture prosthodontics. Part 8. The final phases of denture construction. J. Prosth. Dent., *13*:204, 1963.

Meyer, F. S.: Construction of full dentures with balanced functional occlusion. J. Prosth. Dent., *4*:440, 1954.

Mitchell, L. D., Jr.: Panoramic roentgenography: a clinical evaluation. J.A.D.A., *66*:777, 1963.

Moses, C. H.: Full denture procedure. J. Ontario Dent. Assoc., *20*:494, 1945.

——: Biologic emphasis in prosthodontics. J. Prosth. Dent., *12*:695, 1962.

Nairn, R. I.: Interrelated factors in complete denture construction. J. Prosth. Dent., *15*:19, 1965.

Neil, J. B.: Complete lower denture technique. J. Tennessee Dent. Assoc., *27*:3, 1947.

Pleasure, M. A.: Construction of full dentures in consonance with biologic requirements. New York J. Dent., *27*:22, 1957 (Abstr.).

Pound, E., and Murrell, G. A.: An introduction to denture simplification Phase II. J. Prosth. Dent., *29*:598, 1973.

Roberts, A. L.: Present day concepts in complete denture service. J. Prosth. Dent., *9*:900, 1959.

Sears, V. H.: Dental terminology. J. Prosth. Dent., *3*:592, 1953.

——: Comprehensive denture service. J.A.D.A., *23*:212, 1962.

Stamoulis, S.: Physical factors affecting the retention of complete dentures. J. Prosth. Dent., *12*:857, 1962.

Sussman, B. A.: Procedures in complete denture prosthesis. J. Prosth. Dent., *10*:1011, 1960.

Terrell, W. H.: A precision technique that produces dentures that fit and function. J. Prosth. Dent., *1*:353, 1951.

Updegrave, W. J.: Panoramic dental radiography. Dent. Radiogr. Photogr., 4:75, 1963.

Vaughan, H. C.: Some important factors in complete denture occlusion. J. Prosth. Dent., 6:642, 1956.

Yashizumi, D. T.: An evaluation of factors pertinent to the success of complete denture service. J. Prosth. Dent., *14*:866, 1964.

GLOSSARY OF
Prosthodontic terms*

A

ablation. The surgical removal of a diseased part.

abrasion. The act or result of the grinding or wearing away of a substance, such as a tooth worn by mastication, bruxing, or tooth brushing.

abrasive. A substance used for abrading, grinding, or polishing (may be used as an adjective).

absorption. The taking up of fluids or other substances by the skin, mucous surfaces, absorbent vessels, or dental materials.

abutment. A tooth or portion of an implant used for the support of a fixed or removable dental prosthesis.

  intermediate a. A natural tooth, without other natural teeth in proximal contact, which is used as an abutment, in addition to primary abutments.

  primary a. A tooth used for the direct support of a fixed or removable dental prosthesis.

  subperiosteal implant a. That portion of the implant which protrudes through the mucosa into the oral cavity for the retention or support of a crown or a fixed or removable denture.

accelerator. A catalytic agent used to hasten a chemical reaction (e.g., NaCl or K_2SO_4 added to a mix of plaster of Paris and water to hasten setting).

acrylic resin. Pertains to any of a group of thermoplastic resins made by polymerizing esters of acrylic acid or methacrylic acid. Should be used as in *acrylic resin, acrylic resin denture, acrylic resin tooth,* etc. (See also *resin.*)

adhesion. The physical attraction of unlike molecules for one another.

adjustable anterior guide. An anterior guide the superior surface of which may be varied to provide desired separation of the casts in various eccentric relationships.

adjustable axis face-bow, hinge-bow, kinematic face-bow. A face-bow with caliper ends that can be adjusted to permit location of the (hinge) axis of rotation of the mandible.

adjustable occlusal pivot. An occlusal pivot which may be adjusted vertically by means of a screw or other device.

adjustment. A modification made upon a dental prosthesis in preparation for and/or following its use by the patient. (See also *occlusal adjustment.*)

alginate (irreversible hydrocolloid.) An irreversible hydrocolloid consisting of salts of alginic acid. In dentistry, it is used primarily for making impressions. (See also *hydrocolloid.*)

alloplast. A material originating from a nonliving source which is surgically inserted to replace missing tissue.

alveolar bone. The bone of the maxillae or mandible that surrounds and supports the teeth.

alveolar ridge. The bony ridge (alveolar process) of the maxillae or mandible which contains the alveoli (sockets of the teeth).

alveolus. The cavity in the alveolar process of the maxillae or mandible in which the root of a tooth is held by the periodontal ligament.

anatomic articulation. A rigid or movable junction of bony parts.

anatomic crown. The portion of a natural tooth which extends from its dentinoenamel junction to the occlusal surface or incisal edge.

anatomic teeth. 1. Artificial teeth which duplicate the anatomic forms of natural teeth. 2. Teeth which have prominent pointed or rounded cusps on the masticating surfaces and which are designed to occlude with the teeth of the opposing denture or natural dentition.

anneal. The softening of a metal by controlled heating and cooling. The process makes a metal more easily adapted, bent, or swaged and less brittle.

*Originally published in the July, 1977 issue of The Journal of Prosthetic Dentistry. Reprinted by permission of the C. V. Mosby Company, St. Louis, Missouri.

anterior guidance, incisal guide. That part of an articulator which maintains the incisal guide angle.

anterior guide. That part of an articulator on which the anterior guide pin rests to maintain the vertical dimension of occlusion. The guide influences the degree of separation of the casts in eccentric relationships.

    adjustable a. g. An anterior guide the superior surface of which may be varied to provide desired separation of the casts in various eccentric relationships.

anterior tooth arrangement. The arrangement of anterior teeth for esthetic or phonetic effects.

anterior tooth form. The outline form and other contours of an anterior tooth.

anti-Monson curve. A curve of occlusion which is convex upward.

arch form. The geometric shape of the dental arch (e.g., tapering, ovoid, square, etc.).

arcon. (Adjective.) Used to describe an articulator that contains the condylar path elements in its upper member and its condylar elements in the lower member.

arrow-point tracer, tracer. 1. A mechanical device used to trace a pattern of mandibular movements. 2. A mechanical device with a marking point attached to one jaw and a graph plate or tracing plate attached to the other jaw. It is used to record the direction and extent of movements of the mandible. (See also *gothic arch tracer.*)

arrow-point tracing, gothic arch tracing, needlepoint tracing, stylus tracing. A tracing which resembles an arrowhead or a gothic arch made by means of a device attached to the opposing arches. The shape of the tracing depends upon the relation of the marking point relative to the tracing table. The apex of a properly made tracing is considered to indicate the most retruded, unstrained relation of the mandible to the maxillae, i.e., centric relation.

articulate. The relating of artificial teeth or replicas of natural teeth to each other.

articulation. 1. The placement of teeth on a denture with definite objectives in mind. 2. The setting of teeth on temporary bases.

    anatomic a. A rigid or movable junction of bony parts.

    articulator a. The use of a device which incorporates an artificial temporomandibular joint permitting the orientation of casts in a manner simulating various positions or movements of the mandible.

    dental a. The contact relationship of the maxillary and mandibular teeth when moving into and away from centric occlusion.

    temporomandibular a. The articulation of the condyloid process of the mandible and the interarticular disk with the mandibular fossa of the temporal bone.

articulator. A mechanical device which represents the temporomandibular joints and jaw members to which maxillary and mandibular casts may be attached to simulate jaw movements. (See also *arcon.*)

    adjustable a. An articulator which may be adjusted to permit movement of the casts into recorded eccentric relationships.

articulator articulation. The use of a device which incorporates an artificial temporomandibular joint permitting the orientation of casts in a manner simulating various positions or movements of the mandible.

artificial crown. A fixed restoration of the major part or of the entire coronal part of a natural tooth, usually of gold, porcelain, or acrylic resin.

artificial stone. A gypsum derivative which when combined with water in proper proportions, hardens into a plaster-like form having physical characteristics superior to plaster of Paris for casts, dies, denture processing procedures, etc.

atrophy. A diminution in size of a cell, tissue, organ, or part.

    adipose a. Atrophy due to reduction in fatty tissue.

    bone a. Bone resorption both internally in density and externally in form (viz., of residual ridges).

    muscular a. A wasting of muscular tissue, especially due to lack of use.

    postmenopausal a. A thinning of the oral mucosa following the menopause.

    senile a. The normal diminution of all tissues due to advanced age.

attachment. A mechanical device for the fixation, retention, and stabilization of a dental prosthesis.

    precision a., frictional a., internal a., key and keyway a., parallel a., slotted a. A retainer, used in fixed and removable partial denture construction, consisting of a metal receptacle and a closely fitting part; the former is usually contained within the normal or expanded contours of the crown of the abutment tooth and the latter is attached to a pontic or the denture framework.

autograft. A graft taken from one part of the patient's body and transplanted to another part.

autopolymer. A material which polymerizes without external heat as a result of the addition of an activator and a catalyst.

autopolymer resin, activated resin, cold-curing resin, quick-cure resin, self-curing resin. A resin which can be polymerized by an activator and a catalyst without use of external heat.

autopolymerization. Polymerization without the use of external heat as a result of the addition of an activator and a catalyst.

axis. A straight line around which a body may rotate.

   longitudinal a. (See *sagittal axis*.)

   mandibular a., condylar a., condyle a., hinge a., transverse a. Imaginary line through two mandibular condyles around which the mandible may rotate without translatory movement.

   sagittal a. An imaginary anteroposterior line through a mandibular condyle around which a mandible may rotate in a yawing or pitching motion.

B

backing. A metal support which serves to attach a facing to a prosthesis.

balanced occlusion. An occlusion of the teeth which presents a harmonious relation of the occluding surfaces in all centric and eccentric positions within the functional range of mastication and swallowing. 2. The simultaneous contacting of the maxillary and mandibular teeth on the right and left and in the posterior and anterior occlusal areas in centric and eccentric positions, developed to lessen or limit a tipping or rotating of the denture bases in relation to the supporting structures.

   mechanically b. o. A balanced occlusion without reference to physiologic considerations, as on an articulator.

   physiologically b. o. A balanced occlusion which is in harmony with the temporomandibular joints and the neuromuscular system.

balancing contacts. The contacts between the maxillary and mandibular natural or artificial teeth at the side opposite the working side.

bar. A metal segment of greater length than width which serves to connect two or more parts of a removable partial denture.

   Kennedy b., continuous b. retainer. 1. A metal bar usually resting on lingual surfaces of teeth to aid in their stabilization and act as indirect retainers. 2. A metal bar which contacts lingual surfaces of anterior teeth and aids in retention of a distal-extension partial denture.

   labial b. A major connector located labial to the dental arch joining two or more bilateral parts of a removable partial denture.

   lingual b. A major connector located lingual to the dental arch joining two or more bilateral parts of a mandibular removable partial denture.

   palatal b. A major connector which crosses the palate and unites two or more parts of a maxillary removable partial denture.

Passavant's b., pad, ridge. 1. The bulging of the posterior pharyngeal wall produced by the upper portion of the superior constrictor muscle of the pharynx during the act of swallowing or phonation. 2. A ridge of erectile tissue on the posterior wall of the pharynx.

bar clasp. A clasp having arms which are bar-type extensions from major connectors or from within the denture base; the arms pass adjacent to the soft tissues and approach the point or area of contact on the tooth in a gingivo-occlusal direction.

bar clasp arm. A clasp arm which has its origin in the denture base or major connector. It consists of the arm which traverses the gingival structures and a terminal end which approaches contact with the tooth in a gingivo-occlusal direction.

bar retainer, continuous, Kennedy bar. 1. A metal bar usually resting on lingual surfaces of teeth to aid in their stabilization and to act as indirect retainers. 2. A metal bar which contacts lingual surfaces of anterior teeth and aids in the retention of a distal-extension partial denture.

basal bone. The osseous tissue of the mandible and maxillae, excepting the alveolar processes.

basal seat. That surface of the oral structures which is covered by the denture base.

basal seat area. That surface of the oral mucosa which is covered by the denture base.

basal seat outline. The outline of the entire area to be covered by a denture base appearing on the mucous membrane or on a cast.

basal surface. The surface of the denture the detail of which is determined by a cast from the impression.

basal surface denture, impression surface. That portion of the denture surface which has its contour determined by the impression.

base material. Any substance of which a denture base may be made, such as acrylic resin, vulcanite, polystyrene, metal, etc.

baseplate, record base, temporary base, trial base. A temporary substance representing the base of a denture which is used for making maxillomandibular (jaw) relation records and for the arrangement of teeth.

    stabilized b. (base). A baseplate lined with a plastic material to improve its fit and adaptation.

beam. A term frequently used instead of "bar" referring to a metal structure the length of which exceeds its width and having a curvature which changes under load.

    cantilever b. A beam that is supported by only one fixed support at only one of its ends.

    continuous b. A beam that continues over several supports, with those supports not at the beam ends being equally free supports.

    simple b. A straight beam that has two, and only two, supports—one at either end.

Bennett angle. The angle formed by the sagittal plane and the path of the advancing condyle during lateral mandibular movements as viewed in the horizontal plane.

Bennett movement. The bodily lateral movement or lateral shift of the mandible resulting from the movements of the condyles along the lateral inclines of the mandibular fossae in lateral jaw movements.

bimeter gnathodynamometer, gnathodynamometer. 1. An instrument for measuring the force exerted in closing the jaws. (Dor.) 2. An instrument used for measuring biting pressure.

biology. The science of life or living matter in all its forms and phenomena.

biomechanics, biophysics. 1. The science which deals with the forces which act on living cells of the body. 2. The relationship between the biologic behavior of living structures and the physical influence to which these structures are subjected.

biometry. The science of the application of statistical methods to biologic facts, as the mathematical analysis of biologic data.

biophysics, biomechanics. 1. The science which deals with the forces which act on living cells of the body. 2. The relationship between the biologic behavior of living structures and the physical influence to which these structures are subjected.

    dental b. (biomechanics). The relationship between the biologic behavior of oral structures and the physical influence of a dental restoration.

biopsy. The removal of small amounts of tissue for the purpose of histologic examination and diagnosis.

Bonwill triangle. An equilateral triangle with 4 inch sides, bounded by lines from the contact points of the lower central incisors or by the medial line of the residual ridge of the mandible, to the condyle on either side, and from one condyle to the other.

border. The circumferential margin or edge.

    b. molding, muscle trimming, tissue molding. The shaping of an impression material by the manipulation or action of the tissues adjacent to the borders of an impression.

    b. movement. Any extreme compass of mandibular movement limited by bone, ligaments, or soft tissue.

    b. seal. The contact of the denture border with the underlying or adjacent tissues to prevent the passage of air or other substances.

    b. tissue movements. The action of the muscles and other tissues adjacent to the borders of a denture.

    denture b. 1. The margin of the denture base at the junction of the polished surface and the impression (tissue) surface. 2. The extreme peripheral border of a denture base at the buccolabial, lingual, and posterior limits.

    posterior b. jaw relation. The most posterior relation of the mandible to the maxillae at any specific vertical relation.

    posterior b. movement. Lateral movement of the mandible along the posterior limit of the envelope of motion.

    posterior b. position. The most posterior position of the mandible at any specific vertical relation to the maxillae.

boxing (an impression). The enclosure of an impression by the building up of vertical walls to produce the desired size and form of the base of the cast and to preserve certain details of the impression.

boxing wax. Wax specifically used for boxing impressions.

bracing. The resistance to horizontal components of masticatory force.

bruxism. The forceful grinding of the teeth, other than chewing movements of the mandible, usually performed during sleep.

bruxomania. The grinding of teeth occurring as a neurotic habit during the waking state.

buccal. Pertaining to or adjacent to the cheek.

b. flange. The portion of the flange of a denture which occupies the buccal vestibule of the mouth.

b. surface (of dentures). The side of a denture adjacent to the cheek.

b. vestibule. That portion of the oral cavity which is bounded on one side by the teeth, gingivae, and alveolar ridge (in the edentulous mouth, the residual ridge) and on the other by the cheeks.

buccolingual relationship. The position of a space or tooth in relation to the tongue and the cheek.

bulb, hollow. That portion of a prosthesis made hollow to minimize weight.

butt. 1. To place directly against the tissues covering the alveolar ridge. 2. To bring any two flat-ended surfaces into contact without overlapping, as in a butt joint.

C

Camper's line. The line running from the inferior border of the ala of the nose to the superior border of the tragus of the ear.

capillary attraction. That quality or state which, because of surface tension, causes elevation or depression of the surface of a liquid that is in contact with a solid.

case. 1. An objectional term in prosthodontics. This term should not be used as a synonym for a patient or to refer to a stage of prosthodontic treatment. Specific terms such as "patient," "denture," and "castings" should be used as they apply. 2. A particular instance of disease or injury, as a case of typhoid fever. A case is not synonymous with a patient, for the latter is the human being affected with the disease.

cast. An object formed in or poured into a matrix or impression which is a positive likeness of some desired form.

dental c. A positive likeness of a part or parts of the oral cavity.

diagnostic c., study c., preoperative c. A positive likeness of a part or parts of the oral cavity for the purpose of study and treatment planning.

investment c., refractory c. A cast made of a material that will withstand high temperatures without disintegrating.

master c. A replica of the prepared tooth surfaces (where necessary), residual ridge areas, and/or other parts of the dental arch used to fabricate a dental restoration or prosthesis.

modified c. A master cast that is altered prior to processing a denture base.

casting. 1. An object formed in a mold. 2. The act of forming a casting in a mold.

vacuum c. The casting of a metal in the presence of vacuum.

casting flask, casting ring, refractory flask. A metal tube in which a refractory mold is made for casting metal dental restorations.

casting wax. A composition containing various waxes with controlled properties used in making patterns to determine the shape of metal castings.

cement. 1. A material which, on becoming hard, will usefully fill a space or bind together adjacent objects. 2. A type of filling material, e.g., silicate cement.

cementation. 1. The process of attaching parts by means of a cement. 2. Attaching a restoration to natural teeth by means of a cement.

central bearing. Application of forces between the maxilla and mandible at a single point which is located as near as possible to the center of the supporting areas of the maxillary and mandibular jaws. It is used for the purpose of distributing closing forces evenly throughout the areas of the supporting structures during the registration and recording of maxillomandibular (jaw) relations and during the correction of occlusal errors.

central-bearing point. The contact point of a central-bearing device.

central-bearing tracing device. A device which provides a central point of bearing, or support, between maxillary and mandibular occlusion rims or dentures. It consists of a contacting point which is attached to one occlusion rim or denture and a plate attached to the opposing occlusion rim or denture which provides the surface on which the bearing point rests or moves. It is used for the purpose of distributing closing forces evenly throughout the areas of the supporting structures during the recording of maxillomandibular relations and/or for correction of disharmonious occlusal contacts.

centric. The word "centric" is an adjective and should be used in conjunction with a noun, e.g., centric occlusion, centric position, centric jaw relation.

c. interocclusal record. A record of the centric jaw position (relation).

c. jaw relation. 1. The jaw relation when the condyles are in the most posterior, unstrained position in the glenoid fossae at any given degree of jaw separation from which lateral movement can be made. 2. The most posterior relation of the mandible to the maxillae at the established vertical dimension. 3. The relation of the mandible to the maxillae when the condyles are in their most posterior position in the glenoid fossa from which unstrained lateral movements can be made at the occluding vertical dimension normal for the individual.

c. occlusion. The centered contact position of the occlusal surfaces of the mandibular teeth against the occlusal surfaces of the maxillary teeth.

c. relation record, occluding. A registration of centric relation made at the established occlusal vertical dimension.

cephalometer. An instrument for measuring the head or skull.

cephalostat. A device to fix the head position in relation to a camera or radiographic source.

chew-in record. A record of lateral and protrusive movements of the mandible made upon the occlusal surfaces of an occlusion rim by teeth or mechanical devices (scribing studs).

chewing cycle. A complete course of movement of the mandible during a single masticatory stroke.

chewing force. The degree of force applied by the muscles of mastication during the mastication of food.

clasp. A part of a removable partial denture which acts as a direct retainer and/or stabilizer for the denture by partially encircling or contacting an abutment tooth.

bar c. A clasp having arms which are bar-type extensions from major connectors or from within the denture base; the arms pass adjacent to the soft tissues and approach the point or area of contact on the tooth in a gingivo-occlusal direction.

bar c. arm. A clasp arm which has its origin in the denture base or major connector. It consists of the arm which traverses the gingival structures and a terminal end which approaches contact with the tooth in a gingivo-occlusal direction.

circumferential c. A clasp that encircles a tooth by more than 180 degrees, including opposite angles, and which usually has total contact with the tooth (throughout the extent of the clasp), with at least one terminal being in the infrabulge (gingival convergence) area.

circumferential c. arm. A clasp arm which has its origin in a minor connector and which follows the contour of the tooth in a plane approximately perpendicular to the path of insertion of the partial denture.

continuous c. A metal bar usually resting on the lingual surface of teeth to aid in their stabilization and to act as an indirect retainer.

retentive circumferential c. arm. A circumferential clasp arm which is flexible and engages the infrabulge area of the abutment tooth at the terminal end of the arm.

Roach c. A clasp with arms that are bar-type extensions from major connectors or from within the denture base; the arms pass adjacent to the soft tissues and approach the point or area of contact on the tooth in a gingivo-occlusal direction.

stabilizing circumferential c. arm. A circumferential clasp arm which is relatively rigid and contacts the height of contour of the tooth.

clearance. A condition in which bodies may pass each other without hindrance. Also, the distance between bodies.

interocclusal c. (See *interocclusal distance.*) A condition in which the opposing occlusal surfaces may glide over one another without any interfering projection.

occlusal c. A condition in which the opposing occlusal surfaces may glide over one another without any interfering projection.

cleft-palate impression. An impression of a cleft palate.

cleft-palate prosthesis. A restoration to correct congenital defects in the palate and in related structures if they are involved.

cold-curing resin, activated resin, autopolymer resin, quick-cure resin, self-curing resin. A resin which can be polymerized by an activator and a catalyst without use of external heat.

coloring, extrinsic. Coloring from without, as applying color to the external surface of a prosthesis.

coloring, intrinsic. Coloring from within. The incorporation of pigment within the material of a prosthesis.

comminution of food. The reduction of food into small parts.

compensating curve. The anteroposterior and lateral curvatures in the alignment of the occluding surfaces and incisal edges of artificial teeth which are used to develop balanced occlusion.

complete denture. A dental prosthesis which replaces the entire dentition and associated structures of the maxillae or mandible.

complete denture prosthetics, full denture prosthetics. 1. The replacement of the natural teeth in the arch and their associated parts by artificial substitutes. 2. The art and science of the restoration of an edentulous mouth.

component of force. One of the factors from which a resultant force may be compounded or into which it may be resolved.

components of mastication. The various jaw movements which are made during mastication as determined by the neuromuscular system, the temporomandibular articulations, the teeth, and the food being chewed. The components of the masticatory cycle may be separated (for purposes of analysis or description) into opening components of mastication, closing components of mastication, left lateral components of mastication, right lateral components of mastication, and anteroposterior components of mastication.

components of occlusion. The various factors which are involved in occlusion, such as the temporomandibular joint, the associated neuromusculature, the teeth, and the denture-supporting structures.

compression molding. 1. The act of pressing or squeezing together to form a shape in a mold. 2. The adaptation by pressure of a plastic material to the negative form of a split mold. (See also *injection molding.*)

condylar axis, condyle axis, hinge axis, mandibular axis, transverse axis. An imaginary line through the two mandibular condyles around which the mandible may rotate without translatory movement.

condylar guidance, condylar guide. The mechanical device on an articulator which is intended to produce guidances in articulator movement either similar or identical to those produced by the paths of the condyles in the temporomandibular joints.

condylar guidance inclination, condylar guide inclination. The angle of inclination of the condylar guidance to an accepted horizontal plane.

condylar hinge position. The position of the condyles of the mandible in the glenoid fossa at which hinge axis movement is possible.

condylar inclination, lateral. The direction of the lateral condyle path.

condyle. A rounded projection of bone, usually for articulation with another bone.

    mandibular c. The articular process of the mandible.

    neck of c. That portion of the mandibular ramus to which the condyle is attached.

condyle axis, condylar axis, hinge axis, mandibular axis, transverse axis. An imaginary line through the two mandibular condyles around which the mandible may rotate without translatory movement.

condyle path. The path traveled by the mandibular condyle in the temporomandibular joint area during the various mandibular movements.

    lateral c. p. The path of the condyle in the glenoid fossa when a lateral mandibular movement is made.

connector. A part of a removable partial denture which unites its components.

    major c. A part of a removable partial denture which connects the components on one side of the arch to the components on the opposite side of the arch.

    minor c. The connecting link between the major connector or base of a removable partial denture and other units of the prosthesis, such as clasps, indirect retainers, and occlusal rests.

continuous bar retainer, Kennedy bar. 1. A metal bar usually resting on lingual surfaces of teeth to aid in their stabilization and to act as indirect retainers. 2. A metal bar which contacts lingual surfaces of anterior teeth and aids in the retention of a distal-extension partial denture.

continuous beam. A beam that continues over several supports, with those supports not at the beam ends being equally free supports.

continuous clasp. A metal bar usually resting on the lingual surface of teeth to aid in their stabilization and to act as an indirect retainer.

continuous gum denture. An artificial denture consisting of porcelain teeth and tinted porcelain denture base material fused to a platinum base.

contour. 1. The external shape or form of an object. 2. To create the external shape or form of an object, as that of a denture.

    gingival denture c. The form of the denture base or other material around the necks of the artificial teeth.

    height of c. A line encircling a tooth designating its greatest circumference at a selected position.

contraction (muscle). The development of tension in a muscle in response to nerve stimulation.

isometric c. Muscular contraction in which there is no change in the length of the muscle during contraction.

isotonic c. Muscle contraction in which there is a shortening of the length of the muscle while the muscle maintains a constant tension.

postural c. Maintenance of muscle tension (usually isometric) sufficient to maintain posture, dependent on muscle tone.

coordination. The ability to function harmoniously, as in muscle coordination.

cope. The upper half of a flask in the casting art, hence, applicable to the upper or cavity side of a denture flask.

coping. A thin metal covering or cap.

transfer c. A metallic, acrylic resin, or other covering or cap used to position a die in an impression.

core. 1. A metal casting, usually with a post in the canal of a root, designed to retain an artificial crown. 2. A sectional record, usually of plaster of Paris or one of its derivatives, of the relationships of parts, such as teeth, metallic restorations, or copings.

Costen's syndrome, temporomandibular joint syndrome. Those various symptoms of discomfort, pain, or pathosis stated to be caused by loss of vertical dimension, lack of posterior occlusion, or other malocclusion, trismus, muscle tremor, arthritis, or direct trauma to the temporomandibular joint.

counterdie. The reverse image of a die, usually made of a softer and lower-fusing metal than the metal of the die.

cranial prosthesis. An artificial replacement for a portion of the skull.

crazing. Minute cracks appearing on the surface of plastic, porcelain, or natural teeth.

cross-bite teeth. Posterior teeth designed to accommodate the modified buccal cusps of the maxillary teeth to be positioned in the fossae of the mandibular teeth.

crown. The part of a tooth which is covered with enamel and which normally projects beyond the gum line.

anatomic c. The portion of a natural tooth which extends from its dentinoenamel junction to the occlusal surface or incisal edge.

artificial c. A fixed restoration of the major part or of the entire coronal part of a natural tooth, usually of gold, porcelain, or acrylic resin.

clinical c., extra-alveolar c. The portion of a tooth which extends occlusally or incisally from the junction of the tooth root and the supporting bone.

crown flask, denture flask. A sectional, boxlike metal case in which a sectional mold is made of artificial stone or plaster of Paris for the purpose of compressing and processing dentures or other resinous restorations.

cure. A technical procedure which converts a wax pattern, such as that of a wax trial base, into a solid denture base of another material.

curve. A nonangular deviation from a straight line or surface.

anti-Monson c. A curve of occlusion which is convex upward.

compensating c. The anteroposterior and lateral curvatures in the alignment of the occluding surfaces and incisal edges of artificial teeth which are used to develop balanced occlusion.

c. of Spee. Anatomic curvature of the occlusal alignment of teeth beginning at the tip of the lower canine and following the buccal cusps of the natural premolars and molars, continuing to the anterior border of the ramus, as described by Graf von Spee.

Monson c. The curve of occlusion in which each cusp and incisal edge touches or conforms to a segment of the surface of a sphere 8 inches in diameter with its center in the region of the glabella.

Pleasure c. A curve of occlusion which in transverse cross-section conforms to a line which is convex upward except for the last molars.

reverse c. A curve of occlusion which in transverse cross-section conforms to a line which is convex upward.

curves, milled-in, milled-in paths. 1. Contours carved by various mandibular movements into the occluding surface of an occlusion rim by teeth or studs placed in the opposing occlusion rim. 2. Occlusal curves developed by masticatory or gliding movements of occlusion rims which may be composed of materials that are abrasive. (See also *chew-in record.*)

cusp angle. The angle made by the slopes of a cusp with a perpendicular line bisecting the cusp, measured mesiodistally or buccolingually.

cusp height. The shortest distance between the tip of a cusp and its base plane.

cusp plane. The small imaginary plane in which two buccal cusp tips and the highest lingual cusp are located.

cusp-plane angle. The incline of the cusp plane in relation to the plane of occlusion.

cuspal interference. A condition of tooth contacts which diverts the mandible from a normal path of closure.

cuspless teeth. Teeth designed without cuspal prominences on the occlusal surface.

D

definitive prosthesis. A prosthesis to be used over an extended period of time.

deflective occlusal contact. A condition in which tooth contacts divert the mandible from a normal path of closure. (See also *occlusal disharmony*.)

deformation. The change of form or shape of an object.

deglutition. The act of swallowing.

dental arch. The composite structure of the natural dentition and the residual ridge or the remains thereof after the loss of some or all of the natural teeth.

dental articulation. The contact relationship of the maxillary and mandibular teeth when moving into and away from centric occlusion.

dental biophysics (biomechanics). The relationship between the biologic behavior of oral structures and the physical influence of a dental restoration.

dental cast. A positive likeness of a part or parts of the oral cavity.

dental dysfunction. 1. Abnormal functioning of dental structures. 2. Partial disturbance or impairment of the functioning of a dental organ.

dental engineering. 1. The application of physical, mechanical, and mathematical principles to dentistry. 2. The application of engineering principles to dentistry.

dental geriatrics. 1. Treatment of dental problems peculiar to advanced age. 2. Dentistry for the aged patient.

dental implant. A substance that is placed into the jaw to support a crown or fixed or removable denture.

dental prosthesis. An artificial replacement of one or more teeth and/or associated structures.

dental prosthetic laboratory procedures. The steps in the fabrication of dental prosthesis which do not require the presence of the patient for their accomplishment.

dental senescence. That condition of the teeth and associated structures in which there is deterioration due to aging or premature aging processes.

dentition, natural dentition. The natural teeth, as considered collectively, in the dental arch; may be deciduous, permanent, or mixed.

dentulous. A condition in which natural teeth are present in the mouth.

denture. An artificial substitute for missing natural teeth and adjacent tissues.

acrylic resin d. A denture made of acrylic resin.

basal surface d., impression surface. That portion of the denture surface which has its contour determined by the impression.

complete d. A dental prosthesis which replaces the entire dentition and associated structures of the maxillae or mandible.

continuous gum d. An artificial denture consisting of porcelain teeth and tinted porcelain denture base material fused to a platinum base.

d. base. 1. That part of a denture which rests on the oral mucosa and to which teeth are attached. 2. That part of a complete or removable partial denture which rests upon the basal seat and to which teeth are attached.

d. b., processed. That portion of a polymerized prosthesis covering the oral mucosa of the maxilla and/or mandible to which artificial teeth will be attached with a second processing.

d. b. saddle. 1. That part of a denture which rests on the oral mucosa and to which the teeth are attached. 2. That part of a complete or partial denture which rests upon the basal seat and to which the teeth are attached.

d. b., tinted. A denture base with coloring that simulates the color and shading of natural oral tissues.

d. border. 1. The margin of the denture base at the junction of the polished surface and the impression (tissue) surface. 2. The extreme peripheral border of a denture base at the buccolabial, lingual, and posterior limits.

d. occlusal surface. That portion of the surface of a denture or dentition which makes contact or near contact with the corresponding surface of the opposing denture or dentition.

d., polished surface. That portion of the surface of a denture which extends in an occlusal direction from the border of the denture and includes the palatal surface. It is the part of the denture base which is usually polished, and it includes the buccal and lingual surfaces of the teeth.

duplicate d. A second denture intended to be a copy of the first denture.

esthetic d. A denture which when viewed in the mouth, adds to the patient's charm, beauty, dignity, or naturalness of character.

immediate d. A complete or removable partial denture constructed for insertion immediately following the removal of natural teeth.

implant d. A denture which receives its stability and retention from a substructure which is partially or wholly implanted under the soft tissues of the denture basal seat.

interim d., provisional d., temporary d. A dental prosthesis to be used for a short interval of time for reasons of esthetics, mastication, occlusal support, or convenience or to condition the patient to the acceptance of an artificial substitute for missing natural teeth until more definitive prosthetic therapy can be provided.

partial d. A dental prosthesis which restores one or more but not all of the natural teeth and/or associated parts and which is supported by the teeth and/or the mucosa; it may be removable or fixed.

　　distal-extension p. d. A removable partial denture that is retained by natural teeth only at the anterior end of the denture base segments and in which a portion of the functional load is carried by the residual ridge.

　　fixed p. d. A partial denture that is cemented to natural teeth or roots which furnish the primary support to the prosthesis.

　　p. d. construction. The science and technique of designing and constructing partial dentures.

　　p. d. impression. 1. A negative copy of the partially edentulous dental arch or area made for the purpose of constructing a partial denture. 2. An impression of a part or all of a partially edentulous arch made for the purpose of designing or constructing a partial denture. 3. An impression of a part or all of a partially edentulous arch.

　　removable p. d. A partial denture which can be removed from the mouth and re-placed at will.

　　unilateral p. d. A dental prosthesis restoring lost or missing teeth on one side of the arch only.

transitional d. A removable partial denture serving as a temporary prosthesis to which artificial teeth will be added as natural teeth are lost and which will be replaced after post-extraction tissue changes have occurred. A transitional denture may become an interim denture when all of the natural teeth have been removed from the dental arch.

treatment d. A dental prosthesis used for the purpose of treating or conditioning the tissues which are called upon to support and retain a denture base.

trial d. A setup of artificial teeth so fabricated that it may be placed in the patient's mouth to verify esthetics, to make records, or for any other operation deemed necessary before the completion of the final denture.

denture-bearing area. The surface of the oral structures (basal seat) which is available to support a denture.

denture characterization. Modification of the form and color of the denture base and teeth to produce a more lifelike appearance.

denture construction, partial. The science and technique of designing and constructing partial dentures.

denture curing, denture processing. The process by which the denture-base materials are hardened to the form of a denture in a denture mold.

denture design. A planned visualization of the form and extent of a dental prosthesis arrived at after a study of all factors involved.

denture esthetics. The cosmetic effect produced by a dental prosthesis which affects the desirable beauty, attractiveness, character, and dignity of the individual.

denture flange. 1. The essentially vertical extension from the body of the denture into one of the vestibules of the oral cavity. Also, on the mandibular denture, the essentially vertical extension along the lingual side of the alveololingual sulcus. 2. The buccal and labial vertical extension of a maxillary and mandibular denture base and the lingual vertical extension of the mandibular denture. The buccal and labial denture flanges have two surfaces: the buccal or labial surface and the basal seat surface. The mandibular lingual flange also has two surfaces: the basal seat surface and the lingual surface.

denture flask, crown flask. A sectional, boxlike metal case in which a sectional mold is made of artificial stone or plaster of Paris for the purpose of compressing and processing dentures or other resinous restorations.

denture foundation, tissue-bearing area. That portion of the oral structures which is available to support a denture.

denture foundation area. The surface of the oral structures (basal seat) which is available to support a denture.

denture impression, partial. 1. A negative copy of the partially edentulous dental arch or area made for the purpose of constructing a partial denture. 2. An impression of a part or all of a partially edentulous arch made for the purpose of designing or constructing a partial denture. 3. An impression of a part or all of a partially edentulous arch.

denture packing. Filling and compressing a denture-base material into a mold in a flask.

denture prognosis. An opinion or judgment given in advance of treatment of the prospects for success in the construction of dentures and for their usefulness.

denture prosthetics, complete, full denture prosthetics. 1. The replacement of the natural teeth in the arch and their associated parts by artificial substitutes. 2. The art and science of the restoration of an edentulous mouth.

denture retention. 1. The resistance of the movement of a denture from its basal seat, especially in a vertical direction. 2. A quality of a denture that holds it on its basal seat and/or abutment teeth. (See also *retention of denture.*)

  partial d. r. The fixation of a removable partial denture by the use of clasps, indirect retainers, or precision attachments.

denture service. Those procedures which are involved in diagnosis and in fabrication and maintenance of artificial substitutes for missing natural teeth and associated structures.

denture space. 1. That portion of the oral cavity which is, or may be, occupied by a maxillary and/or mandibular denture(s). 2. The space between and around the residual ridges which is available for dentures.

denture stability. 1. The resistance of a denture to movement on its basal seat. 2. A quality of a denture that permits it to maintain a state of equilibrium in relation to the basal seat and/or abutment teeth.

denture-supporting area. That surface of the oral mucosa which is covered by the denture base.

denture-supporting structures. The tissues (teeth and/or residual ridges) which serve as the foundation for removable partial or complete dentures.

diagnosis. A scientific evaluation of existing conditions.

diagnostic cast, study cast, preoperative cast. A positive likeness of a part or parts of the oral cavity for the purpose of study and treatment planning.

diastema. A space between two adjacent teeth in the same dental arch.

die. The positive reproduction of the form of a prepared tooth in any suitable hard substance, usually in metal or specially prepared artificial stone. (See also *stone die.*)

dimensional stability. The ability of a material to retain its size and form.

direct bone impression. An impression of denuded bone used in the construction of denture implants.

direct retainer. A clasp or attachment applied to an abutment tooth for the purpose of holding a removable denture in position.

direct retention. Retention obtained in a removable partial denture by the use of clasps or attachments which resist removal from the abutment teeth.

displaceability of tissue. 1. The quality of oral tissues which permits them to be placed in other than a relaxed position. 2. The degree to which tissues permit displacement.

distal. Away from the median sagittal plane of the face following the curvature of the dental arch.

  d. end. The posterior extremity of a dental restoration.

distal-extension partial denture. A removable partial denture that is retained by natural teeth only at the anterior end of the denture base segments and in which a portion of the functional load is carried by the residual ridge.

drag. The lower or cast side of a denture flask to which the cope is fitted. The base of the cast is embedded in plaster of Paris or stone with the remainder of the denture pattern exposed to be engaged by the plaster of Paris or stone in the cope.

duplicate denture. A second denture intended to be a copy of the first denture.

durometer. An instrument for measuring hardness.

dynamic relations. Relations of two objects involving the element of relative movement of one object to another, as the relationship of the mandible to the maxillae.

E

eccentric interocclusal record. A record of a jaw position other than centric relation.

eccentric jaw relation. Any jaw relation other than centric relation.

eccentric occlusion. An occlusion other than centric occlusion.

eccentric relation, eccentric position. Any relation of the mandible to the maxillae other than centric relation.

  acquired e. r. An eccentric relation that is assumed by habit in order to bring the teeth together.

edentics. The art, science, and technique used in treating edentulous patients.

edentulate, edentulous. Without teeth, lacking teeth.

edge-to-edge occlusion. An occlusion in which the opposing anterior teeth meet along their incisal edges when the teeth are in centric occlusion.

elastic. Susceptible to being stretched, compressed, or distorted and then tending to assume the original shape.

  e. limit. The greatest stress to which a material may be subjected and still be capable of returning to its original dimensions when the forces are released.

elasticity. The quality which allows a structure or material to return to its original form upon removal of an external force.

  modulus of e. A coefficient found by dividing the unit stress, at any point up to the proportional limit, by its corresponding unit elongation (for tension) or strain.

  physical e. of muscle. The physical quality of muscle of being elastic, that is, yielding to active or passive physical stretch.

  physiologic e. of muscle. The unique biologic quality of muscle of being capable of change and of resuming its size under neuromuscular control.

  total e. of muscle. The combined effect of physical and physiologic elasticity of muscle.

electromyography. The recording of the electric currents set up by muscle activity.

endodontic pin. A metal pin which is placed through the apex of a natural tooth into the bone to stabilize a mobile tooth.

endosseous blade implant. A thin, wedge-shaped metal implant which is placed into the bone to provide an abutment for a fixed or removable denture.

environment. The aggregate of the external conditions and influences affecting the life and development of an organism.

equalization of pressure. The act of equalizing or evenly distributing pressure.

equilibrate. To place in equilibrium.

equilibration. 1. The act or acts of placing a body in the state of equilibrium. 2. The state or condition of being in equilibrium.

  mandibular e. 1. The act or acts performed to place the mandible in equilibrium. 2. A condition in which all of the forces acting upon the mandible are neutralized.

  occlusal e. The modification of occlusal forms of teeth by grinding with the intent of equalizing occlusal stress, producing simultaneous occlusal contacts, or harmonizing cuspal relations.

equilibrator. An instrument or device used in achieving or helping maintain a state of equilibrium.

equilibrium. 1. A state of even adjustment between opposing forces. 2. That state or condition of a body in which any forces acting upon it are so arranged that their product at every point is zero. 3. A balance between active forces and negative resistance.

esthetic denture. A denture which when viewed in the mouth, adds to the patient's charm, beauty, dignity, or naturalness of character.

esthetics. The harmonious components of a restoration, (viz., shape [form], color, and position) which will enhance the appearance of the patient.

  denture e. The cosmetic effect produced by a dental prosthesis which affects the desirable beauty, attractiveness, character, and dignity of the individual.

etiologic factors. The elements or influences that can be assigned as the cause or reason for a disease or lesion.

examination. Scrutiny or investigation for the purpose of making a diagnosis.

extraoral tracing. A tracing made outside the oral cavity.

extrusion. The movement of teeth beyond the natural occlusal plane which may be accompanied by similar movement of their supporting tissues.

F

face form. 1. The outline form of the face. 2. The outline form of the face from an anterior view, sometimes described geometrically as square, tapering, or ovoid and by various combinations of these basic forms.

facebow. 1. A caliper-like device which is used to record the relationship of the maxillae and/or the mandible to the temporomandibular joints. 2. A caliper-like device which is used to record the relationship of the jaws to the temporomandibular joints and to orient the casts on the articulator to the relationship of the opening axis of the temporomandibular joints.

  adjustable axis f., hinge-bow, kinematic f. A face-bow with caliper ends that can be adjusted to permit location of the (hinge) axis of rotation of the mandible.

  f. fork. The part of the face-bow assemblage used to attach the occlusion rim to the face-bow proper.

  f. record. A registration, by means of a face-bow, of the position of the hinge axis and/or the condyles. The face-bow record is used to orient the maxillary and/or mandibular casts to the opening and closing axis of the articulator.

facial profile. 1. The outline form of the face from a lateral view. 2. The sagittal outline form of the face.

festoons. Carvings in the base material of a denture which simulate the contours of the natural tissues which are being replaced by the denture.

final flask closure. The last closure of a flask before curing, after packing of the mold with a denture-base material. Usually, a metal-to-metal contact of the parts of the flask is required.

finish (of a denture). The final perfection of the form of the polished surfaces of a denture.

fistula. A pathologic sinus or abnormal passage resulting from incomplete healing or development of tissue, leading from an internal organ to the surface of the body.

fit. The adaptation of any dental restoration (viz., adaptation of an inlay to the cavity preparation in a tooth or adaptation of a denture to its basal seat.)

fixed partial denture. A partial denture that is cemented to natural teeth or roots which furnish the primary support to the prosthesis.

fixed prosthesis. A restoration or replacement which is attached by a cementing medium to natural teeth, roots, or implants.

fixed support. Support that permits no motion, either of translation or rotation, at the support (bar clamped in vise).

flabby tissue. Excessive movable tissue.

flange. That part of the denture base which extends from the cervical ends of the teeth to the border of the denture.

  buccal f. The portion of the flange of a denture which occupies the buccal vestibule of the mouth.

  denture f. 1. The essentially vertical extension from the body of the denture into one of the vestibules of the oral cavity. Also, on the mandibular denture, the essentially vertical extension along the lingual side of the alveololingual sulcus. 2. The buccal and labial vertical extension of a maxillary and mandibular denture base and the lingual vertical extension of the mandibular denture. The buccal and labial denture flanges have two surfaces: the buccal or labial surface and the basal seat surface. The mandibular lingual flange also has two surfaces: the basal seat surface and the lingual surface.

  f. contour. The design of the flange of a denture.

  labial f. The portion of the flange of a denture which occupies the labial vestibule of the mouth.

  lingual f. The portion of the flange of a mandibular denture which occupies the space adjacent to the tongue.

flask. 1. A metal case or tube used in investing procedures. 2. A sectional metal case in which a sectional mold is made of artificial stone or plaster of Paris for the purpose of compressing and processing dentures or other resinous restorations.

  denture f., crown f. A sectional, boxlike metal case in which a sectional mold is made of artificial stone or plaster of Paris for the purpose of compressing and processing dentures or other resinous restorations.

  refractory f., casting f., casting ring. A metal tube in which a refractory mold is made for casting metal dental restorations.

flask closure. The procedure of bringing the two halves, or parts, of a flask together.

final f. c. The last closure of a flask before curing, after trial packing of the mold with a denture-base material. Usually, a metal-to-metal contact of the parts of the flask is required.

trial f. c. Preliminary closures made for the purpose of eliminating excess denture-base material and ensuring that the mold is completely filled.

flasking. 1. The act of investing in a flask. 2. The process of investing the cast and a wax denture in a flask preparatory to molding the denture-base material into the form of the denture.

foil. An extremely thin, pliable sheet of metal.

gold f. 1. Pure gold rolled into extremely thin sheets. 2. A precious-metal foil used in restoration of carious or fractured teeth.

platinum f. 1. Pure platinum rolled into extremely thin sheets. 2. A precious-metal foil with a high fusing point which makes it suitable as a matrix for various soldering procedures; it is also suitable to provide internal form of porcelain restorations during their fabrication.

tinfoil. 1. Tin rolled into extremely thin sheets. 2. A base-metal foil used as a separating material between the cast and denture-base material during flasking and curing.

force. An influence which when exerted upon a body, tends to set the body into motion or to alter its present state of motion. Force applied to any material causes deformation of that material.

component of f. One of the factors from which a resultant force may be compounded or into which it may be resolved.

masticatory f. The force applied by the muscles of mastication during mastication.

occlusal f. The product of muscular force applied on opposing teeth.

forces of mastication. The motive force created by the dynamic action of the muscles during the physiologic act of mastication.

forward protrusion. A protrusion forward of centric position.

fovea palatinae. Two small pits or depressions in the posterior aspect of the palate, one on each side of the midline, at or near the attachment of the soft palate to the hard palate.

framework. The skeletal portion of a prosthesis (usually metal) around which and to which are attached the remaining portions of the prosthesis to produce the finished restoration (partial denture).

Frankfort plane. A plane passing through the lowest point in the margin of the orbit (the orbitale) and the highest point in the margin of the auditory meatus (the tragion).

free gingival margin. The edge or summit of the free gingival tissue; free gum margin.

free mandibular movements. 1. Any mandibular movements made without tooth interference. 2. Any uninhibited movements of the mandible.

free support. Support that does not permit translation of the beam perpendicular to its axis and presumably offers no restraint to the tendency of the beam to rotate at the support (knife-edge).

free-way space, interocclusal clearance, interocclusal distance, interocclusal gap, interocclusal rest space. The distance between the occluding surfaces of the maxillary and mandibular teeth when the mandible is in its physiologic rest position. This can be determined by calculating the difference between the rest vertical dimension and the occlusal vertical dimension.

frictional attachment, internal attachment, key and keyway attachment, parallel attachment, precision attachment, slotted attachment. A retainer, used in fixed and removable partial denture construction, consisting of a metal receptacle and a closely fitting part; the former is usually contained within the normal or expanded contours of the crown of the abutment tooth and the latter is attached to a pontic or the denture framework.

fulcrum line. An imaginary line around which a removable partial denture tends to rotate.

retentive f. l. 1. An imaginary line connecting the retentive points of clasp arms on retaining teeth adjacent to mucosa-borne denture bases. 2. An imaginary line, connecting the retentive points of clasp arms, around which the denture tends to rotate when subjected to forces, such as the pull of sticky foods.

stabilizing f. l. An imaginary line, connecting occlusal rests, around which the denture tends to rotate under masticatory forces.

full denture prosthetics, complete denture prosthetics. 1. The replacement of the natural teeth in the arch and their associated parts by artificial substitutes. 2. The art and science of the restoration of an edentulous mouth.

full-thickness graft. A transplant of epithelium consisting of skin or mucous membrane with a minimum of subcutaneous tissue.

functional mandibular movements. 1. All natural, proper, or characteristic movements of the mandible made during speech, mastication, yawning, swallowing, and other associated movements. 2. Movements of the mandible which occur during mastication, swallowing, speech, and yawning.

functional occlusal harmony. The occlusal relationship of opposing teeth in all functional ranges and movements that will provide the greatest masticatory efficiency without causing undue strain or trauma upon the supporting tissues.

functional occlusion. The contacts of the maxillary and mandibular teeth during mastication and deglutition.

G

gagging. An involuntary contraction of the muscles of the soft palate or pharynx which results in retching.

gavage. Intranasal feeding by a stomach tube.

generated occlusal path. A registration of the paths of movement of the occlusal surfaces of mandibular teeth on a plastic or abrasive surface attached to the maxillary arch.

geriatrics. That branch of dentistry or medicine which treats all problems peculiar to the aging patient, including the clinical problems of senescence and senility.

   dental g. 1. Treatment of dental problems peculiar to advanced age. 2. Dentistry for the aged patient.

gerodontics. The treatment of dental problems of aging persons or peculiar to advanced age.

gerodontology. The study of the dentition and dental problems in aged or aging persons.

gingiva. The fibrous tissue, covered by mucous membrane, which immediately surrounds a tooth and is continuous with the pericemental ligament.

gingival denture contour. The form of the denture base or other material around the necks of the artificial teeth.

gingival margin, free. The edge or summit of the free gingival tissue; free gum margin.

gingival retraction. The displacement of the marginal gingivae away from a tooth.

gliding occlusion. Used in the sense of designating contacts of teeth in motion. (A substitute for the term *articulation*.)

glossectomy. Partial or total resection of the tongue.

gnathic. Of or pertaining to the jaws.

gnathion. The lowest point of the median line of the mandible.

gnathodynamometer. 1. An instrument for measuring the force exerted in closing the jaws. (Dor.) 2. An instrument used for measuring biting pressure.

gnathology. A science which deals with the masticatory apparatus as a whole, including morphology, anatomy, histology, physiology, pathology, and therapeutics.

gold foil. 1. Pure gold rolled into extremely thin sheets 2. A precious-metal foil used in restoration of carious or fractured teeth.

gothic arch tracer. A tracing which resembles an arrowhead or a gothic arch, made by means of a device attached to the opposing arches. The shape of the tracing depends upon the relative location of the marking point and the tracing table. The apex of a properly made tracing is considered to indicate the most retruded, unstrained relation of the mandible to the maxillae, i.e., centric relation.

gothic arch tracing, arrow-point tracing, needlepoint tracing, stylus tracing. A tracing which resembles an arrowhead or a gothic arch made by means of a device attached to the opposing arches. The shape of the tracing depends upon the tracing table. The apex of a properly made tracing is considered to indicate the most retruded, unstrained relation of the mandible to the maxillae, i.e., centric relation.

graft. A portion of tissue used to replace a defect in the body.

   autograft. A graft taken from one part of the patient's body and transplanted to another part.

   full-thickness g. A transplant of epithelium consisting of skin or mucous membrane with a minimum of subcutaneous tissue.

   heterograft. A graft taken from one species and placed in another.

   homograft. A graft taken from one human subject and transplanted to another.

   split-thickness g. A transplant of epithelium consisting of skin or mucous membrane of a partial thickness that is sectional between the corium and the basement membrane.

guiding planes. Two or more vertically parallel surfaces of abutment teeth so oriented as to direct the path of placement and removal of removable partial dentures.

gums. The fibrous and mucosa covering of the alvolar process or ridges.

gustation. The act of perceiving taste.

H

hamular notch, pterygomaxillary notch. The notch or fissure formed at the junction of the maxilla and the hamular or pterygoid process of the sphenoid bone.

height of contour. A line encircling a tooth designating its greatest circumference at a selected position.

heterograft. A graft taken from one species and placed in another.

high lip line. The greatest height to which the maxillary lip is raised in function.

hinge axis, condylar axis, condyle axis, mandibular axis, transverse axis. An imaginary line through the two mandibular condyles and around which the mandible may rotate without translatory movement.

hinge axis point. A reference point on the skin corresponding with the terminal hinge axis of the mandible.

hinge joint. Ginglymus; a joint which allows motion around an axis.

hinge movement. An opening or closing movement of the mandible on the hinge axis.

hinge position. The orientation of parts in a manner permitting hinge movement between them.

    condylar h. p. The position of the condyles of the mandible in the glenoid fossa at which hinge axis movement is possible.

    mandibular h. p. The position of the mandible in relation to the maxilla at which opening and closing movements can be made on the hinge axis.

    terminal h. p. The position of the mandible in relation to the maxilla from which hinge axis movement can be accomplished.

hinge-bow, adjustable axis face-bow, kinematic face-bow. A face-bow with caliper ends that can be adjusted to permit location of the (hinge) axis of rotation of the mandible.

homograft. A graft taken from one human subject and transplanted to another.

horizontal overlap. The projection of teeth beyond their antagonists in the horizontal direction.

hydrocolloid. The materials listed as colloid sols with water which are used in dentistry as elastic impression materials. Hydrocolloid can be reversible or irreversible.

    irreversible h. (alginate). A hydrocolloid consisting of sols of alginic acid having a physical state which is changed by an irreversible chemical reaction forming an insoluble calcium alginate. (See also *alginate*.)

    reversible h. A hydrocolloid of agar-agar having a physical state that becomes liquid with heat and elastic gel with cooling.

hygroscopic expansion. Expansion due to the absorption of moisture.

hyperplasia. The abnormal multiplication or increase in the number of normal cells in normal arrangement in a tissue. (Dor.)

hypertrophy. An increase in bulk of tissue beyond normal caused by an increase in size but not number of tissue elements.

hypoplasia. Defective or incomplete development. (Dor.)

I

immediate denture. A complete or removable partial denture constructed for insertion immediately following the removal of natural teeth.

implant. A graft or insert set firmly or deeply into or onto the alveolar process that may be prepared for its insertion.

    dental i. A substance that is placed into the jaw to support a crown or fixed or removable denture.

    endosseous blade i. A thin, wedge-shaped metal implant which is placed into the bone to provide an abutment for a fixed or removable denture.

implant abutment, subperiosteal. That portion of the implant which protrudes through the mucosa into the oral cavity for the retention or support of a crown or a fixed or removable denture.

implant denture. A denture which receives its stability and retention from a substructure which is partially or wholly implanted under the soft tissues of the denture basal seat.

    i. d. substructure. The metal framework which is embedded beneath the soft tissues and in contact with the bone for the purpose of supporting an implant denture superstructure.

    i. d. superstructure. The metal framework which is retained and stabilized by the implant denture substructure.

implant substructure (framework), subperiosteal. A skeletal framework of cast metal which fits on the bone under the periosteum.

impression. An imprint or negative likeness of the teeth and/or edentulous areas where the teeth have been removed, made in a plastic material which becomes relatively hard or set while in contact with these tissues. Impressions may be made of full complements of teeth, of areas where some teeth have been removed, or in mouths from which all teeth have been removed. (Impressions are classified according to the materials of which they are made, such as *reversible* and *irreversible hydrocolloid impression, modeling plastic impression, plaster impression, wax impression, silicone impression, Thiokol rubber impression.*)

    cleft-palate i. An impression of a cleft palate.

    direct bone i. An impression of denuded bone used in the construction of denture implants.

    mandibular i., lower i. An impression of the mandibular jaw or dental structures.

    maxillary i., upper i. An impresssion of the maxillary jaw or dental structures.

    partial denture i. 1. A negative copy of the partially edentulous dental arch or area made for the purpose of constructing a partial denture. 2. An impression of a part or all of a partially edentulous arch made for the purpose of designing or constructing a partial denture. 3. An impression of a part or all of a partially edentulous arch.

    preliminary i., primary i. An impression made for the purpose of diagnosis or for the construction of a tray.

    sectional i. An impression that is made in sections.

impression area. That surface which is recorded in an impression.

impression material. Any substance or combination of substances used for making a negative reproduction or impression.

impression surface. That portion of the denture surface which has its contour determined by the impression.

impression technique. A method and manner employed in making a negative likeness.

impression tray. 1. A receptacle into which a suitable material is placed to make an impression. 2. A device which is used to carry, confine, and control an impression material while making an impression.

incisal guidance. The influence of the contacting surfaces of the mandibular and maxillary anterior teeth on mandibular movements.

incisal guide, anterior guidance. That part of an articulator which maintains the incisal guide angle.

incisal guide angle. The angle formed with the horizontal plane by drawing a line in the sagittal plane between incisal edges of the maxillary and mandibular central incisors when the teeth are in centric occlusion.

incisal rest. A rigid extension of a partial denture which contacts an anterior tooth at the incisal edge.

incisive papilla. The elevation of soft tissue covering the foramen of the incisive or nasopalatine canal.

index. 1. A core or mold used to record or maintain the relative position of a tooth or teeth to one another and/or to a cast. 2. A guide, usually made of plaster of Paris, used to reposition teeth or casts or parts in order to reproduce their original positions.

indirect retainer. A part of a removable partial denture which assists the direct retainers in preventing displacement of distal-extension denture bases by functioning through lever action on the opposite side of the fulcrum line.

indirect retention. Retention obtained in a removable partial denture through the use of indirect retainers. (See [*indirect*] *retainer.*)

infrabulge (retention area of a tooth). That portion of the crown of a tooth gingival to the survey line; the height of contour.

initial occlusal contact. The first contact of opposing teeth upon elevation of the mandible toward the maxillae.

injection molding. The adaptation of a plastic material to the negative form of a closed mold by forcing the material into the mold through appropriate gateways. (See also *compression molding.*)

insertion. The intraoral placing of a dental prosthesis.

    path of i. The direction in which a prosthesis is placed upon and removed from the abutment teeth.

interarch distance, interridge distance. 1. The vertical distance between the maxillary and mandibular arches (alveolar or residual) under conditions of vertical dimension which must be specified. 2. The vertical distance between maxillary and mandibular ridges. (See also *reduced interarch distance.*)

interceptive occlusal contact. An initial contact of teeth which stops or deviates the normal movement of the mandible. (See also *occlusal disharmony.*)

intercondylar distance. The distance between the rotational centers of each condyle.

intercuspation. The interdigitation of cusps of opposing teeth.

interdental. Between the proximal surfaces of the teeth of the same arch.

   i. papilla. A projection of the gingiva filling the space between the proximal surfaces of two adjacent teeth.

interdigitation. This refers to teeth and is defined as the act of interlocking or the condition of being interlocked, like the fingers of the folded hand.

interfacial surface tension. The tension or resistance to separation possessed by the film of liquid between two well-adapted surfaces (viz., the thin film of saliva between the denture base and the tissues).

interim denture, provisional denture, temporary denture. A dental prosthesis to be used for a short interval of time for reasons of esthetics, mastication, occlusal support, or convenience or to condition the patient to the acceptance of an artificial substitute for missing natural teeth until more definitive prosthetic therapy can be provided.

intermaxillary relation. Any one of many relations of the mandible to the maxillae, such as centric maxillomandibular relation, eccentric maxillomandibular relation, etc.

intermediary jaw movement. All movements between the extremes of mandibular excursions.

internal attachment, frictional attachment, key and keyway attachment, parallel attachment, precision attachment, slotted attachment. A retainer, used in fixed and removable partial denture construction, consisting of a metal receptacle and a closely fitting part; the former is usually contained within the normal or expanded contours of the crown of the abutment tooth and the latter is attached to a pontic or the denture framework.

internal rest. A rigid metallic extension of a fixed or removable partial denture which contacts an intracoronal preparation in a cast restoration of a tooth.

interocclusal. Between the occlusal surfaces of opposing teeth.

interocclusal distance, free-way space, interocclusal clearance, interocclusal gap, interocclusal rest space. The distance between the occluding surfaces of the maxillary and mandibular teeth when the mandible is in its physiologic rest position. This can be determined by calculating the difference between the rest vertical dimension and the occlusal vertical dimension.

interocclusal record. A record of the positional relation of the opposing teeth or jaws to each other made on occlusal surfaces of occlusion rims or teeth in a plastic material which hardens, such as plaster of Paris, wax, or zinc oxide/eugenol paste.

   centric i. r. A record of the centric jaw position (relation).

   eccentric i. r. A record of a jaw position other than centric relation.

   lateral i. r., lateral checkbite. A record of a lateral eccentric jaw position.

   protrusive i. r. A record of a protruded eccentric jaw position.

interproximal space. The space between adjacent teeth in a dental arch. It is divided into the embrasure occlusal to the contact point and the septal space gingival to the contact point.

interridge distance, interarch distance. 1. The vertical distance between the maxillary and mandibular arches (alveolar or residual) under conditions of vertical dimension which must be specified. 2. The vertical distance between maxillary and mandibular ridges. (See also *reduced interarch distance.*)

intramucosal inserts. Metal inserts with undercuts which are placed into selected surgically prepared locations of the mucosa to enhance the retention of removable dentures.

intraoral. Within the mouth. (Dor.)

   i. tracing. A tracing made within the oral cavity.

invest. To surround, envelop, or embed in an investment material.

investing. The process of covering or enveloping, wholly or in part, an object, such as a denture, tooth, wax form, crown, etc., with a refraction investment material before curing, soldering, or casting.

   vacuum i. The investing of a pattern within a vacuum.

investment. 1. Any material used in dentistry to invest an object. 2. The material used to enclose or surround a pattern of a dental restoration for casting or molding or to maintain the relations of metal parts during soldering.

   refractory i. An investment material which can withstand the high temperatures used in soldering or casting.

investment cast, refractory cast. A cast made of a material that will withstand high temperatures without disintegrating.

irreversible hydrocolloid (alginate). A hydrocolloid consisting of sols of alginic acid having a physical state which is changed by an irreversible chemical reaction forming an insoluble calcium alginate. (See also *alginate.*)

isometric contraction. Muscular contraction in which there is no change in the length of the muscle during contraction.

isotonic contraction. Muscle contraction in which there is a shortening of the length of the muscle while the muscle maintains a constant tension.

J

jaw. A common name for either the maxillae or the mandible.

jaw malposition. Any abnormal position of the mandible.

jaw movement. 1. Movements of the lower jaw. 2. Any changes in position of which the mandible is capable.

    intermediary j. m. All movements between the extremes of mandibular excursions.

jaw relation. Any relation of the mandible to the maxillae.

    centric j. r. 1. The jaw relation when the condyles are in the most posterior, unstrained position in the glenoid fossae at any given degree of jaw separation from which lateral movement can be made. 2. The most posterior relation of the mandible to the maxillae at the established vertical dimension. 3. The relation of the mandible to the maxillae when the condyles are in their most posterior position in the glenoid fossa from which unstrained lateral movements can be made at the occluding vertical dimension normal for the individual.

    eccentric j. r. Any jaw relation other than centric relation.

    median j. r. Any jaw relation when the mandible is in the median sagittal plane.

    posterior border j. r. The most posterior relation of the mandible to the maxillae at any specific vertical relation.

    protrusive j. r. A jaw relation resulting from a protrusion of the mandible.

    rest j. r. The habitual postural jaw relation when the patient is resting comfortably in an upright position and the condyles are in a neutral, unstrained position in the glenoid fossae.

    unstrained j. r. 1. The relation of the mandible to the skull when a state of balanced tonus exists among all the muscles involved. 2. Any jaw relation which is attained without undue or unnatural force and which causes no undue distortion of the tissues of the temporomandibular joints.

jaw relation record. A registration of any positional relationship of the mandible in reference to the maxillae. These records may be of any of the many vertical, horizontal, or orientation relations.

    terminal j. r. r. A record of the relationship of the mandible to the maxilla made at the vertical dimension of occlusion and at the centric relation.

jaw repositioning. The changing of any relative position of the mandible to the maxillae, usually by altering the occlusion of the natural or artificial teeth.

K

Kennedy bar, continuous bar retainer. 1. A metal bar usually resting on lingual surfaces of teeth to aid in their stabilization and to act as indirect retainers. 2. A metal bar which contacts lingual surfaces of anterior teeth and aids in the retention of a distal-extension partial denture.

key and keyway attachment, frictional attachment, internal attachment, parallel attachment, precision attachment, slotted attachment. A retainer, used in fixed and removable partial denture construction, consisting of a metal receptacle and a closely fitting part; the former is usually contained within the normal or expanded contours of the crown of the abutment tooth and the latter is attached to a pontic or the denture framework.

kinematic face-bow, adjustable axis face-bow, hinge-bow. A face-bow with caliper ends that can be adjusted to permit location of the (hinge) axis of rotation of the mandible.

L

labial. 1. Of or pertaining to a lip. 2. Toward a lip.

    l. bar. A major connector located labial to the dental arch joining two or more bilateral parts of a removable partial denture.

    l. flange. The portion of the flange of a denture which occupies the labial vestibule of the mouth.

l. **vestibule.** That portion of the oral cavity which is bounded on one side by the teeth, gingivae, and alveolar ridge (in the edentulous mouth, the residual ridge) and on the other by the lips and cheeks.

lateral. A position either right or left of the midsagittal plane.

l. **checkbite, l. interocclusal record.** A record of a lateral eccentric jaw position.

l. **condylar inclination.** The direction of the lateral condyle path.

l. **condyle path.** The path of the condyle in the glenoid fossa when a lateral mandibular movement is made.

l. **incisor.** The second incisor.

l. **interocclusal record, l. checkbite.** A record of a lateral eccentric jaw position.

l. **movement.** A movement from either right or left of the midsagittal plane.

l. **protrusion.** A protrusion with a lateral component.

l. **relation.** The relation of the mandible to the maxillae when the lower jaw is in a position to either side of centric relation.

line of occlusion. The alignment of the occluding surfaces of the teeth in a horizontal plane. (See *occlusal plane.*)

lingual. Pertaining to the tongue; next to or toward the tongue.

l. **bar.** A major connector located lingual to the dental arch joining two or more bilateral parts of a mandibular removable partial denture.

l. **flange.** The portion of the flange of a mandibular denture which occupies the space adjacent to the tongue.

l. **plate, linguoplate.** A major connector of a removable partial denture extended to contact the lingual surfaces of anterior teeth and in some instances, the lingual surfaces of the posterior teeth.

l. **rest.** A metallic extension of a removable partial denture framework that fits onto a horizontally prepared lingual rest within an abutment tooth which provides denture support and indirect retention.

linguoplate, lingual plate. A major connector of a removable partial denture extended to contact the lingual surfaces of anterior teeth and in some instances, the lingual surfaces of the posterior teeth.

lip line, high. The greatest height to which the maxillary lip is raised in function.

lip line, low. 1. The lowest position of the lower lip during the act of smiling or voluntary retraction. 2. The lowest position of the upper lip at rest.

longitudinal axis. (See *sagittal axis.*)

low lip line. 1. The lowest position of the lower lip during the act of smiling or voluntary retraction. 2. The lowest position of the upper lip at rest.

lower impression, mandibular impression. An impression of the mandibular jaw or dental structures.

M

major connector. A part of a removable partial denture which connects the components on one side of the arch to the components on the opposite side of the arch.

malocclusion. 1. Any deviation from a physiologically acceptable contact of opposing dentitions. 2. Any deviation from a normal occlusion.

mandible. The lower jaw bone.

mandibular anteroposterior ridge slope. The slope of the crest of the mandibular residual ridge from the third molar region to its most anterior aspect in relation to the lower border of the mandible as viewed in profile.

mandibular axis, condylar axis, condyle axis, hinge axis, transverse axis. An imaginary line through the two mandibular condyles around which the mandible may rotate without translatory movement.

mandibular condyle. The articular process of the mandible.

mandibular equilibration. 1. The act or acts performed to place the mandible in equilibrium. 2. A condition in which all of the forces acting upon the mandible are neutralized.

mandibular glide. The side-to-side, protrusive, and intermediate movement of the mandible occurring when the teeth or other occluding surfaces are in contact.

mandibular guide-plane prosthesis. A prosthesis with an extension designed to direct a resected mandible into an occlusal contact relationship with the maxilla.

mandibular hinge position. The position of the mandible in relation to the maxilla at which opening and closing movements can be made on the hinge axis.

mandibular impression, lower impression. An impression of the mandibular jaw or dental structures.

mandibular movement(s). Any movement of the lower jaw.

   free m. m. 1. Any mandibular movements made without tooth interference. 2. Any uninhibited movements of the mandible.

mandibular protraction. A type of facial anomaly in which the gnathion lies anterior to the orbital plane.

mandibular resection. The removal of a portion or all of the mandible.

mandibular retraction. A type of facial anomaly in which the gnathion lies posterior to the orbital plane.

masking. An opaque covering to camouflage the metal parts of a prosthesis.

master cast. A replica of the prepared tooth surfaces (where necessary), residual ridge areas, and/or other parts of the dental arch used to fabricate a dental restoration or prosthesis.

mastication. The process of chewing food for swallowing and digestion.

   components of m. The various jaw movements which are made during mastication as determined by the neuromuscular system, the temporomandibular articulations, the teeth, and the food being chewed. The components of the masticatory cycle may be separated (for purposes of analysis or description) into opening components of mastication, closing components of mastication, left lateral components of mastication, right lateral components of mastication, and anteroposterior components of mastication.

   forces of m. The motive force created by the dynamic action of the muscles during the physiologic act of mastication.

   organ of m. The combination of all the structures involved in speech and in receiving, mastication of, and deglutition of food.

masticatory apparatus. The combination of all the structures involved in speech and in receiving, mastication of, and deglutition of food.

masticatory cycles. The patterns of mandibular movements formed during the chewing of food.

masticatory efficiency. A measure of the comminution of food expended by a person to achieve the same degree of comminution attained by a control subject.

masticatory force. The force applied by the muscles of mastication during mastication.

masticatory movements. 1. Chewing movements. 2. Mandibular movements used for chewing food.

masticatory performance. A measure of the comminution of food attainable under standard testing conditions.

masticatory system. The organs and structures primarily functioning in mastication. They are: jaws, teeth with their supporting structures, temporomandibular articulations, mandibular musculature, tongue, lips, cheeks, and oral mucosa (ADA definition).

maxilla. The irregularly shaped bone that with its fellow maxillae, forms the upper jaw; assists in the formation of the orbit, the nasal cavity, and the palate; and lodges the maxillary teeth.

maxillae. Plural of maxilla.

maxillary impression, upper impression. An impression of the maxillary jaw or dental structures.

maxillary protraction. A type of facial anomaly in which the subnasion lies anterior to the orbital plane.

maxillectomy. The removal of a portion or all of the maxilla.

maxillofacial. Pertaining to the jaws and the face. (Dor.)

   m. prosthetics. That branch of dentistry that provides prostheses to treat or restore tissues of the stomatognathic system and associated facial structures that have been affected by disease, injury, surgery, or congenital defect, providing all possible function and esthetics.

maxillomandibular record, maxillomandibular registration. 1. A record of the relation of the mandible to the maxillae. 2. The act of recording the relation of the mandible to the maxillae.

maxillomandibular relation. Any one of the many relations of the mandible to the maxillae, such as centric maxillomandibular relation, eccentric maxillomandibular relation, etc.

mean foundation plane. The mean of the various irregularities in form and inclination of the basal seat.

mechanically balanced occlusion. A balanced occlusion without reference to physiologic considerations, as on an articulator.

median jaw relation. Any jaw relation when the mandible is in the median sagittal plane.

median line. 1. The intersection of the midsagittal plane with the maxillary and mandibular dental arches. 2. The center line dividing the central body surface into the right and left.

median mandibular point. A point on the anteroposterior center of the mandibular ridge in the median sagittal plane.

mesial. 1. Toward or situated in the middle, as the median line of the body or the center of the dental arch. 2. Situated in the middle; median; toward the middle line of the body or toward the center line of the dental arch. (Dor.)

metal base. A metallic portion of a denture base forming a part or all of the basal surface of the denture. It serves as a base for the attachment of the acrylic resin part of the denture base and the teeth.

metal-insert teeth. Teeth designed to contain metal cutting edges in the occlusal surfaces.

milled-in paths, milled-in curves. 1. Contours carved by various mandibular movements into the occluding surface of an occlusion rim by teeth or studs placed in the opposing occlusion rim. 2. Occlusal curves developed by masticatory or gliding movements of occlusion rims which may be composed of materials that are abrasive. (See also *chew-in record*.)

milling-in. The procedure of refining or perfecting the occlusion of teeth by the use of abrasives between their occluding surfaces while the dentures are rubbed together in the mouth or on the articulator. (See also *selective grinding*.)

minor connector. The connecting link between the major connector or base of a removable partial denture and other units of the prosthesis, such as clasps, indirect retainers, and occlusal rests.

model. An object formed or poured in a matrix or impression with any desired material to create a positive likeness or some other desired form of the object.

modeling plastic, modeling composition, modeling compound. A thermoplastic material usually composed of gum dammar and prepared chalk, used especially for making dental impressions.

modified cast. A master cast that is altered prior to processing a denture base.

modiolus. A point near the corner of the mouth where several muscles of facial expression converge.

modulus of elasticity. A coefficient found by dividing the unit stress, at any point up to the proportional limit, by its corresponding unit of elongation (for tension) or strain.

modulus of resilience. The work or energy required to stress a cubic inch of material (in one direction only) from zero up to the proportional limit of the material, measured by the ability of the material to withstand the momentary effect of an impact load while stresses remain within the proportional limit.

mold. 1. A form in which an object is cast or shaped. 2. The term used to specify the shape of an artificial tooth or teeth.

  mother matrix m. A negative form, usually in sections, used for making positive casts.

Monson curve. The curve of occlusion in which each cusp and incisal edge touches or conforms to a segment of the surface of a sphere 8 inches in diameter with its center in the region of the glabella.

mounting. The laboratory procedure of attaching the maxillary and/or mandibular cast to an articulator.

  split-cast m. 1. A cast with key grooves on its base mounted on an articulator for the purpose of easy removal and accurate replacement. Split remounting metal plates may be used instead of grooves in casts. 2. A means of testing the accuracy of articulator adjustment.

mouth rehabilitation. Restoration of the form and function of the masticatory apparatus to as near normal as possible.

mucobuccal fold. The line of flexure of the mucous membrane as it passes from the mandible or maxillae to the cheek.

mucositis. Inflammation of the surface of the mucous membrane.

mucostatic. 1. The normal, relaxed condition of mucosal tissues covering the jaws. 2. Arresting the secretion of mucus.

muscle contraction. The development of tension in a muscle in response to nerve stimulation.

muscle hypertenseness. Increased muscular tension which is not easily released but which does not prevent normal lengthening of the muscles involved.

muscle, physical elasticity of. The physical quality of muscle of being elastic, that is, yielding to active or passive physical stretch.

muscle, physiologic elasticity of. The unique biologic quality of muscle of being capable of resuming its size under neuromuscular control.

muscle relaxant. A drug which specifically aids in lessening of muscle tension.

muscle spasm. Increased muscular tension and shortness which cannot be released voluntarily and which prevent lengthening of the muscles involved.

muscle spasticity. Increased muscular tension of antagonists preventing normal movement and caused by an inability to relax (a loss of reciprocal inhibition).

muscle, total elasticity of. The combined effect of physical and physiologic elasticity of muscle.

muscle trimming, border molding, tissue molding. The shaping of an impression material by the manipulation or action of the tissues adjacent to the borders of an impression.

mylohyoid region. The region on the lingual surface of the mandible marked by the mylohyoid ridge and the attachment of the mylohyoid muscle.

N

nasion. The point at which the nasofrontal suture is bisected by the midsagittal plane.

natural dentition, dentition. The natural teeth, as considered collectively, in the dental arch; may be deciduous, permanent, or mixed.

neck of the condyle. That portion of the mandibular ramus to which the condyle is attached.

needlepoint tracing, arrow-point tracing, gothic arch tracing, stylus tracing. A tracing which resembles an arrowhead or a gothic arch made by means of a device attached to the opposing arches. The shape of the tracing depends upon the location of the marking point relative to the tracing table. The apex of a properly made tracing is considered to indicate the most retruded, unstrained relation of the mandible to the maxillae, i.e., centric relation.

neutral zone. The potential space between the lips and cheeks on one side and the tongue on the other. Natural or artificial teeth in this zone are subject to equal and opposite forces from the surrounding musculature.

nonanatomic teeth. Artificial teeth with occlusal surfaces which are not anatomically formed but which are designed to improve the function of mastication.

notch, hamular, pterygomaxillary notch. The notch or fissure formed at the junction of the maxilla and the hamular or pterygoid process of the sphenoid bone.

O

obturator. A prosthesis used to close a congenital or acquired opening in the palate.

occlude. 1. To bring together; to shut. 2. To bring or close the mandibular teeth into contact with the maxillary teeth.

occluder. A name given to some articulators.

occluding centric relation record. A registration of centric relation made at the established occlusal vertical dimension.

occluding relation. The jaw relation at which the opposing teeth occlude.

occlusal. 1. Pertaining to the contacting surfaces of opposing occlusal units (teeth or occlusion rims). 2. Pertaining to the masticating surfaces of the posterior teeth.

occlusal adjustment. 1. Any change in the occlusion intended to alter the occluding relation. 2. Any alteration of the occluding surfaces of the teeth or restorations designed to result in a more physiologic condition of teeth, their supporting structures, and the mandibular articulation.

occlusal analysis, occlusion analysis. A systematic examination of the masticatory system with special consideration of the effect of tooth occlusions on the teeth themselves and on their related structures.

occlusal balance. A condition in which there are simultaneous contacts of occluding units on both sides of the opposing dental arches during eccentric movements within the functional range.

occlusal clearance. A condition in which the opposing occlusal surfaces may glide over one another without any interfering projection.

occlusal contact, deflective. A condition in which tooth contacts divert the mandible from a normal path of closure. (See also *occlusal disharmony.*)

occlusal contact, initial. The first contact of opposing teeth upon elevation of the mandible toward the maxillae.

occlusal contact, interceptive. An initial contact of teeth which stops or deviates the normal movement of the mandible. (See also *occlusal disharmony.*)

occlusal correction. The correction of malocclusion.

occlusal curvature. 1. A curved surface which makes simultaneous contact with the major portions of the incisal and occlusal prominences of the existing teeth. 2. The curve of a dentition on which the occlusal surfaces lie.

occlusal disharmony. (See also *occlusal contact, deflective,* and *occlusal contact, interceptive.*) 1. Contacts of opposing occlusal surfaces of teeth which are not in harmony with other tooth contacts and with the anatomic and physiologic control of the mandible. 2. Occlusions which do not coincide with their respective jaw relations.

occlusal equilibration. The modification of occlusal forms of teeth by grinding with the intent of equalizing occlusal stress, producing simultaneous occlusal contacts, or harmonizing cuspal relations.

occlusal force. The product of muscular force applied on opposing teeth.

occlusal form. The form of the occlusal surface of a tooth or a row of teeth.

occlusal harmony. A condition in centric and eccentric jaw relation in which there are no interceptive or deflective contacts of occluding surfaces.

    functional o. h. The occlusal relationship of opposing teeth in all functional ranges and movements that will provide the greatest masticatory efficiency without causing undue strain or trauma upon the supporting tissues.

occlusal path. 1. A gliding occlusal contact. 2. The path of movement of an occlusal surface.

    generated o. p. A registration of the paths of movement of the occlusal surfaces of mandibular teeth on a plastic or abrasive surface attached to the maxillary arch.

occlusal pattern. The form or design of the occluding surfaces of a tooth or teeth. These forms may be based upon natural or modified anatomic or nonanatomic concepts of teeth.

occlusal pivot. An elevation contrived on the occluding surface, usually in the molar region, designed to act as a fulcrum, and to induce a change in mandibular rotation.

    adjustable o. p. An occlusal pivot which may be adjusted vertically by means of a screw or other device.

occlusal plane, plane of occlusion. An imaginary surface which is related anatomically to the cranium and which theoretically touches the incisal edges of the incisors and the tips of the occluding surfaces of the posterior teeth. It is not a plane in the true sense of the word but represents the mean of the curvature of the surface.

occlusal position. The relationship of the mandible and maxillae when the jaw is closed and the teeth are in contact. This position may or may not coincide with centric occlusion.

occlusal pressure. Any force exerted upon the occlusal surfaces of teeth.

occlusal rest. A rigid extension of a partial denture which contacts the occlusal surface of a tooth.

occlusal surface, denture. That portion of the surface of a denture or dentition which makes contact or near contact with the corresponding surface of the opposing denture or dentition.

occlusal system, occlusal scheme. The form or design and arrangement of the occlusal and incisal units of a dentition or the teeth on a denture.

occlusal vertical dimension. The length of the face when the teeth (occlusal rims, central-bearing point, or any other stop) are in contact and the mandible is in centric relation or the teeth are in centric relation.

occlusal wear. Attritional loss of substance on opposing occlusal units or surfaces. (See *abrasion.*)

occlusion. Any contact between the incising or masticating surfaces of the maxillary and mandibular teeth.

    balanced o. 1. An occlusion of the teeth which presents a harmonious relation of the occluding surfaces in all centric and eccentric positions within the functional range of mastication and swallowing. 2. The simultaneous contacting of the maxillary and mandibular teeth on the right and left and in the posterior and anterior occlusal areas in centric and eccentric positions, developed to lessen or limit a tipping or rotating of the denture bases in relation to the supporting structures.

    centric o. The centered contact position of the occlusal surfaces of the mandibular teeth against the occlusal surfaces of the maxillary teeth.

    components of o. The various factors which are involved in occlusion, such as the temporomandibular joint, the associated neuromusculature, the teeth, and the denture-supporting structures.

    eccentric o. Any occlusion other than centric occlusion.

    edge-to-edge o. An occlusion in which the opposing anterior teeth meet along their incisal edges when the teeth are in centric occlusion.

functional o. The contacts of the maxillary and mandibular teeth during mastication and deglutition.

gliding o. Used in the sense of designating contacts of teeth in motion. (A substitute for the term *articulation.*)

line of o. The alignment of the occluding surfaces of the teeth in horizontal plane. (See *occlusal plane.*)

mechanically balanced o. A balanced occlusion without reference to physiologic considerations, as on an articulator.

pathogenic o. An occlusal relationship capable of producing pathologic changes in the supporting tissues.

physiologic o. Occlusion in harmony with functions of the masticatory system.

physiologically balanced o. A balanced occlusion which is in harmony with the temporomandibular joints and the neuromuscular system.

plane of o., occlusal plane. An imaginary surface which is related anatomically to the cranium and which theoretically touches the incisal edges of the incisors and the tips of the occluding surfaces of the posterior teeth. It is not a plane in the true sense of the word but represents the mean of the curvature of the surface.

protrusive o. An occlusion of the teeth when the mandible is protruded.

spherical form of o. An arrangement of teeth which places their occlusal surfaces on an imaginary sphere (usually 8 inches in diameter) with its center above the level of the teeth.

traumatic o. An occlusion of the teeth which is injurious to oral structures.

traumatogenic o. An occlusion of the teeth which is capable of producing injury to oral structures.

working o., working bite relation. The occlusal contacts of teeth on the side to which the mandible is moved.

occlusion analysis, occlusal analysis. A systematic examination of the masticatory system with special consideration of the effect of tooth occlusions on the teeth themselves and on their related structures.

occlusion rim, record rim. Occluding surfaces built on temporary or permanent denture bases for the purpose of making maxillomandibular relation records and arranging teeth.

opening movement. Movement of the mandible executed during jaw separation.

posterior o. m. The opening movement of the mandible about the terminal hinge axis.

orbital exenteration. The removal of the entire contents of the orbit.

organ of mastication. The combination of all the structures involved in speech and in receiving, mastication of, and deglutition of food.

overbite, vertical overlap. 1. The distance teeth lap over their antagonists vertically This term is used especially for the distance the maxillary incisal edges drop below the mandibular ones, but it may be used also to describe the vertical relations of opposing cusps. 2. The extension of the maxillary teeth over the mandibular teeth in a vertical direction when the posterior teeth are in maximum intercuspation. 3. The vertical relationship of the incisal edges of the maxillary incisors to the mandibular incisors when the teeth are in maximum intercuspation.

overclosure, reduced interarch distance. An occluding vertical dimension which results in an excessive interocclusal distance when the mandible is in rest position and in a reduced interridge distance when the teeth are in contact.

overjet, overjut. The projection of the upper anterior and/or posterior teeth beyond their antagonists in a horizontal direction.

P

packing. The act of filling a mold.

denture p. Filling and compressing a denture-base material into a mold in a flask.

palatal bar. A major connector which crosses the palate and unites two or more parts of a maxillary removable partial denture.

palatal incompetency. The inability of an anatomically complete soft palate to effect a functional palatopharyngeal sphincter valve.

palatal insufficiency. An anatomical inadequacy of the soft palate in which the palatopharyngeal sphincter is incomplete.

palatal seal, posterior palatal seal, postpalatal seal. The seal at the posterior border of a denture.

posterior p. s. area. The soft tissues along the junction of the hard and soft palates on which pressure within the physiologic limits of the tissues can be applied by a denture to aid in the retention of the denture.

palatogram. A graphic representation of the area of the palate contacted by the tongue in a specified activity.

palatopharyngeal closure. A sphincteric action sealing the oral cavity from the nasal cavity by the synchronous movement of the soft palate superiorly, the lateral pharyngeal wall medially, and the posterior wall of the pharynx anteriorly.

papilla. Any small, nipple-shaped elevation. (Dor.)

    incisive p. The elevation of soft tissue covering foramen of incisive or nasopalatine canal.

    interdental p. A projection of the gingiva filling the space between the proximal surfaces of two adjacent teeth.

parallel attachment, frictional attachment, internal attachment, key and keyway attachment, precision attachment, slotted attachment. A retainer, used in fixed and removable partial denture construction, consisting of a metal receptacle and a closely fitting part; the former is usually contained within the normal or expanded contours of the crown of the abutment tooth and the latter is attached to a pontic or the denture framework.

parallelometer. 1. An instrument for determining relative parallelism. 2. An apparatus used for making a part or an object parallel with some other part or object or for paralleling attachments and abutments for fixed partial dentures or precision attachments for removable partial dentures.

partial denture. A dental prosthesis which restores one or more but not all of the natural teeth and/or associated parts and which is supported by the teeth and/or the mucosa; it may be removable or fixed.

partial denture construction. The science and technique of designing and constructing partial dentures.

partial denture impression. 1. A negative copy of the partially edentulous dental arch or area made for the purpose of constructing a partial denture. 2. An impression of a part or all of a partially edentulous arch made for the purpose of designing or constructing a partial denture. 3. An impression of a part or all of a partially edentulous arch.

Passavant's pad, bar, ridge. 1. The bulging of the posterior pharyngeal wall produced by the upper portion of the superior constrictor muscle of the pharynx during the act of swallowing or phonation. 2. A ridge of erectile tissue on the posterior wall of the pharynx.

passivity. The quality or condition of inactivity or rest assumed by the teeth, tissues, and denture when a removable partial denture is in place but not under masticatory pressure.

path of insertion The direction in which a prosthesis is placed upon and removed from the abutment teeth.

pathogenic occlusion. An occlusal relationship capable of producing pathologic changes in the supporting tissues.

pathology. The branch of medical science which deals with disease in all its relations, especially its nature and the functional and material changes caused by it. (See also *speech pathology*.)

pathosis. A condition of disease. Not to be called *pathology*.

pattern. A form which is used to make a mold, as for an inlay or partial denture framework.

    occlusal p. The form or design of the occluding surfaces of a tooth or teeth. These forms may be based upon natural or modified anatomic or nonanatomic concepts of teeth.

    wax p. A wax form of a shape which, when invested and burned out, will produce a mold in which the casting is made.

pear-shaped area. A mass of tissue, frequently pear-shaped, which is located at the distal termination of the mandibular residual ridge.

phonetic values. The character or quality of vocal sounds.

phonetics. The science of sounds used in speech.

physiologic occlusion. Occlusion in harmony with functions of the masticatory system.

physiologic rest position. The postural position of the mandible when the patient is resting comfortably in the upright position and the condyles are in a neutral, unstrained position in the glenoid fossae.

physiologically balanced occlusion. A balanced occlusion which is in harmony with the temporomandibular joints and the neuromuscular system.

pickling. The process of cleansing metallic surfaces of the product of oxidation and other impurities by immersion in acid.

plane, cusp. The small imaginary plane in which two buccal cusp tips and the highest lingual cusp are located.

plane, Frankfort. A plane passing through the lowest point in the margin of the orbit (the orbitale) and the highest point in the margin of the auditory meatus (the tragion).

plane motion. The combined motions of translation and rotation of rigid body in which all parts of the body move in parallel planes.

plane of occlusion, occlusal plane. An imaginary surface which is related anatomically to the cranium and which theoretically touches the incisal edges of the incisors and the tips of the occluding surfaces of the posterior teeth. It is not a plane in the true sense of the word but represents the mean of the curvature of the surface.

planes of reference. Planes which act as a guide to the location of other planes.

plaster. A colloquial term applied to dental plaster of Paris.

    p. of Paris. 1. Calcined calcium sulfate in the form of a fine powder. About one half of the water of crystallization has been driven off, and when water is added, it solidifies to a porous mass that is used extensively in dentistry and surgery. (Dor.) 2. The hemihydrate of calcium sulfate which, when mixed with water, forms a paste which subsequently sets.

plastic base. A denture or record base made of a plastic material.

plastic teeth. Artificial teeth fabricated from organic resins.

platinum foil. 1. Pure platinum rolled into extremely thin sheets. 2. A precious-metal foil with a high fusing point which makes it suitable as a matrix for various soldering procedures; it is also suitable to provide internal form of porcelain restorations during their fabrication.

Pleasure curve. A curve of occlusion which in transverse cross-section conforms to a line which is convex upward except for the last molars.

polished surface denture. That portion of the surface of a denture which extends in an occlusal direction from the border of the denture and includes the palatal surface. It is the part of the denture base which is usually polished, and it includes the buccal and lingual surfaces of the teeth.

polishing. 1. (Verb.) Making smooth and glossy, usually by friction; giving luster. 2. (Noun.) The act or process of making a denture or casting smooth and glossy.

polymerization. The forming of a compound from several single molecules of the same substance, the molecular weight of the new compound being a multiple equal to the number of single molecules which have been combined. (Gould.)

pontic. An artificial tooth on a fixed partial denture. It replaces the lost natural tooth, restores its functions, and usually occupies the space previously occupied by the natural crown.

posterior border jaw relation. The most posterior relation of the mandible to the maxillae at any specific vertical relation.

posterior border movement. Lateral movement of the mandible along the posterior limit of the envelope of motion.

posterior border position. The most posterior position of the mandible at any specific vertical relation to the maxillae.

posterior opening movement. The opening movement of the mandible about the terminal hinge axis.

posterior palatal seal, palatal seal, postpalatal seal. The seal at the posterior border of a denture.

posterior palatal seal area. The soft tissues along the junction of the hard and soft palates on which pressure within the physiologic limits of the tissues can be applied by a denture to aid in the retention of the denture.

postpalatal seal, palatal seal, posterior palatal seal. The seal at the posterior border of a denture.

pour hole. An aperture in investment or other mold material leading to the prosthesis space into which prosthetic material is poured.

precision attachment, frictional attachment, internal attachment, key and keyway attachment, parallel attachment, slotted attachment. A retainer, used in fixed and removable partial denture construction, consisting of a metal receptacle and a closely fitting part; the former is usually contained within the normal or expanded contours of the crown of the abutment tooth and the latter is attached to a pontic or the denture framework.

precision rest. A prefabricated, rigid metallic extension of a fixed or removable partial denture which fits intimately into a box-type rest or keyway (female) portion of a precision attachment in a cast restoration of a tooth.

preliminary impression, primary impression. An impression made for the purpose of diagnosis or for the construction of a tray.

premature contact. An initial contact of teeth prior to closure of the mandible to the maxilla. (See *deflective occlusal contact* and *interceptive occlusal contact*.)

prematurity. A condition of tooth contacts which diverts the mandible from a normal path of closure.

preoperative cast, diagnostic cast, study cast. A positive likeness of a part or parts of the oral cavity for the purpose of study and treatment planning.

preoperative records. Any record(s) made for the purpose of study or treatment planning.

pressure area. An area of excessive displacement of tissue.

primary impression, preliminary impression. An impression made for the purpose of diagnosis or for the construction of a tray.

process. 1. (Anatomy.) A marked prominence or projection of a bone. 2. (Dental.) A technical procedure which converts a wax pattern, such as that of a wax trial base, into a solid denture base of another material.

processed denture base. That portion of a polymerized prosthesis covering the oral mucosa of the maxilla and/or mandible to which artificial teeth will be attached with a second processing.

profile. An outline or contour, especially one representing a side view of a human head. (See also *facial profile.*)

profile record. A registration or record of the profile of a patient.

prognosis. A forecast as to the probable result of an attack of disease; the prospect as to recovery from a disease afforded by the nature and symptoms of the case. In denture service, an opinion of the prospects for success of a restoration.

  denture p. An opinion or judgment given in advance of treatment of the prospects for success in the construction of dentures and for their usefulness.

proportional limit. That unit of stress at which deformations are no longer proportional to applied loads.

prosthesis. An artificial replacement of an absent part of the human body.

  cleft-palate p. A restoration to correct congenital defects in the palate and in related structures if they are involved.

  cranial p. An artificial replacement for a portion of the skull.

  definitive p. A prosthesis to be used over an extended period of time.

  dental p. An artificial replacement of one or more teeth and/or associated structures.

  fixed p. A restoration or replacement which is attached by a cementing medium to natural teeth, roots, or implants.

  mandibular guide-plane p. A prosthesis with an extension designed to direct a resected mandible into an occlusal contact relationship with the maxilla.

  postsurgical p. An artificial replacement of a missing part or parts after operation.

  provisional p. An interim prosthesis designed for use for varying periods of time.

  speech p. A prosthesis that assists in the management of speech disorders associated with a congenital or acquired defect of the palate.

  superimposed p. The overlay of artificial teeth on the surfaces of natural teeth to improve occlusion, arch form, and esthetics.

  surgical p. A prosthesis prepared to assist in surgical procedures.

  therapeutic p. A prosthesis used to transport and retain some agent for therapeutic purposes, such as a radium carrier.

prosthetic dentistry, prosthodontia, prosthodontics. 1. That branch of dental art and science pertaining to the restoration and maintenance of oral function by the replacement of missing teeth and structures with artificial devices. 2. The science and art of providing suitable substitutes for the coronal portions of teeth or for one or more lost or missing natural teeth and their associated parts in order that function, appearance, comfort, and health of the patient may be restored. (ADA.)

prosthetic restoration. An artificial replacement of an absent part of the human body.

prosthetic speech aid. A prosthesis used to close a defect in the hard and/or soft palate or to replace lost tissue necessary for the production of intelligible speech.

prosthetics. The art and science of supplying artificial replacements for missing parts of the human body.

  complete denture p., full denture p. 1. The replacement of the natural teeth in the arch and their associated parts by artificial substitutes. 2. The art and science of the restoration of an edentulous mouth.

  maxillofacial p. That branch of dentistry that provides prostheses to treat or restore tissues of the stomatognathic system and associated facial structures that have been affected by disease, injury, surgery, or congenital defect, providing all possible function and esthetics.

  somatoprosthetics. The art and science of prosthetically replacing external parts of the body that are missing or deformed.

prosthetist. An individual involved in the construction of an artificial replacement for any part of the human body.

prosthodontics, prosthodontia, prosthetic dentistry. 1. That branch of dental art and science pertaining to the restoration and maintenance of oral function by the replacement of missing teeth and structures with artificial devices. 2. The science and art of providing suitable substitutes for the coronal portions of teeth or for one or more lost or missing natural teeth and their associated parts in order that function, appearance, comfort, and health of the patient may be restored. (ADA.)

prosthodontist. A dentist engaged in the practice of prosthodontics.

protrusion. A position of the mandible forward of or lateral to centric position.

　forward p. A protrusion forward of centric position.

　lateral p. A protrusion with a lateral component.

protrusive interocclusal record. A record of a protruded eccentric jaw position.

protrusive jaw relation. A jaw relation resulting from a protrusion of the mandible.

protrusive occlusion. An occlusion of the teeth when the mandible is protruded.

protrusive record. A registration of a forward position of the mandible with reference to the maxillae.

protrusive relation. The relation of the mandible to the maxillae when the mandible is thrust forward.

provisional denture, interim denture, temporary denture. A dental prosthesis to be used for a short interval of time for reasons of esthetics, mastication, occlusal support, or convenience or to condition the patient to the acceptance of an artificial substitute for missing natural teeth until more definitive prosthetic therapy can be provided.

provisional prosthesis. An interim prosthesis designed for use for varying periods of time.

psychosomatic. Pertaining to the mind-body relationship; having bodily symptoms of a psychic, emotional, or mental origin. (Dor.)

　p. dentistry. Dentistry which concerns itself with the mind-body relationship.

pterygomaxillary notch, hamular notch. The notch or fissure formed at the junction of the maxilla and the hamular or pterygoid process of the sphenoid bone.

Q

quick-cure resin, activated resin, autopolymer resin, cold-curing resin, self-curing resin. A resin which can be polymerized by an activator and a catalyst without use of external heat.

R

radiogram, radiograph, roentgenogram, roentgenograph. A shadow image record made on a sensitized film or plate by roentgen rays.

rebase. A process of refitting a denture by the replacement of the denture-base material.

reciprocal arm. A clasp arm or other extension used on a removable partial denture to oppose the action of some other part or parts of the prosthesis.

reciprocation. The means by which one part of a prosthesis is made to counter the effect created by another part.

record base, baseplate, temporary base, trial base. A temporary substance representing the base of a denture which is used for making maxillomandibular (jaw) relation records and for the arrangement of teeth.

record rim, occlusion rim. Occluding surfaces built on temporary or permanent denture bases for the purpose of making maxillomandibular relation records and arranging teeth.

reduced interarch distance, overclosure. An occluding vertical dimension which results in an excessive interocclusal distance when the mandible is in rest position and in a reduced interridge distance when the teeth are in contact.

refractory cast, investment cast. A cast made of a material that will withstand high temperatures without disintegrating.

refractory flask, casting flask, casting ring. A metal tube in which a refractory mold is made for casting metal dental restorations.

refractory investment. An investment material which can withstand the high temperatures used in soldering or casting.

registration. The record of desired jaw relations used to transfer these relations to an articulator. (See also *maxillomandibular record.*)

relief. The reduction or elimination of undesirable pressure or force from a specific area under a denture base.

r. area. The portion of the surface of the mouth upon which pressures or forces are reduced or eliminated.

r. chamber. A recess in the impression surface of a denture to reduce or eliminate pressure or forces from that area of the mouth.

reline. To resurface the tissue side of a denture with new base material to make the denture fit more accurately.

removable partial denture. A partial denture which can be removed from the mouth and replaced at will.

residual ridge. The portion of the alveolar ridge and its soft-tissue covering which remains following the removal of teeth.

resin. A broad term used to indicate organic substances, usually translucent or transparent, soluble in ether, etc., but not in water. They are named according to their chemical composition, physical structure, and means for activation or curing. Examples: acrylic resin, autopolymer resin, synthetic resin, styrene resin, and vinyl resin.

acrylic r. A general term applied to a resinous material of the various esters of acrylic acid.

a. r. base. A plastic denture base made of an acrylic resin.

a. r. denture. A denture made of acrylic resin.

a. r. tooth. A tooth made of acrylic resin.

a. r. tray. A tray made of acrylic resin.

autopolymer r., activated r., cold-curing r., quick-cure r., self-curing r. A resin which can be polymerized by an activator and a catalyst without use of external heat.

copolymer r. A synthetic resin which is the product of the concurrent and joint polymerization of two or more different monomers or polymers.

resorption. 1. A loss of tissue substance by physiologic or pathologic means. 2. The reduction of the volume and size of the alveolar portion of the mandible or maxillae.

rest. A rigid (stabilizing) extension of a fixed or removable partial denture which contacts a remaining tooth or teeth to dissipate vertical or horizontal forces.

incisal r. A rigid extension of a partial denture which contacts an anterior tooth at the incisal edge.

internal r. A rigid metallic extension of a fixed or removable partial denture which contacts an intracoronal preparation in a cast restoration of a tooth.

lingual r. A metallic extension of a removable partial denture framework that fits onto a horizontally prepared lingual rest within an abutment tooth which provides denture support and indirect retention.

occlusal r. A rigid extension of a partial denture which contacts the occlusal surface of a tooth.

precision r. A prefabricated, rigid metallic extension of a fixed or removable partial denture which fits intimately into a box-type rest seat or keyway (female) portion of a precision attachment in a cast restoration of a tooth.

r. area, r. seat. That portion of a natural tooth or a cast restoration of a tooth selected or prepared to receive an occlusal, incisal, lingual, internal, or semiprecision rest.

semiprecision r. A rigid metallic extension of a fixed or removable partial denture which fits into an intracoronal preparation in a cast restoration of a tooth.

rest jaw relation. The habitual postural jaw relation when the patient is resting comfortably in an upright position and the condyles are in a neutral, unrestrained position in the glenoid fossae.

rest position. The postural relation of the mandible to the maxillae when the patient is resting comfortably in the upright position and the condyles are in an unstrained position in the glenoid fossae.

rest vertical dimension. The length of the face when the mandible is in rest position. (See also *interocclusal distance.*)

restoration. A broad term applied to any inlay, crown, fixed or removable partial denture, or complete denture which restores or replaces lost tooth structure, teeth, or oral tissues. (See also *prosthetic restoration.*)

retainer. Any type of clasp, attachment, or device used for the fixation or stabilization of a prosthesis.

continuous bar r., Kennedy bar. 1. A metal bar usually resting on lingual surfaces of teeth to aid in their stabilization and to act as indirect retainers. 2. A metal bar which contacts lingual surfaces of anterior teeth and aids in the retention of a distal-extension partial denture.

direct r. A clasp or attachment applied to an abutment tooth for the purpose of holding a removable denture in position.

indirect r. A part of a removable partial denture which assists the direct retainers in preventing displacement of distal-extension denture bases by functioning through lever action on the opposite side of the fulcrum line.

retention. That quality inherent in the prosthesis which resists the force of gravity, the adhesiveness of foods, and the forces associated with the opening of the jaws. (See also *denture retention*.)

direct r. Retention obtained in a removable partial denture by the use of clasps or attachments which resist removal from the abutment teeth.

indirect r. Retention obtained in a removable partial denture through the use of indirect retainers. (See [*indirect*] *retainer*.)

retention arm. An extension which is part of a removable partial denture and which is utilized to aid in the fixation of the prosthesis; a part of a clasp.

retention of denture. The resistance of a denture to dislodgment.

retentive arm. A flexible segment of a removable partial denture which engages an undercut on an abutment and which is designed to retain the denture.

retentive circumferential clasp arm. A circumferential clasp arm which is flexible and engages the infrabulge area of the abutment tooth at the terminal end of the arm.

retentive fulcrum line. 1. An imaginary line connecting the retentive points of clasp arms on retaining teeth adjacent to mucosa-borne denture bases. 2. An imaginary line, connecting the retentive points of clasp arms, around which the denture tends to rotate when subjected to forces, such as the pull of sticky foods.

retrognathic. A retruded position of the mandible in relation to the maxilla.

retromolar pad. A mass of tissue, frequently pear-shaped, which is located at the distal termination of the mandibular residual ridge.

retromylohyoid area. That area in the alveololingual sulcus just lingual to the retromolar pad which extends lingually down to the floor of the mouth and back to the retromylohyoid curtain. It is bounded anteriorly by the lingual tuberosity (the distal end of the mylohyoid ridge).

retromylohyoid space. That area in the alveololingual sulcus just lingual to the retromolar pad bounded anteriorly by the lingual tuberosity, posteriorly by the retromylohyoid curtain, inferiorly by the floor of the alveololingual sulcus, and lingually by the anterior tonsillar pillar.

retrusion. 1. The state of being located posterior to the normal position, as malposition of a tooth posteriorly in the line of occlusion. 2. The backward movement or position of the mandible.

reverse curve. A curve of occlusion which in transverse cross-section conforms to a line which is convex upward.

reversible hydrocolloid. A hydrocolloid of agar-agar having a physical state that becomes liquid with heat and elastic gel with cooling.

ridge. The remainder of the alveolar process and its soft-tissue covering after the teeth are removed.

alveolar r. The bony ridge (alveolar process) of the maxillae or mandible which contains the alveoli (sockets of the teeth).

center of r. The buccolingual midline of the residual ridge.

crest of r. The highest continuous surface of the residual ridge but not necessarily the center of the ridge.

Passavant's r., bar, pad. 1. The bulging of the posterior pharyngeal wall produced by the upper portion of the superior constrictor muscle of the pharynx during the act of swallowing or phonation. 2. A ridge of erectile tissue on the posterior wall of the pharynx.

residual r. The portion of the alveolar ridge and its soft-tissue covering which remains following the removal of teeth.

ridge relation. The positional relation of the mandibular ridge to the maxillary ridge.

ridge slope, mandibular anteroposterior. The slope of the crest of the mandibular residual ridge from the third molar region to its most anterior aspect in relation to the lower border of the mandible as viewed in profile.

Roach clasp. A clasp with arms that are bar-type extensions from major connectors or from within the denture base; the arms pass adjacent to the soft tissues and approach the point or area of contact on the tooth in a gingivo-occlusal direction.

roentgenogram, roentgenograph, radiogram, radiograph. A shadow image record made on a sensitized film or plate by roentgen rays.

root. The portion of the tooth which is covered by cementum and normally is attached to the periodontal ligament and hence to the bone.

rotation. The movement of a rigid body in which the parts move in circular paths with their centers on a fixed, straight line that is called the axis of rotation. In mandibular motion, this is unnatural and can only be demonstrated by manipulation or guidance.

rotation center. A point or line around which all other points in a body move.

rouge. A compound composed of iron oxide for providing a high luster to a polished surface such as gold.

rugae. The irregular ridges in the mucous membrane located in the anterior third of the hard palate.

S

saddle, denture base. 1. That part of a denture which rests on the oral mucosa and to which the teeth are attached. 2. That part of a complete or partial denture which rests upon the basal seat and to which the teeth are attached.

sagittal axis. An imaginary anteroposterior line through a mandibular condyle around which a mandible may rotate in a yawing or pitching motion.

scaffold. A support, either natural or prosthetic, that maintains the contour of tissue.

scribe. To write, trace, or mark by making a line or lines with a pointed instrument.

sectional impression. An impression that is made in sections.

segment. Any of the parts into which a body naturally separates or is divided, either actually or by an imaginary line.

selective grinding. The modification of the occlusal forms of teeth by grinding at selected places marked by spots made by articulating paper.

self-curing resin, activated resin, autopolymer resin, cold-curing resin, quick-cure resin. A resin which can be polymerized by an activator and a catalyst without use of external heat.

semiprecision rest. A ridged metallic extension of a fixed or removable partial denture which fits into an intracoronal preparation in a cast restoration of a tooth.

separating medium. 1. Any coating used upon a surface which serves to prevent another surface from adhering to the first. 2. A material usually coated on impressions to facilitate removal of the cast.

setting expansion. The dimensional increase which occurs concurrently with the hardening of various materials, such as plaster of Paris, dental stone, die stone and dental casting investment, usually amounting to 0.08 to 0.5 per cent.

shade selection, tooth color selection. The determination of the color (hue, brilliance, saturation) of an artificial tooth or set of teeth for a given patient.

shearing stress. The internal induced force that opposes the sliding of one plane on an adjacent plane or the force that resists a twisting action.

shellac bases. Certain resinous materials adapted to maxillary or mandibular casts to form impression trays or record trays.

slotted attachment, frictional attachment, internal attachment, key and keyway attachment, parallel attachment, precision attachment. A retainer, used in fixed and removable partial denture construction, consisting of a metal receptacle and a closely fitting part; the former is usually contained within the normal or expanded contours of the crown of the abutment tooth and the latter is attached to a pontic or the denture framework.

solder. 1. (Noun.) A fusible alloy of metals used to unite the edges or surfaces of two pieces of metal. (Dor.) 2. (Verb.) The act of uniting two pieces of metal by the proper alloy of metals.

somatoprosthetics. The art and science of prosthetically replacing external parts of the body that are missing or deformed.

span length. The length of the beam between two supports.

spatulate. To mix or manipulate with a spatula.

spatulation. The manipulation of material with a spatula in order to mix it into a homogenous mass.

speech aid. Therapy or an instrument, apparatus, or device used to improve speech.

  prosthetic s. a. A prosthesis used to close a defect in the hard and/or soft palate or to replace lost tissue necessary for the production of intelligible speech.

speech pathology. The study and treatment of all aspects of functional and organic speech defects and disorders.

speech prosthesis. A prosthesis that assists in the management of speech disorders associated with a congenital or acquired defect of the palate.

speech science. The broad field dealing with the study, analysis, and measurement of all the components of the processes involved in the production and perception of speech.

spherical form of occlusion. An arrangement of teeth which places their occlusal surfaces on an imaginary sphere (usually 8 inches in diameter) with its center above the level of the teeth.

splint. 1. (Noun.) A prosthesis which maintains hard and/or soft tissue in a predetermined position. 2. A rigid or flexible material (wood, metal, plaster, fabric, or adhesive tape) used to protect, immobilize, or restrict motion in a part. 3. (Verb.) To immobilize, support, or brace.

splinting (of abutments). The joining of two or more teeth into a rigid unit by means of fixed restorations.

split-cast method. 1. A procedure for placing indexed casts on an articulator to facilitate their removal and replacement on the instrument. 2. The procedure of checking the ability of an articulator to receive or be adjusted to a maxillomandibular relation record.

split-cast mounting. 1. A cast with key grooves on its base mounted on an articulator for the purpose of easy removal and accurate replacement. Split remounting metal plates may be used instead of grooves in casts. 2. A means of testing the accuracy of articulator adjustment.

split-thickness graft. A transplant of epithelium consisting of skin or mucous membrane of a partial thickness that is sectional between the corium and the basement membrane.

sprue. Wax or metal used to form the aperture or apertures for molten metal to flow into a mold to make a casting; also, the metal which later fills the sprue hole or holes.

sprue former. The base to which the sprue is attached while the wax pattern is being invested in a refractory investment in a casting flask.

stability. The quality of a denture to be firm, steady, or constant, to resist displacement by functional stresses, and not to be subject to change of position when forces are applied.

    denture s. 1. The resistance of a denture to movement on its basal seat. 2. A quality of a denture that permits it to maintain a state of equilibrium in relation to the basal seat and/or abutment teeth.

    dimensional s. The ability of a material to retain its size and form.

stabilization. The seating or fixation of a fixed or removable denture so that it will not tilt or be displaced under pressure.

stabilized baseplate (base). A baseplate lined with a plastic material to improve its fit and adaptation.

stabilizing circumferential clasp arm. A circumferential clasp arm which is relatively rigid and contacts the height of contour of the tooth.

stabilizing fulcrum line. An imaginary line, connecting occlusal rests, around which the denture tends to rotate under masticatory forces.

staining. Modification of the color of the tooth or denture base.

static relation. Relationship between two parts that are not in motion.

stomatognathic system. The combination of all the structures involved in speech and in the receiving, mastication, and deglutition of food.

stomatology. The study of the structures, functions, and diseases of the mouth.

stone die. A positive likeness in dental stone or improved stone used in the fabrication of a dental restoration.

stress. An internal force that resists an externally applied load or force.

    compressive s. The internal induced force that opposes the shortening of the material in a direction parallel to the direction of the stresses.

    shearing s. The internal induced force that opposes the sliding of one plane on an adjacent plane or the force that resists a twisting action.

    tensile s. The internal induced force that resists the elongation of a material in a direction parallel to the direction of the stresses.

stress-bearing area. 1. The portion of the mouth capable of providing support for a denture. 2. Surfaces of oral structures which resist forces, strains, or pressures brought upon them during function. (See *denture foundation area* and *basal seat*.)

stress breaker. A device which relieves the abutment teeth of all or part of the occlusal forces.

study cast, diagnostic cast, preoperative cast. A positive likeness of a part or parts of the oral cavity for the purpose of study and treatment planning.

stylus tracing, arrow-point tracing, gothic arch tracing, needlepoint tracing. A tracing which resembles an arrowhead or a gothic arch made by means of a device attached to the opposing arches. The shape of the tracing depends upon the location of the marking point relative to the tracing table. The apex of a properly made tracing is considered to indicate the most retruded, unstrained relation of the mandible to the maxillae, i.e., centric relation.

sublingual. Pertaining to the region or structures located beneath the tongue.

    s. crescent. The crescent-shaped area on the floor of the mouth formed by the lingual wall of the mandible and the adjacent part of the floor of the mouth.

    s. fold. The crescent-shaped area on the floor of the mouth following the inner wall of the mandible and tapering toward the molar regions. It is formed by the sublingual gland and submaxillary duct.

submucosal inserts. Metal inserts with undercuts which are placed into selective, surgically prepared locations of the mucosa to enhance the retention of dentures.

subocclusal surface. A portion of the occlusal surface of a tooth which is below the level of the occluding portion of the tooth.

subperiosteal implant abutment. That portion of the implant which protrudes through the mucosa into the oral cavity for the retention or support of a crown or a fixed or removable denture.

subperiosteal implant substructure (framework). A skeletal framework of cast metal which fits on the bone under the periosteum.

substructure (framework), subperiosteal implant. A skeletal framework of cast metal which fits on the bone under the periosteum.

substructure, implant denture. The metal framework which is embedded beneath the soft tissues and in contact with the bone for the purpose of supporting an implant denture superstructure.

sulcus. 1. A furrow, trench, or groove as on the surface of the brain or in folds of mucous membrane. 2. A groove or depression on the surface of a tooth. 3. A groove in a portion of the oral cavity.

superimposed prosthesis. The overlay of artificial teeth on the surfaces of natural teeth to improve occlusion, arch form, and esthetics.

superstructure, implant denture. The metal framework which is retained and stabilized by the implant denture substructure.

support. That location or point at which one of the induced equilibrants to the applied loads is placed.

    fixed s. Support that permits no motion, either of translation or rotation, at the support (bar clamped in vise).

    free s. Support that does not permit translation of the beam perpendicular to its axis and presumably offers no restraint to the tendency of the beam to rotate at the support (knife-edge).

    restrained s. Support that permits no motion perpendicular to the beam axis, but permits some rotation at the support but less than in the free support (fixed partial denture).

supporting area. Those areas of the maxillary and mandibular edentulous ridges which are considered best suited to carry the forces of mastication when the dentures are in function.

suprabulge. That portion of the crown of a tooth which converges toward the occlusal surface of the tooth.

surgical prosthesis. A prosthesis prepared to assist in surgical procedures.

surgical template. A thin, transparent, plastic resin processed base formed to duplicate the tissue surface of an immediate denture and used as a guide for surgically shaping the alveolar process to fit an immediate denture.

survey line. 1. A line produced on a cast of a tooth by a surveyor or scriber marking the greatest height of contour in relation to the chosen path of insertion of a planned restoration. 2. A line drawn on a tooth or teeth of a cast by means of a surveyor for the purpose of determining the positions of the various parts of a clasp or clasps.

surveying. The procedure of locating and delineating the contour and position of the abutment teeth and associated structures before designing a removable partial denture.

surveyor. An instrument used in construction of a removable partial denture to locate and delineate the contours and relative positions of abutment teeth and associated structures.

swage. To shape metal by hammering or adapting it onto a die.

swallowing threshold. 1. The moment the act of swallowing begins after the mastication of food. 2. The critical moment of reflex action initiated by minium stimulation prior to the act of deglutition.

T

technique, technic. A detailed procedure in the fabrication of a prosthesis. (See also *impression technique.*)

teeth. (Plural of tooth.) Organs of mastication.

anatomic t. 1. Artificial teeth which duplicate the anatomic forms of natural teeth. 2. Teeth which have prominent pointed or rounded cusps on the masticating surfaces and which are designed to occlude with the teeth of the opposing denture or natural dentition.

cross-bite t. Posterior teeth designed to accommodate the modified buccal cusps of the maxillary teeth to be positioned in the fossae of the mandibular teeth.

cuspless t. Teeth designed without cuspal prominences on the occlusal surface.

metal-insert t. Teeth designed to contain metal cutting edges in the occlusal surfaces.

nonanatomic t. Artificial teeth with occlusal surfaces which are not anatomically formed but which are designed to improve the function of mastication.

plastic t. Artificial teeth fabricated from organic resins.

set of t. A complete complement of maxillary and/or mandibular teeth as they are carded by the manufacturer in anterior and posterior segments.

tube t. Artificial teeth with an internal, vertical, cylindrical aperture extending from the center of the base upward into the body of the tooth, into which a pin may be placed or cast for the attachment of the tooth to a denture (fixed or removable) base.

zero-degree t. Artificial posterior teeth having no cusp angles in relation to the horizontal occlusal surface.

template. 1. A pattern or mold. 2. A curved or flat surface pattern which is used as an aid in setting teeth.

surgical t. A thin, transparent, plastic resin processed base formed to duplicate the tissue surface of an immediate denture and used as a guide for surgically shaping the alveolar process to fit an immediate denture.

temporary base, baseplate, record base, trial base. A temporary substance representing the base of a denture which is used for making maxillomandibular (jaw) relation records and for the arrangement of teeth.

temporary denture, interim denture, provisional denture. A dental prosthesis to be used for a short interval of time for reasons of esthetics, mastication, occlusal support, or convenience or to condition the patient to the acceptance of an artificial substitute for missing natural teeth until more definitive prosthetic therapy can be provided.

temporomandibular articulation. The articulation of the condyloid process of the mandible and the interarticular disk with the mandibular fossa of the temporal bone.

temporomandibular joint. The union between the temporal bone and the mandible. It is a diarthrodial, ginglymus (sliding-hinge) paired joint.

temporomandibular joint syndrome, Costen's syndrome. Those various symptoms of discomfort, pain, or pathosis stated to be caused by loss of vertical dimension, lack of posterior occlusion, or other malocclusion, trismus, muscle tremor, arthritis, or direct trauma to the temporomandibular joint.

tensile stress. The internal induced force that resists the elongation of a material in a direction parallel to the direction of the stresses.

tension. The state of being stretched, strained, or extended.

interfacial surface t. The tension or resistance to separation possessed by the film of liquid between two well-adapted surfaces (viz., the thin film of saliva between the denture base and the tissues).

terminal hinge position. The position of the mandible in relation to the maxilla from which hinge axis movement can be accomplished.

terminal jaw relation record. A record of the relationship of the mandible to the maxilla made at the vertical dimension of occlusion and at the centric relation.

therapeutic prosthesis. A prosthesis used to transport and retain some agent for therapeutic purposes, such as a radium carrier.

thermal expansion. Expansion caused by heat.

thermoplastic. A characteristic or property of a material which allows it to be softened by the application of heat and to harden upon cooling.

tinfoil. 1. Tin rolled into extremely thin sheets. 2. A base-metal foil used as a separating material between the cast and denture-base material during flasking and curing.

tinted denture base. A denture base with coloring that simulates the color and shading of natural oral tissues.

tissue. 1. The various cellular combinations which make up the body. 2. An aggregation of similarly specialized cells united in the performance of a particular function.

hyperplastic t. Excessive movable tissue. (See *flabby tissue.*)

tissue-bearing area, denture foundation. That portion of the oral structures which is available to support a denture.

tissue displaceability. 1. The quality of oral tissues which permits them to be placed in other than a relaxed position. 2. The degree to which tissues permit displacement.

tissue displacement. The change in the form or position of tissues as the result of pressure.

tissue molding, border molding, muscle trimming. The shaping of an impression material by the manipulation or action of the tissues adjacent to the borders of an impression.

tissue reaction. The response of tissues to altered conditions.

tissue registration. The accurate recording of the shape of tissues by means of a suitable impression material.

tooth arrangement. 1. The placement of teeth on a denture with definite objectives in mind. 2. The setting of teeth on trial bases.

anterior t. a. The arrangement of anterior teeth for esthetic or phonetic effects.

tooth-borne. A term used to describe a prosthesis or part of a prosthesis which depends entirely upon the abutment teeth for support.

tooth-borne base. The denture base restoring an edentulous area which has abutment teeth at each end for support. The tissue which it covers is not used for support.

tooth color selection, shade selection. The determination of the color (hue, brilliance, saturation) of an artificial tooth or set of teeth for a given patient.

tooth form. The characteristics of the curves, lines, angles, and contours of various teeth which permit their identification and differentiation.

anterior t. f. The outline form and other contours of an anterior tooth.

posterior t. f. The distinguishing contours of the occlusal surfaces of the various posterior teeth.

tooth selection. The selection of a tooth or teeth of a shape, size, and color to harmonize with the individual characteristics of a patient.

torque. A rotational force applied to a denture base, tooth, or dental restoration.

toughness. The ability of a material to withstand stresses and strains without breaking.

tracer, arrow-point tracer. 1. A mechanical device used to trace a pattern of mandibular movements. 2. A mechanical device with a marking point attached to one jaw and a graph plate or tracing plate attached to the other jaw. It is used to record the direction and extent of movements of the mandible. (See also *gothic arch tracer.*)

tracing. A line or lines, scribed by a pointed instrument, representing a record of movements of the mandible.

extraoral t. A tracing made outside the oral cavity.

intraoral t. A tracing made within the oral cavity.

needlepoint t., arrow-point t., gothic arch t., stylus t. A tracing which resembles an arrowhead or a gothic arch made by means of a device attached to the opposing arches. The shape of the tracing depends upon the location of the marking point relative to the tracing table. The apex of a properly made tracing is considered to indicate the most retruded, unstrained relation of the mandible to the maxillae, i.e., centric relation.

tracing device. A device which provides a central point of bearing, or support, between maxillary and mandibular occlusion rims or dentures. It consists of a contacting point which is attached to one occlusion rim or denture and a plate attached to the opposing occlusion rim or denture which provides the surface on which the bearing point rests or moves. It is used for the purpose of distributing closing forces evenly throughout the areas of the supporting structures during the recording of maxillomandibular relations and/or for correction of disharmonious occlusal contacts.

transfer coping. A metallic, acrylic resin, or other covering or cap used to position a die in an impression.

transitional denture. A removable partial denture serving as a temporary prosthesis to which artificial teeth will be added as natural teeth are lost and which will be replaced after postextraction tissue changes have occurred. A transitional denture may become an interim denture when all of the natural teeth have been removed from the dental arch.

translatory movement. The motion of a body at any instant when all points within the body are moving at the same velocity and in the same direction.

transverse axis, condylar axis, condyle axis, hinge axis, mandibular axis. An imaginary line through the two mandibular condyles around which the mandible may rotate without translatory movement.

trauma. 1. An injury or wound to a part of the living body caused by the application of external force or by violence. 2. An actual alteration of dental tissues produced by occlusal disharmony.

traumatic. Pertaining to or caused by an injury. (Dor.)

    t. occlusion. An occlusion of the teeth which is injurious to oral structures.

traumatogenic. Capable of producing a wound or injury.

    t. occlusion. An occlusion of the teeth which is capable of producing injury to oral structures.

treatment denture. A dental prosthesis used for the purpose of treating or conditioning the tissues which are called upon to support and retain a denture base.

treatment plan. The sequence of procedures planned for the treatment of a patient following diagnosis.

trial base, baseplate, record base, temporary base. A temporary substance representing the base of a denture which is used for making maxillomandibular (jaw) relation records and for the arrangement of teeth.

trial denture. A setup of artificial teeth so fabricated that it may be placed in the patient's mouth to verify esthetics, to make records, or for any other operation deemed necessary before the completion of the final denture.

trial flask closure. Preliminary closures made for the purpose of eliminating excess denture-base material and ensuring that the mold is completely filled.

try-in. A preliminary insertion of a removable denture wax-up (trial denture) or a partial denture casting or a finished restoration to determine the fit, esthetics, maxillomandibular relation, etc.

tube teeth. Artificial teeth with an internal, vertical, cylindrical aperture extending from the center of the base upward into the body of the tooth, into which a pin may be placed or cast for the attachment of the tooth to a denture (fixed or removable) base.

U

ultimate strength. The greatest unit stress that may be induced in the material in a test to complete rupture.

undercut. 1. That portion of the surface of a residual ridge, cast, tooth, or other object which is inferior to the height of contour and thus would impede the placement or withdrawal of anything closely adapted to the surface of the object. 2. That portion of a tooth which lies between the survey line (height of contour) and the gingivae. 3. The contour of a cross section of a residual ridge or dental arch which would prevent the insertion of a denture. 4. The contour of flasking stone which interlocks in such a way as to prevent the separation of the parts.

unilateral partial denture. A dental prosthesis restoring lost or missing teeth on one side of the arch only.

unstrained jaw relation. 1. The relation of the mandible to the skull when a state of balanced tonus exists among all the muscles invloved. 2. Any jaw relation which is attained without undue or unnatural force and which causes no undue distortion of the tissues of the temporomandibular joints.

upper impression, maxillary impression. An impression of the maxillary jaw or dental structures.

V

vacuum casting. The casting of a metal in the presence of vacuum.

vacuum investing. The investing of a pattern within a vacuum.

vacuum mixing. A method of mixing a material such as plaster of Paris under subatmospheric pressure.

vertical dimension, vertical opening. The length of the face as determined by the amount of separation of the jaws.

    occlusal v. d. The length of the face when the teeth (occlusal rims, central-bearing point, or any other stop) are in contact and the mandible is in centric relation or the teeth are in centric relation.

    rest v. d. The length of the face when the mandible is in rest position. (See also *interocclusal distance*.)

vertical dimension decrease. Decreasing the vertical distance between the mandible and the maxillae by modifications (1) of teeth, (2) of the positions of teeth or occlusion rims, or (3) through alveolar or residual ridge resorption.

vertical dimension increase. Increasing the vertical distance between the mandible and the maxillae by modifications of teeth, the positions of teeth, or occlusion rims.

vertical opening, vertical dimension. The length of the face as determined by the amount of separation of the jaws.

vertical overlap, overbite. 1. The distance teeth lap over their antagonists vertically. This term is used especially for the distance the maxillary incisal edges drop below the mandibular ones, but it may be used also to describe the vertical relations of opposing cusps. 2. The extension of the maxillary teeth over the mandibular teeth in a vertical direction when the posterior teeth are in maximum intercuspation. 3. The vertical relationship of the incisal edges of the maxillary incisors to the mandibular incisors when the teeth are in maximum intercuspation.

vestibule. That portion of the oral cavity which is bounded on one side by the teeth, gingivae, and alveolar ridge (in the edentulous mouth, the residual ridge) and on the other by the lips and cheeks.

   buccal v. That portion of the oral cavity which is bounded on one side by the teeth, gingivae, and alveolar ridge (in the edentulous mouth, the residual ridge) and on the other by the cheeks.

   labial v. That portion of the oral cavity which is bounded on one side by the teeth, gingivae, and alveolar ridge (in the edentulous mouth, the residual ridge) and on the other by lips.

vibrating line. The imaginary line across the posterior part of the palate marking the division between the movable and immovable tissues of the soft palate which can be identified when the movable tissues are moving.

vulcanite. A combination of caoutchouc and sulphur which hardens in the presence of suitable heat and pressure (an obsolete denture-base material).

vulcanize. To produce flexible or hard rubber, as desired, by subjecting caoutchouc, in the presence of sulphur, to heat and high steam pressure in a vulcanizer.

W

warp. Torsional change of shape or outline, such as that which may occur in swaging sheet metal, or the change in shape of a plastic denture base which may occur when internal stresses are released by heating.

wax, boxing. Wax specifically used for boxing impressions.

wax, casting. A composition containing various waxes with controlled properties used in making patterns to determine the shape of metal castings.

wax expansion. A method of expanding the wax patterns to compensate for the shrinkage of gold during the casting process.

wax pattern. A wax form of a shape which, when invested and burned out, will produce a mold in which the casting is made.

waxing. The contouring of a wax pattern or the wax base of a trial denture into the desired form.

whiting. A pure white chalk (calcium carbonate) which has been ground and washed and which is used for polishing dental materials.

work. The product of force acting on a body and the distance of which the point of application of the force moves.

working bite relation, working occlusion. The occlusal contacts of teeth on the side to which the mandible is moved.

working contacts. Contacts of teeth made on the side of the occlusion toward which the mandible is moved.

working occlusion, working bite relation. The occlusal contacts of teeth on the side to which the mandible is moved.

working side. The lateral segment of a denture or dentition on the side toward which the mandible is moved.

X

x ray. A shadow image record made on a sensitized film or plate by roentgen rays.

Z

zero-degree teeth. Artificial posterior teeth having no cusp angles in relation to the horizontal occlusal surface.

ADDENDUM: SPEECH AND HEARING TERMS

acoustic spectrum. The distribution of the intensity levels of the various frequency components of a sound.

adiadochokinesis. Inability to perform rapid alternating movements, such as opening and closing the jaws or lips, raising and lowering the eyebrows, or tapping the finger.

affricate. A fricative speech sound initiated by a plosive. Examples are /ts/ as in /chw/ and /dz/ as in jam.

agnosia. Loss of the function of recognition of individual sensory stimuli; varieties correspond with the several senses.

air conduction. The normal process of conducting sound waves through the ear canal to the drum membrane.

aphasia. Loss of symbolic formulation and expression due to brain lesion (stroke).

aphonia. Loss or absence of voice as a result of the failure of the vocal cords to vibrate properly.

articulation, speech. The production of individual sounds in connected discourse; the movement and placement during speech of the organs which serve to interrupt or modify the voiced or unvoiced air stream into meaningful sounds; the speech function performed largely through the movements of the lower jaw, lips, tongue, and soft palate.

audiogram. A graphic summary of the measurements of hearing loss showing number of decibels loss at each frequency tested.

audiology. The study of the entire field of hearing, including the anatomy and function of the ear, impairment of hearing, and the education or re-education of the person with hearing loss.

audiometer. A device for the testing of hearing; it is calibrated to register hearing loss in terms of decibels.

auditory discrimination. Ability to discriminate between sounds of different frequency, intensity, and pressure-pattern components; ability to distinguish one speech sound from another.

babbling. A stage in the acquisition of speech during which the child carries on vocal play with random production of different speech sounds.

baby talk. A speech defect characterized by substitution of speech sounds similar to those used by the normal speaking child in the early stages of speech development. Same as lalling and infantile speech.

bilabial. Used to describe a consonant sound formed with the aid of both lips, as in /p/, /b/, and /m/.

bone conduction. The transmission of sound waves through the head bones to the inner ear.

cluttering. Rapid, nervous speech marked by omission of sounds or syllables.

conduction deafness. An impairment of hearing due to damage or obstruction of the ear canal, drum membrane, or the ossicular chain in the middle ear; a failure of air vibrations to be adequately conducted to the cochlea.

consonant. A conventional speech sound produced, with or without laryngeal vibration, by certain successive contractions of the articulatory muscles which modify, interrupt, or obstruct the expired air stream to the extent that its pressure is raised.

delayed speech. Failure of speech to develop at the expected age, usually due to slow maturation, hearing impairment, brain injury, mental retardation, or emotional disturbance.

denasality. Pertains to the quality of the voice when the nasal passages are obstructed to prevent adequate nasal resonance during speech.

diadochokinesis. The performance of repetitive movements, such as lowering and raising the mandible, occluding and opening the lips, and tapping with the finger.

dysarthria. A disorder of articulation due to impairment of the part of the central nervous system which directly controls the muscles of articulation.

dyslalia. Defective articulation due to faulty learning or to abnormality of the external speech organs and not due to lesions of the central nervous system.

fricative. Any speech sound produced by forcing an air stream through a narrow opening and resulting in audible high-frequency vibrations. Examples are /f/, /s/, and /v/.

hard-of-hearing. Applied to those whose hearing is impaired but who have enough hearing left for practical purposes.

idioglossia. Imperfect articulation with the utterance of meaningless vocal sounds.

labiodental. A speech sound produced by the contact of the lips with the teeth. Examples are /f/ and /v/.

lalling. A babbling, infantile form of speech.

lateral lisp. Defective production of the sibilant sounds due to excessive escape of air over or around the sides of the tongue.

linguadental. A speech sound produced with the aid of the tongue and teeth. Example is /th/.

lisping. Defective production of the sibilant sounds caused by improper tongue placement or by abnormalities of the articulatory mechanism.

nasality. The quality of speech sounds when the nasal cavity is used as a resonator.

phonation. The production of voiced sound by means of vocal cord vibrations.

phoneme. A group or family of closely related speech sounds, all of which have the same distinctive acoustic characteristics in spite of their differences; often used in place of the term *speech sound*.

plosive. Any speech sound made by creating air pressure in the air tract and suddenly releasing it. Examples are /p/, /d/, and /t/.

sibilant. Accompanied by a hissing sound; especially a type of fricative speech sound called a *sibilant*. Examples are /s/, /z/, /sh/, /ch/, and /dg/.

speech defect. Any deviation of speech which is outside the range of acceptable variation in a given environment.

speech pathology. The study and treatment of all aspects of functional and organic speech defects and disorders.

speech science. The broad field dealing with the study, analysis, and measurement of all the components of the processes involved in the production and reception of speech; sometimes the same as *voice science*.

stuttering. A disturbance of rhythm and fluency of speech by an intermittent blocking, a convulsive repetition, or prolongation of sounds, syllables, words, phrases, or posture of the speech organs.

vowel. A conventional vocal sound produced by certain positions of the speech organs which offer little obstruction to the air stream and which form a series of resonators above the level of the larynx. Distinct from *consonant*.

Index

Page numbers in italics refer to illustrations.

ABRASION OF TEETH, 328, *329*
Abrasive paste, use of, 381
Abutments for tooth-supported complete
    dentures, classification of, 484–488
  noncoping, 484, *484, 485,* 486–488
  preparation for, 492–501
    coping fabrication in, 493, *492, 495*
  selection of, 491, *493*
  submerged vital root, 488
  with attachments, 485–488
  with copings, 484–485
    long cast, *484, 485*
    short cast, *484, 484*
Acme articulator, 55–56, *56*
Acrylic resin, allergic reactions to, 397
  denture base of, preparation and packing,
    365–366
  impression trays of, 188–190, *188, 189*
  record bases of, 238–240, *238*
  polymerization of, 366
  self-curing, 239
  teeth of, 306, 308
Adenoameloblastoma, of the jaw, 153
Adenosine triphosphate, in muscle contraction, 45
Adhesion, 180
Adhesive, denture, 98
Aging, 113–125
  intraoral effects of, 124–125, 328–330
  pathologic changes of, 120–125
  physiologic changes of, 114–118
  psychologic changes of, 118–120
Alginate compound, in denture construction,
    364–365
Alimentation, in geriatric patients, 117
Allergic reactions to denture material, 397
Alveolar process, anatomy of, 2, *2*
  physiology of, 27
  surgery of, 141–144
Alveolar ridge, residual. *See* Residual alveolar
    ridge
Alveolar tubercle, anatomy of, 1, *2*
  impression of, 177, *178*
  surgery of, 145–146, *146,* 439
Alveolectomy, 141–144, *141, 142, 143,* 155–157,
    438–440

Alveoloplasty, 438–440
Alveolotomy, 438–440
Ameloblastoma, 153
Anatomy of stomatognathic system, 1–26
  ideal, for denture support, 106–107, *107, 138*
Anesthesia for dental extraction, 438, 465
Aneurysmal cyst, 153
Antibiotic therapy, postoperative, 167
Aponeurosis, palatine, 13–14, *15*
Arbitrary hinge axis, 250–251
Arcon principle, 84–85
Articular capsule, 22, *22*
Articular disk, 21–22, *21*
Articular tubercles, 19, *20*
Articulating paper, use of, 379, *379*
Articulation, definition of, 217
Articulators, 51–90. *See also* under specific
    models
  arcon principle of, 84–85
  arbitrary type, 54
  average type, 54
  classification of, 53–54
  condyle path of, 84–85
  definitions of, 51
  evaluation of, 82–87
  face-bow of. *See* Face-bow
  four-dimensional, 53
  Hanau remounting technique with, 386–389
  hinge-type, 54
  history of, 54–60, 229–230
  in arrangement of teeth
    for balanced occlusion, 351–357, 383–384
    for neutrocentric occlusion, 349–350
    for organic occlusion, 348
    for trial denture, 339–340
  laboratory remount, 367–368, 463–464
  limitations of, 52–53
  mandibular movements in, 86–87
  maxillomandibular relation records with,
    261–289
    centric, 278–279, 456–457, *458*
    checking accuracy of mountings for, 282–285,
      458–459, *459*
    eccentric, 285–289, *287*
    errors in, 378–379

Articulators (*continued*)
  lateral, 85–86, 289
  models
    current popular, 60–82
    of historic interest, 54–60
  occlusal records with, 265, *265*
    correction of, 381–384, 386–389, 463, 466, *466*
  reline and rebase procedures on, *418*, 417, 422–423, *422*
  requirements of, 51–52
  remount procedure with, 381–384, 386–389, 466, *406*
  selection of, 87–88
  special-type, 54
  uses, 51–52. *See also* specific procedures
Artificial teeth
  acrylic resin, 306, 308
  anterior, definition of, 293
  arrangement of, 311–326
    age considerations in, 328–330
    anterior, 461–463, *462*
    artistic aspects, 334–336
    facial expression and, 241–242, *241*
    for balanced occlusion, 351–357, 383–384
    for immediate complete dentures, 457–458, 461–463, *462*
    for neutrocentric occlusion, 349–350
    for organic occlusion, 348
    for single mandibular denture, 475
    for trial denture, 339–344, *342, 343, 344,* 347–358
    limitations in, 317–321, *318*
    posterior, 457–458
  buccolingual width of, 306
  clicking, 402
  color and shade of, 303–305, 306
  cosmetic aspects of, 334
  cusp of, fossae relations in balanced occlusion and, 383–384
    vs. monoplane, 307–308
  esthetic aspects of, 293, 327–337
    arrangements for, 327, 336
    in immediate complete dentures, 430
    patient dissatisfaction with, 392
    patient requirements for, 95, 118–119, 305, *306,* 334–335
  form of, anterior, 300–303
    occlusal surface, 307–308
    posterior, 307–308
  horizontal overlap of, 317, *318,* 341, *343*
  inclination of, 347–357
  interocclusal distance of, 262
    excessive, 214, *214,* 262, 427
    inadequate, 213–214, *214,* 401
  labioincisal contour, *302*
  material for, 306, 308, 389
    in single complete dentures, 478, *478*
  monoplane, selective grinding of, 388–389
    vs. cusp, 307–308
  personality and, 332–333
  porcelain, 306, 308, 389
  positions of, anatomic guidelines for, 314, 319–320, 323–325
    factors governing, 311–312

  horizontal, 312–321
    in abnormal jaw relations, 316–317, 321
    limitations in, 314, *315*
    natural teeth and, 427–429
    reverse mediolateral relation in, 317, *317*
    vertical, 321–325
  premature contact of, 203, 385–386, 413
  selection of, 292–308
    aids for, 293, *295, 301, 301,* 302
    anterior, 297–306, 461
    face as factor in, 297, 300–303
    in tooth-supported complete dentures, 495–496
    posterior, 306–308
  selective grinding of, 381–384, 385–388
    in reline and rebase procedures, 417, *419*
  size of, 297–307
Atmospheric pressure, 180
Augmentation technique, bone, 169–170
Axis, hinge. *See* Hinge axis.
  opening, 247

BALANCED OCCLUSION. *See* Occlusion, balanced
Barn door hinge articulator, 54, *55*
Baseplates. *See* Record bases
Bearing, cobalt chromium, in tooth-supported complete dentures, 492–493, *494*
Bell's palsy, 104
Bennett movement, 24–25
  effect on cusp path, *221*
  importance of, 204
  recording of, 53, 205, *205*
Bergström arcon articulator, 57, *57,* 84, 85
Biologic denture, 482–483
Blood supply, oral, 28, 120, 396
Bone(s), anatomy, 1–6
  augmentation techniques, 169–170
  blood supply to, 28–29, 120
  effect of aging on, 116
  functional changes and, 27–28
  grafting, 169–170
  pathology of, 152–155
  physiology of, 26–30
  pressure and, 28–29, 430–432, *431, 472, 472, 473*
  regenerative reconstruction of, 27
  resorption of, 28–29, 399, 430–432, *431, 472, 472, 473*
    following surgery, 433
    hypoparathyroidism and, 155
    in unhealed tissue, 429–430, *431,* 439
    prognosis after, 433
  response to metabolic changes, 29–30
  surgical preparation of, 141–145
  tensile stimulation of, 28–29, *29,* 216, *487,* 489
  Wolff's law and, 27, 439
Bone sore mouth, 400
Bonwill articulator, 55, *56*
Bony cyst, 152, *152*
Border(s), denture. *See* Denture borders
Border positions of the mandible, 205–206
Border refining process, 194, *195,* 448, *449*
Bruxism, 11
Buccal corridor, 242
Buccal frenum, *111, 175,* 176

Buccal mucous membrane reflection area, 176
Buccal shelf area, 5, 5, 177, 179
Buccal vestibule, 176
Buccinator muscle, 8, 8, 9
    push-back surgical technique for, 161–162, 161, 162
Buccinator sulcus, surgical extension of, 163, 164
Burning palate, 95, 405
Burning tongue, 95, 403

CAPSULE, articular, 22, 22
Carcinoma, squamous cell, 121, 124
Cardiovascular disease, 104
Cast(s), flasking of, 361–363
    in record base construction, 237–240, 239
    laboratory remount, 367–368
    mounting errors, 379
    outlining, for impression trays, 188–190, 188, 444–445, 445
    plaster remount, 370–371
    positioning teeth in, 313–314, 319–320, 320, 323, 324, 340, 340, 341
    recovery of complete denture from, 368
    wax contouring, 462, 462–463
Ceka-Anchor, 500–501, 500
Cementoma, 153
Central bearing device, in correcting occlusion, 379–381
Centric occlusion. See Occlusion, centric
Centric relation, definitions of, 31–32, 209–211
    records of, 273–288, 411
        functional, 274–275
        graphic, 276–279, 276, 281
        muscle strain and, 33
        tentative, 278–279
        verification of, interocclusal check record in, 279–285, 283, 284, 458–459, 459
        wax occlusion rims in, 271–273, 456–457
Check record, interocclusal, 279–285, 283, 284, 458–459, 459
Cheilitis, commissural, 402
Cheek, biting, 328, 398, 401
    relationship with teeth, 315, 328
Chew-in method
    centric relation, 274–275
    eccentric relation, 286
Chondroma, 153
Circulation, in geriatric patient, 117
Clenching of teeth, muscle kinetics of, 11
Clicking dentures, 402
Closest-speaking space, 265
Clutch for hinge axis location
    in dentulous patient, 249, 249, 250
    in edentulous patient, 249, 250
Cobalt chromium alloys, use of, 169
Cobalt chromium bearing, in tooth-supported complete dentures, 492–493, 494
Coble central-bearing device, 380, 381
Cohesion, 180
Combination syndrome, 164
Condyle, anatomy of, 5, 4, 19, 20, 21
    location of, 249
Condyle path, 25, 206–209
    in articulators, 84–85

Condyloid process, anatomy of, 4, 5, 19, 20
Contouring, wax. See Wax contouring
Congenital deformities, 167
Constrictor muscles, 15, 15
    repositioning, 109, 111
Controlled subatmospheric pressure technique in impression making, 192
Copings, cast metal, disadvantages of, 483, 488
    fabrication, 492, 493, 495
    long, 484, 485
    short, 484, 484
Coronoid process, mandibular, 5, 4
Correlator central-bearing device, 379–381
Cusp(s), paths of, 220–222
    relationship to fossa in balanced occlusion, 383–384
    vs. monoplane, 307–308
Cuspid line, in tooth arrangement, 245, 298–299, 299, 320, 320
Cyst, aneurysmal, 153
    bony, 152, 152
    dentigerous, 140, 140, 152
    dermoid, 151
    follicular, 152, 153
    globulomaxillary, 153
    incisal canal, 153, 153
    nasolabial, 153
    nonodontogenic, 153
    odontogenic, 152–153, 152
    palatal, 153
    periodontal, 152–153
    residual, 152–153
    retention, 150–151, 151

DEFLASKING, 366–367
Deglutition, muscle kinetics in, 11–12, 312
Denar articulators, D5A series, 65–67, 66
    Mark II, 67–68, 67, 86
Denar Field Inspection Gauge, 68, 69
Denar Reference Plane Locator and Marker, 67, 67
Dentatus articulator, 76–77, 77
Dentigerous cysts, 140, 140, 152
Denture(s), additive, 474, 480
    adhesion of, 180
    biologic, 482–483
    borders of. See Denture borders
    cleaning, 97
    contouring, 359–361, 462–463, 463
    deflasking, 366–367
    diagnosis for. See Diagnosis
    esthetic aspects of. See Esthetics
    evaluation of, 375–378, 465–466
    extension of, 191, 191
    finishing, 369
    flasking, 361–363
    former, use of, 269, 479–480, 479, 480, 481
    immediate. See Immediate complete dentures
    impressions for. See Impressions
    in geriatric patients. See Gerodontology
    laboratory procedures for, 359–371, 497
    limitations and disadvantages of, 93–96
    occlusion in. See Occlusion
    overlay, 482–483

Denture(s), (*continued*)
  pain associated with, 39, 46, 96, 98, 120, *398*
  partial, 478–479, *479*
  patient education for, 91–99, 130
    in eating, 96, 312–317
    in use and care, 30, 91–98, 103, 407–408
    Ney mandibular excursion guide for, 279, *280*
  polishing, 369–370
  postoperative treatment plan, 168–170, 466–468
  pressure areas in, 375–378, 408
  problems with, 391–403
    bone, 399–400
    mandibular, 401–402
    maxillary, 401
    mucosa, 393–399
    treating, 400–403, 408–422
  rebase procedures, 412–423
  reline procedures, 412–423
  requirements for, 26, 391–392, 425–426
  retention of, 42–43, 179–180
    excessive, 155–156, 191
  single complete. *See* Single complete dentures
  speaking with, 96, 312–313
  stability of, 95–96, 179, 401–402, 472–473
    evaluation of, 377, 400
  support for, 95. *See also* Anatomy
    deterioration in, 392–400,
      due to immediate complete dentures, 429–
        432
      due to single complete dentures, 472–473,
        472, 473
  preservation of, 30, 179
  surgical preparation for. *See* Surgical
      preparation
  tooth selection. *See* Artificial teeth, selection of
  telescoped, 482–483
  tolerance of, 180
  tooth-supported complete. *See* Tooth-supported
      complete dentures
  transitional, *474, 480*
  treatment, *474, 480*
    immediate claspless, 492, *494*
  trial, arranging teeth for, 339–344, 347–358
    wax contouring of, 344, *344,* 359–361, *360, 361*
Denture adhesives, 98
Denture base, acrylic resin, construction of, 361–
      370
Denture, borders, contouring, 359–361, 462–463,
      463
    facial muscles and, 7–15, 32–33
  evaluation of, 377–378
  overextension, 377–378, 401–402
    lesions due to, 15, *398,* 401, 411
  refining, 194, *195,* 448, *449*
  underextension, 401, 411, 412
Denture mold, 363–366
Denture patient. *See* Patient
Dermoid cyst, 151
Desquamative stomatitis, *437*
Diabetes, 103, *103*
Diagnosis for dentures, 101–135
  immediate complete, 432
  procedures, 125–130, 400, 432
  single complete, 470–474

Diet, inflammatory oral lesions and, 397
  in the geriatric patient, 117–118
Direct check record method, 286, 287–289, *288*
Distobuccal flange, surgical preparation for, 160–
      162
Dough method of record base construction,
      compression molded, 240
  noncompression, 239–240, *239*
Drugs, prosthodontic treatment and, 125–127
Dyskeratosis, *437*
Dysplasia, fibrous, 153, *154, 155*

EATING, 96, 312, 317
Eccentric occlusion, 215
Eccentric relation, balanced occlusion in, 383, *385*
  definition of, 211–212
  records of
    articulator adjustment to, 285–286
    inaccuracy in, 211–212
    methods for, 286–289, *288, 289*
      direct check, 286, 287–289, *289*
      functional, 286
      graphic, 286–287, *287*
Eminentia, angle of, 222
  curves of, *223*
Endocrine gland disturbances, effects of, 397
Envelope, definition of, 206n
Epulis fissuratum, 148, 149, *149*
Esthetics, 430
  patient dissatisfaction with, 392
  patient requirements and, 95, 118–119, 305, *306,*
      334–335, 392
  polished surfaces and, 359
  tooth selection and arrangement for, 293, 327–
      328, 430
Estrogen deficiencies and denture pain, 120
External oblique line, 5, *5*
Exostoses, 145, *145,* 400–401
Extractions, complications after, 438, *438*
  for immediate complete dentures, 465
  healing process, 27, 439

"F" OR "V" AND "S" SPEAKING ANTERIOR TOOTH
      RELATION, 265–269
Face, as consideration in tooth selection, 297,
      300–303
  vertical dimensions of, 212–215
Face-bow, arbitrary type, 252
  articulators designed for use with, 252
  evaluation of, 82–84, 252–255
  functions of, 83, 251, 297
  hinge axis type, 252, *253*
  indications for, 255
  models of, 251–252
  mounting, 257–259, *258,* 455–456, *456*
  transfer procedure for, 83, 255–259, 455–456, *456*
Face-bow record, 256–257, *257*
Facial expression, in geriatric patients, 121
  in maxillomandibular records, 263–264, *264,*
      454–455
  muscles of, 6–9, *8*
    impression making and, 173–175, *173*
    rest position of, 263–264, *264,* 454–455
  tooth position and, 241–242, *241*

Facial measurements in recording vertical
	dimensions of rest, 262–263, *262, 263,* 454,
	454
Fibromas, surgical management of, 151–152, *151,*
	153
Fibrous dysplasia, 153, *154,* 155
Fibrous hyperplasia, 399, 401
	inflammatory, *108, 111,* 124, 148–149
Fibrosarcoma, oral, 124
Flange, distobuccal, 160–162
Flasking of cast, 361–363
Follicular cyst, 152, 153
Food for denture users, 96
Foramen, anterior palatine, 4
	incisal, 3
	mental, 5, *5*
	nasopalatine, 3
Fordyce's spots, 124
Fossa, mandibular, 19, *20*
Fovea, palatina, 176, 178, *178*
Freeway space, 213
Frenectomy, 146–147, *146, 147*
Frenum, buccal, *111, 175,* 176
	labial, *175,* 175–177
	lingual, *175,* 177
		surgical management, 146–147, *146, 147,* 148
Functional method for maxillomandibular
	records, 274–275, 286

Gagging reflex, 402–403
Galetti articulator, 60–61
Gariot hinge joint articulator, 54, *55*
Gaucher's disease, 154
Genial tubercles, 6, *6*
Genioglossus muscle, 12–13
	surgical repositioning of, 109–111
Geniohyoid muscle, 10
	surgical repositioning of, 109, *111*
Geriatric patient. *See also* Gerodontology
	changes in, intraoral, 124–125, 328–330
		pathologic, 120–124
		physiologic, 113–114, 118–120
		psychologic, 114–118
	diet of, 117–118
	facial expression of, 121
	maxillomandibular records for, 116
	tooth arrangement for, 328–330
	tooth selection for, 303, 304
Gerodontology, 110–125
	definition of, 110
	diagnosis in, 122–124
	nutrition and diet in, 117–118
	office furniture and design for, 111–112
	patient classification in, 113–114
	patient communication in, 112–113
Gerontology, definition of, 110
Gliding occlusion, 216
Globulomaxillary cysts, 153
Gnatholator, Granger's, 59, *61*
Gnathology, concepts and philosophies, 229–235
Golgi tendon apparatuses, 37–38, *38*
Graft, bone, 169–170
	mucosal, 159
Granger's Gnatholator, 59, *61*

Granulomas, isolated eosinophilic, 153
Graphic method for maxillomandibular records,
	centric, 276–279, *276, 281*
	eccentric, 286–287, *287*
	lateral, 289
	technique for, 278–279, *277, 278, 279, 281*
Gravity, effect on dentures, 43, 97, 262
Grinding, selective, 381–389, *419*
Guidance, incisal, definition, 353–354, *356*
Gum line, 244–245
Gum soreness, 95–96, 395, 396, 398
Gypsum products in impression-making, 181
Gysi articulators, adaptable, 56
	simplex, 56

Hageman Balancer articulator, 55, *55*
Hairy tongue, 124–125
Halitosis, causes of, *122*
Hamular notch, 176
Hamulus, pterygoid, 2, 4
Hanau articulators, 72–76, *209*
	model **130–28,** 76, *77*
	model **130–30,** 76
	model **158,** 74, *75, 76*
	model H, 72, *72*
		condylar error in, 84, *85*
	remounting technique with, 386–389
	university model **130–21,** 74–76, *76*
House articulator, 62, *63*
Heberden's nodes, 103–104, *104*
Head shape, tooth arrangement and, *321*
Hickok strap, muscle strain and, 33
Hight tracing device, 278, *278*
Hinge axis, 247–251
	arbitrary, 250–251
	location of, 249–250, *249, 250*
	opening, 247
	review of literature on, 247–249
	terminal, 206, 247, 250
		arbitrary point of, 455, *455*
Hydrocolloids in impression making
	irreversible, 182–183
		technique for, 185–187
	reversible, 182
Hygiene, oral, 97, 397
Hyoglossus muscle, 13
Hyperkeratosis, 149–150
Hyperparathyroidism, bone resorption due to, 155
Hyperplasia, fibrous, 399, 401
	inflammatory, *108, 111,* 124, 148–149
Hyperthyroidism, 155
Hypertrophy of mucosa, 108, 397–398, 399, 401

Immediate complete dentures, advantages of,
	426–429
	contraindications to, 437–438
	definitions of, 425
	diagnosis for, 106, 432
	disadvantages of, 429–432
	impressions for, final, 444–452
		preliminary, 443–444
	insertion of, 464–466
	laboratory procedures for, 463–464
	maxillomandibular relation records for, 453, 460

Immediate complete dentures (continued)
  occlusion in, 466, 466
  patient education for, 98
  postoperative evaluation for, 466–468, 467
  preparation for, 441–442
  record base construction for, 452–453
  roentgenographic studies for, 433, 434, 435
  surgical preparation for, 438–440
  tooth arrangement for, 457–458, 461–463, 462
  tooth-supported, 488
Implants, 170
Impressions, 173–201
  anatomic landmarks for, 175–179, 446–447, 447
    interpretation of, 177–179, 178
  borders of, refining, 194–196, 448, 449
  errors in, 413
  facial expression muscles and, 173–175, 173
  final, 190–199
    closed mouth techniques for, 191
    definition of, 173
    equipment for, 194
    for immediate complete dentures, 444–452
    for tooth-supported complete dentures, 494, 496
    mandibular, 194, 195
    maxillary, 194–196, 197
    refining, 195–199
    techniques for, 190–192
    trays for, 188–190
  for reline and rebase procedures, mandibular,
      417–421, 421
    maxillary, 414–417, 415, 416
  masseter groove in, 174–175, 174, 179
  materials for, 18, 180–184, 185
  of labial vestibule, 175, 176, 177
  objectives for, 179–180
  patient position for, 185–186
  preliminary, 185–190
    definition of, 173
    equipment for, 185
    for immediate complete dentures, 443–444
    for tooth-supported complete dentures, 493–
        494, 496
    mandibular, 185, 186, 186, 187
    maxillary, 185, 186–187, 186, 187
  techniques for, 184–185
    mucostatic, 191–192
  terminology, 173
  tissue-bearing areas of, refining, 196–199, 198,
      448–452, 451
  tissue recovery and, 18
Impression trays, acrylic resin, 188–190, 188–189
  for final impressions, 188–190
  for immediate complete dentures, 444–446
  for preliminary impressions, 186–187, 187, 188,
      493
  for tooth-supported complete dentures, 493–494,
      496
  impression compound and zinc-oxide-eugenol
      paste, 192, 195
  stock, 443, 443
Incisal canal cysts, 153, 153
Incisal foramen, 3
Incisal guide angles, lateral, 354
  sagittal, 353, 356

Incisal muscles, 8
Incisive papilla, 176, 178, 178
Inflammation of mucosa, 124, 395, 396, 396, 400–
    401
Infrahyoid muscles, 10
Insertion muscle, 11
Insertion procedures, 375–389
  immediate complete denture, 464–466
  technique for, 375–378
  tooth-supported complete denture, 497–498, 498
Intercondylar distance, 220
Interocclusal check for maxillomandibular
      records, centric, 279–285, 283, 284, 458–459,
      459
  eccentric, 286, 287–289, 289
  materials for, 281–282
Interocclusal distance, 262
  excessive, 214, 214, 262, 427
  inadequate, 213–214, 214, 401
Irish's Dupli-Functional articulator, 59, 60

Jaw(s), adenoameloblastoma of, 153
  malrelated, 167, 316–317
Jaw relation records. See Maxillomandibular
    relations
Joints, diseases of, 103–104, 103, 104

Keagle's procedure for hypermobile soft tissue,
    164–166, 164, 165, 166
Kile Dentograph articulator, 59, 59

Labial frenum, 175–177, 175
Labial vestibule, extension of, 166–167, 166
  impressions of, 175, 176, 177
  surgical preparation of, 158–159, 163–167
Laboratory procedures, 359–371, 497
  for immediate complete dentures, 463–464
Lamina dura, 2
Lateral relations, 85–86, 211, 289
Leukoplakia, 124
Levator palati muscle, 14–15
Lichen planus, 124, 150, 150, 437
Lingual flange, surgical preparation for, 162–163
Lingual frenum, 175, 177
  surgical preparation of, 147, 147, 148
Lingual tuberosity, alveolectomy, 141–142, 141
  anatomy, 6, 6
Lip line, high, 244–245
  low, 242–243, 244
Lips, benign pathology of, 147–148, 149
  characteristics, 108
  muscles of, 7, 9
  neoplasms of, 122
  relationship with anterior teeth, 300, 300, 319
Locks, mechanical, 180
Low viscosity impression materials, 18

Macroglossia, acquired, 125
Magnets, use in dentures, 169
Malar surface, maxillary, 1
Malignancies, oral, 104–105, 105, 106
Mandible, anatomy of, 4–6, 4, 16, 19, 20, 178–179,
    178
  atrophied, 142, 142

Mandible (*continued*)
  border positions of, 205–206
  head of, 4, 5, 19, *20*
  movements of. See Mandibular movements
  physiologic rest position of, 212, 261–262
    vertical dimension of, 212, *213*, 261–262, 453–
      454
  protruded, 123, 299
  reflex closure of, *31*
Mandibular arch, anatomy of, 176–177, *178*
  edentulous, single denture opposing, 477–479,
    478, 479
  mucosa of, 17–18, *17*
  surgical preparation of, 157–163
Mandibular movements, 22–26, 204–209
  and articulator movements, 86–87
  border positions in, 205–206
    definition of, 205
    envelope of motion in, 206, *207*
    muscle spasms and, 46
  classification of, 24–25, 204
  condyle path of, 25, 206–209
  functional range of, 206
  masticatory, 24, 26, 204, *208*, 312
  related to concepts of occlusion, 218, *218, 220,*
    220–224
  somatic nervous system and, 46
  terminology, 204–205, *205*
Mandibular ramus, 4–5, *4*
Massage of abused soft tissue, 409
Masseter groove, 9
  in impression-making, 174–175, *174*, 179
Masseter muscle, 11, *32*
Mastication, mandibular movements in, 24, 26,
  204, *208*, 312
  method of, for denture users, 312, 317
  muscles of, 10–12, *10*, 31–32
  problems in, 392
  teeth contact in, 204
  teeth positions and, 313
Maxilla, anatomy of, 1–3, *2, 16,* 177–178, *178*
  neoplasms of, 124
Maxillary arch, anatomy, 175–176, *175,* 177–178,
  178
  mucosa of, 16–17
  size of, 297–298, *298*
  surgical preparation of, 163–167
Maxillary tuberosity, 1–2
Maxillomandibular records, 261–291
  accuracy of, 52–53, 378–379
  face-bow transfer for, 83, 255–259, 455–456, *456*
  for immediate complete dentures, 453, 460
  for tooth-supported dentures, 495
  in geriatric patient, 116
  muscle properties and, 33, 35
  occlusion rims in, 240–245, 271–273, 282, 456–457
  patient training for, 44, 442
  record bases for, 237
  reflex closure and, *31*
  strained, 386
  unstrained, 386
  verification of, 273, 282–285, 458–459, *459*
Maxillomandibular relations, 209–215
  abnormalities in, 167, 316

centric, definition of, 31–32, 209–211
  recording, 273–288, 411
  verification of, 279–285, *283, 284,* 458–459, *459*
controversy about, 203
eccentric, definition of, 211–212
  recording, 285–289, *287, 288*
  verification of, 286, 287–289, *289*
hinge axis, 247–251
influence of natural teeth on, 203
lateral, 211, 289
  recording, 85–86, 289
occlusion in, vertical dimension of, 213–215,
  214, 264
  recording, 213, 264–273, 457
protrusive, 211
  recording, 287–289, *287, 288,* 459–460, *460*
rest position in, 212, 261–262
  vertical dimension of, 212, *213,* 261–262, 453–
    454
  recording, 262–264, 454–455
tooth selection and, 299
vertical, 212–215, 261–262, 264
  recording, 262–273, 454–457
McCollum Gnathoscope, 59, *60*
Mechanoreceptors, 37–39
Menopause, 105, 403
  signs and symptoms of, *436*
Mental foramen, mandibular, 5, *5*
Mental spines, 6, *6*
Mentalis muscle, 7–8
Midpalatal suture, 2–3, 176, 178, *178*
Minigraph in maxillomandibular records, 64–65,
  65
Mini-grip transfer vise, 65, *65*
Modeling compound in impression-making, 183–
  184, 192–193
Modiolus, 7, 174
Mold, acrylic resin denture base, deflasking, 366
  preparation, 363–365
Mold selector, 297, *298*
Moniliasis, 124
Monson's maxillomandibular articulator, 57, *57*
Mouth breathing, 123
Mucosa, abused, 108, *108, 111,* 392–399, *399*
  due to single complete denture, 476, *476*
  systemic factors in, 407
  treatment of, 407–423
  aging and, 115, *116,* 124
  anatomy of, 15–18, *17*
  autogenous graft of, 159
  basal seat, traumatic lesions of, 396–398
  buccal, reflection area of, 176
  dermatologic diseases and, 104
  diagnosis of, 108–109
  displaceability, 385–386
  excessive denture retention and, 191
  hyperplasia of, surgical management, 148–149
  hypertrophied, 108, 397–398, *399,* 401
  impression-making and, 180–181
  inflammatory reactions of, 124, 395, 396, *396,*
    400–401
  lining, 393
    traumatic lesions of, 398, *398*
  massage of, 409

Mucosa (*continued*)
  mouth breathing and, 123
  pendulous, 108, 142, *142*, 145–146, *146*, 398, *398*, *489*
  physiology of, 393
  shrinkage of, 429–430
  single complete dentures and, 473
  specialized, 393
    traumatic lesions of, 398–399
  stress-bearing, 393, 394–396
  surgical preparation of, 142, *142*, 147–152
  teeth positions and, 312
  tissue conditioners and, 409–412
  tissue rest and, 427, *427*
Muscle(s). *See also* specific names
  abnormal habits, 18
  anatomy of, 6–15, *13*, *17*
  contractions of, 33–35, *34*
    adenosine triphosphate in, 45
  effects of aging on, 115–116
  of facial expression, 6–9, *8*
  physiology of, 30–36
  rest position of, 263–264, *264*, 454–455
  spasms of, 46
Muscle spindle, 37–38, *38*
Muscle tolerance, 180
Muscle tone, 35, 328, *329*
Mucoceles, 150–151
Mucositis, 124
Mucostatic impression technique, 191–192
Mylohyoid line, 5–6, *6*
Mylohyoid muscle, 9–10, 177, 179
  surgical repositioning of, 109, *111*
Myology of stomatognathic system. *See* Muscle(s)
Myxoma, 153

Nasolabial cysts, 153
Nasopalatine foramen, 3
Natural teeth, abrasion of, 328–329, *329*
  appearance of, *294*, *302*
  clenching, 11
  color of, 303–306
  contacting of, 204
  effects of age on, 115, 328–330, *328*, *329*
  extraction of, for immediate complete dentures, 465
    healing process after, 27, 439
    postoperative complications in, 438, *438*
  in artificial tooth arrangement, 313, 427–429
  in retention of prosthesis, 473, *473*
  in vertical dimension of occlusion, 427
  influence on maxillomandibular records, 203
  loss of, 115
    depression due to, 473–474, *474*, 490
  occlusal forms in, 475–477
  opposing mandibular denture, 472–474, *472*, *473*
  opposing mandibular denture, 474–478, *477*, *478*
  retained, surgery of, 139–140
  roots of, submerged vital, 488
  sex-related characteristics of, 330–332
  tensile stimulation of, 28–29, *29*, 216, *487*, 489
  unerrupted, 140, *140*
  vertical overlap in, 428–429
  wear facets on, 428, *428*

with tooth-supported dentures,
    contraindications for, 490–491
    methods of abutment for, 484–488
    minimum retention, 492–498
    positive retention, 498–501
    selection of, 491, *493*
    terminal root, 486, *487*, *488*
Necrosis, radiation, 105, *106*
Needles-House technique for recording centric relation, 274, *275*
Neuritis, peripheral, 120
Neurologic disorders and denture procedures, 104
Neuromuscular perception, maxillomandibular records and, 269–271, *270*
Neutrocentric concept of occlusion, 219, 349–350
Ney articulator, 59–60, *61*
Ney mandibular excursion guide, 279, *280*
Nicotine stomatitis, 124
Niemann-Pick disease, 154
Nociceptive reflex, 39, 46, 97
Nutrition, in the geriatric patient, 117–118

Oblique line, external, 177
Occlusion, balanced, 217–219, 229–230
    bilateral, *352*
    definition of, 215–216, *216*
    gliding, 216
    in centric position, 383, *385*
    in protrusion, *353*, 383, 386
    in static eccentric position, 383, *385*
    selective grinding procedures for, 383–389
  centralized working surfaces in, 350, *351*
  centric, 215, *215*
    long, 386
    verification, 458–459
  concepts of, 216–224, 229–231
  correction of, 381–384, 386–389, 463, 466, *466*
    tooth inclination and, 347–357
    maxillomandibular movement and, 218, *218*, 220, *220*, 221, *223*, 224
  definitions of, 215–216
  disharmony of, causes, 378, 411
    correction of, 379–389
  eccentric, 215
  eminentia and, angle of, *222*
    curves of, *223*
  evaluation of, 273, 279–285, *419*
  gliding, 215
    balanced, 216
  in immediate complete dentures, 466, *466*
  intercondylar distance and, *220*
  interocclusal check record for, 279–285
  interocclusal distance and, 213–214
  intraoral analysis of, 52
  neutrocentric, 219, 349–350
  nonbalanced, 219–224
  organic, 217, 219, 230–231, 235, 348
  protrusive, 386
  recording, 265, *265*
  spherical, 348
  tooth selection and, 307–308
  vertical dimension of, 213–215, *214*
    natural teeth in determining, 427, *427*
    recording, 213, 264–273, 457

Occlusion rims, 240–245
  construction on record base, 452–453, *453*
  contouring, 241–243, *241*
  for tooth-supported complete dentures, 494–495,
    496
  guide lines on, 243–245
  mandibular, 243–245, *243*
  material for, 452
  maxillary, 241–243, *242*
  Needles-House, 274, *275*
  of impression compound, 446, *446*
  Patterson, 274–275, *275*
  wax, in recording maxillomandibular relations,
    271–273, 282, 456–457
Opening axis, 247
Orbicularis oris muscle, *7, 9,* 31
Osteitis deformans, 154
Osteitis fibrosa cystica, 155
Osteoarthritis, 103, *103,* 104
Osteology of stomatognathic system. *See* Bone(s)
Osteoma, 153
Osteoplastoma, 153
Osteoporosis, 29–30
  associated with menopause, 105
  in geriatric patients, 116
Overdenture, 482–483
Overlay denture, 482–483

PAD, retromolar, *17, 17,* 177
Page's Transograph articulator, 58, *58*
Paget's disease, 122, 154
Pain, associated with denture use, 39, 46, 96, 98,
    398
  in geriatric patients, 120
Pain conductors, 39–40
Pain receptors, 39, 47
Pain reflexes, 39, 46, 97
Palatal cysts, 153
Palatal seal, posterior, impressions for, 446–447,
    447
  placement of, *4, 14, 14,* 176
  record base outline of, 460, *461*
Palatal suture, median, *176, 178, 178*
Palatal torus, 3
  surgical management, 144–145, *145*
Palate, bones of, 2–4, *3*
  burning, 95, 405
  hard, 3–4, *17*
  high, 4
  low, 4
  soft, mucosa of, *17, 17*
    muscles of, 13–15, *13, 17*
    posterior seal of, *4, 14, 14,* 176
  traumatic lesions of, 394–395
Palatina fovea, *176, 178, 178*
Palatine aponeurosis, 13–14, *15*
Palatine bones, anatomy of, 3–4
Palatine foramen, anterior, 4
Palatine process, 2–3, *3*
Palatoglossus muscle, 13, *13,* 15
Palsy, Bell's, 104
Panadent articulator, 77–78, *78,* 80
Panadent Quick Analyzer, 78, *79*
Panorex screening, 156, *156*

Pantographs, 230
Pantograms, techniques and interpretation, *231–
    235*
Papilla, incisive, *176, 178, 178*
  retromolar, *17, 17,* 177, 179
Papilloma, 151–152, *151*
Papillomatosis, 148–149, *150*
Parkinson's disease, 104
Partial dentures, 478–479, *479*
Passive techniques in impression making, 191–192
Patient, diagnosis of, 125–131, 106, 432
  dissatisfaction of, 392
  edentulous, condyle path in, 207
    effects of aging on, *29, 111,* 124
    recording maxillomandibular relations in, 64,
        237, 269–271
  education of, 91–99, 130
    in denture use and care, 30, 91–98, 407–408
    in eating, 96, 312–317
    Ney mandibular excursion guide for, 279, *280*
  esthetic requirements of, 95, 118, 305, *306,* 311,
        334–335
  expectations of, 93–96
  geriatric. *See* Geriatric patient; Gerodontology
  ideal, *107*
  instructions for, 92
  mental attitude of, 101–102, 433–436, 473–474,
        474
    of geriatrics, 118–120
    to loss of natural teeth, 473–474, *474,* 490
    to surgical procedures, 137–138
    to tooth-supported dentures, 490
  muscle tolerance of, 180
  position of, for impressions, 185–186
  systemic status of, 102–105, 437–438
  tactile sense of, 263, 273, 454
  training exercises for, 44, 442
  understanding, 92
  vomiting and gagging by, 402–403
  word pronunciation problems of, 96
Patterson technique for recording centric
        relation, 274–275, *275*
Pemphigus, 104, *104*
Periodontal cyst, 152–153
Personnel, auxiliary dental, 336, 339
Personality of patient and prosthodontic
        treatment, 332–333, 392
  in gerodontology, 118–120
Petrotympanic fissure, 19
Pharyngeal muscles, 15, *15*
Phonetics, in recording maxillomandibular
        relations, 263, 273, 454
  patient practice of, 96
Photographs, profile, in maxillomandibular
        records, 264–265, *264*
Physiologic rest position, of mandible, 212, *213,*
        261–262, 453–454
Physiology of stomatognathic system, 26–43
Plaster of Paris in impression making, 181
Polishing, 369–370
Polysulfide in impression making, 183
Porcelain teeth, 306, 308, 389
Posterior nasal spine, 4
Posterior palatal seal. *See* Palatal seal, posterior

Power point technique for recording vertical dimension, 271, *271*

Pre-extraction records, in maxillomandibular records, 264–269

Pressure, areas of, 375–378, 408
  effect on bone, 28–29, 430–432, *431, 472, 472, 473*

Pressure disclosing paste, in evaluating dentures, 375–377, *395, 400*

Profile, facial, in artificial tooth selection, 301, *301, 302*

Proprioceptors, 38

Prosthesis, oral, opposing maxillary denture, 477–478
  retention of, 473, *473*

Protrusive relation, balanced occlusion in, *353,* 383, 386
  definition of, 211
  recording, 287–289, *287, 288,* 459–460, *460*

Pterygoid hamulus, *2, 4*

Pterygoid muscles, 11, *32*

Pterygomandibular ligament, 177, *178*

Pterygomandibular raphe, 14, *15*

Push-back surgical technique, 161–162, *161, 162*

RADIATION THERAPY and denture procedures, 104–105, 472

Radiation necrosis, 105, *106*

Radiography. *See* Roentgenographic studies

Ranulas, 151

Raphe, pterygomandibular, 14, *15*

Realeff, 18, 385

Rebase, definition of, 412–413
  impressions for, 414–417, *415, 416*
  mandibular denture, 417–423, *420, 421*
  maxillary denture, 414–417
  selective grinding in, 417, *419*

Record base, construction of, 239–240, *239,* 452–453, *453*
  for tooth-supported complete dentures, 494–495, *496*
  in maxillomandibular records, 237
  materials for, 237–239

Record, interocclusal check, 279–285, 458–459, *459*

Reflexes, withdrawal, 39, 46–47, 97–98

Reline, definition of, 412–413
  impressions for, 414–417
  mandibular, 417–423, *420, 421*
  maxillary, 414–417
  selective grinding in, 417, *419*

Remount procedure, Hanau technique, 386–389
  laboratory, 367–368, 463–464
  patient, 379–384, 422–423, *422,* 465–466
  selective grinding, 385–389

Residual alveolar ridge, absence of, 108
  management, 155–157, 169–170
  atrophy of, 430
  contours of, loss of, 299
  crests of, shifts in position of, 313–314, *313,* 319, 320–321
  knife-edged, 108, *111,* 399, 400
    surgery of, 142, *142*
  mobile, 163–167, *164, 165*
  mucosa of, 16, 393
  normal structure of, 16

pendulous, 399
preservation of, 30, 179, 472–473, *472, 473*
relations of, 299–230
  classification of, 316–317
resorption of, causes, 28–29, 399–439
  in geriatric patients, *111,* 124
  patterns of, 299
  with single complete dentures, 472–473, *472, 473*
  with tooth-supported complete dentures, 485, *486*
spinous processes, 399
surgical preparation of, 141–145, *141, 142, 143,* 155–157, 438–440
teeth positions on, 312–321
traumatic lesions of, 394–395

Residual cyst, 152–153

Rest position of mandible, 212, 261–262
  vertical dimension of, 212, *213,* 261–262, 453–454
  recording, 262–264, 454–455

Retained dentition, 139–140

Retention cyst, 150–151, *151*
  excessive, 155–156, 191

Retention, denture, 42–43, 179–180

Retromolar pad, 17, *17,* 177

Retromolar papilla, 17, *17,* 177, 179

Retromylohyoid space, 177, 179

Riboflavin deficiency, oral effects, 124, *397*

Ridge, residual alveolar. *See* Residual alveolar ridge

Ridge runners, 411

Roentgenographic studies, for immediate complete dentures, 433, *434, 435*
  in Paget's disease, 122, 154
  in recording maxillomandibular relations, 265
  of denture bearing area, 107, *109*

Roots, submerged, vital, as abutments, 488

Root tips, surgical preparation of, 139–140, *139*

Rubber impression materials, 183

Rugae, 176–178, *178*

SALIVA, adhesion of, 180
  aging effects on, 115
  cohesion of, 180
  denture retention and, 42–43
  excessive, 95
  physiology of, 40–43
  radiation therapy and, 124

Salivary glands, 40–43
  atrophy of, 125

Sclerosing agents, 164

Selective grinding procedures, 381–389, *419*

Selective pressure techniques, in impression making, 192

Sex, tooth characteristics related to, 303, *303,* 330–332

Sharshak's surgical technique for denture seating area, 164

Shellac record base, 238

Silastic implants, 170

Silhouettes, in maxillomandibular records, 265

Silicone, in impression making, 183

Silicone implants for denture support, 170

Simulator articulator, 64–65, *65*

Single complete denture, 470–481
  indications for, 471
  mandibular, to oppose natural teeth, 472–474, 472, 473
  maxillary, to oppose existing denture, 479–481, 479, 480, 481
    to oppose natural teeth, 474–478, 477, 478
    to oppose partially edentulous mandibular arch, 477–479, 478, 479
  preservation of residual alveolar ridge and, 472–473, 472, 473
Skin, aging, 115, 116
  diseases of, 104, 104
Sleep, reflex phenomena during, 97–98
Slidematic face-bow, 68, 69
Smiling line, 244–245
  creation of, 335–336
  effects of age on, 329, 330
Soft palate. See Palate, soft
Somatic nervous system, mandibular movements and, 46
  physiology of, 36–40, 37
  regulation of saliva by, 40–42
  role in denture use, 97
Soreness, gum, 95–96, 395, 396, 398
Speaking, difficulties in, 96
  position of teeth and, 312–313
Speech muscles, innervation of, 41
Sphenomandibular ligament, 22, 23
Spine(s), mental, 6, 6
  posterior nasal, 4
Splints, surgical, 156–157, 157
  postoperative management with, 167–168
  vs. immediate complete denture, 426, 426
Sprinkle-on technique, in impression tray construction, 445–446
  in record base construction, 240, 452–453, 453
Stansbery Tripod articulator, 58–59, 58
Stephens articulator, 60, 62
Stewart articulator, 209
Stomatitis, desquamative, 437
  nicotine, 124
Stomatognathic system, anatomy of, 1–26
  physiology of, 26–43
Stuart articulator, 62–64, 63, 64
Styloglossus muscle, 13
Stylomandibular ligament, 22, 23
Sublingual fold, 177, 179
Submucosa, transitional, 393, 398
Sulcus, buccinator, extension of, 163, 164
  lingual extension of, anterior, 162–163, 163
    posterior, 160, 160, 161
Sulcus slide, mandibular, anterior, 158–159, 158
  reverse anterior, 159, 159
Superior constrictor muscle, 15, 15
  surgical repositioning of, 109, 111
Suprahyoid muscles, 9–10, 9
Surgical procedures, 137–170
  for bone graft, 169–170
  for bony pathology, 152–155
  for congenital deformities, 167
  for immediate complete dentures, 438–440
  for labial vestibule, 158–159, 163–167
  for malrelated jaws, 167

for mandibular arch, 157–163
for maxillary arch, 163–167
for nonpathologic bony conditions, 141–145
for residual alveolar ridge, 141–145, 141, 142, 143, 155–157, 438–440
for soft tissue, 142, 142, 145–152, 147, 148
for specialist, 155–167
postoperative, 167–170
preoperative examination for, 137–139
retained dentition and, 139–140
Surgical splints. See Splints, surgical
Suture, median palatal, 176, 178, 178
Swallowing, 11–12, 312
Swelling, excessive, after extractions, 438, 438
Syndrome, combination, 164

T.M.J. ARTICULATOR, 68–72, 69, 70, 71
T.M.J. Simplex Mandibular Movement Indicator, 71 72
Tactile check record for maxillomandibular relations. See Interocclusal check record for maxillomandibular relations
Tactile sense, in denture patients, 263, 273, 454
Teeth. See Artificial teeth; Natural teeth
Telescoped denture, 482–483
Temporal muscle, 11, 32
Temporomandibular joint, anatomy of, 19–22, 19, 20, 21, 22
  articulation of, 18, 22–26
  condyle path of, 25, 206–209
  definition of, 18
  osteoarthritis of, 104
  receptor reflexes of, 47
Tensor palati muscle, 14
Terminal hinge axis, arbitrary point of, 455, 455
  definition of, 206, 247
  location of, 250
Terminal hinge movement, 210
Terrell's Precision Coordinator, 57, 58
Thiamine deficiency, 120
Tic douloureux, 121, 123
Tissue(s), denture supporting. See Bone; Mucosa soft, abused, 409
Tissue conditioners, 409–412
  limitations of, 410–411, 412
  procedure for, 411
Tissue rest, 427, 427
Tongue, abnormal, 13, 109, 112
  anatomy and function of, 12–13, 12, 177
  biting, 398, 401
  burning, 95, 403
  hairy, 124–125
  lesions of, 124
  macroglossia of, 125
  malignancies of, 105
  training of, for denture stability, 96
  varicose veins of, 125
Tooth arrangement. See Artificial teeth, arrangement of
Tooth indicator, Trubyte, 297, 297, 301–302
Tooth selection. See Artificial teeth, selection of
Tooth-supported complete dentures, abutment in, methods of, 484–488
  advantages of, 488–490

Tooth-supported complete dentures (*continued*)
  classification of, 484–488
  concepts of, 485
  contraindications for, 490–491
  copings for, *483, 484, 485, 488, 492, 493, 495*
  definitions of, 482–484
  denture base for, 494–495, *496*
  immediate, 488
  impressions for, 493–494, *496*
  impression trays for, 493–494, *496*
  indications for, 490
  insertion of, 497–498, *498*
  laboratory procedures for, 497
  maxillomandibular records for, 495
  occlusion rims for, 494–495, *496*
  preparation of retained teeth for, 492–501
    for minimum retention, 492–498
    for positive retention, 498–501
  teeth for, 495–496
  treatment planning for, 491
    preparatory, 491–492
  try-in of, 497
Torus, palatal, 3
  surgical management of, 144–145, *145*
Transitional denture, *474,* 480
Treatment denture, *474,* 480
  immediate claspless, 492, *494*
Trubyte Simplex articulator, 61, *62*
Trubyte tooth indicator, 297, *297,* 301–302, *301*
Tubercle(s), alveolar. *See* Alveolar tubercle,
    maxillary
  articular, 19, *20*
  genial, 6, *6*
Tuberosity, lingual, alveolectomy, 141–142, *141*
  anatomy, 6, *6*
  maxillary, 1–2
Tumors, oral, ameloblastic, 140
  brown, 155
  giant-cell, 153

  in geriatric patient, 121, 122, 123, 124
  odontogenic, 153–154

UNIVERSITY MODEL ARTICULATOR, 74–75, *76*

VEINS, varicose, of tongue, 125
Vertical dimensions, 212–215, *214,* 261–262, *264*
  recording, 262–273, *262, 263,* 454–457, *454*
Vertical relations, occlusion position and,
    213–215, *264*
  recording, 264–273, 457
  rest position and, 212, 261–262
  recording, 262–264, 454–455
Vestibule, buccal, 176
  surgical extension of, 163, *164*
  labial, *175, 176, 177*
  surgical extension, 158–159, 163–167
  lateral posterior, 160–162
Visual aids in denture care and use, 92, *93*
Vitamin B_{12} deficiency, 124
Vomiting, 402–403

WAX, contouring
  muscles and, 7–15
  of occlusion rims, 241–243, *241*
  of trial denture, 344, *344,* 359–361, *360, 361,*
    462–463, *463*
  impression of, 184
  occlusal, 284–285, 381
  speaking, 266, *266*
Whip Mix articulators, 79–82, 86
  model **8500,** 79–81, *80, 81*
  model **8800,** 81, *82*
Whip Mix Quick-Mount Face-bow, 81–82, *82*
Withdrawal reflexes, 39, 46–47, 97–98
Wolff's law, 27, 439

ZINC OXIDE-EUGENOL PASTE, 181–182, 192, *193,* 450
Zygomatico-alveolar crest, 1